EMERGENCY NURSING PROCEDURES

EMERGENCY NURSING PROCEDURES

Third Edition

Jean A. Proehl, RN, MN, CEN, CCRN
Emergency Clinical Nurse Specialist
Dartmouth-Hitchcock Medical Center
Lebanon, New Hampshire

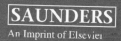
An Imprint of Elsevier

SAUNDERS
An Imprint of Elsevier

11830 Westline Industrial Drive
St. Louis, Missouri 63146

EMERGENCY NURSING PROCEDURES ISBN 0-7216-0341-6

NOTICE

Nursing is an ever-changing field. Standard safety precautions must be followed, but as new research and clinical experience broaden our knowledge, changes in treatment and drug therapy may become necessary or appropriate. Readers are advised to check the most current product information provided by the manufacturer of each drug to be administered to verify the recommended dose, the method and duration of administration, and contraindications. It is the responsibility of the licensed prescriber, relying on experience and knowledge of the patient, to determine dosages and the best treatment for each individual patient. Neither the publisher nor the author assumes any liability for any injury and/or damage to persons or property arising from this publication.

Previous editions copyrighted 1993, 1999

Library of Congress Cataloging in Publication Data

Emergency nursing procedures / [edited by] Jean A. Proehl.—3rd ed.
p. cm.
Previous edition copyrighted 1999
Includes index.
ISBN 0-7216-0341-6
1. Emergency nursing—Handbooks, manuals, etc. 2. Emergency medicine—Handbooks, manuals, etc. I. Proehl, Jean A. II. Adult emergency nursing procedures.
   [DNLM: 1. Emergency Nursing—methods handbooks. WY 49E53 1999]
RT120.E4A285 1999 610.73'61—dc21
DNLM/DLC 98–36264

Executive Editor: Susan R. Epstein
Developmental Editor: Robyn L. Brinks
Publishing Services Manager: John Rogers
Senior Project Manager: Beth Hayes
Design Manager: Bill Drone

Printed in the United States of America

Last digit is the print number: 9 8 7 6 5 4 3 2 1

For my family Jeff, Christopher, and Madeline who listen to injury prevention lectures daily.

And, for emergency nurses who use their heads, hearts, and hands to provide care and comfort every hour of every day, everywhere. Whether you are delivering a baby or extubating a terminally ill patient, I hope this book makes your shift a little easier.

Contributors

Donna York Clark, RN, MS, CFRN, CCRN
Director
Dartmouth-Hitchcock Advanced Response Team
Lebanon, New Hampshire

Lin Courtemanche, RN, CSPI
Director
New Hampshire Poison Information Center
Dartmouth-Hitchcock Medical Center
Lebanon, New Hampshire

Joni Heintzen Daniels, MSN, RN, CEN, CCRN, CFRN, CNS
Chief Nursing Officer
Emtel, Incorporated
Houston, Texas

Patricia A. DeWitt, RN, MSN
Inpatient Cardiac Services Educator
Dartmouth-Hitchcock Medical Center
Lebanon, New Hampshire

Reneé Semonin Holleran, RN, PhD, CEN, CCRN, CFRN, SANE
Clinical Manager
Emergency Department
University of Utah Hospitals and Clinics
Salt Lake City, Utah

Linda A. Hutson, RN, SANE
Assistant Manager
Emergency Department
Mercy Hospital Anderson
Cincinnati, Ohio

Margo E. Layman, MSN, RN, RNC, CN-A
Float Pool Staff Nurse
McKenna Memorial Hospital
New Braunfels, Texas

Kyle Madigan, RN, BSN, CEN, CCRN, CFRN
Training and Education Coordinator
Flight Nurse
California Shock/Trauma Air Rescue
Auburn, California

Mike D. McMahon, RN, BSN
Senior Clinical Specialist
Medtronic Physio-Control
Redmond, Washington

Alexis M. Newton, RN, BSN
Platte Valley Medical Center
Brighton, Colorado

Maureen T. Quigley, MS, ARNP, CEN
Instructor in Surgery
Dartmouth Medical School
Dartmouth-Hitchcock Medical Center
Lebanon, New Hampshire
Nurse Practitioner
Bariatric Surgery Program
Dartmouth-Hitchcock Medical Center
Lebanon, New Hampshire

Ruth Altherr Rench, MS, RN
Senior Clinical Specialist
Genentech, Inc.
Indianapolis, Indiana

Lucinda W. Rossoll, BSN, MS, CEN, CCRN, ARNP
Staff Nurse
Emergency Department
Dartmouth-Hitchcock Medical Center
Lebanon, New Hampshire

Michael Rouse, MSN, CRNA
Flight Nurse
University Air Care
University Hospital
Cincinnati, Ohio

Ruth L. Schaffler, PhD(c), CEN, ARNP
Instructor of Nursing
Pacific Lutheran University
Tacoma, Washington

Daun A. Smith, RN, MS, CEN
Staff Nurse
Emergency Department
Dartmouth-Hitchcock Medical Center
Lebanon, New Hampshire
Associate Professor of Nursing
New Hampshire Community Technical
    College
Claremont, New Hampshire

Deborah A. Upton, RN, BSN, CEN
Clinical Supervisor Emergency Services
Cox Health System
Springfield, Missouri

Teresa L. Will, RN, MSN, CEN
Educator
Community Health Network
Indianapolis, Indiana

Mary E. Wood, RN, MS, CDE, BC-ADM
Diabetes Clinical Nurse Specialist
Dartmouth-Hitchcock Medical Center
Lebanon, New Hampshire

Reviewers

Susan Engman Lazear, RN, MN
Director, Specialists in Medical Education
Woodinville, Washington

Steven A. Weinman, RN, BSN, CEN, EMT
Senior Director–Medical Education and Custom Publishing
Excerpta Medica, Inc./Elsevier Science
Hillsborough, New Jersey
Per Diem Instructor, Emergency and Trauma Care
New York Presbyterian Hospital–Cornell Medical Center
New York, New York

Jennifer A. Williams, RN, MSN, BC, M-S CNS, CCRN
Clinical Nurse Specialist, Emergency Services
Barnes-Jewish Hospital
St. Louis, Missouri

Russell Wilshaw, RN, MS, CEN
Trauma Coordinator
Utah Valley Regional Medical Center
Provo, Utah

Preface

Every day it seems like we're asked to do something new. It may be an innovative, cutting edge intervention, or it may be something routinely done on an inpatient unit (but because there are no inpatient beds available, it now needs to be performed in the Emergency Department [ED]). There is no specialty that sees the variety of patient conditions, ages, and types that we see in the ED. From birth to cardiac arrest, from suture removal to emergency thoracotomy, and from renal to plastic surgery—it all eventually shows up in the ED.

This book is intended to provide you with information that is useful at the bedside. Many new chapters have been added to cover old and new procedures that may now be performed in the ED (extubation, declotting central venous access devices, continuous arteriovenous rewarming, diagnostic bladder ultra sound, etc.). Every effort has been made to make this a comprehensive reference for practicing emergency nurses. Novices will find the basic procedures a helpful review; experienced emergency nurses will appreciate information about new or infrequently performed procedures. The focus is clear, pertinent information to help you perform or assist with procedures. Research findings have been incorporated whenever possible to provide a scientific basis for practice.

This text describes the use of many commercial products; no endorsement of these products is intended. Likewise, omission of products does not imply lack of endorsement. Products are included if they are commonly in use in emergency care based on the experience of the editor and contributors.

Jean A. Proehl, RN, MN, CEN, CCRN

Introduction

This book presents essential information in a standard format about a wide variety of procedures. It is assumed that the reader possesses basic nursing knowledge, and, accordingly, some information is not included in procedures because it is assumed to be part of standard nursing practice. These components of standard nursing practice include, but are not limited to:

- Attending to life-, limb-, or vision-threatening emergencies first
- Verifying the patient's identity and introducing yourself
- Obtaining an appropriate history and physical examination
- Providing age-appropriate care
- Placing the patient in a position of comfort when possible
- Explaining the procedure in lay terminology to the patient
- Providing emotional support
- Obtaining verbal or written consent, or both, as indicated by institutional policy
- Including the family and significant others in explanations, follow-up teaching, and emotional support
- Teaching the patient about prescribed medications
- Draping the patient to provide privacy and warmth
- Washing your hands and maintaining aseptic technique when indicated
- Protecting yourself with personal protective equipment as indicated
- Documenting your assessment findings and interventions and the patient's response to them

Nursing practice varies from state to state and institution to institution. An asterisk (*) has been used throughout the book to indicate portions of a procedure usually performed by a physician or an advanced practice nurse. Some of these tasks are also performed by paramedics, physician's assistants, and nurses in extended roles such as air or ground transport. The use of the asterisk is not intended to prescribe nursing or medical practice, but rather to indicate the usual role delineation in the experience of the editor and contributors. The information about nonnursing components of a procedure helps the nurse anticipate needs and expedite safe patient care.

Jean A. Proehl, RN, MN, CEN, CCRN

Acknowledgments

I would like to gratefully acknowledge the generosity of numerous authors, publishers, and manufacturers who shared illustrations for this book. Good illustrations are essential for explaining procedures, and this book would not be so richly illustrated without the contributions of these individuals and companies. The manufacturers of products provided gratis illustrations and, in some cases, reviewed the content for accuracy as it pertains to their products.

I would also like to acknowledge the contributions of authors to the previous editions; they provided a strong foundation upon which to build and expand for the third edition.

Jean A. Proehl, RN, MN, CEN, CCRN

Contents

Assessment Procedures

Primary Survey

Jean A. Proehl, RN, MN, CEN, CCRN

INDICATION
To rapidly assess and intervene for life-threatening conditions in critically ill or injured patients.

CONTRAINDICATIONS AND CAUTIONS
1. The presence of an environmental hazard, such as fire, noxious fumes, and explosion, that mandates immediate evacuation of the area, takes priority over the primary survey.
2. Do not proceed to the next assessment step until interventions for life-threatening conditions have been implemented.

EQUIPMENT
Towel rolls or other head-support devices
2- to 3-inch cloth adhesive tape
Stethoscope
Flashlight
Other equipment as indicated for resuscitative procedures

PROCEDURAL STEPS
1. Assess airway patency while simultaneously maintaining cervical spine immobilization with manual stabilization. Airway patency is assessed by looking for chest rise and fall, and by listening and feeling for air movement from the nose and mouth. If the airway is partially or completely obstructed, implement the appropriate intervention. Potential interventions include the following and are described elsewhere in this text:

   Procedure 3–Airway Positioning
   Procedure 4–Airway Foreign Object Removal
   Procedure 5–Oral Airway Insertion
   Procedure 6–Nasal Airway Insertion
   Procedure 7–Laryngeal Mask Airway
   Procedure 8–Esophageal Obturator Airway and Esophageal Gastric Tube Airway Insertion
   Procedures 9-13–Endotracheal Intubation
   Procedure 15–Pharyngeal Tracheal Lumen Airway
   Procedure 16–Combitube Airway
   Procedure 17–Cricothyrotomy
   Procedure 18–Percutaneous Transtracheal Ventilation
   Procedure 19–Tracheostomy
   Procedure 31–Pharyngeal Suctioning

2. If the patient is at risk for cervical spine injury, manually immobilize the head or use towel rolls or other lateral head supports with wide cloth tape across the forehead and head supports and down to the backboard or stretcher. Cervical spine immobilization should be maintained until the neck is cleared by x-ray or clinical examination.

3. Assess breathing adequacy by observing the respiratory rate, depth, and difficulty. Briefly auscultate breath sounds bilaterally. Implement pulse oximetry monitoring for all seriously injured or ill patients (see Procedure 23). If respirations are absent or abnormal, implement appropriate interventions. Potential interventions include the following and are described elsewhere in this text:

   Procedure 20–Positioning the Dyspneic Patient
   Procedure 27–General Principles of Oxygen Therapy and Oxygen Delivery
      Devices
   Procedures 31-33–Suctioning
   Procedure 35–Bag-Valve-Mask Ventilation
   Procedure 36–Anesthesia Bag Ventilation
   Procedure 40–Emergency Needle Thoracentesis
   Procedure 41–Chest-Tube Insertion

   Use Flutter valve or occlusive dressing for open pneumothorax (sucking chest wound).

4. Assess circulation by evaluating the radial or carotid pulse for rate and strength. Observe and palpate the skin for warmth, color, and moisture. Check for exsanguinating external hemorrhage, and if present, apply direct pressure to the site. If the circulation is absent or altered, institute electrocardiographic monitoring (see Procedure 58) and implement appropriate interventions, including chest compressions, as indicated. Other potential interventions include the following and are described elsewhere in this text:

   Procedure 51–Positioning the Hypotensive Patient
   Procedure 56–Pericardiocentesis
   Procedure 57–Emergency Thoracotomy and Internal Defibrillation
   Procedures 63-72–Vascular Access
   Procedure 84–Defibrillation
   Procedure 85–Synchronized Cardioversion
   Procedures 88 and 89–Cardiac Pacing

5. Evaluate the neurologic status to determine whether the patient is alert (A), responds to verbal stimuli (V), responds to painful stimuli (P), or is unresponsive to all stimuli (U). Assess pupil size, equality, and reaction to light.

AGE-SPECIFIC CONSIDERATIONS

1. *Airway:* Young infants are obligate nose breathers. Nasal flaring is an indication of respiratory distress. Nasal suctioning is a high-priority intervention in an infant with nasal secretions. Infants also have a proportionately larger tongue, which may obstruct their airway. Displaced dentures may cause airway obstruction in adults, especially the elderly.

2. *Breathing:* The ribs and sternum are more cartilaginous in children; therefore, retractions are common during respiratory distress. Infants rely heavily on diaphragmatic breathing because of poorly developed intercostal muscles; for

this reason, an upright posture is preferred for children in respiratory distress. Because the chest wall of infants and small children is thin, auscultation of breath sounds may be misleading, that is, breath sounds may be transmitted from the opposite side, leading to "equal breath sounds," even in the presence of right mainstem intubation or pneumothorax. A supine position may be poorly tolerated and cause respiratory distress in elderly patients, especially those with significant preexisting pulmonary or cardiac disease.

3. *Capillary refill:* This is an important circulatory assessment in infants and young children. Assess it in a central area, such as the child's forehead or chest. Normal capillary refill is less than 2 seconds. Because capillary refill time increases as part of the aging process, it is not a reliable indicator of systemic perfusion in adults.

COMPLICATIONS
1. Failure to recognize and intervene appropriately for life-threatening conditions before progressing to the next assessment step may result in patient deterioration.
2. Intervening for noncritical conditions, such as extremity fractures, before correcting life-threatening conditions may result in patient deterioration.

PATIENT TEACHING
Do not move until a spinal injury has been ruled out.

PROCEDURE 2

Secondary Survey

Jean A. Proehl, RN, MN, CEN, CCRN

INDICATIONS
1. To rapidly and systematically assess injured patients from head to toe to identify all injuries.
2. To rapidly and systematically assess critically ill patients in whom the etiology of signs and symptoms is unclear.

CONTRAINDICATIONS AND CAUTIONS
1. Do not begin the secondary survey until the primary survey has been completed and resuscitation procedures have been initiated as indicated (see Procedure 1).

2. Continue to monitor airway, breathing, circulatory, and neurologic status during the secondary survey, and interrupt the secondary survey to initiate interventions for life-threatening conditions as indicated.
3. Prioritize and initiate interventions for injuries or conditions discovered in the secondary survey *after* the entire head-to-toe examination is complete.

EQUIPMENT

Stethoscope
Pulse oximeter
Cardiac monitor
Blood pressure cuff or noninvasive blood pressure monitor
Thermometer
Blanket

PROCEDURAL STEPS

1. Maintain cervical spine stabilization for trauma patients as initiated in the primary survey.
2. Remove all clothing to facilitate a complete patient assessment. Cover the patient to preserve the body temperature.
3. Obtain blood pressure, pulse, and respirations. Temperature determination may be deferred until the secondary survey is completed, but it should be performed as quickly as possible in the very old, in the very young, and in those with potential hypothermia or hyperthermia.
4. Initiate cardiac (see Procedure 58) and pulse oximetry monitoring (see Procedure 23).
5. If the patient is conscious, obtain information about painful areas by instructing him/her to report any tenderness elicited by palpation. Obtain a brief history of the mechanism of the injury; the history of the present illness; any chronic diseases, allergies, or pertinent immunizations; current medications (prescription, over the counter, and herbal); and any recent use of alcohol or illicit drugs.
6. Inspect the head and face for wounds, deformities, discolorations, or bloody/serous drainage from the nose or ears. Palpate the entire head and face for wounds, deformities, or tenderness. In the conscious and cooperative patient, evaluate extraocular movements, gross vision, and dental occlusion. Note any unusual odors, for example, gasoline, fruity breath, or ethanol.
7. If necessary, remove the anterior portion of the cervical collar while another person maintains manual immobilization of the head and neck. Inspect the anterior neck for wounds, jugular venous distention, discolorations, or deformities. Palpate the anterior neck for deformities, crepitus, tenderness, or tracheal deviation (best palpated in the notch above the manubrium). Gently palpate the posterior neck from the base of the skull to the upper back for wounds, deformities, tenderness, or muscle spasm.
8. Inspect the anterior and lateral chest for wounds, deformities, discolorations, respiratory expansion, symmetry, and paradoxical movement. Palpate the anterior and lateral chest for deformities, tenderness, or crepitus. Auscultate breath sounds to determine whether they are present and equal bilaterally, and note any abnormal sounds, such as crackles and wheezes. Auscultate heart sounds to determine whether they are clear or muffled.

9. Inspect the abdomen for wounds, discolorations, or distention. Auscultate all quadrants for the presence of bowel sounds. Gently palpate the abdomen for tenderness, guarding, rigidity, or masses (palpate the areas that are known to be painful last).
10. Inspect the pelvic area and genitalia for wounds, deformities, discolorations, or bleeding from the urinary meatus, vagina, or rectum. Palpate for pelvic tenderness, crepitus, or instability by gently pressing in on the anterosuperior iliac crests bilaterally and pushing down on the pubic symphysis. Palpate femoral pulses for presence and equality.
11. Inspect all extremities for wounds, deformities, or discolorations. Palpate all extremities for tenderness, deformities, muscle spasm, and distal pulses. If the patient is conscious, determine gross motor and sensory function by having the patient wiggle toes and fingers and asking whether he/she can feel your touch.
12. In the injured patient, obtain assistance to maintain cervical spine alignment and support injured extremities while logrolling the patient to the side. Avoid rolling the patient onto an injured extremity if possible. In some patients, it may be necessary to roll the patient to both sides to assess the posterior surfaces adequately. Inspect the posterior surfaces for wounds, deformities, or discolorations. Palpate all posterior surfaces for wounds, deformities, or muscle spasm.
13. *In male trauma patients, perform a rectal examination to assess sphincter tone and the prostate.

AGE-SPECIFIC CONSIDERATIONS
1. Infants and young children have immature thermoregulatory capability and are susceptible to iatrogenic hypothermia. Elderly patients may have less subcutaneous fat and lose body heat easily. Keep them covered and provide warming as indicated.
2. The normal range for vital signs in children varies by age (Table 2-1). The heart and respiratory rates may be altered by fear, pain, and anxiety, in addition to physiologic problems, such as hypoxia and hypovolemia. In children, blood pressure may be maintained in the presence of significant hypovolemia. Therefore, other assessments of circulatory status (heart rate, capillary refill, skin color, and so forth) should be monitored closely. In older patients, the decreased sensitivity of baroreceptors, decreased response to β stimulation, and medications may prevent a compensatory tachycardia in response to decreased systemic perfusion.
3. Pediatric patients should be weighed as soon as possible because medication doses, fluid resuscitation, and other interventions are influenced by the child's size.

COMPLICATIONS
1. Failure to recognize and intervene appropriately for life-threatening conditions that develop or worsen during the secondary survey may result in patient deterioration.

*Indicates portions of the procedure that are usually performed by a physician or an advanced practice nurse.

TABLE 2-1
NORMAL VITAL SIGNS BY AGE

Age	Heart Rate	Systolic Blood Pressure	Respiratory Rate
Preterm newborn	120-180	40-60	55-65
Term newborn	90-170	52-92	40-60
1 month	110-180	60-104	30-50
6 months	110-180	65-125	25-35
1 year	80-160	70-118	20-30
2 years	80-130	73-117	20-30
4 years	80-120	65-117	20-30
6 years	75-115	76-116	18-24
8 years	70-110	76-119	18-22
10 years	70-110	82-122	16-20
12 years	60-110	84-128	16-20
14 years	60-105	84-136	16-20

2. In the injured patient, failure to maintain spinal alignment and immobilization throughout the secondary survey may result in trauma to the spinal cord.
3. Failure to complete the secondary survey and prioritize interventions before initiating them may result in patient deterioration.
4. Intervening for noncritical problems, such as extremity fractures, before correcting life-threatening conditions may result in patient deterioration.

PATIENT TEACHING
Do not move until spinal injury has been ruled out.

Airway Procedures

Airway Positioning

Donna York Clark, RN, MS, CFRN, CCRN

INDICATION

To establish and maintain a patent airway or to relieve a partial or total airway obstruction due to displacement of the tongue into the posterior pharynx and/or the epiglottis at the level of the larynx. These positions are indicated for unconscious patients who do not have an adequate airway.

CONTRAINDICATIONS AND CAUTIONS

1. In an unconscious trauma patient or a patient with a known or suspected neck injury, the head and neck should be maintained in a neutral position without neck hyperextension. Use the jaw-thrust or chin-lift maneuver to open the airway in this situation (AHA, 2001).
2. Positioning alone may be insufficient to achieve and maintain an open airway. Additional interventions, such as suctioning, oral/nasal airway insertion, and intubation, may be indicated.

PROCEDURAL STEPS

1. Place the patient in a supine position.
2. For the head-tilt/chin-lift maneuver, lift the chin forward to displace the mandible anteriorly while tilting the head back with a hand on the forehead (Figure 3-1). This maneuver results in hyperextension of the neck and is contraindicated when a neck injury is suspected or known to be present.
3. If the head-tilt/chin-lift maneuver is unsuccessful or contraindicated, use either the jaw-thrust or the chin-lift maneuver.
   Jaw-thrust maneuver: Lift the mandible forward with your index fingers while pushing against the zygomatic arches with your thumbs (Figure 3-2). Your thumbs provide counterpressure to prevent movement of the head when the mandible is pushed forward.
   Chin-lift maneuver: Place one hand on the forehead to stabilize the head and neck. Grab the mandible between the thumb and index finger of the other hand. Lift the mandible forward (Figure 3-3).
4. Reassess airway patency after any maneuver.

AGE-SPECIFIC CONSIDERATIONS

1. For the head-tilt/chin-lift maneuver in the infant, place one hand on the infant's forehead and tilt the head gently back into a neutral position. The neck should be slightly extended. This is known as the "sniffing position" (Figure 3-4). Hyperextension of an infant's neck may cause airway compromise or obstruction. Place fingers under the bony part of the lower jaw at the chin and lift the mandible upward and outward. Use caution not to close the

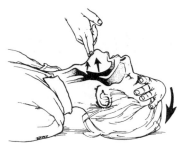

FIGURE 3-1 Head-tilt/chin-lift. (From American Heart Association. [1994]. *Textbook of basic life support for healthcare providers.* Dallas: Author [p. 4-4], reproduced with permission. Copyright American Heart Association.)

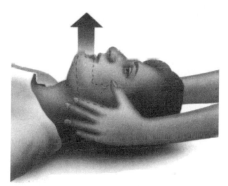

FIGURE 3-2 Jaw thrust. (From Emergency Nurses Association. [2000]. *Trauma nursing core course: Provider manual,* 5th ed. Des Plaines, IL: Author [p. 364].)

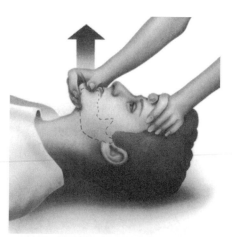

FIGURE 3-3 Chin lift. (From Emergency Nurses Association. [2000]. *Trauma nursing core course: Provider manual,* 5th ed. Des Plaines, IL: Author [p. 364].)

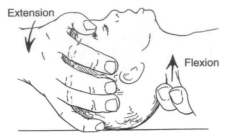

FIGURE 3-4 Sniffing position. (From American Academy of Pediatrics & American College of Emergency Physicians. [1998]. *Advanced pediatric life support: The pediatric emergency medicine course.* Elk Grove Village, IL: Authors [p. 63].)

mouth or push on the soft tissues under the chin because these maneuvers may obstruct the airway.

2. Children presenting with symptoms of epiglottitis, such as high fever, drooling, and respiratory distress, should not be forced into a supine position, which could completely obstruct the airway. Allow the child to maintain a position of comfort until definitive airway management is available.

COMPLICATIONS

1. If the airway remains obstructed, suctioning should be completed, and then an oropharyngeal or nasopharyngeal airway should be inserted. (See Procedures 5, 6, and 31.)
2. Injury to the spinal cord may occur if the head and/or neck are moved in patients with cervical spine injuries.
3. If your fingers press deeply into the soft tissue under the chin, blood vessels or the airway could be obstructed.

REFERENCES

American Heart Association (AHA). (2001). The systematic ACLS approach. In *ACLS Provider Manual*. Dallas: Author.

Airway Foreign Object Removal

Donna York Clark, RN, MS, CFRN, CCRN

Abdominal thrusts are also known as the Heimlich maneuver.

INDICATION

To relieve upper airway obstruction caused by foreign objects. Signs and symptoms of airway obstruction are characterized by some or all of the following:

1. Sudden inability to speak
2. Universal sign for choking: clutching the neck (AHA, 2001a)
3. Noisy airflow (high-pitched sounds) during inspiration
4. Accessory muscle use during respiration and increasing work of breathing
5. A weak or ineffective cough or an inability to cough
6. Absence of spontaneous respirations or cyanosis
7. Infants or children with a sudden onset of respiratory distress associated with coughing, gagging, stridor, or wheezing (ACEP/AAP, 1998)

CONTRAINDICATIONS AND CAUTIONS

1. In the conscious patient, a voluntary cough generates the greatest airflow and may relieve the obstruction. Do not interfere with the patient's attempts to cough up the obstruction.
2. Chest thrusts should not be used in the patient who has a chest injury, for example, flail chest, cardiac contusion, or sternal fractures
3. In the advanced stages of pregnancy or in the markedly obese, chest thrusts are recommended (AHA, 2001a).
4. Correct hand placement is essential for avoiding injury to underlying organs during delivery of abdominal thrusts.

EQUIPMENT

Oral suction, if available

Magill or Kelly forceps and laryngoscope (optional for the removal of a foreign object that can be visualized in the upper airway)

PATIENT PREPARATION

1. The patient may be sitting, standing, or supine.
2. Suction any blood or mucus you can visualize in the patient's mouth.
3. Remove broken or loose-fitting dentures.
4. Be prepared to perform more definitive airway management, such as cricothyrotomy (see Procedure 17).

13

PROCEDURAL STEPS

1. Stand behind the sitting or standing patient and wrap your arms around the abdomen. If the patient is supine, kneel and straddle the patient's thighs.
2. Hand placement is as follows:
   a. For the standing or sitting patient, make a fist with one hand and cover the fist with your other hand. Hand placement on the patient's abdomen should be below the xiphoid process and above the navel (Figure 4-1) (AHA, 2001a).
   b. For the supine patient, place one hand over the other, with the heel of the bottom hand against the patient's abdomen below the xiphoid process and above the navel (Figure 4-2) (AHA, 2001a).
3. Thrust quickly, compressing the abdomen inward and upward.
4. If necessary, repeat the abdominal thrusts several times to relieve airway obstruction. Assess the airway frequently to determine the success of the maneuver.
5. For the pregnant or obese patient, the chest thrust may be performed. The patient may be supine, sitting, or standing. Put one hand directly over the other and position the bottom hand at the midsternal area above the xiphoid process (mid-nipple line, the same position used in the external cardiac massage). Thrust straight down toward the spine. If necessary, repeat chest thrusts several times to relieve airway obstruction (Figure 4-3).
6. *For complete obstruction, where ventilation is not possible and thrusts ineffective, use Magill forceps with direct laryngoscopy to facilitate removal of the obstruction (Walls, 2000).

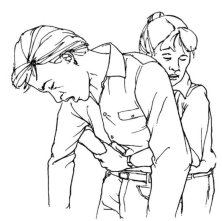

FIGURE 4-1 Abdominal thrusts for the standing or sitting victim of choking. (From American Heart Association. [1994]. *Textbook of basic life support for healthcare providers.* Dallas: Author [p. 4-17], reproduced with permission. Copyright American Heart Association.)

---

*Indicates portions of the procedure usually performed by a physician or an advanced practice nurse.

AGE-SPECIFIC CONSIDERATIONS
Infant (<1 Year)

1. Straddle the infant in the prone position over the rescuer's forearm, with the head lower than the trunk. Support the infant's head by holding the jaw (Figure 4-4).
2. Deliver up to five forceful back blows between the shoulder blades by using the heel of your hand.

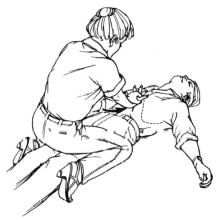

FIGURE 4-2 Abdominal thrusts for the supine, unconscious victim of choking. (From American Heart Association. [1994]. *Textbook of basic life support for healthcare providers.* Dallas: Author, [p. 4-18], reproduced with permission. Copyright American Heart Association.)

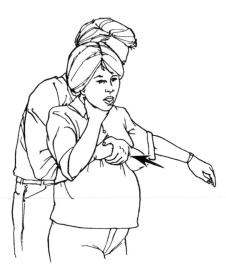

FIGURE 4-3 Chest thrusts for the pregnant or obese victim of choking. (From American Heart Association. [1994]. *Textbook of basic life support for healthcare providers.* Dallas: Author, [p. 4-19], reproduced with permission. Copyright American Heart Association.)

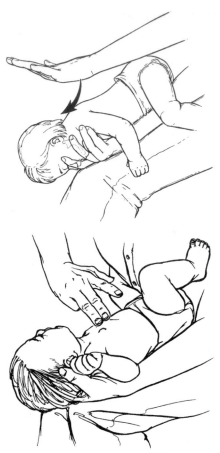

FIGURE 4-4 Back blows (*top illustration*) and chest thrusts (*bottom illustration*) for foreign body obstruction in an infant. (From American Heart Association. [1994]. *Textbook of basic life support for healthcare providers.* Dallas: Author, [p. 6-2], reproduced with permission. Copyright American Heart Association.)

3. Turn the infant supine, supporting the head and neck and positioning on the thigh.
4. Give up to five quick downward chest thrusts. To find the correct finger location, place the index finger just below the level of the infant's nipples. Place the middle fingers on the sternum, adjacent to the index finger (AHA, 2001b; AHA, 2001c; ACEP/AAP, 1998).
5. Steps 1 through 4 are continued until the object is expelled or there is a loss of consciousness.
6. If the infant loses consciousness, open the airway and remove the foreign object if it is visible. Blind finger sweeps should be avoided in infants and children, because the foreign object can be pushed farther back into the airway.

7. *For complete obstruction, in which ventilation is not possible, use Magill forceps with direct laryngoscopy to facilitate removal of the obstruction (ACEP/AAP, 1998).

Child (1 to 8 Years)

1. For the standing or sitting patient, place your arms under the axillae, encircling the victim's torso. Place your hands against the patient's abdomen, slightly above the navel and below the xiphoid process (AHA, 2001a; AHA, 2001b). Exert upward thrusts until the foreign object is expelled or the patient loses consciousness.
2. For the supine patient, kneel beside or straddle the victim's hips. Place your hands above the navel and below the xiphoid process (AHA, 2001a; AHA, 2001b). Quick upward thrusts are directed toward the midline and should not be directed to either side of the abdomen. If a foreign object is visible, remove it by using a finger sweep.
3. Back blows are not recommended for patients above the infant age range.
4. Blind finger sweeps should be avoided in infants and children, because the foreign object can be pushed farther back into the airway.
5. *For complete obstruction, in which ventilation is not possible, use Magill forceps with direct laryngoscopy to facilitate removal of the obstruction (ACEP/AAP, 1998).

COMPLICATIONS

1. Abdominal pain, ecchymosis
2. Nausea, vomiting
3. Fractured ribs
4. Injury to underlying abdominal or chest organs

REFERENCES

American College of Emergency Physicians (ACEP) and American Academy of Pediatrics (AAP). (1998). *APLS: The pediatric emergency medicine course.* Dallas: Author.

American Heart Association. (2001a). *Basic life support for healthcare providers.* Dallas: Author.

American Heart Association. (2001b). *ACLS provider manual.* Dallas: Author.

American Heart Association. (2001c). *Advanced pediatric life support: instructors manual.* Dallas: Author.

Walls, R. (2000). Foreign body in the adult airway (pp. 190-194). In Walls, R., Luten, R., Murphy, M., & Schneider, R. (Eds.), *Manual of emergency airway management.* Philadelphia: Lippincott Williams & Wilkins.

*Indicates portions of the procedure usually performed by a physician or an advanced practice nurse.

Oral Airway Insertion

Donna York Clark, RN, MS, CFRN, CCRN

The oral airway is also known as an oropharyngeal airway.

INDICATION
To maintain airway patency for patients in the following situations:
1. An unconscious spontaneously breathing patient with an airway obstruction caused by an impaired gag reflex and a loss of tone to the submandibular muscles.
2. Unsuccessful airway opening by other maneuvers, such as the head tilt, the chin lift, and the jaw thrust.
3. A patient ventilated by a bag-valve-mask device. The oral airway elevates the soft tissues of the posterior pharynx, easing ventilation and minimizing gastric insufflation.
4. An orally intubated patient who bites/clenches the endotracheal tube; the oral airway is used as a bite block.
5. An unconscious patient during suctioning, to facilitate the removal of a patient's oral secretions (AHA , 2001; Greenlee, 2001).

CONTRAINDICATIONS AND CAUTIONS
1. Insertion of an oral airway in a conscious or semiconscious patient stimulates the gag reflex and may stimulate airway spasm or cause the patient to vomit (McGee & Vender, 1996; AHA, 2001).
2. Incorrect placement of an oral airway may compress the tongue into the posterior pharynx and cause further obstruction (Urocher & Hopson, 2004).
3. An airway that is too small may push the tongue into the oropharynx and cause an obstruction, and an airway that is too large may obstruct the trachea (McGee & Vender, 1996).
4. Failure to clear the oropharynx of foreign material before insertion of the airway may result in aspiration.
5. To avoid vomiting and aspiration, the oropharyngeal airway should be removed immediately after the patient regains a gag reflex.

EQUIPMENT
Oropharyngeal suction equipment
Oropharyngeal airway
Tongue blade

PATIENT PREPARATION
1. Place the patient in a supine position.
2. Suction blood, secretions, or other foreign material from the patient's oropharynx. See Procedure 31.

TABLE 5-1

ORAL AIRWAY SIZING BY AGE

Age	Size
Premature neonate	000
Newborn	00
Infant	0
1-3 yr	1
3-8 yr	2
9-18 yr, large child, small adult	3
Medium adult	4
Large adult	5, 6

From Boggs, R.L., Wooldrige-King, M. (1993). *AACN procedure manual for critical care*, 3rd ed. (p. 3). Philadelphia: W.B. Saunders.

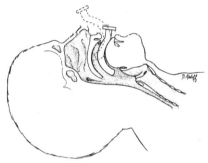

FIGURE 5-1 Correct placement of oropharyngeal airway. (From Rosen, P., & Sternbach, G.L. [1983]. *Atlas of emergency medicine,* 2nd ed. [p. 7]. Baltimore: Williams & Wilkins.)

3. Select the appropriately sized oropharyngeal airway. Table 5-1 lists usual airway sizes by age. Align the tube on the side of the patient's face and choose an airway that extends from the corner of the mouth to the tragus of the ear (Luten, 2000) or from the lips to the angle of the jaw (Greenlee, 2001).

PROCEDURAL STEPS

1. Use a tongue blade to depress and displace the tongue forward. Insert the airway with the curve pointing up into the oropharynx.
2. As an alternative procedure, insert the airway upside down (with the curve pointing toward the back of the patient's head) into the mouth. As the tip of the airway reaches the posterior wall of the pharynx, rotate the airway 180 degrees to the proper position.
3. The distal tip of the airway should lie between the base of the tongue and the back of the throat. The flange of the tube should sit comfortably on the lips (Figure 5-1).
4. Reassess the airway patency and auscultate the lung for equal and clear breath sounds during ventilation.

AGE-SPECIFIC CONSIDERATION

For pediatric patients, depress and displace the tongue forward with a tongue blade and insert the airway (described in step 1 above). Do *not* insert an upside-down airway and then rotate it (described in step 2 above), because this technique may injure the soft tissue of the oropharynx (Eichelberger et al, 1998).

COMPLICATIONS

1. Trauma to the lips, tongue, teeth, and oral mucosa
2. Vomiting and aspiration (Greenlee, 2001)
3. Laryngospasm (McGee & Vender, 1996)
4. Complete airway obstruction (AHA, 2001)

REFERENCES

American Heart Association (AHA). (2001). The advanced ACLS skills (pp. 19-40). In *Textbook of advanced cardiac life support*. Dallas: Author.

Boggs, R.L. & Wooldridge-King, M. (1993). *AACN procedurel manual for critical care:* 3rd ed. Philadelphia: W.B. Saunders.

Eichelberger, M., Ball, J., Pratsch, G., & Clark, J. (1998). Equipment and procedures for management of ABCs (pp. 47-74). In *Pediatric Emergencies*, 2nd ed. Old Tappan, New Jersey: Brady/Prentice Hall.

Greenlee, K.K. (2001). Oropharyngeal airway insertion (pp. 31-35). In Lynn-McHale, D.H. & Carlson, K.K. (Eds.), *AACN procedure manual for critical care*, 3rd ed. Philadelphia: W.B. Saunders.

Luten, R. (2000). The pediatric patient (pp. 143-152). In Walls, R., Luten, R., Murphy, M., & Schneider, R. (Eds.), *Manual of emergency airway management*. Philadelphia: Lippincott Williams & Wilkins.

McGee, J. & Vender, J. (1996). Nonintubation management of the airway: mask ventilation (pp. 228-254). In Benumof, J.L. (Ed.), *Airway management principles and practice*. St. Louis: Mosby.

Urocher, D. & Hopson, L. (2004). Basic airway mangement and decision-making (pp. 53-68). In Roberts, J. & Hedges, J. (Eds.), *Clinical procedures in emergency medicine*, 4th ed. Philadelphia: W.B. Saunders.

Nasal Airway Insertion

Donna York Clark, RN, MS, CFRN, CCRN

Nasal airways are also known as nasopharyngeal airways and nasal trumpets.

INDICATIONS

The nasal airway is indicated in the following situations:
1. There is a question of patency of the posterior nasopharynx with intact upper airway reflexes.
2. Bag-valve-mask ventilation is ineffective, and the nasopharyngeal airway may facilitate ventilation. The nasal airway may be used in combination with the oropharyngeal airway in this setting.
3. Insertion of an oropharyngeal airway is technically difficult or impossible because of massive trauma around the mouth, such as mandibulomaxillary wiring.
4. To decrease soft tissue trauma when frequent nasotracheal suctioning is necessary (Schneider, 2000; AHA, 2001; Bledsoe, 2003; Greenlee, 2001).

CONTRAINDICATIONS AND CAUTIONS

1. The insertion of a nasal airway may stimulate the gag reflex and cause the patient to vomit.
2. If the tube is too long, it may enter the esophagus and cause gastric insufflation and hypoventilation (AHA, 2001).
3. Epistaxis may occur and may lead to aspiration of blood.
4. Nasal airways should not be used in patients who have extensive facial trauma or a basilar skull fracture (Bledsoe, 2003).

EQUIPMENT

Nasopharyngeal suction equipment
Water-soluble lubricant or anesthetic jelly
Nasopharyngeal airway

PATIENT PREPARATION

1. Place the patient in a supine position or high Fowler's position.
2. Select the nostril that appears to be the largest and most open. Assess the nasal passages for trauma, foreign body, septal deviation, or polyps.
3. Prepare suction equipment for use.

PROCEDURAL STEPS

1. Select appropriately sized nasal airway. Use the largest airway that will pass easily through the naris. Measure the length of the nasopharyngeal airway from the tip of the nose to the tragus of the ear (Luten, II, 2000; Hubble & Hubble, 2002; McGee & Vender, 1996) (Table 6-1).

21

2. Vasoconstriction of the mucous membranes may be indicated. Agents commonly prescribed for this purpose include phenylephrine (Neo-Synephrine) or cocaine spray or liquid (McGee & Vender, 1996).
3. Lubricate the tube with water-soluble gel or anesthetic ointment (McGee & Vender, 1996).
4. Pass the airway along the floor of the nostril with the bevel facing the nasal septum (Figure 6-1). Direct the airway posteriorly and rotate it slightly toward the ear until the flange rests against the nostril. Note that all nasal airways have a bevel that is angled for insertion into the right naris. The airway may be used in the left nares. Place the airway in the left naris with the bevel facing the nasal septum. The nasopharyngeal airway curvature will be opposite of the natural nasal curvature. Once the airway tip has reached the correct position, rotate the airway 180 degrees (Hubble & Hubble, 2002).
5. If resistance is met, a slight rotation of the tube may facilitate passage as the device reaches the hypopharynx (AHA, 2001).
6. Reassess the airway patency.

TABLE 6-1
NASOPHARYNGEAL AIRWAY SIZING

Large adult	8.0-9.0 i.d.
Medium adult	7.0-8.0 i.d.
Small adult	6.0-7.0 i.d.

i.d., Internal diameter in millimeters
From American Heart Association. (1997). *Textbook of advanced cardiac life support.* Dallas: Author, p. 22.

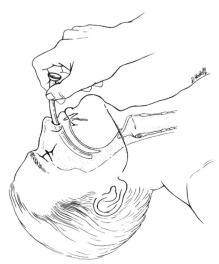

FIGURE 6-1 Correct placement of nasopharyngeal airway. (From Rosen, P., & Sternbach, G.L. [1983]. *Atlas of emergency medicine,* 2nd ed. Baltimore: Williams & Wilkins, p. 9.)

COMPLICATIONS

1. Epistaxis
2. Aspiration
3. Hypoxia secondary to aspiration or improper placement
4. Extreme caution should be used when a nasopharyngeal airway is placed in patients with basilar skull or facial fractures because penetration of the cranial vault may occur.

REFERENCES

American Heart Association (1997). *Textbook of advanced cardiac life support* [p. 22]. Dallas: Author.

American Heart Association (AHA). (2001). The advanced ACLS skills (pp 19-40). In *Textbook of advanced cardiac life support*. Dallas: Author.

Bledsoe, B., Porter, R., & Cherry, R. (2003). *Essentials of paramedic care*. Old Tappan, NJ: Brady/Prentice Hall.

Greenlee, K.K. (2001). Nasopharyngeal airway insertion (pp. 27-30). In Lynn-McHale, D.H. & Carlson, K.K. (Eds.), *AACN procedure manual for critical care*, 3rd ed. Philadelphia: W.B. Saunders.

Hubble, M.W. & Hubble, J.P. (2002). Airway and ventilation management (pp. 303-448). *Principles of advanced trauma care*. Albany, NY: Delmar Thompson Learning.

Luten, R. (2000). The pediatric patient (pp. 143-152). In Walls, R., Luten, R., Murphy, M., & Schneider, R. (Eds.), *Manual of emergency airway management*. Philadelphia: Lippincott Williams & Wilkins.

McGee, J. & Vender, J. (1996). Nonintubation management of the airway: mask ventilation (pp. 228-254). In Benumof, J.L. (Ed.), *Airway management: principles and practice*. St. Louis: Mosby.

Schneider, R. (2000). Basic airway management (pp. 43-157). In Walls, R., Luten, R., Murphy, M., & Schneider, R. (Eds.) *Manual of emergency airway management*. Philadelphia: Lippincott Williams & Wilkins.

Laryngeal Mask Airway

Donna York Clark, RN, MS, CFRN, CCRN

The laryngeal mask airway (LMA) resembles an endotracheal tube with a spoon-shaped mask at one end. The spoon-shaped mask has an inflatable collar that forms a seal around the larynx (Figure 7-1) (Murphy, 2000; Bledsoe, 2003).

The LMA has gained popularity in use in situations in which tracheal intubation is not possible. In adult Advanced Cardiovascular Life Support (ACLS), the LMA is recommended as a Class IIa device, defined as "Interventions are acceptable, safe, and useful. Considered within standard of care." This airway is an adjunct and can be used if tracheal intubation is not possible (AHA, 2001a). In Pediatric Advanced Life Support (PALS), the LMA is classified as a Class Indeterminate device, defined as "Interventions can still be recommended for use,

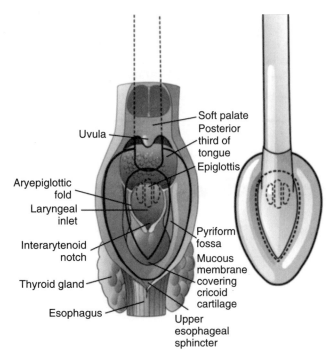

FIGURE 7-1 Dorsal view of the laryngeal mask airway (LMA) showing position in relation to pharyngeal anatomy. (From Brain, A.I.J., Denman, W.T., & Goudsouzian, N.G. [1996]. *Laryngeal mask airway instruction manual.* San Diego, CA, reprinted courtesy Gensia Automedics, Inc.)

but reviewers must acknowledge that research quantity/quality fall short of supporting a final class decision. Indeterminate is limited to promising interventions." The airway may be used, depending on the situation at the time of the arrest (AHA, 2001b).

The LMA is manufactured solely by Laryngeal Mask Company Limited. (San Diego, CA) Four types of LMA devices are produced: the LMA Classic (a reusable LMA), the LMA Unique (a disposable LMA designed as the classic), the LMA Fastrach (designed to facilitate tracheal intubation with an endotracheal tube), and the LMA ProSeal (LMA, 2002).

In October 2000, LMA North America introduced a new product named the LMA-ProSeal. This product is described as the next generation of airway management for the operating room and is designed to do the following (LMA, 2002; Brain, et al., 2000; Keller, et al., 2000):
- Improve the laryngeal seal without increasing mucosal pressures
- Separate the respiratory and alimentary tracts
- Provide higher airway seal pressures for use with positive-pressure ventilation

This ProSeal product is intended for use in the operating room; however, given the crossover of practice, the author and editor believed that introducing this product to the readers was necessary. However, the procedure for the placement and use of this product is beyond the scope of this chapter.

INDICATIONS

1. The LMA is used as an alternative to a face mask in bag-valve-mask ventilation. The LMA is not intended to be used instead of intubation (Murphy, 2000; Bledsoe, 2003; Urocher & Hopson, 2004).
2. In an emergency, the LMA may serve as a temporary route for gas exchange in failed intubation scenarios until definitive airway control is achieved (Pollack, 2001; Murphy, 2000).

CONTRAINDICATIONS AND CAUTIONS

1. The LMA does not constitute definitive airway control. It does *not* protect the airway from gastric content aspiration and should be used only in a patient with an empty stomach.
2. The LMA is not indicated for patients with decreased pulmonary compliance, because the low-pressure seal that is formed around the larynx may not allow adequate ventilation (Murphy, 2000).

EQUIPMENT

LMA (Table 7-1 provides sizing information)
Water-soluble lubricant
Syringe
Tonsil-tip suction
Bag-valve ventilation system
Oxygen source and connecting tubing
Tape or securing device
For intubating LMA (Fastrach): Accompanying silicone-tipped endotracheal tube

TABLE 7-1

LARYNGEAL MASK AIRWAY SIZING AND CUFF INFLATION VOLUMES

Patient Weight	Recommended LMA Size	Maximum Cuff Inflation Volume
<5 kg	1	Up to 4 ml
5-10 kg	1.5	Up to 7 ml
10-20 kg	2	Up to 10 ml
20-30 kg	2.5	Up to 14 ml
>30 kg	3	Up to 20 ml
Normal and large adults	4	Up to 30 ml
Large adults	5	Up to 40 ml

Modified from Brain, A.I.J., Denman, W.T., Goudsouzian, N.G. (1996). *Laryngeal mask airway instruction manual.* San Diego, CA, reprinted courtesy Gesnia Automedics, Inc.

PATIENT PREPARATION (for LMA Classic, LMA Unique, and LMA Fastrach)

1. Preoxygenate the patient with a bag-valve-mask.
2. Administer sedation as prescribed. Deep sedation or an unconscious state is required for LMA use (Murphy, 2000).
3. Position the patient with the head extended and the neck flexed (except in patients with potential cervical spine injury). During LMA insertion, it may be helpful to push the patient's head from behind to maintain this position.

PROCEDURAL STEPS (for LMA Classic, LMA Unique)

1. *Inflate the cuff to check for leaks and deflate it to form a spoon shape (Figure 7-2).
2. *Coat the posterior surface of the LMA with a water-soluble lubricant.
3. *Grasp the LMA by positioning your index finger in the crease between the airway tube and the laryngeal mask (Figure 7-3).
4. *Insert the LMA with the cuff tip gliding against the posterior pharyngeal wall.
5. *Using your index finger to push the LMA, apply slight backward (toward the ears) pressure and follow the anatomic curve (Figure 7-4).
6. *Advance the mask until resistance is noted at the hypopharynx (Figure 7-5).
7. *Remove the index finger while applying slight pressure to the airway tube for the prevention of dislocation.
8. *Inflate the cuff with air; the volume varies with the LMA size (see Table 7-1). During inflation, release the LMA to ensure that placement is maintained as the cuff expands (Figure 7-6).
9. Assess the LMA placement. The following signs indicate an appropriate placement:
   a. A slight outward movement of the airway tube with cuff inflation
   b. A slight swelling at the cricoid region
   c. No visible cuff in the oral cavity
   d. Equal bilateral breath sounds and chest rise and fall
   e. Pulse oximetry readings that indicate adequate oxygenation

---

*Indicates portion of the procedure usually performed by a physician or an advanced practice nurse.

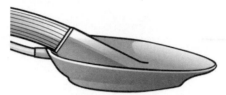

FIGURE 7-2 LMA cuff properly deflated for insertion. (From Brain, A.I.J., Denman, W.T., & Goudsouzian, N.G. [1996]. *Laryngeal mask airway instruction manual.* San Diego, CA, reprinted courtesy Gensia Automedics, Inc.)

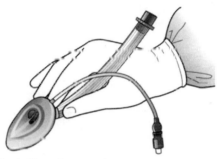

FIGURE 7-3 Method for holding the LMA for insertion. (From Brain, A.I.J., Denman, W.T., & Goudsouzian, N.G. [1996]. *Laryngeal Mask airway instruction manual.* San Diego, CA, reprinted courtesy Gensia Automedics, Inc.)

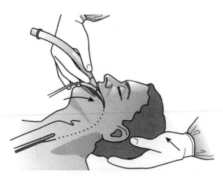

FIGURE 7-4 To facilitate LMA introduction into the oral cavity, gently press the middle finger down on the jaw. (From Brain, A.I.J., Denman, W.T., & Goudsouzian, N.G. [1996]. *Laryngeal mask instruction manual.* San Diego, CA, reprinted courtesy Gensia Automedics, Inc.)

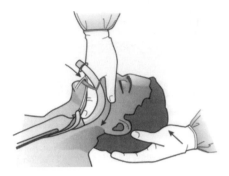

FIGURE 7-5 Maintaining pressure with the finger on the tube in the cranial direction, advance the mask until definite resistance is felt at the base of the hypopharynx. (From Brain A.I.J., Denman, W.T., & Goudsouzian, N.G. [1996]. *Laryngeal mask airway instruction manual.* San Diego, CA, reprinted courtesy Gensia Automedics, Inc.)

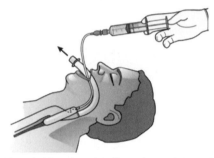

FIGURE 7-6 Inflation without holding the tube allows the mask to seat itself optimally. (From Brain A.I.J., Denman, W.T., & Goudsouzian, N.G. [1996]. *Laryngeal mask airway instruction manual.* San Diego, CA, reprinted courtesy Gensia Automedics, Inc.)

10. Ventilate the patient with a bag-valve system and supplemental oxygen.
11. Secure the LMA with tape or a securing device; a bite block may be used (LMA, 2002).

PROCEDURAL STEPS (for Intubating LMA [Fastrach])

1. *Deflate the cuff of the mask and apply a water-soluble lubricant to the posterior surface. Distribute the lubricant over the anterior hard palate.
2. *Place the curved metal tube in contact with the chin and the mask tip flat against the palate before advancing (Figure 7-7).
3. *Rotate the mask into place with a circular motion, maintaining pressure against the palate and the posterior pharynx (Figure 7-8).
4. *Inflate the mask. Without holding the tube or handle, inflate cuff to a pressure of 60 cm H_2O (Murphy, 2000).

Intubating through the Intubating LMA (Fastrach)

1. *Validate endotracheal tube (ETT) cuff integrity.

---

*Indicates portion of the procedure usually performed by a physician or an advanced practice nurse.

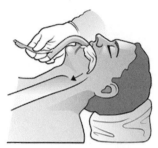

FIGURE 7-7 Insert the intubating LMA with the curved metal tube in contact with the chin and the mask tip flat against the palate. (From LMA North America. [2002]. Available at www.lmana.com/prod/components/products.)

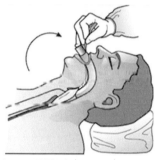

FIGURE 7-8 Advance the intubating LMA and rotate the mask into place with a circular motion, maintaining pressure against the palate and posterior pharynx. (From LMA North America. [2002]. Available at www.lmana.com/prod/components/products.)

2. *Deflate the ETT cuff, lubricate the ETT, and pass it through the intubating LMA tube. Rotate and move the ETT up and down to ensure adequate distribution of water-soluble lubricant.
3. *Advance the ETT to the 15-cm depth indicator. This position signifies passage of the tip of the ETT through the epiglottic opening of the LMA (Figure 7-9).
4. *Use the handle to gently lift the device 2-5 cm. A slight resistance is felt as the ETT is advanced (Figure 7-10).
5. *Advance until intubation is complete.
6. Inflate the ETT cuff and confirm intubation.
7. *Remove the LMA. Remove the connector and gently ease the intubating LMA out over the ETT into the oral cavity while using the stabilizer rod to hold ETT in position as the LMA is pulled over the tube (Figure 7-11).
8. *Remove the stabilizer rod and hold onto the ETT at the level of the incisors (Figure 7-12).
9. *Remove the intubating LMA completely.
10. Replace the ETT connector (Fig 7-13).
    (LMA, 2002; Murphy, 2000, Levitan et al, 2000; Rosenblatt & Murphy, 1999.)

---

*Indicates portion of the procedure usually performed by a physician or an advanced practice nurse.

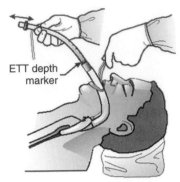

FIGURE 7-9 Advance the endotracheal tube (ETT) to the 15-cm depth indicator. (From LMA North America. [2002]. Available at www.lmana.com/prod/components/products.)

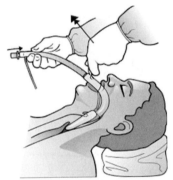

FIGURE 7-10 Use the handle to gently lift the device 2-5 cm as the ETT is advanced. (From LMA North America. [2002]. Available at www.lmana.com/prod/components/products.)

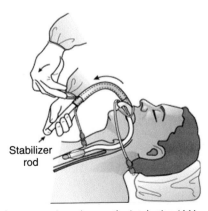

FIGURE 7-11 Remove connector and gently ease the intubating LMA out over the ETT into the oral cavity while using the stabilizer rod to hold the ETT in position as the LMA is pulled over the tube. (From LMA North America. [2002]. Available at www.lmana.com/prod/components/products.)

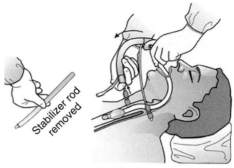

FIGURE 7-12 Remove the stabilizer rod and hold onto the ETT at the level of the incisors. (From LMA North America. [2002]. Availabe at www.lmana.com/prod/components/products.)

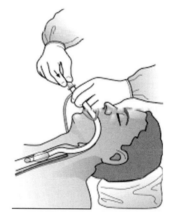

FIGURE 7-13 Replace the ETT connector. (From LMA North America. [2002]. Available at www.lmana.com/prod/components/products.)

AGE-SPECIFIC CONSIDERATION

An appropriately sized LMA is effective for use in infants and children of all weights (see Table 7-1) (LMA, 2002; Luten, 2000).

COMPLICATIONS (LMA, 2002; Urocher & Hopson, 2004)

1. Air leak
2. Laryngospasm
3. Desaturation
4. Severe hypercarbia
5. Regurgitation, aspiration
6. Sore throat
7. Laryngeal hematoma
8. Hypoglossal nerve injury

REFERENCES

American Heart Association (AHA). (2001a). *ACLS provider manual.* Dallas: Author.

American Heart Association (AHA). (2001b). *Instructor's manual: pediatric advanced life support.* Dallas: Author.

Bledsoe, B., Porter, R., & Cherry, R. (2003). *In Essentials of paramedic care.* New Jersey: Brady/Prentice Hall.

Brain, A.I.J., Denman, W.T., Goudsouzian, N.G. (1996). Laryngeal mask airway instruction manual. San Diego, CA.

Brain A.I.J., Verghese C., & Strube P.J. (2000). The LMA ProSeal: a laryngeal mask with an oesophageal vent. *British Journal of Anaesthesia 84*(5), 650-654.

Keller C., Brimacombe J., Kleinsasser A., & Loeckinger A. (2000). Does the ProSeal laryngeal mask airway prevent aspiration of regurgitated fluid? *Anesthesia and Analgesia 91*(4), 1017-1020.

Levitan R., Ochroch E., Stuart S., & Hollander J. (2000). Use of the intubating laryngeal mask airway by medical and nonmedical personnel. *American Journal of Emergency Medicine 18*(1), 12-16.

LMA North America. (2002). www.lmana.com/prod/components/products.

Luten, R. (2000). The pediatric patient (pp. 143-152). In Walls, R., Luten, R., Murphy, M., & Schneider, R. (Eds.), *Manual of emergency airway management.* Philadelphia: Lippincott Williams & Wilkins.

Murphy, M. (2000). Special devices and techniques for managing the difficult or failed airway (pp. 68-88). In Walls, R., Luten, R., Murphy, M., & Schneider, R. (Eds.), *Manual of emergency airway management.* Philadelphia: Lippincott Williams & Wilkins.

Pollack, C. (2001). The laryngeal mask airway: a comprehensive review for the emergency physician. *The Journal of Emergency Medicine 20*(1), 53-66.

Rosenblatt W.H., & Murphy M. (1999). The intubating laryngeal mask: use of a new ventilating-intubating device in the emergency department. *Annals of Emergency Medicine 33*(2), 234-238.

Urocher, D. & Hopson, L. (2004). Basic airway management and decision-making (pp. 53-68). In Roberts, J. of Hedges, J. (Eds.), *Clinical procedures in emergency medicine,* 4th ed. Philadelphia: W.B. Saunders.

Esophageal Obturator Airway and Esophageal Gastric Tube Airway Insertion

Donna York Clark, RN, MS, CFRN, CCRN

The esophageal obturator airway (EOA) and the esophageal gastric tube airway (EGTA) are classed with an indeterminate recommendation by the American Heart Association. The American Heart Association (AHA) states "the evidence is lacking for inclusion of these devices in the guidelines" (AHA, 2001). However, these two airways are discussed in some paramedic and emergency medical technician (EMT) intermediate-provider curricula and are used in the provision of emergency medical care in several areas of the country (Bledsoe et al, 2003).

The EOA and the EGTA are adjuncts that may be used instead of endotracheal tubes. Both airways are rigid, cuffed, plastic tubes that are blindly inserted into the esophagus. Placement of the cuffed tube into the esophagus prevents vomiting and aspiration, and insufflation of air into the stomach during ventilation is minimized. Ventilation of the lungs is provided through a mask, which is sealed over the mouth and nose (Urocher & Hopson, 2004).

The EOA is a blind tube that is placed into the esophagus (Figure 8-1). Ventilation is delivered through holes near the proximal end of the tube. Although this tube seals the esophagus and prevents vomiting and aspiration, there is no mechanism to vent or empty the stomach. This limitation has resulted in esophageal perforation and stomach rupture (Pons, 1988; Semonin-Holleran, 1996).

The EGTA is an improved version of the EOA. The EGTA is an open tube that incorporates a gastric tube for venting and evacuating the stomach contents (Figure 8-2). Ventilation is delivered through a separate port in the mask. This modification prevents the high gastric pressures that lead to esophageal perforation and gastric rupture when the EOA is used (Pons, 1988; Bledsoe et al, 2003).

INDICATION

To secure the airway in adult patients without a gag reflex. Most sources believe that the EOA and EGTA are becoming obsolete. However, the following advantages have been discussed (Bledsoe et al, 2003):

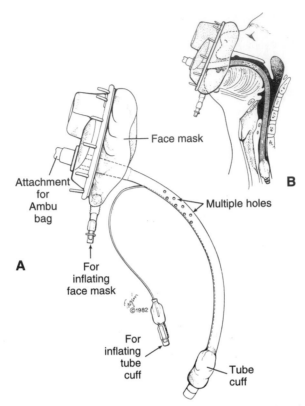

FIGURE 8-1 A, The esophageal obturator airway (EOA). **B,** The EOA in place. (From McCabe, C.J. [1989]. Pre-hospital medical care. In Wilkins, Jr., E.W. [Ed.], *Emergency medicine: Scientific foundations and current practice,* 3rd ed. [p. 3]. Baltimore: Williams & Wilkins.)

1. Minimal training is required for insertion.
2. Minimal skill is required for use.
3. Both can be inserted blindly without visualization of the glottis.
4. Insertion requires minimal movement of the cervical spine.

CONTRAINDICATIONS AND CAUTIONS

1. Most sources consider endotracheal intubation to be the most effective method of airway protection (Walls, 2000). The EOA and EGTA are being replaced in the field by the Combitube (Procedure 16). The laryngeal mask airway is also considered a significant adjunct in emergency airway management (Procedure 7).
2. Absolute contraindications for the use of the EOA or EGTA include the following (Bledsoe et al, 2003; Semonin-Holleran, 2003):
   a. Patient height of less than than 5 feet
   b. Intact gag reflex
   c. Known esophageal disease
   d. Ingestion of corrosive substances
3. Facial trauma may make it difficult to achieve an adequate seal with the mask.

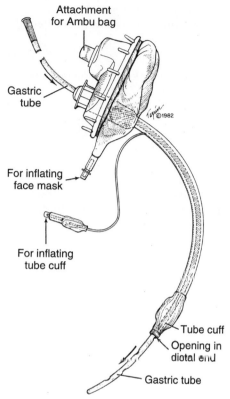

FIGURE 8-2 The esophageal gastric tube airway (EGTA). (From McCabe, C.J. [1989]. Pre-hospital medical care. In Wilkins, Jr., E.W. [Ed.], *Emergency medicine: Scientific foundations and current practice,* 3rd ed. [p. 4]. Baltimore: Williams & Wilkins.)

EQUIPMENT

EOA or EGTA
Stethoscope
Tonsil-tip suction
Bag-valve-mask with reservoir
Oxygen source and connecting tubing
Pulse oximeter
Limb restraints (if indicated)

PATIENT PREPARATION

1. If possible, place the patient in a supine position. Place the head in a neutral position or in the sniffing position unless contraindicated by a potential spinal injury or other condition. Provide manual stabilization of the head if cervical spine immobilization is indicated.
2. Initiate supplemental ventilation and/or oxygenation using a bag-valve-mask.

3. Hyperventilate/hyperoxygenate the patient.
4. Restrain the patient as indicated to prevent accidental extubation.

PROCEDURAL STEPS
1. Inflate the cuff to test for air leaks and then deflate it.
2. Attach the mask to the EOA or EGTA tube.
3. Turn on the suction and place the tonsil tip next to the patient's head.
4. Grasp the patient's lower jaw and elevate it slightly.
5. Insert the EOA or EGTA into the patient's mouth with the curve of the tube directed toward the feet.
6. Advance the tube until the mask is flush against the face.
7. Inflate the cuff with 35 ml of air.
8. Maintain the head in the sniffing position and seal the mask on the face.
9. Attach the bag-valve-mask to the port on the mask and initiate ventilation.
10. Check for correct tube placement by assessing epigastric sounds and bilateral breath sounds.
11. Secure the tube.
12. If an EGTA is used, insert the gastric tube through the lumen of the EGTA and attach it to low suction.

AGE-SPECIFIC CONSIDERATIONS
1. The EOA and EGTA are not recommended for individuals shorter than 5 feet.
2. These airways are not recommended for persons younger than 16 years of age (Mageau, 1997; Bledsoe et al, 2003).

COMPLICATIONS
1. Esophageal perforation (Semonin-Holleran, 2003; Pons, 1988).
2. Gastric rupture (this complication may be decreased with the use of the EGTA).
3. Complete airway obstruction caused by kinking of the tube or overinflation of the distal balloon in the esophagus. Obstruction is caused by anterior displacement of the trachea.
4. Inadvertent, unrecognized endotracheal intubation. Inaccurate placement of any airway device, including the endotracheal tube, has serious consequences. This complication is not limited to the EOA or EGTA.
5. Aspiration of vomitus or blood. This complication is neither caused nor prevented by use of the EOA or the EGTA.

REFERENCES
American Heart Association. (2001). *ACLS provider manual*. Dallas: Author.
Bledsoe, B., Porter, R., & Cherry, R. (2003). *Essentials of paramedic care*. New Jersey: Brady/Prentice Hall.
Mageau, A. (1997). Airway management and oxygen therapy (pp. 69-95). In Krupa D. (Ed.), *Flight nursing core curriculum*. Park Ridge, IL: National Flight Nurses Association.
Pons, P.T. (1988). Esophageal obturator airway. *Emergency Medicine Clinics of North America*, 6, 693-698.

Semonin-Holleran, R. (Ed.) (2003). *Air and Surface patient transport: principles and practice*, 3rd ed. St. Louis: Mosby.

Urocher, D. & Hopson, L. (2004). Basic airway management and decision-making (pp. 53-68). In Roberts, J. & Hedges, J. (Eds.), *Clinical Procedures in emergency medicine*, 4th ed. Philadelphia: W.B. Saunders.

Walls, R. (2000). Airway management in the prehospital setting (pp. 195-201). In Walls, R., Luten, R., Murphy, M., & Schneider, R. (Eds.), *Manual of emergency airway management*. Philadelphia: Lippincott Williams & Wilkins.

PROCEDURE 9

General Principles of Endotracheal Intubation

Donna York Clark, RN, MS, CFRN, CCRN

Endotracheal intubation refers to the procedure of inserting a tube directly into the trachea. The endotracheal tube (ET or ETT) may be placed through the nose or the mouth. Methods of insertion include visual (using laryngoscopy), blind (through the nose), or digital (also blind). Details of oral and nasal intubation procedures are included in Procedures 11 and 12.

INDICATION

The purpose of intubation is to secure a patent and effective airway. Intubation is the preferred means of airway control because it has the following benefits (Walls, 2000; AHA 2001; Benumof, 1996):
1. Protects the trachea and lungs from aspiration of gastric contents, saliva, or blood and fluid into the upper airway
2. Provides an airway for mechanical ventilation
3. Allows direct access to the lungs for removal or suctioning of secretions
4. Allows tracheal administration of emergency medications for rapid absorption through the pulmonary tree (AHA, 2001)

CONTRAINDICATIONS AND CAUTIONS

1. There are no absolute contraindications to endotracheal intubation; however, the procedure should be considered carefully when it is performed in

a patient with the following (Walls, 2000; Benumof, 1996, Lutes & Hopson, 2004):

   a. Intact gag reflex
   b. Potential or actual cervical spine injury
   c. Head trauma, increased intracranial pressure, or both
   d. Facial fractures

2. Epiglottitis complicates any intubation attempt because of the potential for laryngospasm and complete airway obstruction. Ideally, intubation of the patient with epiglottitis should be performed in the most controlled setting with the most skilled intubator. Contingency planning should include set up for the performance of a surgical airway (Sack & Brock, 2002).

3. Specific precautions exist for each method of endotracheal intubation. These are discussed in the procedures devoted to nasal and oral intubation (Procedures 12 and 11, respectively).

EQUIPMENT

Endotracheal tubes
   1-5 mm, uncuffed; 6-9 mm, cuffed
Laryngoscope handle
Laryngoscope blades
   Curved (sizes 1-4)
   Straight (sizes 1-4)
Stylets to fit each size of endotracheal tube
10-ml syringe for inflating the cuff of the tube
Lubricating or lidocaine jelly for nasal intubation
Benzocaine, cocaine, or phenylephrine hydrochloride (Neo-Synephrine)
   drops or spray for nasal intubation (optional)
Medications as prescribed for paralysis and sedation (see Procedure 10)
Tube securing device (commercially manufactured or ties or tape)
Stethoscope
Bag-valve-mask with reservoir connected to 100% oxygen
Additional supportive equipment:
   Suction, complete with tonsil and catheter tips
   Extra laryngoscope bulbs and batteries
   Carbon dioxide detector for tube position confirmation (optional)
   Pulse oximeter to monitor oxygen saturation during intubation and to
      help confirm tube placement (optional)
   Limb restraints

PATIENT PREPARATION

1. Preoxygenate the patient with 100% oxygen by using a nonrebreather oxygen mask or a bag-valve-mask as indicated.
2. Administer sedatives, paralytic agents, or topical anesthesia as prescribed (see Procedure 10).
3. Restrain the patient as indicated to prevent accidental extubation.

PROCEDURAL STEPS
Intubate

*The specific steps of intubation depend upon the method of insertion used. See Procedures 11 and 12 for specific directions for oral and nasal intubation.

Confirm Tube Placement

A number of methods may be employed to confirm the correct endotracheal tube placement (AHA, 2001; Danzl, 2001; Walls, 2000; Salem & Baraka, 1996):

1. *Epigastric sounds/chest rise:* With the first ventilation, auscultate over the epigastric area while observing for chest rise (AHA, 2001). The presence of burping sounds over the epigastrium in the absence of chest rise suggests esophageal placement. Remove the tube immediately and hyperventilate the patient before attempting intubation again.

2. *Breath sounds:* Auscultate the right and left axilla, then the right and left anterior chest. Unilaterally absent or decreased breath sounds (usually on the left) suggest that the tube was advanced into a mainstem bronchus. Withdraw the tube slightly and reassess until breath sounds are equal bilaterally

3. End-tidal carbon dioxide detection and/or monitoring also helps confirm tube placement (see Procedure 26). These devices are recommended as a secondary technique of tube confirmation in patients with adequate perfusion (AHA, 2001). If the patient is poorly perfused or in cardiac arrest, there may be minimal CO_2 expiration even when the tube is properly placed.

4. *Esophageal detector devices.* These devices are attached to the ETT and suction is applied with a bulb or syringe device. If the ETT is in the esophagus, the tissue will collapse around the tube when suction is applied and there will be resistance to filling of the bulb or syringe. If the ETT is in the trachea, the bulb or syringe will fill with air easily. These devices are recommended for secondary confirmation of tube placement for the patient in cardiac arrest (AHA, 2001).

5. Direct visualization of the tube passing through the cords with the laryngoscope.

6. *Bag-valve compliance:* Ventilation of the stomach is easier than ventilation of the lungs, whereas tube obstruction, bronchospasm, or tension pneumothorax makes ventilation more difficult.

7. Condensation in the ETT tube on exhalation suggests that the tube is positioned in the trachea.

8. Transillumination of the neck using a lighted stylet: If the neck glows after intubation with the lighted stylet, the tube is placed correctly in the trachea (Murphy, 2000).

9. *Pulse oximetry:* Maintenance of adequate oxygen saturation helps confirm tube placement.

10. Presence of gastric contents in the endotracheal tube: Material resembling food present in the tube may indicate esophageal intubation.

---

*Indicates portions of the procedure usually performed by a physician or an advanced practice nurse.

11. Cuff palpation may be used to verify the appropriate placement within the trachea in reference to the carina and the bronchi. After the cuff is inflated, and with the patient's head in a neutral position, gently palpate at the suprasternal notch while holding the pilot balloon in your other hand. Advance or withdraw the tube slightly. When the pilot balloon is maximally distended in response to pressure at the suprasternal notch, the tube is appropriately positioned within the trachea (Pollard & Lobato, 1995).

12. Chest x-ray documentation of the tube location in the trachea just above the carina.

Secure the Endotracheal Tube

To prevent accidental extubation, the endotracheal tube must be secured carefully. Although several techniques can be used for this maneuver, many principles apply to all of them:

1. A bite block or oral airway should be inserted after oral intubation to prevent the patient from biting the tube and occluding the airway.
2. To allow suctioning and mouth care, the mouth must not be completely occluded by tape, ties, or other devices.
3. The method used should prevent the accidental advancement or withdrawal of the tube.
4. When possible, the method used should minimize pressure points on the skin to prevent long-term complications.
5. When tape or ties are used, they should encircle the head completely for maximum security.
6. When possible, the markings on the tube should be noted at the patient's teeth and documented so that movement of the tube can be checked visually.
7. The commonly employed methods include commercial tube–securing devices (follow manufacturer's directions), tape, and ties.

Tape

a. Tear off approximately 24 inches of 1-inch adhesive tape.
b. Split the tape in half for the last 4 inches at each end.
c. Slide the tape under the middle of the neck, adhesive side up.
d. Bring each end of the tape alongside the patient's head and wrap the split ends securely around the tube. Split the tape further if necessary.

Tube Ties or Umbilical Tape

a. Cut off about 24 inches of umbilical tape.
b. Place the tape under the patient's neck. Center the length of the tape under the middle of the neck.
c. Bring the ends alongside the head and wrap them once around the ET tube (Figure 9-1, A).
d. Tie a secure overhand knot around the tube, and then wrap the ends around the tube again (Figure 9-1, B).
e. Tie another firm overhand knot, and then a square knot, to complete the procedure (Figure 9-1, C).

8. Reconfirm the tube position after it has been secured.

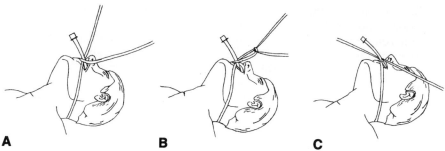

A   **B**   **C**

FIGURE 9-1 Steps for securing the endotracheal tube using tube ties.

TABLE 9-1

USUAL ENDOTRACHEAL TUBE SIZE BY AGE AND WEIGHT

Age	Weight (kg)	Endotracheal Tube Size (Internal Diameter)
Premature	1.5-2.0	3.0
Newborn 3 months	3-6	3.5
6-12 months	7-10	4.0
2 years	12	5.0
4 years	16	5.5
6 years	20	6.0
8 years	25	6.5
10 years	34	6.5 (cuffed)
12 years	40	6.5-7.0 (cuffed)
14 years	50	7.0 (cuffed)

Age-Specific Considerations

1. Several methods exist for estimating the correct tube size (Table 9-1), usually by age and weight. Other methods include the following:

   a. Estimates based on the size of the patient's little finger: Men usually require a 7.0- to 8.5-mm tube, whereas women usually require a 7.0- to 8.0-mm tube (Pollard & Lobato, 1995). Nasal intubation generally requires a tube that is 0.5 mm smaller than the tube used for oral intubation.

   b. The following formula may be used to calculate the appropriately sized endotracheal tube for children 2 years of age or older (Cole, 1957; Luten, 2000): 16 + age in years/4 = endotracheal tube size

   c. Size estimate based on a child's length: This is facilitated by using a length-based (Broselow) resuscitation tape (Luten, 2000).

2. The depth to which the endotracheal tube should be advanced into the trachea varies with the age and size of the patient. Adult women usually require a depth (from the central incisors) of 17-23 cm, and adult men require 19-25 cm (Pollard & Lobato, 1995). The following formula estimates the required length of the oral tracheal tube from lip to midtrachea for children 1 year of age and older (Manley, 1997): airway length (cm) = age/2 + 12

3. Oral intubation is the preferred method for intubation in the pediatric population (Luten, 2000).
4. Children younger than 8 years are generally intubated with uncuffed endotracheal tubes (Luten, 2000). The narrowest region of the airway in children is the cricoid cartilage. This area forms a physiologic cuff around the uncuffed endotracheal tube (Luten, 2000).
5. In infants and small children, transmittal of breath sounds across the chest may result in "equal" breath sounds, even in the presence of mainstem bronchus intubation or pneumothorax. A chest x-ray study is indicated to help ascertain appropriate position of the tube.
6. Take care to maintain neutral head position in intubated infants and toddlers. Because the airway is shorter and the tubes are uncuffed in this population, head movement may result in significant tube movement. Flexion may withdraw the tube resulting in extubation. Extension may advance the tube into the right mainstem bronchus.
7. Esophageal detector devices are unreliable in children < 1 year old, morbidly obese patients, and patients in late pregnancy. There is insufficient evidence to support their use in children at this time (AHA/ILCOR, 2000).

COMPLICATIONS
1. Esophageal intubation: This is a serious complication, because the patient's lungs are not ventilated and gastric distention may occur. Gastric distention increases the risk of vomiting and may decrease the tidal volume.
2. Dislodgment of the tube: Frequent reassessment of the tube position is necessary, especially after the patient is moved.
3. Damage to teeth, nasal mucosa, posterior pharynx, or larynx (depending on the method of insertion).

PATIENT TEACHING
1. You will not be able to speak while the tube is in place.
2. Swallowing may help diminish gagging.
3. Do not move or manipulate the tube in any way.

REFERENCES
American Heart Association. (2001). *Textbook of Advanced Cardiac Life Support,* Dallas: Author.
American Heart Association & International Liaison Committee on Resuscitation (AHA/ILCOR). (2000). Guidelines 2000 for cardiopulmonary resuscitation and emergency cardiovascular care: international consensus on science. *Circulation, 102* (suppl), I1-I384.
Benumof, J.L. (1996). Indications for tracheal intubation (pp. 261-276). In Benumof J.L. (Ed.), *Airway management: principles and practice.* St. Louis: Mosby.
Cole, F. (1957). Pediatric formulas for the anesthesiologist. *American Journal of Disease in Children, 94,* 472.
Danzl, D. (2001). Endotracheal intubation (pp. 4-19). In Rosen, P., Chan, T., Vilke, G., & Sternbach, G. (Eds.), *Atlas of emergency procedures.* St. Louis: Mosby.
Luten, R. (2000). The pediatric patient (pp. 143-152). In Walls, R., Luten, R., Murphy, M., & Schneider, R. (Eds.), *Manual of emergency airway management.* Philadelphia: Lippincott Williams & Wilkins.

Lutes, M. & Hopson L.R. (2004). Tracheal intubation (pp. 69-99). In Roberts, J. & Hedges, J. (Eds.), *Clinical procedures in emergency medicine*, 4th ed. Philadelphia: W.B. Saunders.

Manley, L. (1997). Essentials of airway management for the injured child. *International Journal of Trauma Nursing, 3*(1), 27-30.

Murphy, M. (2000). Special devices and techniques for managing the difficult or failed airway (pp. 68-81). In Walls, R., Luten, R., Murphy, M., & Schneider, R. (Eds.) *Manual of Emergency Airway Management*. Philadelphia: Lippincott Williams & Wilkins.

Pollard, R.J., & Lobato, E.B. (1995). Endotracheal tube location verified reliably by cuff palpation. *Anesthesia and Analgesia, 81*, 135-138.

Sack, J.L. & Brock, C.D. (2002). Identifying acute epiglottitis in adults. High degree of awareness, close monitoring are key. *Postgraduate Medicine, 112*(1), 81-2, 85-6.

Salem, M.R., & Baraka, A. (1996). Confirmation of tracheal intubation (pp. 351–359). In Benumof J.L. (Ed.), *Airway management: principles and practice*. St. Louis: Mosby.

Walls, R. (2000). The decision to intubate (pp. 3-7). In Walls, R., Luten, R., Murphy, M., & Schneider, R. (Eds.) *Manual of emergency airway management*. Philadelphia: Lippincott Williams & Wilkins.

PROCEDURE 10

Rapid Sequence Intubation

Donna York Clark, RN, MS, CFRN, CCRN

The information in this procedure should be used in conjunction with the information in Procedures 9 and 11.

Rapid sequence intubation is also known as RSI, crash intubation, paralytic intubation, and neuromuscular blockade intubation.

INDICATIONS

1. To facilitate intubation of a critically ill or injured patient, when the ability of the patient to protect his or her airway is in question and trismus or a gag reflex is present (Walls, 2000).
2. To augment intubation of combative head-injured patients (Semonin-Holleran, 2003).
3. To minimize the risk of aspiration in nonfasting patients with complex airway emergencies (Walls, 2000).

CAUTIONS AND CONTRAINDICATIONS

1. Neuromuscular blocking agents (NMBAs) are the foundation of emergency airway management. They allow placement of the oral endotracheal tube while minimizing potential complications, such as aspiration. There are two classes of NMBAs. One class is the noncompetitive depolarizing agents, of which succinylcholine is the most common. The second class is the competitive, nondepolarizing NMBAs, which is made up of two categories of agents: benzylisoquinolone compounds and aminosteroid compounds. Benzylisoquinolone compounds include atracurium, and aminosteroid compounds include vecuronium and pancuronium (Schneider, 2000a).

2. The most common method of RSI uses succinylcholine. Succinylcholine is absolutely contraindicated in patients who have a family history of malignant hypertension, burn injuries that are greater than 24 hours old, or crush injuries greater than 7 days old. These patients are at risk for developing life-threatening hyperkalemia (Schneider, 2000a). There are many other conditions in which succinylcholine must be given with care, if at all. Consult your pharmacist or medication reference material for details.

3. Penetrating eye injuries are considered relative contraindications to RSI because of the increased intraocular pressure resulting from some of the medications; alternatives may need to be considered (Biehl, 2001; Kelly et al., 1993).

4. RSI requires rapid administration of several medications. Keeping the medications, needles, and syringes together in a kit facilitates rapid administration. Box 10-1 lists a sample inventory.

EQUIPMENT (Walls, 2000; Schneider, 2000a; Schneider, 2000b)
Endotracheal intubation and ventilation supplies (see Procedure 9)
Cricothyrotomy supplies (see Procedure 17)
Syringes and needles

BOX 10-1
SAMPLE INVENTORY LIST OF AN ASI KIT

Medications (two of each with noted expressions)
Atropine 1-mg prefilled syringe
Lidocaine 100-mg prefilled syringe
Succinylcholine 200-mg vial
Vecuronim 10-mg vial
Rocuronium 50-mg vial
Pancuronium 10-mg vial
Midazolam 5-mg vial
Fentanyl 250-fg vial
Etomidate 40-mg vial
Thiopental 500-mg syringe kit (1 each)
Ketamine 500-mg vial
Sterile water 10-ml vial
Normal saline 10-ml vial (4 each)

Syringes/Needles
Four 1-ml TB syringes with attached needle
Four 3-ml syringes with attached needle
Three 6-ml syringes with attached needle
Six 12-ml syringes
Two 20-ml syringes
Ten 18-G needles

Miscellaneous
Alcohol wipes
Preprinted medication labels
Calculator
Rapid sequence induction worksheets
Plastic locks

Courtesy Emergency Department, Dartmouth-Hitchcock Medical Center, Lebanon, NH.

Premedication(s) as prescribed:
  Lidocaine (1.0-1.5 mg/kg)
  Atropine (0.02 mg/kg)
Induction agent(s), such as:
  Etomidate (0.2 mg/kg)
  Thiopental (3-7 mg/kg)
  Midazolam (0.1-0.3 mg/kg)
Neuromuscular blocking agent(s), such as:
  Succinylcholine (1-1.5 mg/kg)
  Vecuronium (0.1-0.25 mg/kg)

PATIENT PREPARATION

1. Complete a brief neurologic assessment.
2. Maintain the patient in a supine position with spinal immobilization, if indicated.
3. Preoxygenate the patient with 100% oxygen. If possible, avoid bag-valve-mask ventilation to prevent gastric distention, which increases the risk of vomiting and aspiration.
4. Initiate an intravenous line.
5. Attach cardiac and oxygen saturation monitors.
6. Draw up all pharmacologic agents in individual syringes and label clearly. A worksheet can help with dosing and sequencing of medications (Figure 10-1).

PROCEDURAL STEPS (Walls, 2000; O'Connor & Levine, 2001; Hopson & Dronen, 2004).

1. Administer premedications as prescribed:
   a. Give lidocaine to attenuate the increase in intracranial pressure associated with intubation. Lidocaine is usually used in patients with head injuries (Walls, 2000). Administer the lidocaine approximately 90 seconds before administering succinylcholine.
   b. Give atropine to minimize the bradycardic impact of succinylcholine for children younger than 10 years of age (Schneider, 2000c) or bradycardic adults.
   c. Give vecuronium or another nondepolarizing paralytic agent at one tenth of the paralytic dose. This is a defasciculating dose and may be used when succinylcholine is the prescribed paralytic.
2. As soon as the defasciculating dose is administered or the patient begins to lose consciousness (Hopson & Dronen, 2004), apply cricoid pressure, that is, the Sellick maneuver. Cricoid pressure is applied by placing your thumb and index finger on the cricoid cartilage. Firmly press the cricoid cartilage backward to occlude the esophagus. This helps prevent regurgitation and may improve visualization of the vocal cords. Maintain cricoid pressure throughout the procedure until the endotracheal tube placement is verified and the cuff is inflated.
3. Administer the induction agent of choice.
4. Administer the neuromuscular blocking agent of choice.
5. *Orally intubate the patient.

---

*Indicates portions of the procedure usually performed by a physician or an advanced practice nurse.

Rapid Sequence Induction Worksheet

Estimated Patient Weight _____ kg

PRE-MEDICATIONS	0 MINUTES

Atropine _____ mg IV
Pediatric = 0.02 mg/kg, min dose of 0.1 mg,
Always used in patients < 5 y.o.
Adult = 0.5 mg (only for bradycardic adults)

Lidocaine _____ mg IV
Adult & *Pediatric = 1 mg/kg*

Defasciculating Dose
Vecuronium, Pancuronium, or Rocuronium
Use 1/10 of the dose listed below

_____ mg IV

Not used in children < 5 y.o.
Apply cricoid pressure until ET cuff inflated

SEDATION	2 MINUTES

Midazolam _____ mg IV
Adult & *Pediatric = 0.1 mg/kg*

Fentanyl _____ mcg IV
Adult & *Pediatric = 2 mcg/kg*
Administer slowly over 3-5 minutes

Etomidate _____ mg IV
Pediatric = Not studied in children <10 y.o.
Adult = 0.3 mg/kg

Thiopental _____ mg IV
Adult & *Pediatric = 3 mg/kg*
Administer slowly over 30-60 seconds

Ketamine _____ mg IV
Adult & *Pediatric = 2 mg/kg*

PARALYSIS

Succinylcholine _____ mg IV
Pediatric = 2 mg/kg
Adult = 1 mg/kg

Vecuronium _____ mg IV
Adult & *Pediatric = 0.1 mg/kg*

Rocuronium _____ mg IV
Adult & *Pediatric = 1 mg/kg*

Pancuronium _____ mg IV
Adult & *Pediatric = 0.1 mg/kg*

FIGURE 10-1 Sample RSI worksheet. (Courtesy Emergency Department, Dartmouth-Hitchcock Medical Center, Lebanon, NH.)

6. Verify the endotracheal tube placement, inflate the cuff, and ventilate the patient with 100% oxygen while manually maintaining the tube placement (see Procedure 9).
7. Release the cricoid pressure. Have suction immediately available in case of regurgitation when the cricoid pressure is released.
8. Secure the endotracheal tube.
9. Administer long-acting paralytic agents as prescribed. Pharmacologically paralyzed patients also require sedation and/or analgesia.
10. Decompress the stomach with a gastric tube (see Procedure 101).
11. If intubation is unsuccessful and an alternative airway must be established, consider needle cricothyrotomy (see Procedure 18) or surgical cricothyrotomy (see Procedure 17).

AGE-SPECIFIC CONSIDERATIONS

1. Most sources recommend that children between 5 and 10 years of age receive premedication with atropine to prevent bradycardia associated with intubation and the administration of RSI agents (Luten, 2000).
2. A defasciculating dose of a nondepolarizing paralytic agent is not used in children because dosing errors may result in earlier than intended paralysis.
3. Surgical cricothyrotomy is not recommended in children younger than 12 years of age because of the size of the cricothyroid membrane; needle cricothyrotomy is the procedure of choice (Luten, 2000).

COMPLICATIONS

Complications are related to the medications administered or to the intubation procedure (see Procedure 9).

PATIENT TEACHING

1. We have given you medications that relax your muscles temporarily so the machine can breathe for you. We are here to take care of you and keep you safe.
2. See Procedure 9.

REFERENCES

Biehl, J. (2001). Military and civilian penetrating eye trauma: anesthetic complications. *American Association of Nurse Anesthetists Journal, 69*(1), 31-37.

Hopson, R.L. & Dronen, S. (2004). Pharmacologic adjuncts to intubation (pp. 100-114). In Roberts, J & Hedges, J. (Eds.), *Clinical Procedures in Emergency Medicine*, 4th ed. Philadelphia: W.B. Saunders.

Kelly, R.E., et al. (1993). Succinylcholine increases intraocular pressure in the human eye with extraocular muscles detached. *Anesthesiology, 79*, 948-952.

Luten, R. (2000). The pediatric patient (pp. 143-152). In Walls, R., Luten, R., Murphy, M., & Schneider, R. (Eds.), *Manual of emergency airway management*. Philadelphia: Lippincott Williams & Wilkins.

O'Connor, R. & Levine, B. (2001). Airway management in the trauma setting (pp. 52-74). In Ferrera, P., Colucciello, S., Marx, J., Verdile, V., Gibbs, M. (Eds.), *Trauma management: an emergency medicine approach*. St. Louis: Mosby.

Schneider, R. (2000a). Muscle relaxants (pp. 121-128). In Walls, R., Luten, R., Murphy, M., & Schneider, R. (Eds.), *Manual of emergency airway management*. Philadelphia: Lippincott Williams & Wilkins.

Schneider, R. (2000b). Sedatives and induction agents (pp. 129-134). In Walls, R., Luten, R., Murphy, M., & Schneider, R. (Eds.), *Manual of emergency airway management*. Philadelphia: Lippincott Williams & Wilkins.

Schneider, R. (2000c). Drugs for special clinical circumstances (pp. 135-139). In Walls, R., Luten, R., Murphy, M., & Schneider, R. (Eds.), *Manual of emergency airway management*. Philadelphia: Lippincott Williams & Wilkins.

Semonin-Holleran, R. (Ed.). (2003). *Air and Surface patient transport: principles and practice*, 3rd ed. St. Louis: Mosby.

Walls, R. (2000). Rapid sequence intubation (pp. 8-15). In Walls, R., Luten, R., Murphy, M., & Schneider, R. (Eds.), *Manual of emergency airway management*. Philadelphia: Lippincott Williams & Wilkins.

PROCEDURE 11

Oral Endotracheal Intubation

Donna York Clark, RN, MS, CFRN, CCRN

The information in this procedure should be used in conjunction with the information found in Procedure 9.

INDICATIONS

To place an endotracheal tube via the mouth. The oral route is usually used for comatose, apneic, sedated, or chemically paralyzed patients. Indications include the following:

1. To maintain an adequate, patent airway
2. To facilitate mechanical ventilation
3. To provide a route for pulmonary secretion evacuation
4. To provide a route for medication administration for a patient in cardiac arrest

CONTRAINDICATIONS AND CAUTIONS

There are no absolute contraindications to oral intubation; however, the procedure should be considered carefully and performed when the patient has the following:

1. An intact gag reflex.
2. Potential or actual cervical spine injury. Laryngoscopy is known to cause spinal movement (Aprahamian et al., 1984). Many studies have examined the impact of orotracheal intubation on cervical spine movement and resulting neurologic sequelae. No conclusive data have been published that clearly state the safety of endotracheal intubation in the presence of a cervical spinal

injury; however, there is literature supporting the safety of this procedure (O'Connor & Levine, 2001; Danzl, 2001; Gibbs, 2000).

EQUIPMENT
See Procedure 9.

PATIENT PREPARATION
1. Place the patient in the supine position with the head in the sniffing position unless there is a potential cervical spine injury. Provide manual stabilization of the head if spinal movement is contraindicated.
2. Initiate hyperventilation with 100% oxygen using a bag-valve-mask (see Procedure 35).
3. Apply cardiac and oxygen saturation monitors (see Procedures 23 and 58).
4. Administer sedative, paralytic agents, or topical anesthesia as prescribed (see Procedure 10).
5. Restrain the patient as indicated to prevent accidental extubation (see Procedure 192).

PROCEDURAL STEPS
1. Ensure that all larnygoscopic equipment is in appropriate working order. Inflate the endotracheal tube cuff to test for air leaks and deflate after testing.
2. Insert the stylet into the endotracheal tube and apply a water-soluble lubricant to allow easy advancement of the tube. Confirm appropriate placement of the stylet within the endotracheal tube. Ensure that the stylet has not been advanced beyond the end of the tube.
3. Turn on the suction and place the tonsil-tip suction next to the patient's head.
4. *Insert the laryngoscope with your left hand. The patient's tongue should be swept to the left side and the laryngoscope inserted and lifted up and away from the intubator (Figure 11-1). Be careful not to rock the laryngoscope against the patient's teeth! Advance the laryngoscope blade under the epiglottis when using a straight blade or into the vallecula when using a curved blade.
5. *Visualize the epiglottis and the vocal cords (Figure 11-2).
6. If the cords are not visible, downward cricoid pressure (also known as the Sellick maneuver) may move the glottis into view (Benumof, 1996). This maneuver is performed by placing your index finger and thumb on the cricoid membrane and applying posterior pressure to occlude the esophagus. The cricoid pressure may also prevent aspiration of emesis by occluding the esophagus during intubation (Sellick, 1961). If applied, cricoid pressure should be maintained until tube placement is verified and the cuff inflated.
7. *Using the right hand, pass the endotracheal tube through the cords. The tube should be advanced until the cuff moves forward 1-2 cm through the cords.
8. *Remove the laryngoscope while maintaining a grip on the endotracheal tube.
9. *Remove the stylet.
10. Verify correct endotracheal tube placement and secure the tube as described in Procedure 9.

---

*Indicates portions of the procedure usually performed by a physician or an advanced practice nurse.

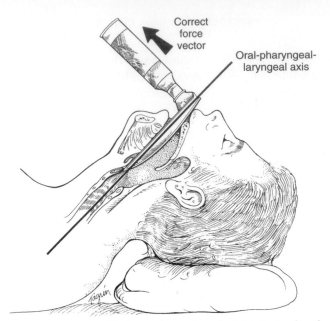

FIGURE 11-1 The laryngoscope is lifted up and away from the intubator to align the airway structures. (From Cullen, D.J. [1989]. Orotracheal intubation. In Wilkins, Jr., E.W. [Ed.], *Emergency medicine: scientific foundations and current practice,* 3rd ed. [p. 990]. Baltimore: Williams & Wilkins.)

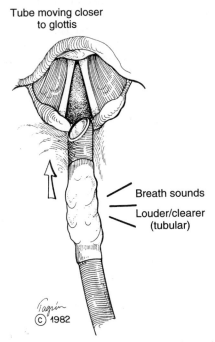

FIGURE 11-2 After the cords are visualized, the tube should be advanced through the cords until the cuff disappears. (From Cullen, D.J. [1989]. Orotracheal intubation. In Wilkins, Jr., E.W. [Ed.], *Emergency medicine: scientific foundations and current practice,* 3rd ed. [p. 993]. Baltimore: Williams & Wilkins.)

11. Inflate the cuff and instill air until an adequate seal is attained; 10-15 ml of air are usually required. Ventilate the patient with 100% oxygen.

AGE-SPECIFIC CONSIDERATIONS

Oral intubation is the preferred method of intubation in the pediatric population (Luten, 2000).

COMPLICATIONS

See Procedure 9.

PATIENT TEACHING

See Procedure 9.

REFERENCES

Aprahamian, C., et al. (1984). Experimental cervical spine injury model: evaluation of airway management and splinting techniques. *Annals of Emergency Medicine, 13,* 584-587.

Benumof, J.L. (1996). Conventional (laryngoscopic) orotracheal and nasotracheal intubation (single-lumen tube) (pp. 261–276). In Benumof J.L. (Ed.), *Airway management: principles and practice.* St. Louis: Mosby.

Danzl, D. (2001). Endotracheal intubation (pp. 4-7). In Rosen, R., Chan, T., Vilke, G., & Sternbach, G. (Eds.) *Atlas of emergency procedures.* St. Louis: Mosby.

O'Connor, R. & Levine, B. (2001). Airway management in the trauma setting (pp. 52-74). In Ferrera, P., Colucciello, S., Marx, J., Verdile, V., & Gibbs, M (Eds.), *Trauma management: an emergency medicine approach.* Mosby: St. Louis.

Gibbs, M (2000). The trauma patient (pp. 153-158). In Walls, R., Luten, R., Murphy, M., & Schneider, R. (Eds.), *Manual of emergency airway management.* Philadelphia: Lippincott Williams & Wilkins.

Luten, R. (2000). The pediatric patient (pp. 105-111). In Walls, R., Luten, R., Murphy, M., & Schneider, R. (Eds.), *Manual of emergency airway management.* Philadelphia: Lippincott Williams & Wilkins.

Sellick, B.A. (1961). Cricoid pressure to control regurgitation of stomach contents during induction of anesthesia. *Lancet, 2,* 404-408.

PROCEDURE 12

Nasotracheal Intubation

Donna York Clark, RN, MS, CFRN, CCRN

The information in this procedure should be used in conjunction with the information in Procedure 9.

INDICATION

Nasotracheal intubation is becoming obsolete and being replaced by oral intubation with the use of neuromuscular blockade in most settings (Walls & Luten, 2000). Some investigators support the use of the nasotracheal intubation technique in the prehospital environment because of the time required to complete oral intubation with the use of neuromuscular blockade (Rhee & O'Malley, 1994).

CONTRAINDICATIONS AND CAUTIONS

The only absolute contraindication to blind nasotracheal intubation is apnea. Relative contraindications include the following:

1. Suspected facial, nasal, or basilar skull fractures. Many sources cite head trauma as a contraindication to nasal intubation because of concerns that the endotracheal tube will pass through the cribriform plate into the brain (Danzl, 2001). However, there is only one documented case of endotracheal tube penetration into the brain (Horellou et al., 1978).
2. Concurrent coagulopathy, anticoagulant therapy, or thrombolytic therapy, which increases the risk of epistaxis (Danzl, 2001).
3. Obstructions of the nose or posterior nasopharynx, including trauma, tumor, and foreign body (Walls & Luten, 2000; Danzl, 2001).

EQUIPMENT

See Procedure 9.

PATIENT PREPARATION

1. Place the patient in the supine position, with the head in the sniffing position unless there is a potential cervical spine injury. Provide manual stabilization of the head if spinal movement is contraindicated.
2. Initiate preoxygenation with 100% oxygen via nonrebreather mask or bag-valve-mask (see Procedures 27 and 35). Avoid bag-valve-mask ventilation when spontaneous ventilations are ample (Danzl, 2001).
3. Apply cardiac and oxygen saturation monitors (see Procedures 23 and 58).
4. Administer sedatives or topical anesthesia as prescribed.
5. Restrain the patient as indicated to prevent accidental extubation (see Procedure 192).

PROCEDURAL STEPS

1. Ensure that equipment is in appropriate working order. Inflate the endotracheal tube cuff to test for air leaks and deflate after testing. Liberally apply a water-soluble lubricant to the endotracheal tube.
2. Turn on the suction and place the tonsil-tip suction next to the patient's head.
3. *Insert the endotracheal tube through the naris with the bevel facing the septum. Advance the tube along the floor of the nasal passage, directing it toward the bottom of the ear. Resistance will be felt at the posterior pharyngeal wall. Rotate the tube a quarter turn to place the short aspect of the bevel in the superior position. Gentle pressure should facilitate entry to the poste-

---

*Indicates portions of the procedure usually performed by a physician or an advanced practice nurse.

rior oropharynx. Advance the tube until it reaches the glottis, usually heralded by a cough or gag. Retract the tube slightly (Figure 12-1) (Danzl, 2001).

4. *Listen to the breath sounds to develop a sense of timing and rhythm. Advance the tube through the glottis on inspiration while applying cricoid pressure (Danzl, 2001).

5. *Continue to listen for breath sounds through the tube. If breath sounds are clearly audible and air movement is felt, hold the tube in position. If breath sounds are absent through the tube and no air movement is felt, you may assume the tube has entered the esophagus. Retract the tube to the posterior pharynx and reattempt intubation.

6. Verify the appropriate endotracheal tube placement and secure the tube as described in Procedure 9.

7. Inflate the cuff and instill air until an adequate seal is obtained; 10-15 ml of air are usually required. Ventilate the patient with 100% oxygen.

AGE-SPECIFIC CONSIDERATION

Nasotracheal intubation is not a method of choice for the pediatric patient; because of the small size of the nasal passages, the procedure is difficult, and the small size often prevents the placement of an endotracheal tube that is large enough to be effective (Luten, 2000).

COMPLICATIONS

See Procedure 9. Complications specific to the nasotracheal route include the following (Walls & Luten, 2000):

1. Nasal bleeding during the intubation procedure or after extubation
2. Turbinate disruption or retropharyngeal perforation

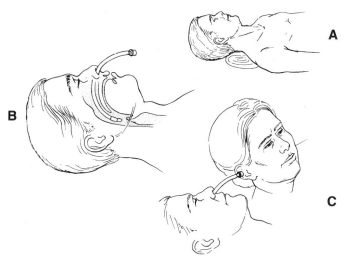

FIGURE 12-1 A, Place the patient in the sniffing position. **B,** Advance the tube along the floor of the nasal cavity. Continue advancing until the glottis is reached. **C,** Listen to the respiratory pattern; the tube is advanced on inspiration. (From Rosen, P., & Sternbach, G.I. [1983] *Atlas of emergency medicine,* 2nd ed. [p. 17]. Baltimore: Williams & Wilkins, with permission.)

3. Laryngeal injury or spasm
4. Sinusitis

PATIENT TEACHING
See Procedure 9.

REFERENCES
Danzl, D. (2001). Nasotracheal intubation (pp. 16-17). In Rosen, R., Chan, T., Vilke, G., & Sternbach, G. (Eds.), *Atlas of emergency procedures*. St. Louis: Mosby.

Horellou, M.D., Mathe, D., & Feiss, P. (1978). A hazard of naso-tracheal intubation. *Anaesthesia*, *33*, 73-74.

Luten, R. (2000). The pediatric patient (pp. 105-111). In Walls, R., Luten, R., Murphy, M., & Schneider, R. *Manual of emergency airway management*. Philadelphia: Lippincott Williams & Wilkins.

Rhee, K., & O'Malley, R. (1994). Neuromuscular blockade-assisted oral intubation versus nasal endotracheal intubation in the prehospital care of injured patients. *Annals of Emergency Medicine, 23*, 37-42.

Walls, R., & Luten, R. (2000). Awake intubation techniques (pp. 63-67). In Walls, R., Luten, R., Murphy, M., & Schneider, R. *Manual of emergency airway management*. Philadelphia: Lippincott Williams & Wilkins.

PROCEDURE 13

Retrograde Intubation

Donna York Clark, RN, MS, CFRN, CCRN

The information in this procedure should be used in conjunction with the information in Procedure 9.

Retrograde intubation is also known as retrograde transtracheal intubation (RTI), retrograde guide for endotracheal intubation, guided blind oral intubation, and translaryngeal guided intubation. Retrograde intubation (RI) is performed by puncturing the cricothyroid membrane, feeding a wire retrograde between the vocal cords, and exiting through the nose or the mouth. The tube is passed over this guide wire and advanced through the glottis (Murphy, 2000).

INDICATIONS
1. To facilitate emergent intubation when visualization of the vocal cords is not possible because of anatomic alterations, secretions, or blood (Killeen, 2001).

2. To facilitate intubation in patients with restricted range of motion of the head or neck because of anatomic variance or trauma (Murphy, 2000; Williams & Sahni, 2001; Guggenberger & Lenz, 1988).
3. To facilitate tracheal intubation when other routes have failed or significant difficulty is anticipated (Murphy, 2000; Sanchez & Pallares, 1996).

CONTRAINDICATIONS AND CAUTIONS

1. Infection at the area of insertion is an absolute contraindication.
2. Relative contraindications include the following (Murphy, 2000; Sanchez & Pallares, 1996):

   Apneic patient not able to be effectively ventilated with a bag-valve device

   Unfavorable anatomy

   Laryngotracheal disease

   Coagulopathies

EQUIPMENT

1 extra stiff wire guide: 110 cm long

1 radiopaque catheter

1 syringe (10-20 ml)

1 18-G introducer needle

1 catheter introducer needle

(Prepackaged kits with the equipment listed above are available.)

Scissors

Laryngoscope

Magill forceps

Bag-valve-mask system

Oxygen source/delivery system

Suction with tonsil-tip adapter

PATIENT PREPARATION

1. Place the patient in the supine position with the neck extended and maintain the neck in the neutral position. Provide manual stabilization of the head if spinal movement is contraindicated.
2. Initiate preoxygenation with 100% oxygen via a nonrebreather mask or bag-valve-mask (see Procedures 27 and 35). Administer oxygen via nasal cannula throughout the procedure.
3. Apply cardiac and oxygen saturation monitors (see Procedures 23 and 58).
4. Administer sedatives as prescribed.
5. Restrain the patient as indicated to prevent accidental extubation (see Procedure 192).

PROCEDURAL STEPS

1. *Palpate the cricothyroid membrane.
2. *Infiltrate the cricothyroid area with local anesthetic if indicated.

---

*Indicates portions of the procedure usually performed by a physician or an advanced practice nurse.

3. *Puncture the cricothyroid membrane with the introducer needle and direct it cephalad.
4. *Insert the wire through the introducer needle and direct it cephalad (Figure 13-1) (Killeen, 2001, Mariani, 1992).
5. *Advance the wire through the vocal cords and into the oropharynx (Figure 13-2) (Killeen, 2001; Mariani, 1992).
6. *Use a laryngoscope to visualize the wire.
7. *Use the Magill forceps to grasp the wire and draw it out through the mouth.
8. *Insert the cephalad end of the wire through the Murphy eye (side hole) of the endotracheal tube (outside to inside) and out the proximal end of the tube.
9. *Place slight tension on the wire and advance the endotracheal tube through the glottic opening (Figure 13-3) (Killeen, 2001; Mariani, 1992).
10. After the advancement of the endotracheal tube to the level of the cricothyroid membrane, cut the wire at the skin (*be sure to retain a grasp on the wire as it is being cut*) or pull the wire through and advance the tube into the trachea (Figure 13-4) (Killeen, 2001; Mariani, 1992).

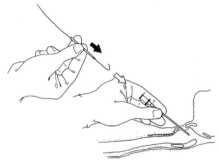

FIGURE 13-1 Insertion of needle and guide wire in cephalad direction. (From Mariani, P. [1992]. Endotracheal intubation. In Jastremski M.S., Dumas M., & Peñalver L. [Eds.]. *Emergency procedures* [p. 84]. Philadelphia: W.B. Saundersn.)

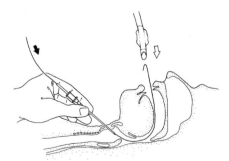

FIGURE 13-2 Advance the endotracheal tube over the wire. (From Mariani, P. [1992]. Endotracheal intubation. In Jastremski M.S., Dumas M., Peñalver L. [Eds.]. *Emergency procedures* [p. 85]. Philadelphia: W.B. Saunders.)

---

*Indicates portions of the procedure usually performed by a physician or an advanced practice nurse.

11. Verify the appropriate endotracheal tube placement and secure the tube as described in Procedure 9.
12. Inflate the cuff and instill air until an adequate seal is obtained; 10-15 ml of air is usually required. Ventilate the patient with 100% oxygen.

AGE-SPECIFIC CONSIDERATIONS

Airway management in the pediatric patient is challenging because of immature structures. Little current literature is available addressing the efficacy of retrograde intubation in the pediatric population. Orotracheal intubation is still the procedure of choice in children (Luten, 2000). Some older sources consider ret-

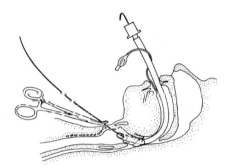

FIGURE 13-3 Advance the endotracheal tube into the airway. (From Mariani, P. [1992]. Endotracheal intubation. In Jastremski M.S., Dumas M., Peñalver L. [Eds.]. *Emergency procedures* [p. 85]. Philadelphia: W.B. Saunders.)

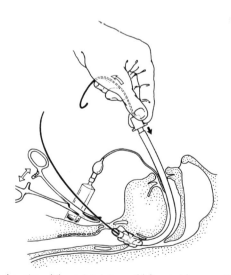

FIGURE 13-4 Retract the wire while maintaining mild forward force on the tube. Alternatively, cut the wire at skin level. (From Mariani, P. [1992]. Endotracheal intubation. In Jastremski M.S., Dumas M., & Penalver L. [Eds.]. *Emergency procedures* [p. 87]. Philadelphia: W.B. Saunders.)

rograde intubation a valuable adjunct to pediatric airway management (Audenaert et al., 1991; Schwartz & Singh, 1992; Sanchez & Pallares, 1996).

COMPLICATIONS

Complications specific to retrograde intubation include the following (Sanchez & Pallares, 1996; Wijesinghe & Gough, 2000; Murphy, 2000):

1. Bleeding of the nasopharynx and oropharynx
2. Localized subcutaneous emphysema (Powell & Ozdil, 1967)
3. Guide wire breakage requiring surgical removal of the broken segment of wire
4. Pneumothorax
5. Trigeminal nerve damage

PATIENT TEACHING

See Procedure 9.

REFERENCES

Audenaert, S.M., et al. (1991). Retrograde assisted fiber optic tracheal intubation in children with difficult airways. *Anesthesia and Analgesia, 73,* 660-664.

Guggenberger, H., & Lenz, G. (1988). Training in retrograde intubation. *Anesthesiology, 69,* 292.

Killeen, J. (2001). Retrograde intubation (pp. 10-11). In Rosen, R., Chan, T., Vilke, G., Sternbach, G. (Eds.), *Atlas of emergency procedures.* St. Louis: Mosby.

Luten, R. (2000). The pediatric patient (pp. 143-152). In Walls, R., Luten, R., Murphy, M., Schneider, R.(Eds.), *Manual of emergency airway management.* Philadelphia: Lippincott Williams & Wilkins.

Mariani, P. (1992). Endotracheal intubation (pp. 55-87). In Jastremski M.S., Dumas M., Peñalver L. (Eds.), *Emergency procedures.* Philadelphia: W.B. Saunders.

Murphy, M. (2000). Special devices and techniques for managing the difficult or failed airway (pp. 68-81). In Walls, R., Luten, R., Murphy, M., Schneider, R. (Eds.), *Manual of emergency airway management.* Philadelphia: Lippincott Williams & Wilkins.

Powell, W., Ozdil, T. (1967). A translaryngeal guide for tracheal intubation. *Anesthesia and Analgesia, 46,* 231-234.

Sanchez, A., Pallares, V. (1996). Retrograde intubation technique (pp. 320-341). In Benumof J.L. (Ed.), *Airway management principles and practice* St. Louis: Mosby.

Schwartz, D., Singh, J. (1992). Retrograde wire guided direct laryngoscopy in a 1 month old infant. *Anesthesiology, 77,* 602-608.

Wijesinghe, H.S., Gough J.E. (2000). Complications of a retrograde intubation in a trauma patient. *Academic Emergency Medicine, 712,* 67-71.

Williams, J.B., Sahni, R.. (2001). Performance of retrograde intubation in a multiple-trauma patient. *Prehospital Emergency Care, 5*(1), 49-51.

Extubation

Donna York Clark, RN, MS, CFRN, CCRN

INDICATIONS

1. It is appropriate to consider extubation (removal of the endotracheal tube) when the indications for intubation are no longer present. Extubation is indicated when there has been a resolution of the indication for intubation as well as hemodynamic stability (Henneman et al., 1999).
2. Extubation is also appropriate when ventilatory support is being withdrawn in anticipation of a patient's death.

CONTRAINDICATIONS AND CAUTIONS

Except when ventilatory support is being withdrawn pending death, extubation is contraindicated when the patient is deemed unable to protect his/her own airway or is unable to effectively ventilate without the assistance of mechanical ventilation. It is critical that a careful patient assessment is completed before removal of the endotracheal tube. Assessment findings must include the following:

1. Level of consciousness: awake and following commands
2. Adequate spontaneous respirations. Respiratory rate: in adults, respiratory rate < 35 during spontaneous breathing. In infants and children, regular respiratory rates consistent with age (Durbin et al., 1999). Not requiring high levels of positive airway pressure or inspired oxygen to maintain adequate arterial blood oxygenation. The American Association of Respiratory Care suggests positive end-expiratory pressure (PEEP) ≤ 10 cm H_2O and FIO_2 ≤ 0.40 (Durbin et al., 1999).
3. Ability to protect airway, positive gag and swallow reflexes
4. Hemodynamic stability
5. Effective respiratory muscle strength
6. Difficulty encountered when originally placing the endotracheal tube. If intubation was difficult, the health care team should develop a contingency plan for airway access should extubation fail.

EQUIPMENT

Suction set-up
Suction catheter/tonsil tip suction
30-ml syringe
Bag-valve-mask
Oxygen set-up
Pulse oximeter
Equipment to reintubate the patient if indicated (see Procedure 9)

PROCEDURAL STEPS (Greenlee, 2001)

1. To prevent aspiration, ensure that stomach contents have been evacuated.
2. Suction endotracheal tube, mouth, and oropharynx.
3. Elevate the head of the bed.
4. Instruct the patient to take a deep breath.
5. Deflate the endotracheal tube cuff.
6. Remove endotracheal tube at maximum inspiration (DHMC, 2002).
7. Suction the oropharynx as needed (see Procedure 31).
8. Apply supplemental oxygen as indicated (see Procedure 27).
9. Listen for stridor and auscultate bilateral breath sounds.
10. Monitor patient for adequate breathing and oxygenation (see Procedure 23).

AGE-SPECIFIC CONSIDERATIONS

Evaluation of the ratio of dead space V(D) to tidal volume V(T) has been found to be predictive of successful extubation in pediatric patients. Hubble and colleagues (2000) described a dead space/tidal volume ratio of less than or equal to 0.50 to be reliably predictive of successful extubation. These authors suggested that routine V(D)/V(T) monitoring of pediatric patients may permit earlier extubation and reduce unexpected extubation failures.

COMPLICATIONS

Extubation may fail, and the patient may require reintubation. Extubation may fail for the following reasons (St. John, 1998):

1. Airway obstruction/acute laryngeal edema
2. Aspiration
3. Respiratory muscle fatigue
4. Exacerbation of heart failure/pulmonary edema

REFERENCES

Dartmouth-Hitchcock Medical Center (DHMC), Department of Respiratory Care. (2002). *Extubation protocol.* Lebanon, NH: Author.

Durbin, C.G., Campbell, R.S., & Branson, R.D. (1999). Clinical practice guidelines: Removal of the endotracheal rube. *Respiratory Care, 44*(1), 85-90.

Greenlee, K. (2001). Performing extubation and decannulation. (pp. 24-26). In Lynn-McHale, D. & Carlson, K. (Eds.), *AACN procedure manual for critical care,* 4th ed. Philadelphia: W.B. Saunders.

Henneman, E., Ellstrom, K., & St. John, R. (1999). Airway management. In *AACN protocols for practice: care of the mechanically ventilated patient series.* Aliso Viejo, CA: American Association of Critical Care Nurses.

Hubble, C.L., Gentile, M.A., Tripp, D.S., Craig, D.M., Meliones, J.N., & Cheifetz, I.M. (2000). Deadspace to tidal volume ratio predicts successful extubation in infants and children. *Critical Care Medicine, 28,* 2034-2040.

St. John, R.E. (1998). The pulmonary system (pp. 1-136) In Alspach, J. (Ed.), *American Association of Critical Care Nurses core curriculum for critical care nursing,* 5th ed. Philadelphia: W.B. Saunders.

Pharyngeal Tracheal Lumen Airway

Donna York Clark, RN, MS, CFRN, CCRN

The pharyngeal tracheal lumen airway (Gettig Pharmaceutical Instrument Company, Spring Mills, PA) is classed with an indeterminate recommendation in the American Heart Association (AHA). The AHA states that "the evidence is lacking for inclusion of this device in the (ACLS) guidelines" (AHA, 2001). However, the pharyngeal tracheal lumen airway (PtL) is discussed in some paramedic and emergency medical technician (EMT) intermediate provider educational material and is used in the provision of emergency medical care in a few areas of the country (Bledsoe et al., 2003; Haskell, 2002). In many areas, the PtL is being replaced by the Combitube because of its ease of use (Rumball & MacDonald, 1997).

INDICATIONS
1. To establish an airway and ventilate a patient in respiratory arrest.
2. To establish an airway when tracheal intubation is unsuccessful or personnel trained in tracheal intubation are not available; placement of a PtL airway does not require the use of a laryngoscope.

CONTRAINDICATIONS AND CAUTIONS (Gettig Pharmaceutical
Instrument Company, 2002)
1. The PtL airway should not be used in children younger than 14 years of age, conscious or semiconscious patients, patients with known or suspected caustic poisoning, and patients with known esophageal disease.
2. Immediately remove the PtL airway if the gag reflex returns or the patient regains consciousness.
3. Improper tightening of the neck strap may result in leakage around the oral cuff.
4. If a patient does not seem to be responding to the PtL airway, or if its effectiveness is in question, remove the PtL airway and try a different airway device.
5. The PtL is a single-patient, short-term device.
6. Performing cuff inflation to verify cuff integrity before the PtL is inserted is not recommended because it may weaken the cuff.

EQUIPMENT
Oxygen source
PtL airway
Suction set-up with catheters
Gastric tube

61

Bag-valve-mask
Water-soluble lubricant

PATIENT PREPARATION

1. Place the patient in a supine position with the neck hyperextended, unless a cervical spine injury is suspected. If such an injury is suspected, leave the neck in a neutral position.
2. Remove dentures if present and suction the oropharynx if necessary.

PROCEDURAL STEPS (Gettig Pharmaceutical Instrument Company, 2002)

1. Ensure that both cuffs of the PtL airway are completely deflated.
2. Coat the tube with a water-soluble lubricant.
3. Insert your thumb deep into the patient's mouth. Grasp the tongue and the lower jaw between your thumb and index finger and lift straight upward.
4. In your other hand, hold the PtL airway so that it curves in the same direction as the natural curve of the pharynx. Insert the tip into the mouth and advance it carefully behind the tongue until the teeth strap touches the patient's teeth. There will be a modest resistance when making the right-angle bend at the back of the pharynx. Do not use force. If the tube does not advance, either redirect it or withdraw it and start over.
5. When the tube is at the proper depth, flip the neck strap over the patient's head. Tighten the strap with the hook and loop closures on both sides.
6. Inflate both cuffs simultaneously by directing a sustained breath into the No. 1 inflation valve (Figure 15-1). (NOTE: Make sure that the white cap is closed.) Pressure on the patient's cheeks may increase the pressure in the cuffs and improve the seal.
7. Ventilate immediately with a bag-valve-mask into the No. 2 green tube while observing for the rise and fall of the patient's chest, indicating that the No. 3 tube is in the esophagus (Figure 15-2). Then continue ventilating via the green tube with high-flow oxygen and a bag-valve-mask. The provider must verify breath sounds by auscultating the anterior and lateral areas of the chest and over the epigastric region.
8. If the patient's chest does not rise when ventilating into the No. 2 green tube, the No. 3 tube may have entered the trachea. Remove the stylet from tube No. 3 and ventilate through tube No. 3 with a bag-valve-mask and high-flow oxygen. Assess breath sounds and chest rise to confirm the placement of the No. 3 tube in the trachea.
9. Once the airway is in place, decompress the stomach by placing an 18-French gastric tube or suction catheter into the nonairway tube (either No. 3 or No. 2).
10. If adequate ventilations are verified but an air leak is present, tighten the teeth strap; this maneuver will ensure that the PtL is placed against the teeth. Alternatively, increase the cuff pressure via the No. 1 inflation valve (Gettig Pharmaceutical Instrument Company, 2002).
11. To replace the PtL airway with an endotracheal tube if the patient is being ventilated through the No. 2 green tube:
    a. Decompress the stomach as described in step 9 above.
    b. Hyperventilate the patient.

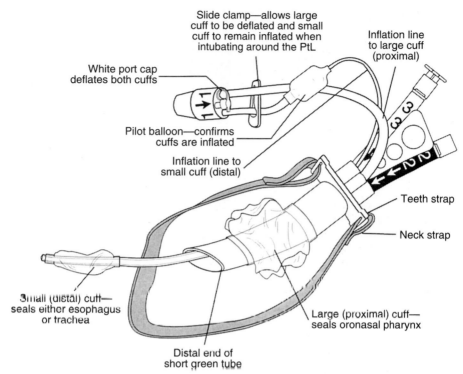

Slide clamp—allows large
cuff to be deflated and small
cuff to remain inflated when
intubating around the PtL

Inflation line
to large cuff
(proximal)

White port cap
deflates both cuffs

Pilot balloon—confirms
cuffs are inflated

Inflation line to
small cuff (distal)

Teeth strap

Neck strap

Small (distal) cuff—
seals either esophagus
or trachea

Large (proximal) cuff—
seals oronasal pharynx

Distal end of
short green tube

FIGURE 15-1 PtL airway. (Courtesy Gettig Pharmaceutical Instrument Company, Spring Mills, PA.)

    c. Pinch the pilot balloon inflation line with the plastic slide clamp (see Figure 15-1). Open the white cap on the No. 1 inflation valve. The large oral cuff will deflate to the atmospheric pressure and will deflate further when one orally sucks out air through the uncapped port of the No. 1 inflation valve.

    d. Insert the laryngoscope and quickly intubate the trachea around the PtL airway.

    e. An alternative is to deflate both cuffs by opening the No. 1 inflation valve. Remove the PtL airway and intubate the patient.

12. To replace the PtL airway with an endotracheal tube if the patient is being ventilated through the No. 3 tube:

    a. Pass a tube-changing stylet through the No. 3 tube.

    b. Deflate cuffs by opening the No. 1 inflation valve and removing the PtL airway.

    c. Insert the proper size of endotracheal tube over the stylet to reintubate the patient.

    d. An alternative is to deflate both cuffs by opening the inflation valve. Remove the PtL airway and intubate the patient.

13. To remove the PtL airway if the patient regains consciousness or the gag reflex returns, turn the patient to the side and open the white port cap on the

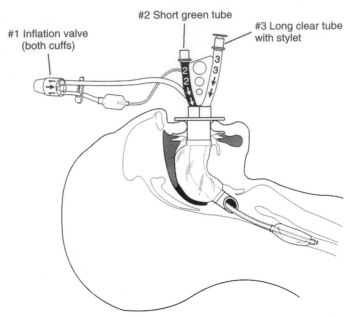

FIGURE 15-2 PtL airway in place. (Courtesy Gettig Pharmaceutical Instrument Company, Spring Mills, PA.)

No. 1 inflation valve to deflate both cuffs. Pull out the PtL airway and discard. Have suction available.

AGE-SPECIFIC CONSIDERATION

The PtL is designed for use on patients ranging from a small 14-year-old girl to a large man (Gettig Pharmaceutical Instrument Company, 2002).

COMPLICATIONS

1. The PtL airway may not seal the esophagus adequately; therefore, aspiration is always possible.
2. Inadequate ventilation may occur.
3. Assessing tube placement and deciding through which lumen to ventilate may be difficult (Pepe et al., 1993; McMahon et al., 1992; Hunt et al., 1989).

REFERENCES

American Heart Association (AHA). (2001). *Advanced cardiac life support provider manual.* Dallas: Author.

Bledsoe, B., Porter, R., & Cherry, R. (2003). In *Essentials of Paramedic Care.* New Jersey: Brady/Prentice Hall.

Gettig Pharmaceutical Instrument Company. (2002). *PtL airway: instructions.* Spring Mills, PA: Author.

Haskell, G. H. (2002). Prehospital airway devices. Available at www.emedicine.com/emerg/topic705.htm

Hunt, R.C., Sheets, C.A., & Whitley, T.W. (1989). Pharyngeal tracheal lumen airway training: failure to discriminate between esophageal and endotracheal modes and failure to confirm ventilation. *Annals of Emergency Medicine, 18*, 947-952.

McMahan, S., Ornato, J.P., Racht, E.M., & Cameron, J. (1992). Multi-agency, prehospital evaluation of the pharyngeo-tracheal lumen (PTL) airway. *Prehospital Disaster Medicine, 7*(1),13-18.

Pepe, P.E., Zachariah, B.S., & Chandra, N.C. (1993). Invasive airway techniques in resuscitation. *Annals of Emergency Medicine, 22*, 393–403.

Rumball, C.J. & MacDonald, D. (1997). The PTL, Combitube, laryngeal mask, and oral airway: a randomized prehospital comparative study of ventilatory device effectiveness and cost-effectiveness in 470 cases of cardiorespiratory arrest. *Prehospital Emergency Care, 1*(1), 1-10.

PROCEDURE 16

Combitube Airway

Donna York Clark, RN, MS, CFRN, CCRN

The Combitube and the Combitube SA (small adult) are products of the Kendall Company (Mansfield, MA). The Combitube esophageal tracheal double lumen airway is an emergency airway adjunct that combines the functions of the endotracheal tube and an esophageal obturator. The Combitube has two lumens that permit ventilation whether positioned in the esophagus or the trachea (Kendall Company, 1998).

INDICATION

The Combitube is indicated when emergency airway management is required and endotracheal intubation is not possible or permitted. In many situations, particularly pre-hospital, personnel trained in tracheal intubation may not be available. Placement of the Combitube does not require use of a laryngoscope (Agro et al., 2001; Birnbaumer & Pollack, 2002).

CONTRAINDICATIONS AND CAUTIONS (Kendall Company, 1998)

The Combitube is contraindicated in the following situations:
1. Responsive patients with an intact gag reflex.
2. Patients with known esophageal disease or who have ingested caustic chemicals.

3. Patients with laryngeal foreign bodies/pathologies resulting in upper airway obstructions (Murphy, 2000).
4. Combitube: Individuals less than 5 feet (152 cm) tall (use Combitube SA).
5. Combitube SA: Individuals less than 4 feet (122 cm) tall.

EQUIPMENT
Oxygen source
Combitube airway
Suction set-up and 12-French suction catheter (a 10-French suction catheter for the Combitube SA)
140-ml syringe (included with airway)
20-ml syringe (included with airway)
Bag-valve-mask
Water-soluble lubricant

PATIENT PREPARATION
1. Ensure that the airway is patent and ventilate the patient with a bag-valve-mask and supplemental oxygen.
2. Assess tube cuff integrity by inflating each lumen's cuff with air; the pharyngeal cuff (blue pilot balloon) is inflated with 100 ml of air, and the esophageal cuff (white pilot balloon) receives 15 ml of air (Kendall Company, 1998).
3. In presence of mouth/oropharyngeal trauma, remove sharp pieces and ensure that the cuffs do not tear upon placement.
4. Suction oropharynx if indicated (Procedure 31).

PROCEDURAL STEPS (Kendall Company, 1998)
Placing the Combitube
1. Ensure that both cuffs of the Combitube are completely deflated.
2. Lubricate the tube with a water-soluble lubricant.
3. Place the patient in a supine position, lift the tongue and jaw upward with one hand.
4. With the other hand, hold the Combitube airway with the curve in the same direction as the anatomic curve of the pharynx. Insert the tip into the patient's mouth and guide it gently behind the tongue until the two black (alveolar) rings on the tube are between the teeth. **Do not use force.** If the tube does not advance, either redirect it or withdraw it and reattempt insertion.
5. Inflate the upper or pharyngeal (blue) cuff (Figure 16-1) with 100 ml of air (85 ml for the Combitube SA). During inflation, the pharyngeal cuff adjusts to fill and seal the pharynx by pressing against the back of the tongue and closing the soft palate in an upward fashion. The Combitube is anchored against the posterior end of the hard palate by the pharyngeal cuff.
6. Inflate the distal (white) cuff with 15 ml of air (12 ml for the Combitube SA).
7. Immediately ventilate through the longer blue tube with a bag-valve-mask while observing the rise and fall of the chest. The presence of chest movement indicates that the distal end is in the esophagus (Figure 16-1). Continue ventilating via the blue tube with high-flow oxygen and a bag-valve-mask. Verify bilateral breath sounds by auscultating over the epigastric area and the anterior and lateral chest.

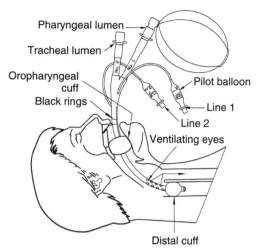

Pharyngeal lumen

Tracheal lumen

Oropharyngeal cuff

Black rings

Pilot balloon

Line 1

Line 2

Ventilating eyes

Distal cuff

FIGURE 16-1 Combitube airway, distal portion in the esophagus. (Courtesy the Kendall Company. [1998]. *Combitube and Combitube SA product literature.* Mansfield, MA.)

8. If the chest does not rise with ventilation through the longer blue tube, the distal portion may have entered the trachea. In this case, attempt ventilation through the shorter, clear tube. Assess the breath sounds and the chest rise to confirm the placement of the distal portion in the trachea. Positioning in the trachea is rare (Murphy, 2000).

9. If the distal portion of the Combitube is confirmed to be in the esophagus, decompress the stomach by placing a suction catheter or a nasogastric tube through the shorter, clear tube.

Replacing the Combitube With an Endotracheal Tube

1. To replace the Combitube with when ventilating through the longer, blue tube:
   a. Decompress the stomach as described in step 9 on p. 67.
   b. Hyperventilate the patient.
   c. Withdraw all the air from the pharyngeal cuff (blue) by using the 140-ml syringe. (Lutes & Hopson, 2004).
   d. Position the Combitube to the left side of the mouth. Insert the laryngoscope and intubate the trachea quickly with the Combitube still in place.
   e. Deflate the distal cuff by withdrawing 15 ml of air (12 ml for the Combitube SA) by syringe. Withdraw the Combitube (Hoak & Koestner, 1997).
   f. An alternative is to deflate both cuffs, remove the Combitube airway, and intubate the patient (Lutes & Hopson, 2004).

2. To replace the Combitube airway when ventilating through the shorter, clear tube:
   a. Hyperventilate the patient.
   b. Pass a tube-changing stylet through the shorter, clear tube.
   c. Deflate both cuffs by using the appropriate syringes and remove the Combitube airway.

    d. Insert the proper size of endotracheal tube over the stylet to reintubate the patient.
3. To remove the Combitube airway if the patient regains consciousness or the gag reflex returns, turn the patient to the side (if possible) and remove all the air from the pharyngeal and distal cuffs by syringe. Pull out the Combitube airway and discard. Be prepared to suction the patient as indicated.

AGE-SPECIFIC CONSIDERATIONS

The Combitube should not be used in a patient shorter than 5 feet. The Combitube SA may be used in patients 4 feet to 5 feet 6 inches tall (Kendall Company, 1998).

COMPLICATIONS

1. Inability to seal the esophagus adequately, leading to risk of aspiration
2. Inadequate ventilation
3. Difficulty determining placement and deciding which tube to use for ventilation
4. Perforation of the vallecula, pyriform recess, and esophagus (Murphy, 2000)

REFERENCES

Agro, F., Frass, M., Benumof, J., Kraft, P., Urtubia, R., Gaitini, L., & Giuliano, I. (2001). The esophageal tracheal Combitube as a non-invasive alternative to endotracheal intubation: A review. *Minerva Anestesiologica, 67*, 863-874.

Birnbaumer, D. & Pollack, C. (2002). Troubleshooting and managing the difficult airway. *Seminars in Respiratory and Critical Care Medicine, 23*(1):3-9.

Hoak, S., & Koestner, A. (1997). Esophageal tracheal Combitube in the emergency department. *Journal of Emergency Nursing, 23*, 347-350.

Kendall Company. (1998). *Combitube and Combitube SA product literature.* Mansfield, MA: Author.

Lutes, M. & Hopson L.R. (2004). Tracheal intubation (pp. 69-99). In Roberts, J. & Hedges, J. (Eds.), *Clinical procedures in emergency medicine*, 4th ed. Philadelphia: W.B. Saunders.

McGill, J. & Clinton, J. (1998) Tracheal intubation (pp.15-43). In Roberts, J. & Hedges, J. (Eds.) *Clinical procedures in emergency medicine*, 3rd ed. Philadelphia: WB Saunders.

Murphy, M. (2000). Special devices and techniques for managing the difficult or failed airway (pp. 68-81). In Walls, R., Luten, R., Murphy, M., & Schneider, R. *Manual of Emergency Airway Management.* Lippincott Williams & Wilkins: Philadelphia.

Cricothyrotomy

Donna York Clark, RN, MS, CFRN, CCRN

Cricothyrotomy (also known as cricothyroidotomy or "crich") is a surgical procedure that creates an opening through the cricothyroid membrane in which a cuffed endotracheal or tracheostomy tube is placed to secure an airway.

INDICATIONS

To establish an airway when intubation or ventilation by other means has failed or total upper airway obstruction is present (Walls & Vissers, 2000; Walls, 2001). Examples include the following:

1. Massive midfacial trauma
2. Anatomic variants
3. Ongoing severe oral or glottic area bleeding
4. Mechanical upper airway obstruction
   a. Oral or pharyngeal edema from infection or lesions
   b. Anaphylaxis
   c. Chemical inhalation injuries or burns
   d. Occult foreign bodies

CONTRAINDICATIONS AND CAUTIONS

There are no absolute contraindications.

1. Relative contraindications include crush injuries to the larynx, pre-existing laryngeal tumor or stricture, tracheal transection, anterior neck hematoma or infections, and coagulopathies (Walls, 2001).
2. Surgical cricothyrotomy is generally not recommended for children younger than 10 years of age because of poor landmarks and small size of the cricothyroid space. These factors increase the risk for damage to the cricoid cartilage, which is the only circumferential support to the upper trachea (Luten, 2000; Melker & Florete, 1996).

EQUIPMENT

Sterile gloves
Masks
Antiseptic solution
Local anesthetic (with epinephrine)
Syringe and needles for local anesthesia
Bag-valve-mask with supplemental oxygen source
Surgical cricothyrotomy
   Gauze dressings
   Sterile drapes
   No. 11 scalpel
   Hemostat or tracheal spreader
   Mayo scissors

Tracheal hook
Tape or ties to secure tube
Tracheostomy tube (No. 4 Shiley) or endotracheal tube (5-6 mm)
  Melker technique (also known as the Seldinger technique or percutaneous cricothyrotomy)
    Melker tray (contains a guide wire, dilator, 6-mm uncuffed tube, needles, syringe, No. 11 blade)

PATIENT PREPARATION

1. Place the patient in a supine position with the neck in a neutral position.
2. Cleanse the anterior neck with antiseptic solution.

PROCEDURAL STEPS

Surgical Technique

1. *Drape the neck with sterile towels.
2. *Anesthetize the area with a local anesthetic if the patient is conscious.
3. *Manually stabilize the thyroid cartilage and incise vertically over the lower half of the cricothyroid membrane (Figure 17-1).
4. *Open the incision with the hemostat or tracheal spreader.
5. *Insert a cuffed endotracheal tube or tracheostomy tube into the cricothyroid membrane incision, directing the tube distally into the trachea.
6. Inflate the cuff and ventilate the patient.
7. Observe for chest expansion and auscultate the chest for adequate ventilation.
8. Secure the endotracheal or tracheostomy tube with tape or ties and document the centimeter measurement at the skin line.
9. Place a sterile dressing around the incision area.

Melker Technique

NOTE: The Melker emergency cricothyrotomy catheter set is designed to establish an emergency airway access by utilizing a percutaneous entry (Seldinger) technique via the cricothyroid membrane with a subsequent dilatation of the tracheal entrance tract and with passage of an airway catheter.

1-3. Follow steps 1-3 as outlined on p. 70.
4. *Place a 6-ml syringe containing saline solution on the 18-G catheter and the introducer needle.
5. *Advance the 18-G catheter and the introducer needle through the incision and into the cricothyroid membrane at a 45-degree angle in the caudad direction. The proper placement is confirmed by the aspiration of the syringe with free air return (Figure 17-2).
6. *Remove the syringe and the needle, leaving the catheter in place. Advance the guide wire through the catheter and several centimeters into the airway (Figure 17-3).
7. *Remove the catheter, leaving the guide wire in place (Figure 17-4).
8. *Advance the dilator and the airway catheter over the wire and through the cricothyroid membrane (Figure 17-5).

---

*Indicates portions of the procedure usually performed by a physician or an advanced practice nurse.

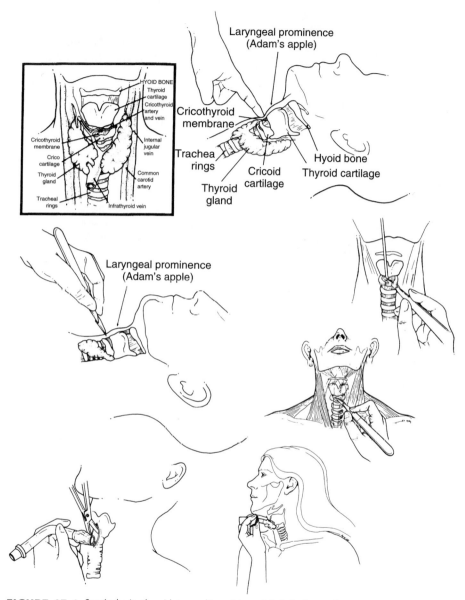

FIGURE 17-1 Surgical cricothyroidotomy. (From Mace, S.E. & Hedges, J. [2004], Cricothyrotomy and translaryngeal jet ventilation [p. 120]. In Roberts J.R. & Hedges J.R. [Eds.]. *Clinical procedures in emergency medicine,* 4th ed. Philadelphia: W.B. Saunders.)

9. *Once the airway catheter is in place, remove the guide wire and the dilator simultaneously (Figure 17-6).
10. Ventilate the patient and follow steps 7-9 as outlined above.

*Indicates portions of the procedure usually performed by a physician or an advanced practice nurse.

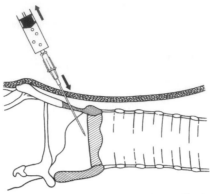

FIGURE 17-2 Advance the 18-G catheter and introducer needle through the incision into the cricothyroid membrane at a 45-degree angle in the caudad direction. Proper placement is confirmed by the aspiration on the syringe with free air return. (From Cook Critical Care. [1988]. *Melker emergency cricothyroidotomy catheter sets* [p. 6]. Bloomington, IN: Author.)

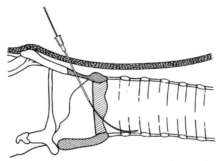

FIGURE 17-3 Remove the syringe and needle leaving the catheter. Advance the guide wire through the catheter into the airway several centimeters. (From Cook Critical Care. [1988]. *Melker emergency cricothyroidotomy catheter sets* [p. 7]. Bloomington, IN: Author.)

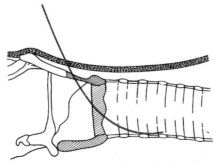

FIGURE 17-4 Remove the catheter leaving the guide wire in place. (From Cook Critical Care. [1988]. *Melker emergency cricothyroidotomy catheter sets* [p. 8]. Bloomington, IN: Author.)

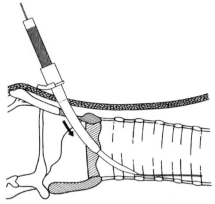

FIGURE 17-5 Advance the dilator and airway catheter over the wire through the cricothyroid membrane. (From Cook Critical Care. [1988]. *Melker emergency cricothyroidotomy catheter sets* [p. 10]. Bloomington, IN: Author.)

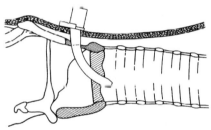

FIGURE 17-6 Once airway catheter is in place, remove guide wire and dilator simultaneously. (From Cook Critical Care. [1988]. *Melker emergency cricothyroidotomy catheter sets* [p. 11]. Bloomington, IN: Author.)

AGE-SPECIFIC CONSIDERATION

In children younger than 10 years of age, the small larynx lies much higher, at the C2-3 level, rather than at the C5-6 level, as in adults. A 12-or 14-G over-the-needle catheter (see Procedure 18) is safer than a surgical cricothyrotomy (Luten, 2000; Melker & Florete, 1996).

COMPLICATIONS

1. Creation of a false passage into the subcutaneous tissues
2. Asphyxia
3. Aspiration, usually blood
4. Hemorrhage or hematoma formation
5. Laceration or trauma of either the trachea or the esophagus
6. Mediastinal emphysema
7. Vocal cord hoarseness or paralysis

PATIENT TEACHING

1. You will not be able to speak while the tube is in place.
2. Report any air leak at the incision site or any respiratory difficulty.
3. Do not touch the tube or the incision site.

REFERENCES

Cook Critical Care. (2000). *Melker emergency cricothyroidotomy catheter sets*. Bloomington, IN: Author.

Luten, R. (2000). Pediatric airway techniques (pp. 105-111). In Walls, R., Luten, R., Murphy, M., & Schneider, R. (Eds.), *Manual of Emergency Airway Management*. Philadelphia: Lippincott Williams & Wilkins.

Melker, R. & Florete, O. (1996) Percutaneous dilatational cricothyrotomy and tracheostomy. In Benumof J.L. (Ed.), *Airway management principles and practice*. St. Louis: Mosby.

Walls, R. & Vissers, R. (2000). Surgical airway techniques (pp. 89-104). In Walls, R., Luten, R., Murphy, M., & Schneider, R. (Eds.) *Manual of emergency airway management*. Philadelphia: Lippincott Williams & Wilkins.

Walls, R. (2001). Cricothyrotomy (pp. 24-29). In Rosen, R., Chan, T., Vilke, G. & Sternbach, G. (Eds.), *Atlas of emergency procedures*. St. Louis: Mosby.

PROCEDURE 18

Percutaneous Transtracheal Ventilation

Donna York Clark, RN, MS, CFRN, CCRN

Percutaneous transtracheal ventilation (PTV) is also known as needle cricothyrotomy, jet insufflation, percutaneous translaryngeal ventilation, and percutaneous tracheal ventilation.

INDICATION

PVT is an emergency technique that provides a temporary avenue for gas exchange until a definitive airway can be secured (Walls & Vissers, 2000; Benumof, 1996). PTV is an appropriate intervention for emergency nonsurgical ventilation control when intubation has been unsuccessful and mask ventilation is inadequate. PTV is considered a temporary airway to allow effective gas delivery until a more stable airway can be placed (Bledsoe et al., 2003). This is the surgical airway of choice for patients younger than 12 years of age (Walls & Vissers, 2000).

CONTRAINDICATIONS AND CAUTIONS

1. PTV does not provide complete control of the airway, and aspiration may occur (Walls & Vissers, 2000).
2. Because carbon dioxide accumulates, this technique is recommended only until a definitive airway can be secured (Bramwell, 2001).
3. The catheter may kink easily or dislodge after placement into the trachea. Constant monitoring of the ventilation is necessary (Metz et al., 1996).
4. Tracheal suctioning cannot be performed through the catheter (Bledsoe et al., 2003).
5. The patient must be able to exhale passively through the nose or mouth.

EQUIPMENT

Antiseptic solution
14-G or larger over-the-needle catheter or commercially available needle cri-
    chothyrotomy device
3-ml syringe
2 ml saline for injection (optional)
Regulating valve connected to a high-pressure oxygen source
Suction equipment (pharyngeal)
Oral and nasal airways
3.0 endotracheal tube adaptor (optional, for use with a bag-valve-mask)

PATIENT PREPARATION

1. Place the patient in a supine position with the neck in neutral alignment.
2. Cleanse the anterior neck with an antiseptic solution.
3. Prepare the suction equipment and maintain immediate availability.
4. Restrain or sedate the patient, or do both as indicated to prevent accidental dislodgment of the catheter.
5. If possible, the patient should have nasal and oral airways placed to facilitate exhalation (see Procedures 5 and 6) (Walls & Vissers, 2000).

PROCEDURAL STEPS

1. *Locate the cricothyroid membrane (Fig. 18-1).
2. *Pass the over-the-needle catheter (with syringe attached) at a 45-degree angle caudally, and cannulate the trachea through the cricothyroid membrane. Air will be aspirated into the syringe when the entrance to the trachea has been attained. Saline in the syringe makes it easier to see air bubbles when aspirating (Figure 18-2) (Bramwell, 2001; Walls & Vissers, 2000).
3. *Remove the syringe and needle while manually stabilizing the catheter. Advance the catheter caudally into the trachea (Figure 18-3).
4. *Reconfirm the endotracheal placement by aspirating air.

---

*Indicates portions of the procedure usually performed by a physician or an advanced practice nurse.

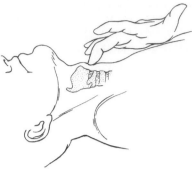

FIGURE 18-1 Locating the cricothyroid membrane. (From Rosen, P., & Sternbach, G.L. [1983]. *Atlas of emergency medicine*, 2nd ed. [p. 21]. Baltimore: Williams & Wilkins.)

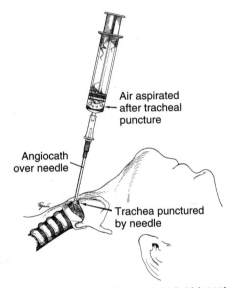

Air aspirated after tracheal puncture

Angiocath over needle

Trachea punctured by needle

FIGURE 18-2 Tracheal cannulation. (From Wilkins, Jr., E. W. [Ed.] [1989]. *Emergency medicine: scientific foundations and current practice*, 3rd ed. [p. 999]. Baltimore: Williams & Wilkins.)

5. For most adults, attach the catheter hub to the jet ventilator device. Table 18-1 lists the appropriate initial pressures based on the patient's weight.
6. There is no standard ventilatory device for PTV. The method described here can be accomplished with commonly available equipment. Other options include the use of intermittent high-pressure oxygen delivery by attaching noncollapsible tubing to an oxygen source at one end and to the catheter at the other. A regulating valve or a commercially available system (e.g., the Shrader blow gun) is attached to a high-pressure oxygen supply and placed within the system to allow for intermittent oxygen delivery (Figure 18-4). The customary frequency of inflation is once every 5 seconds (12 breaths per

TABLE 18-1
SUGGESTED VENTILATORY PARAMETERS

Weight	Pressure	Tidal Volume
12 kg	5 psi	234 cc
20 kg	15 psi	390 cc
30 kg	25 psi	585 cc
40 kg	35 psi	780 cc
>50 kg	50 psi	975 cc

psi, Pounds per square inch.
From Klofas, E. (1991). *Needle cricothyrostomy and percutaneous transtracheal ventilation (PTTV)*. Policy 300.44. Santa Clara County, CA: Central Fire Department.

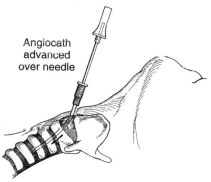

Angiocath
advanced
over needle

FIGURE 18-3 Catheter placement in trachea. (From Wilkins, Jr., E.W. [Ed.] [1989]. *Emergency medicine: scientific foundations and current practice*, 3rd ed. [p. 1000]. Baltimore: Williams & Wilkins.)

minute), and the duration for this method is 1 second or less (Walls & Vissers, 2000). The chest rise is a good indicator of adequate inflation. If a high-pressure oxygen source is not available, ventilation may be attempted with a bag-valve-mask via the adaptor from a 3.0-mm endotracheal tube. Remove the adaptor from the endotracheal tube, insert it into the catheter, attach a bag-valve-mask, and ventilate (Figure 18-5). This method is less effective than a high-pressure oxygen source, and ventilation may be very difficult, if not impossible.

7. Secure the catheter by holding it manually at all times, being careful not to bend or kink it.

8. Auscultate the patient's chest to assess ventilation. Visualize the chest for rise and fall as oxygen is delivered. Exhalation is passive from the glottis and, ultimately, from the mouth and nose (Benumof, 1996).

AGE-SPECIFIC CONSIDERATION

In children 12 years of age or younger, PTV is the procedure of choice for surgical airway management (Walls & Vissers, 2000).

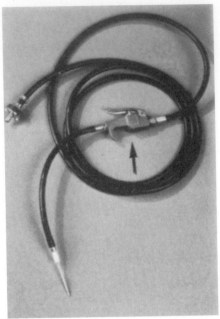

FIGURE 18-4 A high-pressure oxygen delivery device. (From Jorden, R.C. [1988]. Percutaneous transtracheal ventilation [PTTV]. *Emergency Medicine Clinics of North America, 6*, 749.)

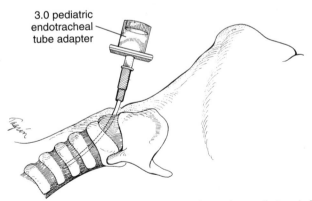

3.0 pediatric endotracheal tube adapter

FIGURE 18-5 Catheter attached to endotracheal tube adaptor for ventilation via bag-valve-mask. This technique is less effective than a high-pressure oxygen delivery system. (From Wilkins, Jr., E.W. [Ed.] [1989]. *Emergency medicine: scientific foundations and current practice*, 3rd ed. [p. 1001]. Baltimore: Williams & Wilkins.)

COMPLICATIONS

1. Subcutaneous or mediastinal emphysema, or both (Benumof, 1996)
2. Hemorrhage at the site of the needle puncture (Bramwell, 2001)
3. Posterior tracheal wall or esophageal puncture (Bledsoe et al., 2003)

4. Pneumothorax (rare) (Bledsoe et al., 2003; Benumof, 1996)
5. Inadequate ventilation, which may lead to hypoxia, hypotension, and so on.
6. Carbon dioxide retention
7. Obstruction or kinking of the catheter

REFERENCES

Benumof, J.L. (1996). Transtracheal jet ventilation via percutaneous catheter and high pressure source (pp. 454-474). In Benumof J.L. (Ed.), *Airway management: principles and practice.* St. Louis: Mosby.

Bledsoe, B., Porter, R., & Cherry, R. (2003). *Essentials of paramedic care.* New Jersey: Brady/Prentice Hall.

Bramwell, K.J. (2001). Needle cricothyrotomy (pp. 22-23). In Rosen, R., Chan, T., Vilke, G. & Sternbach, G. (Eds.), *Atlas of emergency procedures.* St. Louis: Mosby.

Klofas, E. (1991). *Needle cricothyrostomy and percutaneous transtracheal ventilation (PTTV).* Policy 300.44. Santa Clara County, CA: Central Fire Department.

Metz, S., Parmet, J.L. & Levitt, J.D. (1996). Failed emergency transtracheal ventilation through a 14-gauge intravenous catheter. *Journal of Clinical Anesthesia, 8,* 58-62.

Walls, R. & Vissers, R. (2000). Surgical airway techniques (pp. 89-104). In Walls, R., Luten, R., Murphy, M., & Schneider, R. *Manual of emergency airway management.* Philadelphia: Lippincott Williams & Wilkins.

Breathing Procedures

Tracheostomy

Donna York Clark, RN, MS, CFRN, CCRN

A tracheostomy is also known as a "trach" or a surgical airway.

INDICATIONS

To establish a definitive airway under the following conditions:
1. Inability to perform endotracheal intubation or cricothyrotomy (Davidson & Magit, 1996)
2. Severe laryngotracheal trauma or laryngeal fracture (Murphy, 2000)
3. Epiglottitis, neoplasm, space abscess, or foreign body in the pharynx that prevents endotracheal intubation (Davidson & Magit, 1996)
4. Need for a definitive airway after a cricothyrotomy (surgical or needle) has been performed. Usually, tracheostomy is performed in the operating room in this circumstance

CONTRAINDICATIONS AND CAUTIONS

1. Complications in the emergency setting are usually due to haste, inadequate lighting, equipment problems, and management of a patient who is struggling to breathe.
2. The complexity of this procedure mandates that it be performed by an appropriately trained professional.
3. Patients with suspected neck injuries require spinal immobilization. This precludes optimal positioning for a tracheostomy.
4. Universal precautions need to be employed by all involved personnel because blood is likely to splatter during the procedure.

EQUIPMENT

Sterile gloves
Masks
Protective goggles
Antiseptic solution
Scalpel blades, nos. 15 and 11
Local anesthetic
5-ml syringe with an 18-G needle and a 27-G needle for anesthesia
Tracheostomy tube with an obturator (size 6, 7, or 8 for adults)
Metzenbaum scissors
Scissors (sharp and blunt)
Tissue forceps (with and without teeth)
Mosquito forceps
Tracheal dilator and hook
Kelly clamps
Retractors

Adhesive tape
Gauze dressings
Suction equipment, pharyngeal and tracheal
Bag-valve-mask
High-flow oxygen source
3-0, 4-0 silk suture

PATIENT PREPARATION

1. When possible, the patient should be ventilated through an endotracheal tube, a cricothyrotomy, or another method until the tracheostomy is completed.
2. Unless there is a potential cervical spine injury, place the patient in a supine position with the neck in extension and provide support under the shoulders by using a blanket or small pillow (Figure 19-1). Provide manual stabilization of the head if spinal movement is contraindicated.
3. Cleanse the skin from the mandible to below the clavicles with antiseptic solution.
4. *Drape the chest and the neck.
5. *Infiltrate the skin with a local anesthetic (optional).
6. Restrain or sedate the patient as indicated.
7. Bleeding may be significant during exposure of the trachea. Prepare the tracheal and pharyngeal suction equipment and ensure immediate availability.

PROCEDURAL STEPS

1. *Make a midline skin incision vertically to expose the strap muscles (Figure 19-2).
2. *Retract the strap muscles laterally to expose the pretracheal fascia and thyroid isthmus (Figure 19-3).
3. *Clamp the thyroid isthmus and bluntly dissect to divide the isthmus and expose the trachea. Transect the thyroid isthmus and ligate it by means of sutures (Figure 19-4) (Davidson & Magit, 1996). Bleeding may be significant, so be prepared to suction.
4. *Incise through the tracheal rings to enter the trachea (Figure 19-5). Take care to control the depth of penetration to minimize the risk of injury to the posterior trachea and the esophagus (Davidson & Magit, 1996).
5. Suction the tracheal secretions.

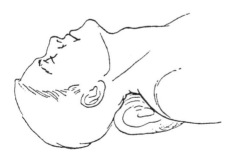

FIGURE 19-1 Patient positioning for tracheostomy. (From Rosen, P., & Sternbach, G.L. [1983]. *Atlas of emergency medicine,* 2nd ed. [p. 7]. Baltimore: Williams & Wilkins.)

---

*Indicates portions of the procedure usually performed by a physician or an advanced practice nurse.

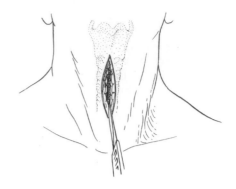

FIGURE 19-2 Midline incision. (From Rosen, P., & Sternbach, G.L. [1983]. *Atlas of emergency medicine*, 2nd ed. [p. 25]. Baltimore: Williams & Wilkins.)

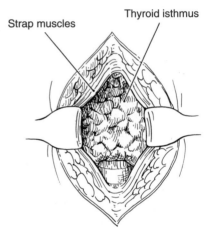

FIGURE 19-3 The thyroid isthmus exposed. (From Rosen, P., & Sternbach, G.L. [1983]. *Atlas of emergency medicine*, 2nd ed. [p. 25]. Baltimore: Williams & Wilkins.)

6. *Insert the tracheal tube and the obturator (Figure 19-6). Remove the obturator, inflate the cuff with 5-8 ml of air, and ventilate the patient with a bag-valve-mask. Auscultate the lungs to assess the tube placement and verify the tube position with a chest x-ray.
7. Tie the tracheostomy tube in place around the neck with tracheostomy tape (Figure 19-7).
8. Clean and dress the insertion site.
9. Deliver humidified oxygen as soon as possible (Sheldon et al., 2001).

AGE-SPECIFIC CONSIDERATIONS
1. The tracheostomy procedure is not different for the pediatric patient; however, careful attention to nearby vascular structures is necessary.
2. Pulmonary edema is an additional potential complication in the pediatric population (Derkay & Buescher, 1996).

---

*Indicates portions of the procedure usually performed by a physician or an advanced practice nurse.

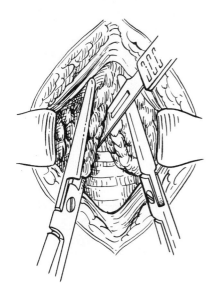

FIGURE 19-4 The trachea exposed. (From Rosen, P., & Sternbach, G.L. [1983]. *Atlas of emergency medicine,* 2nd ed. [p. 25]. Baltimore: Williams & Wilkins.)

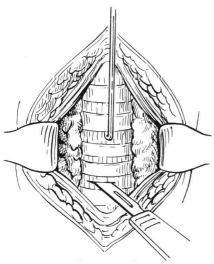

FIGURE 19-5 Tracheal entry. (From Rosen, P., & Sternbach, G.L. [1983]. *Atlas of emergency medicine,* 2nd ed. [p. 25]. Baltimore: Williams & Wilkins.)

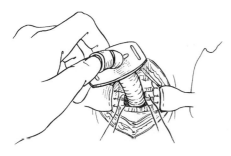

FIGURE 19-6 Insertion of tracheal tube and obturator. (From Rosen, P., & Sternbach, G.L. [1983]. *Atlas of emergency medicine,* 2nd ed. [p. 27]. Baltimore: Williams & Wilkins.)

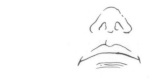

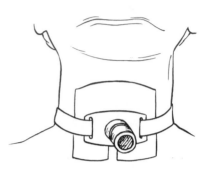

FIGURE 19-7 Tracheostomy tube tied in place. (From Rosen, P., & Sternbach, G.L. [1983]. *Atlas of emergency medicine,* 2nd ed. [p. 27]. Baltimore: Williams & Wilkins.)

COMPLICATIONS
1. Cardiopulmonary arrest secondary to hypoxia
2. Hemorrhage and injury to the thyroid gland, esophagus, laryngeal nerve, great vessels, or trachea
3. Pneumothorax
4. False passage of the tube into the pleura, esophagus, or surrounding vessels
5. Bradycardia or hypotension secondary to hypoxia
6. Subglottic stenosis (late)

PATIENT TEACHING
1. Report any respiratory difficulty or tubing disconnections immediately.
2. Do not touch or move the tube.
3. You will not be able to speak with the tube in place.

REFERENCES
Davidson, T.E., & Magit, A.E. (1996). Surgical airway (pp. 513-530). In Benumof, J.L. (Ed.), *Airway management: principles and practice*. St. Louis: Mosby.
Derkay, C.S., & Buescher, S. (1996). Pediatric ear, nose and throat procedures (pp. 427-445). In Taeusch, H.W., Christiansen, R.O., & Buescher, E.S. (Eds.), *Pediatric and neonatal tests and procedures*. Philadelphia: W.B. Saunders.
Murphy, M. (2000). The distorted airway and upper airway obstruction (pp. 169-171). In Walls, R., Luten, R., Murphy, M, Schneider, R. *Manual of Emergency Airway Management*. Lippincott Williams & Wilkins: Philadelphia.
Sheldon, G., Fakhry, S. Messick, W. & Rutherford (2001). Respiratory failure and ventilator management (pp. 107-135). In Baker, R., & Fischer, J. (Eds.) *Mastery of surgery*, volume 1. Philadelphia: Lippincott Williams & Wilkins.

Positioning the Dyspneic Patient

Teresa L. Will, RN, MSN, CEN

INDICATION

To facilitate spontaneous respirations and maintain optimal oxygenation in patients with moderate-to-severe respiratory distress

CONTRAINDICATIONS AND CAUTIONS

This position can be used only if the patient is responsive and has an unobstructed airway.

PROCEDURAL STEPS

1. Raise the head of the bed to an upright position at a 90-degree angle.
2. Support the patient's feet with a footboard if available. Consider using the knee gatch on the stretcher to maintain the patient's position. (The knee gatch should be used for only a limited time because of pressure created on the popliteal vessels.) This position is commonly known as high Fowler's position (Figure 20-1).
3. An alternative to the high Fowler's position is the orthopneic position, in which the patient is seated on the edge of the bed with the feet dangling, or the patient is seated in bed with an overbed table placed across the lap. The table is raised to a comfortable level and padded with a pillow or blankets. This is of particular benefit for patients with respiratory distress related to chronic obstructive pulmonary disease (COPD). This position is also known as the tripod position. In addition, this position may help relieve dyspnea related to pulmonary edema (Figure 20-2).

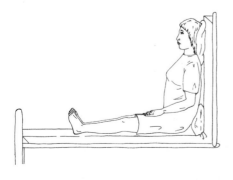

FIGURE 20-1 High Fowler's position.

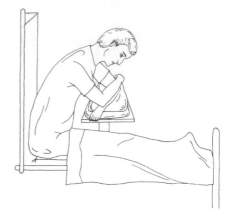

FIGURE 20-2 Orthopneic position.

AGE-SPECIFIC CONSIDERATIONS

1. It is particularly important to allow the pediatric patient to assume a position of comfort, for example, sitting on the caregiver's lap. This will decrease anxiety and facilitate spontaneous respirations. Even if it is not possible for the child to sit on the caregiver's lap, it is extremely important to allow the caregiver to be present to help alleviate the anxiety of the child.
2. Infants and children will often assume a tripod position on their own to facilitate breathing when in respiratory distress.

PATIENT TEACHING

Ease of respiration is of the utmost importance. The patient will assume a position of comfort naturally. Allow the patient to assume the position of choice.

PROCEDURE 21

Drawing Arterial Blood Gases

Teresa L. Will, RN, MSN, CEN

Arterial blood gases are also known as ABGs.

INDICATIONS

1. To evaluate acute respiratory distress and assist in determining therapeutic interventions

2. To document the existence and severity of a problem with oxygenation or carbon dioxide exchange
3. To analyze acid-base balance
4. To evaluate the effectiveness of respiratory interventions, for example, continuous ventilatory assistance or oxygen therapy

CONTRAINDICATIONS AND CAUTIONS
Proceed with caution and avoid arterial sticks in the following circumstances:
1. Previous surgery in the area (e.g., cutdown or femoral artery surgery)
2. Patients on anticoagulants or with known coagulopathy
3. Skin infection or other damage to the skin (e.g., burns) at the puncture site
4. Decreased collateral circulation
5. Severe atherosclerosis
6. Serious injury to the extremity
7. Thrombolytic therapy or a candidate for the same
8. Femoral punctures are contraindicated in patients with femoral grafts or cellulitis.

EQUIPMENT
Syringe (1- to 3-ml size)
20- to 25-G needle with a clear hub (smaller gauge should be used for a radial puncture)
23- or 25-G butterfly needle (for pediatric patients)
Stopper (cap) for a syringe
(Most of the above equipment is usually available in a prepackaged kit [Figure 21-1].)
Antiseptic pledgets
Heparin, 1:1000 (if the syringe is not preheparinized)
Gauze dressings
Ice
Local anesthetic (optional)

PATIENT PREPARATION
1. Select the puncture site on the basis of the clinical situation, how rapidly the sample must be obtained, and the circulatory status of the patient. The preferred site in most patients is the radial artery. The second most commonly used site is the brachial artery (Barnes, 1994). The femoral artery is most frequently used in critically ill or injured patients; however, this site should be avoided because of its potential for complications (e.g., hematoma or hemorrhage, because bleeding is more difficult to control).
2. If the radial artery is chosen as the puncture site, it is optional to check for the patency of the collateral circulation to the hand by performing a modified version of Allen's test. Some sources dispute the reliability and accuracy of Allen's test (McGregor, 1987; Stead & Stirt, 1985; Williams & Schenken, 1987). If used, it is performed as follows:
   a. Elevate the patient's hand and arm for several seconds. Have the patient open and close the fist several times. Occlude both the radial and the ulnar arteries simultaneously until blanching occurs (Figure 21-2). If the patient

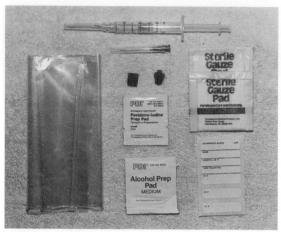

FIGURE 21-1 Typical equipment found in a prepackaged ABG kit. The syringe is preheparinized.

is unconscious or uncooperative, elevate the hand above the level of the heart and squeeze it until blanching occurs.

b. While maintaining pressure over the arteries, ask the patient to open the fist and relax the hand.

c. Release pressure from the ulnar artery while maintaining pressure on the radial artery. Observe the hand or palm closely for immediate flushing, which indicates the patency of the ulnar artery. The entire hand should regain color within 5-10 seconds. A flushed hand within 15 seconds indicates adequate collateral circulation, and the radial artery may be used for arterial puncture. If the hand remains blanched for longer than 15 seconds, there is inadequate collateral circulation, and that radial artery should not be used (Barnes, 1994).

3. Position the extremity:

a. *Radial:* Stabilize the wrist over a small rolled towel or washcloth. The wrist should be dorsiflexed about 30 degrees.

b. *Brachial:* Place a rolled towel under the patient's elbow while hyperextending the elbow. Rotate the patient's wrist outward.

c. *Femoral:* Rotate the leg slightly outward. Choose a site near the inguinal fold, approximately 2 cm below the inguinal ligament.

PROCEDURAL STEPS

1. Prepare the syringe (if not preheparinized). Draw up 1-2 ml of heparin and rotate the syringe to coat the barrel and fill the dead space of the syringe and needle. Holding the syringe upright, expel the excess heparin and air bubbles from the syringe.

2. Palpate the pulse and determine the point of maximal impulse.

3. Local anesthesia may be useful in particularly anxious patients. Inject approximately 0.2-0.3 ml of anesthetic subcutaneously on either side and above the artery. Aspirate before injecting the anesthetic to avoid injecting it into the vessel. Wait 3-4 minutes to allow for effective anesthesia to be in place.

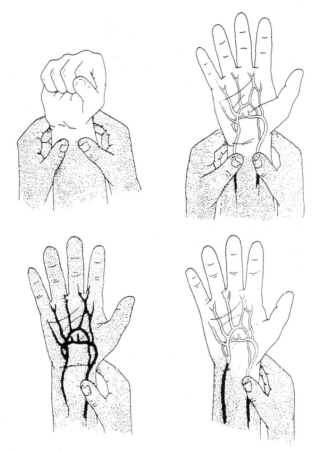

FIGURE 21-2 Allen's test. (From May, H.L. [Ed.]. [1984]. *Emergency medical procedures* [p. 84]. New York: John Wiley & Sons.) **A,** Elevate the patient's hand and arm for several seconds. Ask the patient to make a fist. Using your thumbs (or index and middle fingers), apply direct pressure over the radial and ulnar arteries simultaneously. **B,** While maintaining pressure over the arteries, ask the patient to open the fist and relax the hand. Note the blanched appearance of the palm. **C,** Release pressure from the ulnar artery while maintaining pressure on the radial artery. Observe the hand or palm closely for immediate flushing, indicating patency of the ulnar artery. The entire hand should regain color within 5-10 seconds. **D,** If the hand remains blanched for longer than 10-15 seconds, the radial artery should not be used.

4. Cleanse the overlying skin with an antiseptic solution.
5. Use the index finger of your free hand to palpate the arterial pulse just proximal to the puncture site (Figure 21-3). An alternative technique is to bracket above and below the arterial pulsation with two fingers of one hand and perform the puncture between the two fingers (Figure 21-4).
6. Grasp the syringe as if holding a pencil. Direct the needle with the bevel up, and puncture the skin slowly at approximately a 45- to 60-degree angle to the radial or brachial artery (90 degrees to the femoral artery). Watch the needle hub constantly for the appearance of blood.

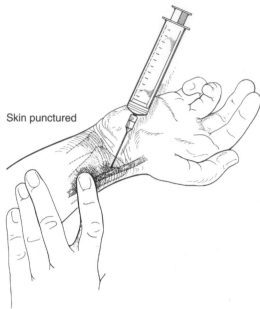

Skin punctured

FIGURE 21-3 Radial artery puncture. The index finger of one hand is used to palpate the arterial pulse just proximal to the puncture site. (From McCabe, C.J. Radial arterial puncture. In Wilkins E.W., Jr. [Ed.] [1989]. *Emergency medicine: scientific foundations and current practice,* 3rd ed. [p. 1013]. Baltimore: Williams & Wilkins.)

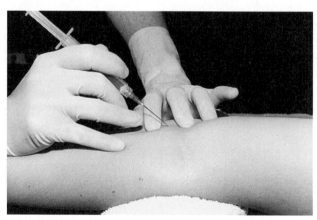

FIGURE 21-4 Brachial artery puncture. Two fingers of one hand may be used to bracket the artery and stabilize it.

7. When blood appears, stop advancing the needle and allow the blood to flow freely into the syringe. The blood should fill the syringe without aspiration, except in patients with severe hypotension. In these patients, red arterial blood should appear spontaneously in the needle hub. At this time, gentle aspiration may be used to obtain the sample. Some ABG syringes have a vented plunger that must be occluded if aspiration is necessary.

8. If the puncture is unsuccessful, both walls of the artery may have been pierced. Withdraw the needle slightly until the tip reenters the artery and blood flows into the syringe. If the needle fails to enter the artery and a good pulse is still present, withdraw the needle to just above the bevel and redirect it to the point of maximal impulse.

9. The disappearance of a pulse usually indicates an arterial spasm or hematoma formation. If this occurs, withdraw the needle immediately, apply direct pressure, and select another site.

10. Obtain a sample of 1-2 ml. Remove the needle from the artery. Immediately apply direct pressure to the puncture site with dry gauze for at least 5 minutes (longer for patients on anticoagulants or with clotting disorders). The next three steps should be performed by an assistant.

   a. Prepare the blood sample for the laboratory by immediately expelling all air bubbles. With the syringe upright, finger tap the air bubbles to the top of the syringe and expel them into a gauze dressing or alcohol pledget to catch the drops of blood.

   b. Stick the needle into a rubber stopper, or remove the needle with forceps, and cap the syringe with a rubber plug. Gently rotate the syringe between your hands to mix the heparin and the blood.

   c. Label the syringe. Indicate the concentration of oxygen the patient was receiving and the patient's temperature. An elevated temperature can significantly increase the partial pressure of oxygen (PO_2). Place the syringe on ice and immediately take it to the laboratory for analysis.

11. Place a dry, sterile gauze over the puncture site and secure it firmly with tape. Check the circulation and pulses of the extremity every 15 minutes for 1 hour.

AGE-SPECIFIC CONSIDERATIONS

1. The preferred site for pediatric patients is the radial artery (Aloan & Hill, 1997; Kilpatrick et al., 1995).

2. The brachial artery is larger than the radial artery and may therefore be easier to palpate in a small child (Evans & Bishop-Kurylo, 1996).

3. The femoral artery should be used only as a third choice, because this site has a greater risk for complications (Evans & Bishop-Kurylo, 1996; Kilpatrick et al., 1995). Avoid the more proximal arteries, such as brachial and femoral, because of the risk of ischemia should a thrombus occur (Sullivan, 1999).

4. EMLA cream, a topical anesthetic, may be used in infants greater than 3 months of age and children. EMLA cream is applied about 60 minutes before the arterial puncture and lasts about 90 minutes.

5. Use a 23- or 25-G butterfly needle attached to a syringe. Both the needle and the syringe must be heparinized and the heparin must be fully expelled (Evans & Bishop-Kurylo, 1996).

6. Draw approximately 0.5-1 ml of blood for blood gas analysis. Additional blood may be drawn for other laboratory tests if needed.

COMPLICATIONS

1. Compression neuropathies may occur secondary to hematomas caused by arterial punctures. Patients on anticoagulants are at greater risk (Simon & Brenner, 2002).

2. If air bubbles are not removed from the sample, the PO_2 can increase and yield inaccurate test results.
3. The blood sample may clot if the heparin and blood are not mixed adequately.
4. Thrombosis may occur with repeated puncture of the same site.
5. Arterial spasm or hematoma formation may cause impaired circulation to the extremity, especially in the brachial artery, because it has no collateral circulation (Simon & Brenner, 2002).
6. Nerve injury may occur with inadvertent puncture of the nerve.
7. Arterial punctures are at greater risk of bleeding if the patient has a partial thromboplastin time (PTT) greater than 72 seconds or an international normalized ratio (INR) greater than 2.2 or a platelet count of less than 50,000.
8. Screening the patient for medications such as heparin, warfarin, or thrombolytics or glycoprotein IIB/IIIA inhibitors within 12 hours may assist in preventing large hematomas. If the patients is taking any of these medications, carefully consider the necessity for the arterial puncture and hold pressure for 10 minutes or longer in these patients.

PATIENT TEACHING
1. Do not rub the puncture site.
2. Report any bleeding, pain, numbness, or tingling following the arterial puncture.

REFERENCES

Aloan, C.A., & Hill, T.V. (Eds.). (1997). *Respiratory care of the newborn and child*, 2nd ed. Philadelphia: Lippincott-Raven.

Barnes, T.A. (1994). Core textbook of respiratory care practice. St. Louis: Mosby.

Evans, T.C., & Bishop-Kurylo, D. (1996). Pediatric procedures. *Topics in Emergency Medicine*, *18* (2), 30-45.

Kilpatrick, F., et al. (1995). Arterial and capillary blood gas analysis (pp. 114-129). In Barnhart, S.L., & Czervinske, M.P. (Eds.), *Perinatal and pediatric respiratory care*. Philadelphia: W.B. Saunders.

McGregor, A.D. (1987). The Allen test: an investigation of its accuracy by fluorescein angiography. *Journal of Hand Surgery (British)*, *12*, 82-85.

Simon, R.R., & Brenner, R.E. (2002). *Emergency procedures and techniques*, 4th ed. Baltimore: Williams & Wilkins.

Stead, S.W., & Stirt, J.A. (1985). Assessment of digital blood flow and palmar collateral circulation. *International Journal of Clinical Monitoring and Computing*, *2*, 29-34.

Sullivan, M. (1999). Arterial puncture. In *The Resident Medical Officers On line Handbook. Capital Coast Health*. Dunedin School of Medicine. University of Otago. Retrieved Sept. 11, 2002, from *http://medmic02.wnmeds.ac.nz/groups/rmo/arterial_puncture0.html*.

Williams, T., & Schenken, J.R. (1987). Radial artery puncture and the Allen test. *Annals of Internal Medicine*, *106*(1), 164-165.

Capillary Blood Gases

Jean A. Proehl, RN, MN, CEN, CCRN

Capillary blood gases are also known as cap gases, CBGs, or mixed venous gases.

INDICATION
To obtain a capillary blood specimen for blood gas analysis when arterial access is unavailable or frequent sampling is indicated. Capillary blood gas values do not vary from arterial blood gas values to a degree of clinical significance when the samples are properly collected from normotensive patients (Curley & Thompson, 2001; Escalante-Kanashiro & Tataleán-Da-Fieno, 2000; Murphy & Harrison, 2001).

CONTRAINDICATIONS AND CAUTIONS
1. Collection and analysis may be adversely affected in the presence of poor peripheral perfusion secondary to peripheral vasoconstriction, hypothermia, or hypoperfusion (Escalante-Kanashiro & Tataleán-Da-Fieno, 2000).
2. Use a proper size of lancet (3 mm) to avoid too deep a puncture.
3. Avoid bruised or inflamed sites for sampling. Repetitive sampling from the same site may cause inflammation or scarring and should be avoided.

EQUIPMENT
Antiseptic solution or pledgets
2×2 inch gauze pad
Adhesive strip
3-mm lancet or skin-puncturing device used for blood glucose determination
1 blood-collecting pipette
Seal for pipette (cap or clay)
Heparin solution (1:1000), approximately 0.05 ml
2 metal fleas
Magnet
Label
Plastic bag
Ice

PROCEDURAL STEPS
1. Warm the area to be punctured for approximately 5-7 minutes before drawing the blood. This "arterializes" the capillary and increases the accuracy of the analysis. Warming can be accomplished with a chemical pack specifically manufactured for this purpose or a warm moist towel. If a towel is used, be sure it is not hot enough to burn the patient.
2. Instill heparin into the pipette to coat the walls. Be careful not to leave extra heparin in the pipette; a coating of the inner wall is all that is necessary.

3. Cleanse the site with antiseptic solution and perform the puncture.
4. Wipe away the first drop of blood with gauze and then completely fill the heparinized pipette with blood, making sure that no air bubbles enter the tube. Place the tip of the capillary tube as close to the puncture site as possible to decrease exposure to environmental oxygen.
5. Seal one end of the pipette with the cap or with clay.
6. Insert two metal fleas into the open end. Run the magnet up and down along the length of the pipette to move the fleas through the blood sample and mix with the heparin.
7. Seal the open end of the pipette with a cap or with clay.
8. Label the pipette, place it in a bag on ice, and send it to the laboratory immediately. Document the FIO_2 and temperature.

AGE-SPECIFIC CONSIDERATIONS

For infants, punctures to the lateral or medial aspect of the heel are used to obtain capillary gases. The preferred sites for older children and adults are the finger or the earlobe.

COMPLICATIONS

1. Inability to obtain enough blood
2. Obtaining a contaminated blood sample. Usually, a blood sample becomes contaminated with interstitial fluid when the area is "milked" for blood or if all the air bubbles are not removed.
3. Clotted sample from improper mixing
4. Infection or scarring at the puncture site
5. Inaccurate results if analysis of the specimen is delayed. Consult your laboratory for specimen handling and transport requirements.

REFERENCES

Curley, M.A.Q., & Thompson, J.E. (2001). Oxygenation & ventilation (pp. 233-308). In Curley M.A.Q., & Maloney-Harmon, P.A. (Eds.), *Critical care nursing of infants and children*, 2nd ed. Philadelphia: W.B. Saunders.

Escalante-Kanashiro, R., & Tataleán-Da-Fieno, J. (2000). Capillary blood gases in a pediatric intensive care unit. *Critical Care Medicine, 28*(1), 224-226.

Murphy, R., & Harrison, M. (2001). Toward evidence based emergency medicine: best BETs from the Manchester Royal Infirmary. Capillary blood gases in COPD. *Emergency Medicine Journal, 18*(2), 117.

Pulse Oximetry

Mike D. McMahon, RN, BSN

Pulse oximetry is also known as "pulse ox," "O_2 sat," or SpO_2.

INDICATION

To monitor oxygen saturation (SpO_2) quickly and noninvasively in patients who are at risk for hypoxemia. The SpO_2 notation indicates the arterial oxygen saturation by pulse oximetry rather than by arterial blood gas analysis. This abbreviation is used because blood analysis and oximetry readings may give different readings owing to machine capabilities and patient status. The waveform that accompanies the reading is called a plethysmograph or "pleth."

CONTRAINDICATIONS AND CAUTIONS

There is no absolute contraindication for pulse oximetry; however, in some situations, data may be misinterpreted:

1. SpO_2 is a measurement of oxygen saturation, not a measurement of ventilation or acid-base status (Keogh, 2002).
2. Patient motion may interfere by mimicking a vascular waveform. Newer devices (Masimo SET, Nellcor, Oxismart) have reduced errors as a result of movement through the use of improved software algorithms.
3. At about 90% saturation level, small changes in SpO_2 can represent a large change in the patient's partial pressure of arterial oxygen (PaO_2) (Schneider, 1999). Readings below 70% should be considered unreliable (Scanlan, 1999).
4. Anemia.
5. Elevated carboxyhemoglobin levels (secondary to carbon monoxide exposure or heavy cigarette smoking) and methemoglobinemia result in falsely elevated SpO_2 readings. Pulse oximetry measures the percentage of occupied binding sites on the hemoglobin molecule without differentiating oxygen from other substances. Carbon monoxide and methemoglobin have a higher binding affinity with hemoglobin than with oxygen, so they displace oxygen from the binding sites.
6. Administration of intravenous dyes (methylene blue, indigo, carmine) results in a falsely low SpO_2, because these dyes also absorb light at a wavelength similar to that of hemoglobin.
7. Shock, cardiac arrest, excessive vasoconstriction due to hypothermia, peripheral vascular disease, and low-flow states result in poor tissue perfusion, and the oximeter cannot detect hemoglobin binding accurately in this situation.
8. An arterial line or direct arterial compression of an extremity to which a sensor is applied (e.g., a blood pressure cuff, tourniquet, pneumatic antishock garment [PASG]) results in blood flow that cannot be detected.
9. Exposure of the oximeter's photo detector to bright external light can result in false data.

EQUIPMENT

Pulse oximeter
Appropriate sensor (probe) (Figure 23-1)

PATIENT PREPARATION

Remove nail polish if possible, because some colors, especially blue (Hamlin & Pronovost, 2000) interfere with pulse oximetry. If the nail polish cannot be removed rapidly and the oximeter cannot detect SpO_2 accurately, try to mount the probe side by side on a finger. This technique may also be useful for patients with extremely long fingernails.

PROCEDURAL STEPS

1. Select an appropriate sensor for patient size and placement site (see Figure 23-1).
2. Apply the sensor to the site. Accurate readings depend on the proper placement of the sensor. Sensors contain both red and infrared light sources and a photo detector. The saturation is determined by the ratio of red to infrared as sensed by the photo detector. To ensure the accuracy of the readings, it is important to place the two light sources directly opposite the photo detector.
3. If you are unable to obtain readings, assess the following:
   a. Circulation in the extremity, capillary refill, color, and temperature
   b. Sensor position in which both light sources pass through the pulsating arterial bed and reach the photo sensor
   c. Ambient light sources in the room (e.g., surgical lamps, fiber optic lights, fluorescent lights, infrared heating lamps, direct sunlight), because the photo detector cannot differentiate bright external lights from those transmitted from the sensor light source
   d. Dirt or blood on the sensor at the light source or at the photo detector site
   e. Patient movement
4. Troubleshooting options:
   a. Change the site, the type of sensor, or both. In low-flow states, move the pulse oximeter probe to a better-perfused area, such as the nose or the earlobe, to help yield better readings.
   b. Reposition the sensor to ensure that the light sources are opposite the photo detector.
   c. Decrease the ambient light by turning off the external light sources, shutting the blinds, or covering the sensor with a dry washcloth or a blanket.
   d. Replace the probe with a new one (disposable) or clean the probe (nondisposable).
5. If the oximetry reading does not correlate with the patient's clinical presentation, assess the pulse rate apically or radially and compare it with the pulse reading on the oximeter. If the readings differ, repeat steps 4 a through d or obtain an arterial blood gas reading.
6. Vasoconstriction may alter the SpO_2 waveform and numerical number (Murphy & Thompson, 2002). Consider shock as a cause of decreasing values.

QUICK SENSOR APPLICATION REFERENCE

DURASENSOR® DS-100A adult digit oxygen transducer

- For patients who weigh over 40 kg (88 lbs).
- Short-term monitoring only.
- Preferred site is index finger.
- Alternate sites are smaller fingers. *No thumbs or toes!*
- For low-motion environments.
- Accuracy specifications: ± 3 digits (70–100% SaO$_2$) ± 1 S.D
- Reusable durable sensor.
- Change sensor site every 4 hours.
- Never tape sensor shut.

OXISENSOR™ R-15 adult nasal oxygen transducer

- For patients who weigh over 50 kg (110 lbs)
- Only site for application is across nasal bridge.
- For no-motion environments.
- Accuracy specifications: ± 3.5 digits (80–100% SaO$_2$) ± 1 S.D.
- For one time use only—may *not* be reapplied.
- Requires skin preparation prior to sensor application. (Preparation solution enclosed.)

OXISENSOR D-25 adult digit oxygen transducer

- For patients who weigh over 30 kg (66 lbs).
- Preferred application site is index finger.
- Alternate sites include thumb, great toe or smaller finger.
- Accuracy specifications: ± 2 digits (70–100% SaO$_2$) ± 1 S.D. ± 3 digits (50–69% SaO$_2$) ± 1 S.D.
- May be reused as long as adhesive quality is adequate to maintain proper placement without slippage.
- Site must be inspected every 8 hours.

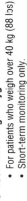

OXISENSOR D-20 pediatric digit oxygen transducer

- For patients who weigh 10–50 kg (22–110 lbs).
- Preferred application site is index finger.
- Alternate sites include thumb, great toe or smaller digit.
- Accuracy specifications: ± 2 digits (70–100% SaO$_2$) ± 1 S.D.; ± 3 digits (50–69% SaO$_2$) ± 1 S.D.
- May be reused as long as adhesive is adequate to maintain proper placement without slippage.
- Site must be inspected every 8 hours.

OXISENSOR I-20 infant digit oxygen transducer

- For patients who weigh 1–20 kg (2.2–44 lbs).
- Preferred application site is great toe.
- Alternate sites include thumb or other digits.
- Use supplied additional tape to secure the I-20 to the patient's foot or hand.
- Accuracy specifications: ± 2 digits (70–100% SaO$_2$) ± 1 S.D. (in neonatal population); ± 3 digits (70–95% SaO$_2$) ± 1 S.D.
- Limited reuse with adhesive dots supplied with I-20.
- Site must be inspected every 8 hours.

OXISENSOR N-25 neonatal oxygen transducer

- For patients who weigh under 3 kg (6.6 lbs) or over 40 kg (88 lbs).
- Preferred application site for neonates is around ball of foot.
- Alternate site for neonates is across palm of hand.
- Accuracy specifications in neonatal population: ± 3 digits (70–95% SaO$_2$) ± 1 S.D.
- Limited reuse with adhesive dots supplied with N-25.
- Site must be inspected every 8 hours.

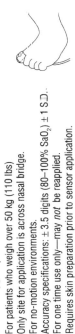

Warning: Carefully read the Directions for Use provided with each NELLCOR sensor for descriptions, complete instructions, warnings, cautions, and specifications.

FIGURE 23-1 Appropriate placement of various types of pulse oximeter probes. (Courtesy of Nellcor Puritan Bennett Inc., Pleasanton, CA.)

AGE-SPECIFIC CONSIDERATIONS

1. Pulse oximetry probes may be placed around the entire foot or hand of a small infant (Figure 23-1).
2. Pulse oximetry is accurate in the presence of fetal hemoglobin (which is normally present in neonatal patients) (Baker et al., 1998).
3. Pediatric patients are more likely to cause false alarms due to inadvertent movement (Miyasaka, 2002).
4. Specific problems related to a newborn in the delivery room are as follows (Kopotic & Lindner, 2002):
   a. Low perfusion secondary to transitional circulation
   b. High ambient lighting, which may be found in the delivery room

COMPLICATIONS

1. False high or false low readings (see Contraindications and Cautions)
2. Reaction to the latex in some adhesive probes
3. Skin breakdown (Check the site every 8 hours and change it as indicated.)

PATIENT TEACHING

Hold the extremity where the sensor is placed as still as possible to obtain an accurate reading.

REFERENCES

Hedges, J.R., Baker, W.E., Lanoix, R., & Field, D.L. (2004). Use of monitoring devices for assessing ventilation and oxygenation. (pp. 82-107). In Roberts, J.R. & Hedges, J.R. (Eds.). *Clinical procedures in emergency medicine*, 4th ed. Philadelphia: W.B. Saunders.

Hamlin, M.P., & Pronovost, P.J. (2000). Blood gases: pathophysiology and interpretation (pp. 140-150). In Tintinalli, J.E., Kelen G.D., & Stapczynski, J.S. (Eds.), *Emergency medicine*. New York: McGraw-Hill.

Keogh, B.F. (2002). When pulse oximetry monitoring of the critically ill is not enough. *Anesthesia and Analgesia*, *94*, S96-99.

Kopotic, R.J., & Lindner, W. (2002). Assessing high-risk infants in the delivery room with pulse oximetry. *Anesthesia and Analgesia*, *94*, S31-36.

Miyasaka, K. (2002). Pulse oximetry in the management of children in the PICU. *Anesthesia and Analgesia*, *94*, S44-46.

Murphy, M.F., & Thompson J. (2002). Monitoring the emergency patient (pp. 28-33). In Marx, J.A. et al. (Eds.), *Rosen's emergency medicine: concepts and clinical practice*, 5th ed. St. Louis: Mosby.

Scanlan, C.L. (1999). Analysis and monitoring of gas exchange (pp. 337-369). In Scanlan, C.L., Wilkins, R.L., & Stoller, J.K. (Eds.), *Egan's fundamentals of respiratory care*. St. Louis: Mosby.

Schneider, S. (1999). Acute respiratory insufficiency: overview (pp. 556-571). In Schwartz, G.R. (Ed.), *Principles and practice of emergency medicine*. Baltimore: Williams & Wilkins.

Websites for more information
www.nellcor.com
www.masimo.com

Assessing Pulsus Paradoxus

Teresa L. Will, RN, MSN, CEN

Pulsus paradoxus is also known as paradoxical pulse.

INDICATION

To assess hemodynamic status in conditions that may cause a greater-than-normal decline in left ventricular outflow during inspiration. Pulsus paradoxus is an exaggeration of the normal drop in systolic blood pressure that occurs during inspiration. Conditions that result in pulsus paradoxus include cardiac tamponade, pericarditis, asthma, chronic obstructive pulmonary disease (COPD), severe congestive heart failure, tension pneumothorax, mechanically ventilated patients with large tidal volume, and superior vena cava syndrome (Barach, 2000).

CONTRAINDICATIONS AND CAUTIONS

1. Surgical procedures or disease processes that prevent blood pressure readings in both of the upper extremities (e.g., amputation, mastectomy, extra-anatomic bypass, and dialysis fistula)
2. Severe dysrhythmias, severe hypotension, and irregular respirations prevent accurate measurement of pulsus paradoxus.
3. A patient must be removed from a ventilator before this procedure is performed.

EQUIPMENT

Blood pressure cuff and stethoscope

PROCEDURAL STEPS

1. Assess the patient for any irregular cardiac rhythms.
2. Observe the patient for normal respirations. Do not ask the patient to breathe normally, because you may make the patient aware that respirations are being monitored and cause alteration of the respiratory pattern.
3. Obtain a baseline blood pressure and note the systolic finding.
4. Reinflate the blood pressure cuff slightly higher than the previous systolic reading.
5. Deflate the cuff slowly while observing the respiratory pattern. Listen for the first systolic Korotkoff sound, which can be heard during expiration. Note the systolic reading.
6. Continue to deflate the cuff slowly while listening for sounds as you continue to monitor the respiratory pattern. Note the systolic reading again when you hear the first sound during inspiration. Repeat steps 4 through 6 to validate accuracy.
7. Wait 60 seconds with cuff fully deflated between blood pressure measurements to avoid venous congestion.

8. The difference in mm Hg between the first Korotkoff sound during expiration and the first Korotkoff sound during inspiration is the measurement of the paradoxical pulse. For example, if the first Korotkoff sound on expiration is heard at 150 mm Hg and the first Korotkoff sound during inspiration is heard at 130 mm Hg, then the paradoxical pulse is said to be 20 mm Hg.
9. A difference of 10 mm Hg or less is considered to be normal (Handerhan, 1993).

REFERENCES

Barach, P. (2000). Pulsus parodoxus. *Hospital Physician*, *36*(1), 49-50.
Handerhan, B. (1993). Pulsus paradoxus: no paradox at all. *American Journal of Nursing*, *93*(6), 24D.

PROCEDURE 25

Peak Expiratory Flow Measurement

Teresa L. Will, RN, MSN, CEN

Peak expiratory flow measurement is also known as peak flow, peak expiratory flow rate, and PEFR.

INDICATION

To assess peak expiratory flow rate in obstructive airway diseases (especially asthma) and to evaluate response to bronchodilator therapy. Peak flow is the most commonly used objective value that can be assessed at the bedside; a declining value indicates that the patient's condition is deteriorating or not responding to therapy (Novak & Tokarski, 2002).

CONTRAINDICATIONS AND CAUTIONS

1. Patients who are severely short of breath or who are hemodynamically unstable should not be further stressed by attempting to perform this procedure.
2. Recent eye surgery in which straining is contraindicated.

EQUIPMENT

Peak flowmeter

Disposable mouthpiece (if necessary)

PATIENT PREPARATION

1. If possible, place the patient in a sitting position with the legs dangling to maximize diaphragmatic excursion.
2. Loosen any tight or restrictive clothing.

PROCEDURAL STEPS

1. Insert the mouthpiece into the flowmeter (Figure 25-1).
2. Make sure the indicator is reset to zero.
3. Give the patient the following instructions:
   a. Hold the flowmeter in the correct position.
   b. Do not block the openings.
   c. Do not obstruct the scale.
   d. Inhale deeply.
   e. While holding a breath, place the mouth firmly around the mouthpiece and seal the circumference with the lips.
   f. Exhale through the mouth as forcefully as possible. If exhaled air leaks through the nose, use a nose clip or pinch the nose closed.
4. Read the peak expiratory flow measurement.
5. Have the patient perform the procedure three times.
6. Document the highest value of the three.
7. The normal range for adults is 350-750 L/min, based on the age and height of the person (Figure 25-2). A peak flow of 50%-80% of the patient's personal best indicates a moderate exacerbation; less than 50% is a severe exacerbation (Novak & Tokarski, 2002).

AGE-SPECIFIC CONSIDERATIONS

1. Peak flow measurements may be obtained in children as soon as they are able to understand the instructions to perform the test. This usually occurs between 5 and 6 years of age.

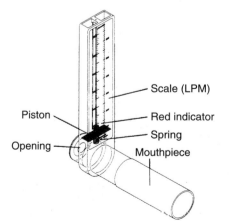

Scale (LPM)

Piston

Red indicator

Spring

Opening

Mouthpiece

FIGURE 25-1 Peak flowmeter. (From *Assess peak flowmeter: instructions for use.* Courtesy Health Scan Products Inc., Cedar Grove, NJ.)

NORMAL PREDICTED AVERAGE PEAK EXPIRATORY FLOW (liters per minute)

The National Asthma Education and Prevention Program recommends that a patient's "personal best" be used as his/her baseline peak flow. "Personal best" is the maximum peak flow rate that the patient can obtain when his/her asthma is stable or under control. The following tables are intended as guidelines only.

NORMAL MALES*

Age (Years)	Height					
(in) (cm)	60" 152	65" 165	70" 178	75" 191	80" 203
20	554	575	594	611	626
25	580	603	622	640	656
30	594	617	637	655	672
35	599	622	643	661	677
40	597	620	641	659	675
45	591	613	633	651	668
50	580	602	622	640	656
55	566	588	608	625	640
60	551	572	591	607	622
65	533	554	572	588	603
70	515	535	552	568	582
75	496	515	532	547	560

NORMAL FEMALES*

Age (Years)	Height					
(in) (cm)	55" 140	60" 152	65" 165	70" 178	75" 191
20	444	460	474	486	497
25	455	471	485	497	509
30	458	475	489	502	513
35	458	474	488	501	512
40	453	469	483	496	507
45	446	462	476	488	499
50	437	453	466	478	489
55	427	442	455	467	477
60	415	430	443	454	464
65	403	417	430	441	451
70	390	404	416	427	436
75	377	391	402	413	422

NORMAL CHILDREN AND ADOLESCENTS†

Height (in) (cm)	Males & Females	Height (in) (cm)	Males & Females
43　109	147	55　140	307
44　112	160	56　142	320
45　114	173	57　145	334
46　117	187	58　147	347
47　119	200	59　150	360
48　122	214	60　152	373
49　124	227	61　155	387
50　127	240	62　157	400
51　130	254	63　160	413
52　132	267	64　163	427
53　135	280	65　165	440
54　137	293	66　168	454

* Nunn, AJH, Gregg I: Brit Med J 298:1068-70, 1989.
† Polgar G, Promadhat V: Pulmonary Function Testing in Children: Techniques and Standards. Philadelphia, W.B. Saunders Company, 1971.
NOTE: All tables are averages and are based on tests with a large number of people. The peak flow rate of an individual can vary widely. Individuals at altitudes above sea level should be aware that peak flow readings may be lower than those at sea level, which are provided in the tables.

FIGURE 25-2 Peak expiratory flow measurement chart. (From Assess peak flowmeter: instructions for use. Courtesy Health Scan Products Inc., Cedar Grove, NJ.)

2. Pediatric normal measurements are based on the patient's height (see Figure 25-2).

COMPLICATIONS
1. Bronchospasm and increased dyspnea
2. Inaccurate reading because of poor effort by the patient

PATIENT TEACHING
1. Keep a daily log of your peak expiratory flow when you initially start using the meter in order to establish your normal baseline. Peak expiratory flow numbers vary with gender, age, and height. Each person may have a personal best that is higher or lower than the average. When you become short of breath, using the peak flowmeter to help you decide whether you need to use your rescue inhaler or seek further medical care. If the peak expiratory flow is between 50%-80% of your personal best, use your rescue inhaler. If the peak expiratory flow is less than 50% of your personal best, seek emergency medical care (Klements, 2001).
2. Report any increase in shortness of breath, faintness, or dizziness.

REFERENCES
Klements, E.M. (2001). Monitoring peak flow rates as a health promoting behavior in managing and improving asthma. *Clinical Excellence for Nurse Practitioners*, 5(3), 147-151.
Novak, R.M., & Tokarski, G.F. (2002). Asthma (pp. 938-956). In Marx, J. et al. (Eds.), *Rosen's emergency medicine: concepts and clinical practice*, 5th ed. St. Louis: Mosby.

PROCEDURE 26

End-Tidal Carbon Dioxide Detection and Monitoring

Mike D. McMahon, RN, BSN

End-tidal carbon dioxide ($EtCO_2$) detection is also known as capnometry, capnography, and $EtCO_2$. Some of the devises to measure $EtCO_2$ include Easy Cap II, Pedi-CAP, Fenem device, and STAT Cap.

Capnometry is the numerical measurement of CO_2 in expired air. Capnography is the capnometry value over time, and capnagram is the CO_2 waveform. $EtCO_2$ is the numerical value of CO_2 at the end of the exhalation phase of breathing.

CO_2 is the by-product waste of metabolism and used by the body to control pH levels. The following formula shows the importance in the body's ability to excrete CO_2:

$$CO_2 + H_2O \longleftrightarrow H_2CO_3 \longleftrightarrow H^+ + HCO_3^-$$

The CO_2 and H_2O are excreted through the lungs, allowing the body to quickly adjust the pH. The lungs are capable of removing 10,000 mEq of carbonic acid (H_2CO_3) in a day, compared with 100 mEq of acid removed by the kidneys (West, 2000).

Most of the CO_2 produced through metabolism is expired by the lungs and can be used as a measurement of ventilatory effort. Because of the function of the lungs in the excretion of CO_2, detection of CO_2 in expired gas aids in verifying the position of an endotracheal tube (American Heart Association [AHA], 2000). In a patient with effective ventilatory support, the CO_2 levels can be used to assess pulmonary and systemic blood circulation. Additionally, capnometry may be used to determine the effectiveness of pulmonary response to treatments.

In the emergency department, capnometry may be performed by means of a disposable device that shows color change to levels of CO_2, or by sensors that measure the content of CO_2 in the flow of air from breathing.

The disposable device houses a nontoxic chemical indicator that reacts to the presence of at least 4% CO_2 by temporarily changing color. This device attaches to the end of the endotracheal tube (ETT) and allows connection to a ventilator or a resuscitation bag. In the presence of CO_2, the device will change color with every breath.

Capnometry may also be performed with a capnometer that measures exhaled CO_2 in intubated or nonintubated patients. There are two basic types of sensors that measure the level of CO_2 in the patient's breath: mainstream and sidestream. Mainstream CO_2 devices use a sensor that is most commonly attached to the endotracheal tube. The sensor projects infrared beams across the ET tube and compares the adsorbed waveform with waveforms that have not been exposed to CO_2. Sidestream capnometry devices use a tube and pump to withdraw air from the patient's airway and measure the collected gas inside a separate device. This makes sidestream use more applicable for the nonintubated patient. The sampling tubes can be placed inline to an ET tube or may resemble an oxygen cannula and be placed in the patient's oral/nasal area. Sidestream sampling rates can be up to 100 cc/min, and low-flow technologies, such as Microstream devices, sample down to a rate of 30 cc/min. Both types can be used on the adult patient, whereas consideration should be given to the pediatric patient, who may be compromised by the additional air draw with the higher flow devices.

INDICATIONS

1. To help confirm ETT placement. The AHA (2000) lists $EtCO_2$ as a secondary procedure for confirmation of ETT placement. Unrecognized esophageal intubation has a significant impact on morbidity and mortality. Caplan et al. (1997) reviewed the American Society of Anesthesiologists' closed-claims database and found that more than half of the injuries could have been prevented by the use of capnography and/or pulse oximetry.
2. To help monitor the ETT position during patient transport.

3. To monitor continued ETT and airway patency. Secretions can build up and restrict airflow (Danzl, 2000).
4. To monitor respiratory effectiveness during sedation (Miner et al., 2002).
5. To assess the effectiveness of cardiopulmonary resuscitation (CPR) and return of spontaneous circulation. $EtCO_2$ drops suddenly when cardiac circulation is halted and returns rapidly with the return of the patient's circulation. Grmec & Klemen (2001) found that patients who had $EtCO_2$ values of 10 mm Hg or less during the entire course of cardiac arrest treatment were unable to be revived.
6. In mechanically ventilated patients, the numerical value and shape of the CO_2 waveform can be used to detect hypoventilation and hyperventilation, CO_2 rebreathing, and ETT dislodgement, as well as for assistance in weaning (Yacoub & Dubaybo, 1999).
7. To guide ventilator efforts in patients with head injuries. Low CO_2 values resulting from hyperventilation can cause cerebral vasoconstriction to the point of ischemia. The goal is to keep $PaCO_2$ values in the range of 30-35 mm Hg (Biros & Heegaard, 2002).
8. To confirm placement of a gastric tube (Burns et al., 2001).
9. To assist in the monitoring of patients suspected of having large pulmonary embolism (Weigand et al., 2000). Low levels of $EtCO_2$ may present in the initial stage due to restricted blood flow into the lungs. As the embolism is treated, $EtCO_2$ levels should begin to return to expected normal levels.
10. Future uses may include diagnosis of obstructive and restrictive airway disease on the basis of the shape of the $EtCO_2$ waveform (Murphy & Thompson, 2002).

CONTRAINDICATIONS AND CAUTIONS

1. During cardiopulmonary arrest, CO_2 values may not be detectable because of the lack of circulation. With effective CPR, $EtCO_2$ levels can be in the range of 1-10 mm Hg during exhalation and may be detected by a CO_2 device.
2. Colorimetric detectors are reliable for breath-to-breath CO_2 sensing for up to 2 hours (Nellcor, 2001).
3. A false-positive detection of CO_2 may occur in esophageal intubation if the patient has recently ingested carbonated beverages or antacids; however, this CO_2 washes out in 5-6 breaths (Yacoub & Dubaybo, 1999).
4. The contamination of a colorimetric device by gastric contents or drugs delivered endotracheally alters the reliability of the device (Nellcor, 2000).
5. The Easy Cap II device has 25 ml of dead space and should not be used for patients who weigh less than 15 kg (33 lb) (Nellcor, 2000).
6. Altered end-tidal CO_2 values can be detected in the presence of mainstream bronchus intubation. Other parameters, such as equality of breath sounds and chest rise, should also be assessed.
7. Water vapor in the ETT can affect measurements by mainstream technology and cause clogging in the sidestream tube. Mainstream sensors are heated to remove moisture from the area where the infrared beam is used. Sidestream devices use a hydrophilic filter in the tubing to prevent water from entering the sensor chamber.
8. High levels of oxygen or nitrous oxide can interfere with the specific infrared wavelengths used by the sensors. Current models have become much more specific in wavelength detection, reducing the risk of error in these situations.

ENDOTRACHEAL INTUBATION

Equipment

End-tidal CO_2 colorimetric detector, or $EtCO_2$ device
Bag-valve-mask

Procedural Steps Using Colorimetric Device

1. Accomplish endotracheal intubation as outlined in Procedures 9 through 13.
2. Attach the colorimetric device between the endotracheal tube and the bag-valve-mask.
3. Administer 6 breaths via the bag-valve system.
4. Evaluate the exhaled CO_2 content via the color change of the device (indicated by the color yellow in the Nellcor devices).
5. If CO_2 is present, continue ventilation, constantly assessing the color changes of the device. The color should change with each ventilation or expiration (purple to yellow with the Nellcor devices). If there is no indication of CO_2, or if other indicators of ETT placement are negative or questionable, remove the endotracheal tube, hyperventilate the patient with a bag-valve-mask, and reattempt intubation.

Procedural Steps Using Infrared-Sensing Devices

1. If using a mainstream device, attach the sensor to the ETT, with the sidestream device attached the connection to the end of the ETT (Figure 26-1).
2. Observe the display for $EtCO_2$ waveforms and associated numerical values (Figure 26-2).
3. Administer 6 breaths to wash out any gastric CO_2 content.

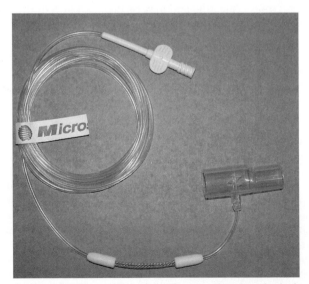

FIGURE 26-1 Microstream $EtCO_2$ sampling adapter for use with endotracheal tubes. The adapter fits between the endotracheal tube and the bag-valve or ventilator. (Photograph courtesy M. McMahon.)

4. Patients who are in respiratory arrest show elevated levels of CO_2 on the monitor; those in cardiac arrest with CPR will be in the range of 2-10 mm Hg.
5. If there is no indication of CO_2, or if other indicators of ETT placement are negative or questionable, remove the endotracheal tube, hyperventilate the patient with a bag-valve-mask, and reattempt intubation.

GASTRIC TUBE PLACEMENT

Properly placed gastric tubes should have an $EtCO_2$ reading of 0 mm Hg. Burns et al. (2001) presented a study utilizing $EtCO_2$ as a method for confirming placement of gastric tubes. The following procedural steps are abbreviated from their paper.

Equipment
$EtCO_2$ device
Gastric tube

Procedural Steps
1. The $EtCO_2$ device is connected to the proximal end of the gastric tube before insertion.
2. As the tube is advanced (Procedure 101), the $EtCO_2$ value is observed for any increase.
3. Values greater than 10-15 mm Hg require the user to remove the tube.
4. If the value is below 10 mm Hg, wait for three breaths from the patient. If the values drop down to 0 mm Hg, the tube may remain in place.
5. If the $EtCO_2$ value remains above 0, then the tube should be removed and reinsertion attempted.
6. Other methods of confirming tube placement, such as auscultation and withdrawal of gastric fluids, are still required.

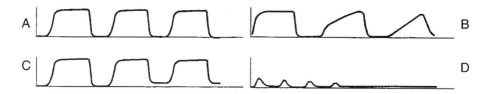

FIGURE 26-2 $EtCO_2$ waveforms (capnograms). **A,** Normal CO_2 waveform. The $EtCO_2$ measurement is taken at the end of the plateau just before the downward movement of the waveform. Normal value range is 35-45 mm Hg. **B,** CO_2 waveform showing obstruction. The second complex displays a "shark fin" type appearance. This waveform can be seen in patients with obstructive lung disease (asthma) or with a mechanical obstruction in the patient's airway or ventilator circuit. **C,** CO_2 waveform showing rebreathing. The waveform is moving off the baseline, the $EtCO_2$ value may also increase. This waveform may be caused by improper mechanical ventilator setup. It also occurs in patients who are using a bag for rebreathing. **D,** CO_2 waveform showing endotracheal tube (ETT) in the esophagus. The $EtCO_2$ value rapidly drops to zero. This occurs in acute esophageal intubations and if the ETT becomes dislodged. This waveform may also occur in patients who have no pulmonary circulation during CPR.

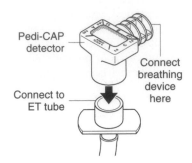

FIGURE 26-3 Connecting the Pedi-CAP to the endotracheal tube. (From *Pedi-CAP pediatric end-tidal CO₂ detector: directions for use.* Courtesy Nellcor Puritan Bennett Inc., Pleasanton, CA.)

AGE-SPECIFIC CONSIDERATION

For children who weigh less than 15 kg (33 lb), the Pedi-CAP (Figure 26-3) by Nellcor is indicated, because it has only 3 ml of dead space (Nellcor, 2000). Practitioners need to be aware that up to 100 ml/min of air is removed by some sidestream devices.

COMPLICATIONS

1. Increased airway resistance is encountered if the Pedi-CAP is used on patients who weigh more than 15 kg (33 lb). Excessive dead space is encountered if the Easy Cap is used on patients who weigh less than 15 kg (33 lb).
2. There are significant complications related to esophageal intubation (see Procedure 9).

REFERENCES

American Heart Association (AHA). (2000). Guidelines 2000 for cardiopulmonary resuscitation and emergency cardiovascular care. *Circulation, 102* (suppl. I).

Biros, M.H., & Heegaard, W. (2002). Head (pp. 28-33). In Marx, J.A. et al. (Eds.), *Rosen's emergency medicine: concepts and clinical practice.* St. Louis: Mosby.

Burnes, S.M., Carpenter, R., & Truwit, J.D. (2001). Report on the development of a procedure to prevent placement of feeding tubes into the lungs using end-tidal CO₂ measurements. *Critical Care Medicine, 29,* 936-939.

Caplan, R.A. et al. (1997). Adverse anesthetic outcomes arising from gas delivery equipment. *Anesthesiology, 87,* 731-733.

Danzl, D.F. (2000). Tracheal intubation and mechanical ventilation (pp. 85-97). In Tintinalli, J.E., Kelen, G.D., & Stapszynski, J.S. (Eds.), *Emergency medicine.* New York: McGraw-Hill.

Grmec, Š., & Klemen, P. (2001). Does the end-tidal carbon dioxide (EtCO₂) concentration have prognostic value during out-of-hospital cardiac arrest? *European Journal of Emergency Medicine, 8,* 263-269.

Miner, J.R., Heegaard, W., & Plummer, D. (2002). End-tidal carbon dioxide monitoring during procedural sedation. *Academic Emergency Medicine, 9,* 275-280.

Murphy, M.F., & Thompson J. (2002). Monitoring the emergency patient (pp. 28-33). In Marx, J.A. et al. (Eds.), *Rosen's emergency medicine: concepts and clinical practice,* 5th ed. St. Louis: Mosby.

Nellcor (Division of Tyco). (2000). Easy Cap II CO₂ Detectors (data sheet). Pleasanton, CA: Author.

Nellcor (Division of Tyco). (2001). CO₂ Detection (data sheet). Pleasanton, CA: Author.

Weigand, U.K.H., Kurowski, V., Giannitsis, E., Katus, H.A., Djonlagic, H. (2000). Effectiveness of end-tidal carbon dioxide tension for monitoring of thrombolytic therapy in acute pulmonary embolism. *Critical Care Medicine, 28,* 3588-3592.

West, J.B. (2000). *Respiratory physiology: the essentials.* Philadelphia: Lippincott Williams & Wilkins.

Yacoub, G.S., & Dubaybo, B.A. (1999). Evaluation of pulmonary function in the emergency department (pp. 593-600). In Schwartz, G.R. (Ed.). *Principles and practice of emergency medicine.* Baltimore: Williams & Wilkins.

Oxygen Therapy

General Principles of Oxygen Therapy and Oxygen Delivery Devices

Reneé Semonin. Holleran, RN, PhD, CEN, CCRN, CFRN, SANE

INDICATION

To provide supplemental oxygen to patients with adequate spontaneous respirations, but inadequate oxygenation

CONTRAINDICATIONS AND CAUTIONS

1. In ill or injured patients, oxygen is never contraindicated. Insufficient oxygen administration, leading to hypoxia, is the major risk. Hypoxia can lead to cardiac dysrhythmias and damage to organs, including the brain and kidneys. Supplemental oxygen should be administered to maintain an oxygen saturation greater than 90% (Murphy et al., 2001).

2. Oxygen-induced hypoventilation must always be considered as a possible hazard with patients who have carbon dioxide (CO_2) retention. Approximately 12% of breathless patients are at risk for CO_2 retention; in this scenario, excessive oxygen administration could lead to hypercapnic respiratory failure and acidosis. Causes of chronic CO_2 retention include chronic obstructive pulmonary disease (COPD), cystic fibrosis, sedation or narcosis from medications, severe kyphoscoliosis, neuromuscular disease affecting respiratory muscles, gross obesity, and extensive previous chest disease. In these patients, oxygen therapy should be titrated to maintain an oxygen saturation between 90% and 92% until blood gas results are available to guide further therapy (Murphy et al., 2001). Venturi masks are often used to precisely control fraction of inspired oxygen (FIO_2) in this population.

3. The primary physical hazard of oxygen therapy is fire. Oxygen supports combustion. Smoking should not be permitted in the room, and spark-producing appliances and volatile or flammable substances, such as gasoline and alcohol, should be removed from the immediate vicinity. Patients may need to be searched to ensure that they do not have any matches or lighters on their person.

4. Oxygen masks may cause some care problems in patients who have facial burns or patients who need frequent nursing care to the facial area. Gastric tubes may interfere with the tight seal of the mask.

5. Aspiration is a potential hazard when a mask is in place. Special caution must be used with patients who have an impaired gag reflex or a depressed level of consciousness. Elevating the head of the bed may decrease this risk.

6. The concentration of oxygen delivered is variable and depends on the flow rate, ventilatory pattern, and anatomic dead space.
7. Masks require a tight-fitting seal to provide accurate, high-oxygen concentrations. The tight seal may be uncomfortable and irritating to the skin.
8. Masks interfere with the patient's speech and must be removed while the patient is eating.
9. All oxygen delivery devices should be monitored to ensure that they are providing the appropriate amount of oxygen. For example, if the bag attached to a partial rebreathing mask is allowed to collapse, more exhaled air can enter the reservoir and increase inhaled CO_2 concentration (Lynn-McHale & Carlson, 2000).

EQUIPMENT

Appropriate oxygen delivery device (Table 27-1)
Oxygen delivery system (tubing, connectors)
Flowmeter (regulator must be used for cylinder systems)
Nut and tailpiece ("Christmas tree adapter," green nipple connector)
Oxygen source
Humidification set-up for selected patients

PATIENT PREPARATION

1. Explain no-smoking instructions to the patient and visitors.
2. When not contraindicated, allow patient to assume a position of comfort (Nettina, 2001).

PROCEDURAL STEPS

1. Attach the flowmeter to the oxygen source.
2. Attach the nut and tailpiece to the flowmeter. If the patient requires humidified oxygen, attach the humidifier to the flowmeter. Humidification is not necessary for short-term use.
3. Attach the flared vinyl tip of the oxygen tubing to the tailpiece or humidifier.
4. Adjust the oxygen to the flow rate as directed by the equipment recommendations to deliver the prescribed amount of oxygen. The float ball in the flowmeter should be positioned so that the flow rate line is in the middle of the ball.
5. Check to ensure that oxygen is flowing freely through the cannula or mask.
6. For nonrebreather masks, the reservoir bag must be prefilled with oxygen before it is placed on the patient. When using an oxygen mask with a bag, adjust the flow of the oxygen to prevent collapse of the bag, even during deep inspiration (Smith et al., 2000).
7. Place the mask on the patient's face or insert the cannula prongs into the nostrils. Mold the malleable metal nose strip (on oxygen masks) to the patient's nose. Monitor the mask to ensure that the side ports of the mask do not become blocked.
8. Pad straps with gauze or cotton as needed to prevent discomfort or irritation.
9. When delivering medication through a mask, ensure that medication is misting. If humidification is being used, periodically check and drain tubing as needed.

TABLE 27-1

OXYGEN DELIVERY DEVICES

Delivery Device	Indications	Advantages	Disadvantages
Nasal cannula	• Flow rates of 1-6 L/min provide 22%-45% oxygen concentration	• Patient can eat and talk without removing the cannula • Convenient and comfortable for all ages	• Can be easily dislodged • May become plugged with nasal secretions • Patient must have patent nasal passages • Flow rates greater than 6 L/min should not be used because of the discomfort this causes the patient
Simple face mask	• Flow rates of 5-8 L/min provide 40%-60% oxygen concentration	• Effective for mouth breathers or patients who have nasal obstruction	• Use a flow rate of at least 5 L/min to prevent the rebreathing of carbon dioxide
Partial rebreather mask	• Flow rates of 8-12 L/min deliver 50%-80% oxygen concentration	• Delivers a high concentration of oxygen	• Reservoir bag must be kept from kinking and obstructing the flow of oxygen • The bag should never completely collapse
Nonrebreather mask	• Flow rates of 10-15 L/min deliver 60%-80% oxygen concentration • This mask should be for short-term use when the highest possible oxygen concentration is required	• Delivers highest concentration of oxygen short of mechanical ventilation	• Some nonrebreather masks have one of the valves removed from the side exhalation ports, allowing the patient to inhale through the side port if oxygen flow should be interrupted; this results in a mask that is little more than a partial breather mask • The reservoir bag should never completely collapse

TABLE 27-1
OXYGEN DELIVERY DEVICES—cont'd

Delivery Device	Indications	Advantages	Disadvantages
Nonrebreather mask—cont'd			• Suffocation is possible if the oxygen flow is obstructed and the mask is tightly sealed, unless the mask is equipped with a spring-valve mechanism that can open when the patient inspires.
Air-entrainment mask (also known as Venti mask or Venturi mask)	• To provide precise oxygen concentrations of 24%-50%	• Allows inhalation of a constant oxygen concentration, regardless of the rate or depth of respiration • Oxygen concentration can be changed by changing the dilution jets or resetting the dial	• Not useful for oxygen concentrations greater than 50% • Air-entrainment ports must never be blocked • Bubble humidifiers often result in activation of the pressure-release valve
Tracheal collar (also known as puritan collar or tracheostomy collar)	• To deliver oxygen, humidity, and medications to patients with tracheostomies	• Used in conjunction with large-volume aerosol systems; provides oxygen concentrations of 28%-100% • High humidity • Open port allows suctioning without removing the mask	• Observe the patient to be sure that mist escapes the oxygen delivery device during inspiration because inadequate flow is the most common problem • Water from condensation may collect in the tubing and drain into the tracheostomy

Illustrations drawn by Esther Slabach. Used with permission.

AGE-SPECIFIC CONSIDERATIONS

1. Allow an alert child to remain in the position of comfort.
2. Decrease a child's anxiety by allowing the parents to remain in the room. Allow the caregiver to hold the child when not contraindicated by the child's condition.
3. Introduce the airway equipment in a nonthreatening manner. Allow the caregiver to hold the oxygen delivery device to decrease the child's anxiety.
4. Use alternative methods of delivery if a child is upset by one method. A drinking cup with oxygen supply tubing inserted into the bottom of the cup is a nonthreatening manner of directing the oxygen.
5. All devices listed in Table 27-1 are available in pediatric sizes.

COMPLICATIONS

1. The nasal mucosa may become excessively dry. Standard humidification equipment delivers only 20%-40% of humidity to the patient (Flynn & Bruce, 1993).
2. The mask or cannula may be easily dislodged.
3. Masks are of standard sizes and may not fit all patients comfortably and snugly.
4. Facial irritation may result because the mask is too tight or the plastic rubs.
5. Some patients may complain of a feeling of suffocation if the mask covers both the mouth and the nose. A mask may also make the patient feel hot.
6. A mask must be removed for the patient to eat, drink, expectorate, or blow the nose.

PATIENT TEACHING

1. No smoking while oxygen is in the room.
2. Remove the mask only to eat, blow the nose, expectorate, or vomit. Replace the mask immediately. The mask may be replaced with a nasal cannula for eating.
3. Explain the proper position of the mask and the importance of a snug fit.

REFERENCES

Flynn, J.M., & Bruce, N.P. (1993). *Introduction to critical care skills*. St. Louis: Mosby.

Lynn-McHale, D.J., & Carlson, K. (Eds.) (2000). *AACN procedure manual for critical care*, 4th ed. Philadelphia: W.B. Saunders.

Murphy, R., Mackway-Jones, K., Sammy, I. et al. (2001). Emergency oxygen therapy for the breathless patient. Guidelines prepared by North West Oxygen Group. *Emergency Medical Journal, 18*, 421-423.

Nettina, S.M. (Ed.). (2001). *Lippincott manual of nursing practice*. Philadelphia: Lippincott.

Smith, A., Duell, D., & Martin, B. (2000). *Clinical nursing skills: basic to advanced skills*. Upper Saddle River, NJ: Prentice Hall Health.

Application and Removal of Oxygen Tank Regulators

Reneé Semonin Holleran, RN, PhD, CEN, CCRN, CFRN, SANE

Oxygen tanks are also known as D cylinder, E cylinder, H cylinder, K cylinder, and so forth. Regulators are also known as adjustable regulator, regulator or flowmeter, or control valve (a regulator reduces the cylinder pressure to a working pressure before the oxygen enters the flowmeter; the flowmeter controls and measures the liter flow of oxygen to the patient). Sealing washers are also known as O-rings or gaskets. E-cylinders are the most common tanks used in the emergency department. C-cylinders are generally used for transport.

INDICATIONS
Oxygen cylinders are used to provide oxygen in the following situations:
1. During the transportation of patients
2. When no piped oxygen source is available

CONTRAINDICATIONS AND CAUTIONS
1. Secure oxygen cylinders in support stand to avoid damage during transport and storage. The pressurized oxygen may turn the cylinder into a "torpedo" if damage occurs to the regulator.
2. Cylinders are heavy and cumbersome to handle. A full E-cylinder weighs approximately 16 lb (White, 1996). However, some sizes of tanks are available in aluminum. Do not drag, slide, or roll a cylinder. Use a portable carrier to move it to the point of use.
3. Never drop a cylinder or allow it to strike another surface.
4. To prevent fire, never permit oil, grease, or other highly flammable materials to come in contact with oxygen cylinders, valves, regulators, or fittings.
5. To prevent an accidental readjustment of oxygen flow, never drape anything over the cylinder or the regulator.
6. Use only the proper wrench or key to open or close the post valve, that is, a key that has a circular opening. Keys that have a hexagonal opening of approximately 1 inch should be discarded. Use of an incorrectly shaped key can loosen the retaining nut on the stem of the cylinder and may result in serious injury or death of the patient.
7. Oxygen tanks should be stored according to hospital policies and procedures based on Joint Committee on Accreditation of Healthcare Organizations (JCAHO) guidelines.

EQUIPMENT
A cylinder of oxygen (E-cylinder is the most commonly used size in the emergency setting) (Figure 28-1)

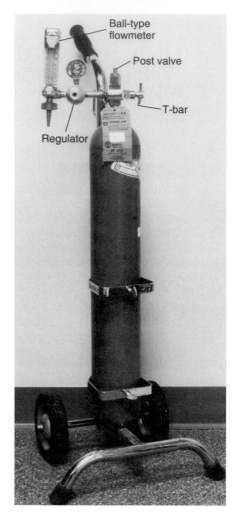

FIGURE 28-1 An E-cylinder in a portable stand with a regulator and a flowmeter attached.

Regulator with flowmeter and cylinder pressure gauge (pin index safety system compatible with an oxygen cylinder [Figure 28-2])

Nut and tailpiece ("Christmas tree," nipple) adapter

Wrench or key (some cylinder posts may have a regulator knob, and these do not require a wrench)

PROCEDURAL STEPS
Application of Regulator

1. Secure the cylinder in a support stand or assigned location on the stretcher or transport cart.
2. Remove the protective seal from the post valve.
3. Turn the post-valve outlet away from any personnel. Warn anyone present that a loud noise is going to occur. Turn the post valve open (counterclock-

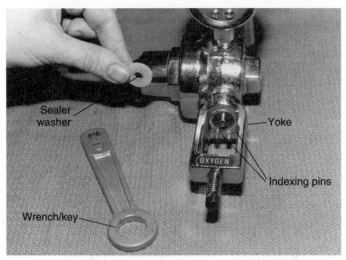

FIGURE 28-2 A sealing washer is usually provided with the dust cover. Note the two indexing pins, which indicate the appropriate regulator for an E-cylinder. Do not force regulator connectors onto cylinders or alter the indexing.

wise) and close it quickly with the key. This action produces a "whooshing" sound. That clears (cracks) the valve and eliminates any dust or foreign materials. If you have difficulty remembering which direction to turn the key, the saying "righty-tighty, lefty-loosey" may help.

4. Place the yoke on the cylinder, making sure the fittings are compatible and the gasket or sealing washers are in place (see Figure 28-2).
5. Tighten the yoke securely with an appropriate wrench or "T-bar" (Figure 28-2 and 28-3).
6. Turn the flowmeter off.
7. Slowly open the post valve until the pressure-gauge needle stops rising. Usually, one full turn is sufficient. The pressure gauge on a full E-cylinder reads 2200 lb per square inch (psi).
8. Assess the system for any audible leaks. If a leak is heard, turn the post valve off and bleed all pressure from the regulator. Retighten the connections.
9. Check the pressure gauge to ascertain whether cylinder pressure is adequate for a sufficient supply of gas. Do not use the cylinder for transporting a patient if the pressure gauge reads below 500 psi. To calculate the approximate amount of oxygen left in a tank at a given flow rate, the following formula may be used (McPherson, 1995):

minutes of O_2 = cylinder gauge pressure (psi) × cylinder factor // flow rate (L/min)

Table 28-1 lists the cylinder factor for the most common cylinder sizes.
10. Connect the desired form of patient oxygen delivery device (see Procedure 27).
11. Open the flowmeter to register desired flow rate. If you are using the "ball-type" flowmeter, the middle of the ball should be at the desired level (see Figure 28-3).

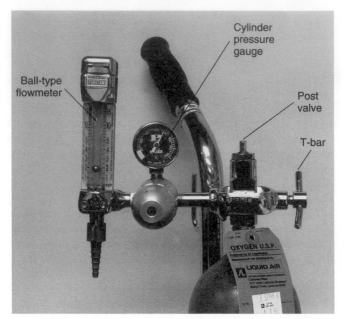

FIGURE 28-3 A close-up view of a regulator and a ball-type flowmeter on an E-cylinder.

TABLE 28-1

TIME AT 2 L/MIN PER OXYGEN CYLINDER TYPE*

Cylinder Type	Volume (L)	Cylinder Factor	Hours O$_2$ at 2 L/min
D	356	0.16	3.0
E	622	0.28	5.0
H, K	6600	3.0	55.0

*Values are approximate. Volume is for a full tank.

12. When the cylinder is not in use, turn the post valve off and bleed the system by turning the flowmeter open until the pressure gauge reads "0."

Removal of Regulator
1. Secure the cylinder in an upright position.
2. Turn the post valve off with an appropriate key or wrench.
3. Open the flowmeter to bleed the system until the pressure gauge reads "0."
4. Loosen the yoke and remove the regulator.
5. Label the tank "empty" or "in use" and store it in a rack.

COMPLICATIONS
1. Ball-type flowmeters are constructed to be used in an upright position (see Figure 28-3). Laying them on their side affects the accuracy of their reading but not the accuracy of the actual flow. An obstruction to the flow (e.g.,

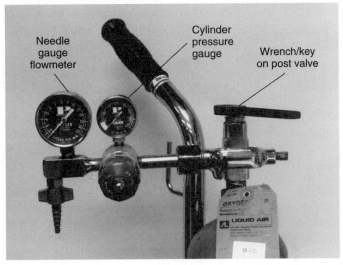

FIGURE 28-4 A close-up view of a regulator and needle-gauge flowmeter on an E-cylinder.

crimped or pinched tubing) causes the ball to drop to the actual flow reaching the patient.

2. Needle-gauge flowmeters may be used in any position without affecting the accuracy of their reading (Figure 28-4). An obstruction to the flow causes the gauge to register higher than the actual flow being delivered to the patient.

3. A cylinder containing less than 500 psi should not be used when transporting patients.

REFERENCES

McPherson, S.P. (1995). *Respiratory care equipment*, 5th ed. St. Louis: Mosby.

White, G.C. (1996). *Equipment theory for respiratory care*, 2nd ed. Albany, NY: Delmar Publishers.

Noninvasive Assisted Ventilation

Reneé Semonin Holleran, RN, PhD, CEN, CCRN, CFRN, SANE

Noninvasive assisted ventilation (NIAV) provides an alternative method to assisting an acutely ill patient's ventilations without having to place either an endotracheal tube or a tracheotomy tube into the patient's airway. The advantages of NIAV include the following (Mak, 2002):
- Allowing respiratory muscles to rest by augmenting each breath by inspiratory pressure or volume support
- Improving tidal volumes by applying pressure or increasing volume support
- Improving expiratory airflow by applying a degree of positive expiratory pressure that reduces the dynamic airways compression and hyperinflation
- Timing breaths to compensate for the lack of central drive
- Allowing the administration of higher levels of fraction of inspired oxygen (FIO_2) without causing excessive respiratory depression

Noninvasive assisted ventilation is used in chronic obstructive pulmonary disease (COPD) and acute hypercapnic respiratory failure (may also be referred to as AHRF) NIAV can help avoid endotracheal intubation, reduce a patient's breathlessness, allow a patient to eat and drink, decrease the complications that occur with intubation and mechanical ventilation, decrease the need for sedation and neuromuscular blockade in order to tolerate mechanical ventilation, and decrease the length of hospitalization.

There are two techniques that can be used to accomplish this. The first is by using a device to expand the thorax by negative pressure. The second uses a technique to inflate the patient's chest using positive pressure applied through a mask. Positive pressure can be applied through a face mask (face mask mechanical ventilation; continuous positive airway pressure [CPAP] mask) or through nasal mask ventilation.

INDICATIONS
1. To provide short-term (1- to 4-day) mechanical ventilatory support to patients presenting with respiratory failure to avoid intubation and complications arising from intubation. Patients who are candidates for NIAV generally present as tachypneic, tachycardic, and possibly diaphoretic, with paradoxic respirations and increased work of breathing. The patient should be alert and able to cooperate, protect his or her airway, and understand that intubation is the probable alternative to this mode of ventilation.
2. To reduce respiratory muscle fatigue by supporting inspiratory effort, reducing the work of breathing, and providing rest to the respiratory musculature.

3. To reduce dyspnea, tachypnea, and hypercapnia associated with an exacerbation of COPD and AHRF (Mak, 2002; Brochard et al., 1995; Wysocki et al., 1995).
4. To correct gas exchange through the application of either positive end-expiratory pressure (PEEP) alone or in conjunction with inspiratory positive airway pressure (IPAP), pressure support ventilation (PSV), or pressure control ventilation (PCV). PEEP or CPAP improves gas exchange by increasing the functional residual capacity of the lung through alveolar recruitment. PEEP or CPAP decreases the need for intubation in patients with acute congestive heart failure (CHF) (Bersten et al., 1991).
5. To treat purely hypercapnic respiratory failure with associated respiratory muscle fatigue. NIMV is significantly less successful in avoiding intubation in patients whose mechanism of failure (other than CHF) is primarily hypoxemia (Wysocki et al., 1995). Patients presenting with an exacerbation of COPD generally have acute hypercapnia superimposed on chronic respiratory failure. Patients presenting with CHF may demonstrate either hypoxia or a combination of hypoxia and hypercapnia.
6. To facilitate the weaning of ventilator-dependent COPD patients who have failed to complete the conventional weaning process for extubation (Tebal et al., 1996).

CONTRAINDICATIONS AND CAUTIONS
1. Immediate need for intubation to preserve life
2. Unstable cardiac status
3. Inability to protect or clear the airway of copious secretions, altered level of consciousness, or absent gag reflex
4. Facial trauma, surgery, or malformation that precludes an effective seal mask
5. Ability and willingness to cooperate are essential for an effective NIAV trial.

PATIENT PREPARATION
1. Position the patient in an upright position, with the head of the bed raised at least 30 degrees. The patient's position in bed may affect the seal of the mask, and thereby the synchrony of the patient-ventilator interface.
2. Place the patient on a cardiac monitor (see Procedure 58) and a pulse oximeter (see Procedure 23).
3. The choice of either a nasal mask or a full-face mask for the delivery of NIAV rests with the caregiver. This choice depends on the caregiver's experience and comfort with the various masks and associated ventilators, and the patient's ability to adapt to the patient-ventilator interface. A properly fitting, self-sealing, clear mask is essential to the successful management of patients receiving NIAV. Most air leaks occur at the nasal bridge area (both nasal and full-face masks) or the corners of the mouth (full-face mask) and are caused by a mask that is too large. A smaller mask may solve the leakage problem. In the acute care setting, many of the caregivers in the studies cited used a full-face mask (Fernandez et al., 1993; Wysocki et al., 1993) to deliver NIAV. Nasal masks provide some advantages over full-face masks, including better comfort, ease of use, less dead space, and decreased risk of inadvertent aspiration. However, nasal ventilation may have some serious drawbacks for the critically ill patient, including the inadvertent loss of significant gas volume through the mouth and patient-ventilator dyssyn-

chrony secondary to this volume loss. Closing the mouth during nasal ventilation is mandatory. Patients in acute respiratory failure may in fact respond better to a full-face mask simply because they do not have to concentrate on breathing with a closed mouth. Synchrony with the ventilator is a key factor in reducing the work of breathing.

4. When beginning the initial trial of NIAV, the mask should be held in place rather than strapped in order to accustom the patient to the closed system. The patient should be "talked through" this initial phase to reduce the anxiety associated with NIAV. At this time, the respiratory therapist or nurse should remain at the bedside for extended periods to alleviate the anxiety associated with NIAV and to titrate the ventilator settings to best meet the patient's needs.

5. If the total system pressure (PSV, IPAP, PCV plus PEEP, or CPAP) exceeds 20 cm of water (H_2O), a gastric tube may be necessary to prevent gastric distention (see Procedure 101).

6. In most clinical settings, NIAV is delivered intermittently, with breaks of several minutes given to patients every 1-2 hours. Depending on the clinical scenario, the patient takes a break from the NIAV with a specific type of oxygen delivery system (e.g., a nonrebreathing mask for the CHF patient, or a precise concentration Venturi mask for the COPD patient). Most often, the first day of treatment has the greatest duration of ventilation. On subsequent days, the duration of ventilation is gradually reduced, depending on the clinical status of the patient.

7. In all types of NIAV (CPAP, bilevel positive airway pressure [BiPAP], NIAV with a ventilator), improvement in gas exchange and arterial blood gas results, and reduction in work of breathing should occur within 1-2 hours of initiation of treatment. Patients who do not demonstrate these improvements are at significant risk of failing the NIAV trial and may require intubation.

CPAP
Equipment

Humidification system
Oxygen blender, flow generator, high-flow flowmeter
Large-bore tubing
3-L intermittent mandatory ventilation bag setup to act as a reservoir
CPAP valve
Low-pressure disconnect alarm with tubing
One-way valve to prevent rebreathing
Adaptors as necessary to assemble the unit
Tight-fitting CPAP mask with adjustable head straps

Many commercial CPAP systems are available. CPAP and BiPAP systems are commonly administered through ventilators. Figure 29-1 represents a schematic of a general system, but not one system in particular.

Procedural Steps

1. Attach the appropriate CPAP valve to the expiratory housing of the CPAP mask. Some valves come preset to a certain level, whereas some are adjustable. It is common to start with 5 cm H_2O of CPAP.

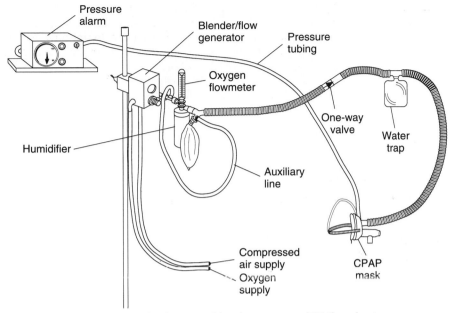

FIGURE 29-1 Continuous positive airway pressure (CPAP) mask setup.

2. Adjust the flow of gas on the CPAP setup so the reservoir bag remains inflated throughout the respiratory cycle.
3. Adjust the disconnect alarm 2-3 cm H_2O below the CPAP level. Temporarily detach the system from the patient to test the alarm function.
4. Monitor the level of CPAP delivered via a pressure manometer and the delivered fraction of inspired oxygen (FIO_2) via an oxygen analyzer.
5. Assess and document the patient's response to CPAP. Monitor the patient's vital signs, work of breathing, and oxygen saturation (pulse oximetry). If CPAP does not achieve the desired response, consult the physician and respiratory therapist regarding an increase in the level of CPAP or a change to a system that delivers IPAP in addition to CPAP.

BiPAP
Equipment
The BiPAP system provides time-cycled, pressure-limited ventilation. This device is capable of delivering different pressures during inspiration (IPAP) and expiration (EPAP) (Figure 29-2).

BiPAP ventilator circuit
Humidifier
Nasal mask
Adjustable nasal mask straps
T in device for oxygen flow
Oxygen tubing

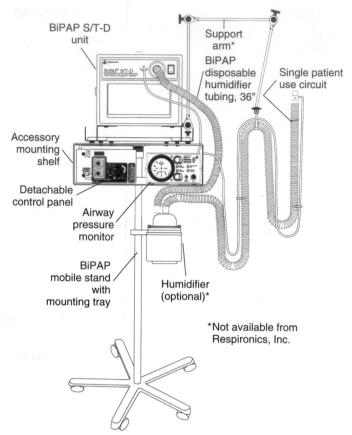

FIGURE 29-2 Commercially available bilevel positive airway pressure (BiPAP) unit. (From *The Complete BiPAP S/T-D Hospital System* [1992]. Courtesy Respironics Inc., Pittsburgh, PA.)

Procedural Steps

1. Set the bleed-in oxygen flow rate to achieve the desired FIO_2. Monitor FIO_2 via an in-line oxygen analyzer. A disadvantage of some BiPAP systems is inexact and varying FIO_2 delivery, particularly when high FiO_2 levels are required.

2. Initially, set the level of IPAP to accustom the patient to positive-pressure ventilation. Typical initial settings would be 5 cm H_2O of IPAP over 5 cm H_2O of PEEP (or EPAP, depending on the manufacturer's designation). Gradually increase the IPAP level as clinical needs demand. Reassess the mask seal. At higher levels of IPAP, leaks around the mask are more frequent. A leak may require reseating the mask, tightening the mask straps, and repositioning the patient (Figure 29-3).

3. Assess the patient-ventilator interface for synchrony. The patient should receive inspiratory support (IPAP) on each spontaneous breath. If the patient is a mouth breather and is wearing a nasal mask, the patient's efforts may not be synchronous and fully supported by the ventilator. If the patient is unable to synchronize with the machine, consider switching to a full-face mask. If

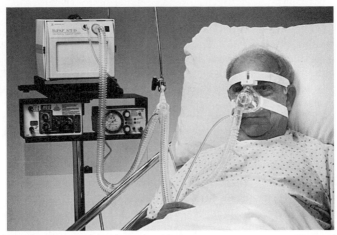

FIGURE 29-3 Correctly fitted nasal mask. (Courtesy Respironics Inc., Pittsburgh, PA.)

you do not have the capability to do full-face mask ventilation with the BiPAP unit, consider switching to noninvasive mechanical ventilation (NIMV) with a mechanical ventilator with PSV and PCV modes.

NONINVASIVE VENTILATION VIA A MECHANICAL VENTILATOR
Equipment
Mechanical ventilator capable of pressure support and pressure-control modes of ventilation

Self-sealing full-face mask

Adjustable head straps

Procedural Steps

1. Pressure-regulated modes of ventilation (PSV, PCV) are the most common modes of ventilation used in NIMV. Volume-targeted modes (synchronized intermittent mandatory ventilation [SIMV] assist control volume cycled) have been used successfully; however, some authors have cited better patient tolerance for pressure-regulated modes of ventilation (Foglio et al., 1994).

2. Start with low PSV levels to accustom the patient to positive-pressure breathing. Typical initial PSV levels are 5 cm H_2O. Gradually increase the PSV level until adequate tidal volume and chest excursion have been achieved.

3. Should large air leaks around the mask interfere with the synchrony of the patient-ventilator interface, you may choose to switch to the PCV mode, which is time limited, and therefore inspiration will always terminate when the inspiratory time is reached. Adjust the inspiratory time to a comfortable level for the patient.

4. Most mechanical ventilators have several types of alarms. These include high and low pressure, high and low minute volume, high respiratory rate, low tidal volume, low PEEP, and a general disconnect alarm. The alarm limits depend on the patient's status.

AGE-SPECIFIC CONSIDERATIONS

1. NIAV has been used on pediatric patient populations as young as 4 years of age (Padman et al., 1994). These populations include patients with cystic fibrosis, asthma, and various neuromuscular diseases. NIAV has also been used in the pediatric setting as a treatment for atelectasis.
2. Generally, pediatric patients start at lower levels of CPAP, IPAP, and PSV than do adult patients.
3. Nasal CPAP is routinely used for infants in the neonatal intensive care unit. Indications include low gestational age, immature lung, atelectasis, and unresolved spells of apnea and bradycardia.

COMPLICATIONS

1. Decreased cardiac output due to reduced venous return secondary to increased intrathoracic pressure. Patients may be particularly sensitive to this phenomenon if they are hypovolemic.
2. Pneumothorax secondary to increased intrathoracic pressure.
3. Gastric insufflation due to air swallowing or total inspiratory pressures greater than 20 cm H_2O.
4. Potential for aspiration due to a tight-fitting mask and gastric insufflation.
5. Conjunctivitis secondary to gas leakage around the bridge of the nose.
6. Respiratory failure secondary to the failure of NIAV to reverse respiratory muscle fatigue and correct gas exchange.

PATIENT TEACHING

1. Instruct the patient to remain in a stable, upright position to avoid creating leaks in the seal of the mask.
2. Demonstrate how to remove the mask quickly in the event of vomiting.
3. Immediately report:
   Sudden increased difficulty in breathing
   Nausea or vomiting
4. Hydration and mouth care are important when using NIAV. Instruct the patient to drink fluids as well as keep mouth moist (Nettina, 2001).

REFERENCES

Bersten, A.D., et al. (1991). Treatment of severe cardiogenic pulmonary edema with continuous positive airway pressure delivered by facemask. *New England Journal of Medicine, 325,* 1825-1830.

Brochard, L., et al. (1995). Noninvasive ventilation for acute exacerbations of chronic obstructive lung disease. *New England Journal of Medicine, 333* (13), 817–822.

Fernandez, R., et al. (1993). Pressure support ventilation via facemask in acute respiratory failure in hypercapnic COPD patients. *Intensive Care Medicine, 19,* 456-461.

Foglio, K., Clini, E., & Vitacca, M. (1994). Different modes of noninvasive, intermittent positive pressure ventilation (IPPV) in acute exacerbations of COLD patients. *Monaldi Archives for Chest Disease, 49,* 556-557.

Mak, V. (2002). Non-invasive assisted ventilation (NIPPV/NIAV) in the management of acute hypercapnic failure secondary to COPD. *Chest Medicine On-line. www.priory.com/cmol/niav1.htm. Accessed 6/30/02.*

Nettina, S.M. (Ed.). (2001). *Lippincott Manual of Nursing Practice.* Philadelphia: Lippincott.

Padman, R., Lawless, S., & Von Nessen, S. (1994). Use of BiPAP by nasal mask in the treatment of respiratory insufficiency in pediatric patients: preliminary investigation. *Pediatric Pulmonology, 17*, 119-123.

Tebal, L., Marks, P., & Benzo, R. (1996). Non-invasive mechanical ventilation: the benefits of the BiPAP system. *West Virginia Journal of Medicine, 92* (1), 18-21.

Wysocki, M., et al. (1993). Noninvasive pressure support ventilation in patients with acute respiratory failure. *Chest, 103*, 907-913.

Wysocki, M., et al. (1995). Noninvasive pressure support ventilation in patients with acute respiratory failure: a randomized comparison with conventional therapy. *Chest, 107*, 761-768.

PROCEDURE 30

T-Piece

Reneé Semonin Holleran, RN, PhD, CEN, CCRN, CFRN, SANE

The T-piece is also known as a T-piece aerosol nebulizer, "tee" piece, or Briggs adaptor.

INDICATIONS
1. To assist with weaning from a ventilator while providing humidification and oxygen to patients with endotracheal or tracheostomy tubes and spontaneous breathing patterns that meet the following parameters (Lynn-McHale & Carlson, 2001):
   Vital capacity (VC) $\geq$15 ml/kg
   Negative inspiratory pressure (NIP) ≤ -20 cm H_2O
   Positive expiratory pressure (PEP) $\geq$30 cm H_2O
   Tidal volume (VT) $\geq$5 ml/kg
2. To provide humidification and oxygen to patients with endotracheal or tracheostomy tubes and spontaneous breathing patterns.

CONTRAINDICATIONS AND CAUTIONS
1. Patients who are obtunded without spontaneous respirations or who do not meet minimum spontaneous parameters require mechanical ventilation.
2. The aerosol temperature at the patient end of the circuit should be at body temperature (optional for normothermic patients requiring short-term use).
3. Tubing must be checked and drained of excess water frequently. A water trap may be included in the circuit and is recommended if extended use is anticipated. The water trap is placed in the lowest portion of the aerosol tubing.

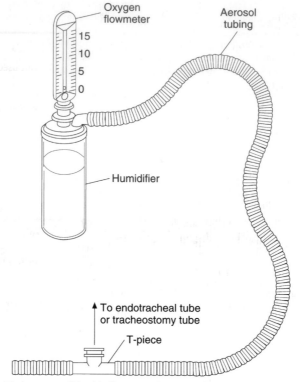

FIGURE 30-1 T-piece setup (bleed-in flowmeter, heater, and water trap not shown).

EQUIPMENT

Heated aerosol (optional)
Oxygen analyzer
T-piece setup (Figure 30-1)
Flowmeters (air or O_2)

PROCEDURAL STEPS

1. Assemble the aerosol nebulizer and make sure the humidifier is filled with sterile water to the appropriate mark.
2. Connect the flowmeter to the oxygen source and attach the nebulizer.
3. Set the fraction of inspired oxygen FIO_2 of the O_2 blender or humidifier and plug in the heating element if one is being used.
4. Turn the primary flowmeter to 14 L/min of oxygen. Analyze the FIO_2 with an oxygen analyzer and label the flowmeters with the proper L/min settings. To maintain adequate flow, Table 30-1 can be used. Always run the flowmeter by powering the nebulizer at 14 L/min or greater and/or adjust the bleed until the desired FIO_2 is obtained.

TABLE 30-1
FLOWMETER USE IN T-PIECE SETUP

FIO$_2$	Nebulizer Power Flow Required	Bleed-in Desired
.21	Air flowmeter	Not used
.22-.27	Air flowmeter	O$_2$ flowmeter
.28-.45	O$_2$ flowmeter	Not used
.45-.80	O$_2$ flowmeter	O$_2$ flowmeter

5. Check to see that mist is visible at the T-piece. If it is not visible, the unit may be faulty or the flow rate may not be high enough. Attach the T-piece to the endotracheal or tracheostomy tube.

It is important to maintain a high-flow system. If the patient's inspiratory flow rate exceeds the output of the nebulizer, the resultant flow deficit will result in room-air entrainment and a decreased FIO$_2$. To ensure a high-flow system, the Venturi should never be turned higher than the 40% setting. Any FIO$_2$ greater than 0.40 must be achieved by bleeding in additional flow to the system. This guarantees the patient at least 40 L/min total flow. Be sure to analyze for proper FIO$_2$ after setup and equipment changes.

The heating element should be checked to ensure that it is functioning properly. The humidifier should be warm, not hot, to the touch.

COMPLICATIONS

1. FIO$_2$ changes can result from unsecured flowmeter controls and entrainment port handles.
2. Inadequate oxygen flow can impede the production of the mist.
3. Aspiration of water can occur if the tubing is not drained.
4. Excessive condensate can also block oxygen flow.
5. Excessive condensate can also contribute to the possibility of bacterial growth and aerosolization of bacteria into the patient's lungs.
6. Patients being weaned from a mechanical ventilator may not be able to tolerate a T-piece and may require reconnection to the ventilator.

REFERENCES

Lynn-McHale, D.J., & Carlson, K.K. (2001). *AACN Procedure Manual for Critical Care*, 4th ed. Philadelphia: W.B. Saunders.

Suctioning

Pharyngeal Suctioning

Teresa L. Will, RN, MSN, CEN

Pharyngeal suctioning is also known as oropharyngeal suctioning, Yankauer suctioning, nasopharyngeal suctioning, or tonsillar suctioning.

INDICATIONS
1. To clear the airway of secretions, foreign matter, or blood in patients incapable of clearing their own oropharynx or nasopharynx. Pharyngeal suctioning may be used with conscious or unconscious and intubated or nonintubated patients.
2. To stimulate coughing and deep breathing in the nonintubated patient.

CONTRAINDICATIONS AND CAUTIONS
1. Oropharyngeal secretions may be thick (e.g., blood or vomit). Use a large-bore suction catheter, a tonsillar-pharyngeal suction-tip device (Yankauer), or the suction connecting tubing alone for more effective airway clearance.
2. Excessive suctioning may traumatize the pharyngeal tissue and cause bleeding, swelling, or localized inflammation. Using a beveled tip and limiting suctioning to 10-15 seconds per attempt help decrease adverse effects.
3. Hypoxemia may result from prolonged suctioning.
4. Suctioning may cause coughing, gagging, or both, which increase intracranial pressure and should be avoided in patients with head injuries. If gagging leads to vomiting, aspiration and respiratory compromise may occur.
5. Suctioning may stimulate the vagal response, leading to bradycardia and hypotension.
6. If possible, use the less traumatic oropharyngeal route rather than the nasopharyngeal approach.
7. Excessive bleeding may occur in patients who have bleeding disorders or who are receiving anticoagulant therapy. Observe for bleeding and use lower suction pressures in this population.
8. If epiglottitis is suspected, nasopharyngeal suctioning is contraindicated, because it may induce hypoxemia or occlusion of the airway.
9. Pharyngeal suctioning is considered a clean procedure. Regular examination gloves should be worn during the procedure.
10. If both nasopharyngeal and oropharyngeal suctioning are necessary, suction the nares first because they are considered cleaner than the mouth (Curley & Thompson, 2001).

EQUIPMENT
Portable or wall continuous-suction unit with regulator
Suction canister

Suction connecting tubing
Tonsillar or pharyngeal suction tip or bulb syringe
Suction catheter with an age-appropriate size of French whistle tip with a
    vent port or Y connector
30-60 ml of tap water to clear the connecting tubing and suction tip
Container to hold water (an emesis basin works well)
Water-soluble lubricant for a catheter inserted via the nasopharyngeal route
Emesis basin
Tissues
Supplemental oxygen source and oxygen delivery device
Examination gloves

PATIENT PREPARATION

1. For optimal airway alignment, place the patient in semi-Fowler's position. The sniffing position maximizes alignment of the airway for nasopharyngeal suctioning. Pharyngeal suctioning may be performed in any position.
2. The patient may feel breathless during the 10- to 15-second procedure. A high-flow oxygen mask may be set up for use between suctioning. Instruct the patient to use the oxygen mask and take deep breaths until he or she feels comfortable.
3. Warn the patient that the suctioning procedure may stimulate the gag or cough reflex. Provide an emesis basin and tissues.

PROCEDURAL STEPS

1. Assemble the suction canister and attach it to the suction unit.
2. Attach the connecting tubing to the suction canister.
3. Select an appropriate catheter or suction device. To prevent hypoxia and trauma, the suction catheter for the nasopharyngeal route should not be greater than half the diameter of the naris to be suctioned.
4. Set the suction gauge between 120 and 200 mm Hg. Full suction assists in the rapid removal of a large amount of fluid or debris from the oropharynx. Occlude the suction tubing to test the level of suction as measured by the suction gauge.

Oropharyngeal Route

1. Attach the catheter or pharyngeal suction tip to the connecting tubing.
2. Insert the catheter or pharyngeal suction tip into the back of the mouth without applying suction. If using a Yankauer tip, gently sweep the posterior pharynx while applying suction for 10-15 seconds.
3. If using a catheter, insert it into the area on either side of the glottis. Apply suction intermittently for 10-15 seconds, gently rotating as you withdraw the catheter.
4. Flush the catheter by aspirating water through the connecting tubing.

Nasopharyngeal Route

1. Nasopharyngeal suctioning is used when the oral route is not accessible (e.g., with clenched teeth or oral trauma).

2. Assess for nasal patency by inspecting each naris for any obstruction, such as polyps, structural deformity, or trauma. Occlude each naris and ask the patient to inhale to determine which side is most patent. Use the most patent naris for suctioning.

3. Attach the suction catheter to the connecting tubing. Apply a small amount of water-soluble lubricant to the catheter.

4. Instruct the patient to use supplemental oxygen before the procedure and take deep breaths for 30 seconds.

5. Without applying suction, gently insert the lubricated catheter medially into the naris. As you slide the catheter to the back of the naris, instruct the conscious patient to assume the sniffing position. This position assists in passage of the catheter through the larynx and enhances access to the pharyngeal area. Slide the catheter through the naris until resistance is met or coughing is stimulated. If coughing is stimulated, pull back on the catheter slightly.

6. Apply suction intermittently for a maximum of 10-15 seconds and rotate the catheter slightly while withdrawing.

7. Flush the catheter by aspirating water through the connecting tubing.

8. Offer supplemental oxygen after suctioning.

9. If frequent suctioning is required, a nasopharyngeal airway may be inserted to decrease mucosal trauma and to act as a guide for the catheter. See Procedure 6.

Bulb Syringe

1. Depress the bulb syringe and gently advance into the nose or to the area of pooled secretions and debris in the oropharynx. Release the large bulb syringe to aspirate secretions and debris.

2. Depress bulb syringe into a basin to dispose of secretions and debris.

3. Flush the bulb syringe by aspirating and expelling water until clear.

4. Repeat steps 1-3 until the airway is clear.

AGE-SPECIFIC CONSIDERATIONS

1. To prevent hypoxia and mucosal damage, decrease suction to 60-80 mm Hg for infants, 80-100 mm Hg for children 1-8 years old, and 120-150 mm Hg for children older than 8 years (Curley & Thompson, 2001).

2. Hyperventilate and hyperoxygenate children and neonates to prevent effects of hypoxemia.

3. Children are especially prone to vagal stimulation, so premedication with atropine may be necessary.

4. A bulb syringe is usually used only for infants.

COMPLICATIONS

1. Infection is a potential complication of nasopharyngeal suctioning when the correct technique is not used. A new catheter must be used each time for nasopharyngeal suctioning, because contamination of the tracheobronchial area is possible.

2. A catheter or pharyngeal suction tip for the oropharynx may be used repeatedly for the same patient unless it is grossly contaminated or becomes clogged with large debris.

3. Excessive suctioning may create irritation to the upper airway and result in bleeding or edema, which may further compromise the airway patency.

PATIENT TEACHING
1. Cough when possible to assist in clearing the airway.
2. Report any respiratory difficulty.
3. For a conscious patient with excessive oral secretions, a tonsil tip may be set up and the patient instructed on how to suction himself or herself.

REFERENCES

Curley, M.A.Q., & Thompson, J.E. (2001). Oxygenation and ventilation (pp. 233-308). In Curley, M.A.Q., & Maloney-Harmon, P.A. (Eds.), *Critical care nursing of infants and children*, 2nd ed. Philadelphia: W.B. Saunders.

PROCEDURE 32

Nasotracheal Suctioning

Teresa L. Will, RN, MSN, CEN
and Jean A. Proehl, RN, MN, CEN, CCRN

INDICATIONS
1. To maintain airway patency, maximize oxygenation, and reduce lower airway resistance in the nonintubated patient through removal of secretions.
2. To stimulate coughing in the weak or debilitated patient who is unable to clear secretions without assistance.
3. To obtain a sputum specimen when the patient is unable to do so without assistance.

CONTRAINDICATIONS AND CAUTIONS
1. To prevent hypoxia and tissue trauma, select a suction catheter no more than one half the diameter of the naris to be suctioned.
2. Suctioning may exacerbate increased intracranial pressure or severe hypertension and should be performed with caution in patients with these conditions.
3. Hypoxia may occur during suctioning, particularly in patients with a history of pulmonary or cardiac disease.
4. Continuous suction may cause trauma to mucosa. Suction should be applied no longer than 10-15 seconds.
5. Nasotracheal suction should not be used for patients with severe facial or head trauma. There is risk of penetration of the cranial vault by the suction catheter.

6. Use caution in patients with narrow or obstructed nares and in those who are anticoagulated or who have bleeding disorders.

EQUIPMENT
Portable or wall continuous-suction unit with regulator
Suction canister
Suction-connecting tubing
Water-soluble lubricant
Sterile-suction catheter (14 French is the standard size for adults; 10 French is the standard size for children)
Sterile water or 0.9% saline solution to flush tubing
Sterile container for flush solution
Sterile gloves
Oxygen source with oxygen mask or nasal cannula
Towels
Emesis basin and tissues
Option: Commercially prepared suction catheter kits are also available.

PATIENT PREPARATION
1. For optimal airway alignment, place the patient in semi-Fowler's position. In the supine position, place the head in a neutral position. If possible, have the patient blow his or her nose to clear the nasal passages. If copious secretions are in the mouth, suction the mouth and pharynx first to clear these secretions before nasotracheal suctioning.
2. Obtain baseline assessments of breath sounds, skin color, heart rate, and oxygen saturation. Monitor skin color, oxygen saturation, and heart rate during the procedure.
3. Provide an oxygen source before and after suctioning. If a nasal cannula is being used, the prongs may be adjusted so that one naris continues to receive oxygen.
4. Inform the patient that a brief feeling of breathlessness is normal during the procedure.
5. Inform the patient that the procedure may stimulate the gag or cough reflex. Provide an emesis basin and tissues. Encourage the patient to expectorate any mucus produced.
6. Drape towels over the patient's chest to prevent contamination by secretions.
7. Measure from the nose to the sternal notch with the catheter. Do not contaminate the sterile catheter while measuring. This will give a rough estimate of how far to advance the catheter to reach the lower airway.

PROCEDURAL STEPS
1. Assemble the suction canister and attach it to the wall or a portable suction unit. Attach the connecting tubing to the suction canister.
2. Set the suction pressure between 80 and 100 mm Hg. Full suction is not recommended. Pressures greater than 100 mm Hg increase trauma to the area and are no more effective in removing secretions (Boggs, 1993). Occlude the suction tubing to test the level of suction being delivered, as measured by the suction gauge.
3. Examine both nares and choose a patent one. Avoid using a naris that is partially blocked by polyps, hemorrhage, or a deviated nasal septum. To prevent

hypoxia and trauma, the suction catheter for the nasotracheal route should not be greater than one half of the internal diameter of the naris.

4. Preoxygenate the patient with high-flow oxygen for 2 minutes before suctioning; alternatively, place the prong of a nasal cannula in the opposite naris, or have an assistant hold an oxygen mask with high-flow oxygen to the mouth. Ask patients to take slow, deep breaths through the mouth during the procedure. Preoxygenation is a key method of preventing a decrease in the patient's baseline oxygenation status.
5. Dispense a small amount of water-soluble lubricant onto a sterile field, such as the inside of the catheter package.
6. Put on sterile gloves.
7. Attach the sterile suction catheter to the connecting tubing.
8. Hold the suction catheter in your dominant hand, which must remain sterile. Your other hand, which controls the suction control vent, is considered clean.
9. Apply a water-soluble lubricant to the suction catheter.
10. Gently advance the catheter through the nasal passage in a medial, downward direction. Never apply suction upon insertion of the catheter.
11. Have the patient open his or her mouth and extend the tongue to prevent retraction of the tongue when the gag reflex is stimulated
12. Have the patient take slow, deep breaths or cough gently. Coughing assists in opening the glottis, which permits insertion of the catheter into the trachea.
13. When the patient coughs, advance the suction catheter until resistance is met or spontaneous coughing is noted.
14. When resistance is met, withdraw the catheter 2-3 cm and apply suction intermittently for 10 seconds. Gently rotate the catheter while withdrawing it.
15. Withdraw the suction catheter to the epiglottis area or to the point at which spontaneous coughing or gagging is absent. When secretions are excessive, necessitating repeat suction, do not withdraw the catheter beyond the epiglottis. This prevents having to traverse the nasal passages again. Discontinuation of suctioning is heavily dependent on the patient's tolerance of the procedure.
16. Reoxygenate the patient with high-flow oxygen for at least 2 minutes before repeating the procedure.
17. Flush the catheter by aspirating sterile water or saline solution through the tubing.

Alternative Method

1. Pass an unconnected suction catheter through the naris to the point of the epiglottis. Listen at the end of the suction catheter for breath sounds. Advance the catheter 1-2 cm until coughing is stimulated, and then advance the catheter quickly into the trachea. Attach the catheter to connecting tubing and proceed to suction, or
2. Advance the catheter until no breath sounds are heard. Withdraw the catheter 1-2 cm. Ask the patient to cough, and pass the catheter into the tracheal area. To verify tracheal entry, listen for breath sounds or watch for condensation in the catheter. Proceed with suctioning (Kersten, 1989).

AGE-SPECIFIC CONSIDERATIONS

1. To prevent hypoxia, hyperinflate and hyperoxygenate infants and children before nasotracheal suctioning (Smith Wenning et al., 1995).

2. To prevent retinopathies in children younger than 6 months of age, consider using less than 100% oxygenation. Use a fraction of inspired oxygen (FIO_2) 10%-15% greater than maintenance for preoxygenation. One hundred percent oxygen is appropriate for children older than 6 months (Smith-Wenning et al., 1995).
3. Monitor the heart rate in children during the suctioning procedure, because vagal stimulation may create bradycardia. Bradycardia is usually reversed quickly with the administration of supplemental oxygen and the cessation of the suctioning procedure. To prevent bradycardia, premedication with atropine may be considered.

COMPLICATIONS
1. Infection of the lower respiratory tract is a potential complication, because the catheter is contaminated when it is passed through the nasopharyngeal area.
2. The patient may refuse to allow the procedure to be repeated because it is very uncomfortable.
3. Prolonged suctioning may deplete the residual volume of the lung and lead to alveolar collapse, or atelectasis and hypoxia. Hypoxia can be decreased by providing adequate preoxygenation and postoxygenation and limiting suctioning to 10-15 seconds.
4. Suctioning may stimulate a vagal response, resulting in hypotension or bradycardia.
5. Forcing the suction catheter or inserting it repeatedly may result in mucosal damage and bleeding or local inflammation of the nasopharynx or trachea. Passing the catheter during inspiration is essential to avoid mucosal damage.
6. Laryngospasm, bronchospasm, and bronchoconstriction may occur.

PATIENT TEACHING
1. Cough and breathe deeply, to assist in clearing the airway.
2. Increase fluid intake to loosen and thin secretions by adequate hydration.
3. Good oral hygiene decreases the risk of infection or bacterial colonization.

REFERENCES
Boggs, R. (1993). Airway management (pp. 2-54). In Boggs, R., & Wooldridge-King, M. (Eds.), *AACN procedure manual for critical care*, 3rd ed. Philadelphia: W.B. Saunders.
Kersten L. (1989). *Comprehensive respiratory nursing*. Philadelphia: W.B. Saunders.
Smith-Wenning, K., et al. (1995). Neonatal and pediatric respiratory care (pp. 991-1055). In Scanlon, C. et al. (Eds.), *Egan's fundamentals of respiratory care*, 6th ed. St. Louis: Mosby.

Endotracheal or Tracheostomy Suctioning

Teresa L. Will, RN, MSN, CEN
and Jean A. Proehl, RN, MN, CEN, CCRN

Endotracheal suctioning is also known as ET suctioning.

INDICATIONS
1. To maintain patency of an artificial airway
2. To remove secretions via an endotracheal or tracheostomy tube, which may obstruct the airways and cause hypoxia, pneumonia, bronchitis, or atelectasis. The need for suctioning may be indicated by decreasing oxygen saturation, audible gurgling, or restlessness.
3. To obtain a sputum specimen for laboratory analysis
4. To stimulate a deep cough reflex in patients who are sedated or neurologically impaired in order to mobilize secretions to the larger airways

CONTRAINDICATIONS AND CAUTIONS
1. Suctioning may exacerbate increased intracranial pressure or severe hypertension.
2. Do not deflate the endotracheal tube or tracheostomy cuff before suctioning. The inflated cuff assists in preventing aspiration of any contents into the lungs if the gag reflex is stimulated and vomiting occurs. Positioning the patient with the head of the bed elevated 30 degrees during and after suctioning may minimize aspiration risk.
3. To prevent hypoxia, suctioning should not exceed 10 seconds per attempt (Chulay, 2001).
4. For patients receiving mechanical ventilation with positive end-expiratory pressure (PEEP), a PEEP adapter may be added to the bag-valve-mask device to prevent interruption of pressure support.
5. Suctioning should be based on individual need and should not be a scheduled procedure. Limiting suctioning prevents excessive mucosal damage and decreases exposure to bacterial colonization.
6. Instillation of saline to loosen secretions is not effective and may decrease arterial oxygenation (Chulay, 2001). Saline may also promote bacterial colonization of the lower airways (Curley & Thompson, 2001).

EQUIPMENT
Portable or wall continuous-suction unit with regulator
Suction canister

Suction connecting tubing

Sterile suction catheter with intermittent suction-control vent or closed-suction system device (see Alternative Technique section)

Sterile gloves

Sterile container

Sterile water or saline solution

Bag-valve-mask or anesthesia bag connected to a high-flow oxygen source

Option: Commercially prepared, disposable suction catheter kits are available.

PATIENT PREPARATION

1. Endotracheal or tracheostomy suctioning may be accomplished in any position; however, the Fowler's position with neutral head alignment is optimal. If the patient is combative or uncooperative, restraints or sedation may be necessary to perform the procedure safely.
2. Obtain baseline assessments of breath sounds, skin color, heart rate, and oxygen saturation. Monitor skin color, oxygen saturation, and heart rate during the procedure.
3. Warn the patient that suctioning may stimulate uncontrolled coughing or brief periods of breathlessness.
4. To maintain patency in the patient who is unconscious and has an endotracheal tube inserted through the mouth, insert a bite block so that the tube is not kinked or bitten.

PROCEDURAL STEPS

1. If possible, obtain assistance before suctioning. To maximize oxygen delivery, one person should hyperventilate and hyperoxygenate the patient while another person suctions. One-handed bagging usually does not achieve adequate tidal volume in an adult patient. The ventilator may also be used (Chulay, 2001).
2. Assemble the suction canister and attach it to the wall or a portable suction unit. Attach the connecting tubing to the suction canister. Be sure that all the connections are tight or the suction may not function.
3. Set the suction gauge between 100 and 120 mm Hg (Chulay, 2001). Occlude the suction tubing to test the level of suction being delivered, as measured by the suction gauge.
4. Select a suction catheter that is no larger than half the diameter of the endotracheal or tracheostomy tube.
   Tracheostomy-Specific Method: If the patient has a double-walled tracheostomy, remove the inner cannula and place it in a saline-filled basin during the procedure. The inner cannula may be cleaned with hydrogen peroxide and a pipe cleaner. Rinse it in saline and shake it dry before re-inserting it (Figure 33-1).
5. Attach the suction catheter to the connecting tubing. Hold the suction catheter in your dominant hand, which must remain sterile. Use your other hand to control the suction vent. This hand is considered clean.
6. Use the ventilator to hyperventilate and hyperoxygenate the patient or have your assistant hyperventilate the patient with 100% oxygen via the bag-valve-mask for 30 seconds or at least 5-6 hyperinflations (Chulay, 2001).

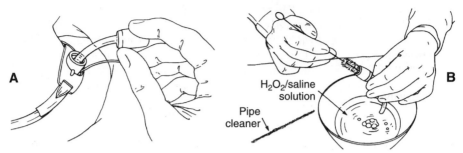

FIGURE 33-1 A, Remove inner cannula; the cannula may need to be turned counterclockwise to release locking mechanism. **B.** Clean inner cannula. (From Kersten, L. (1989). *Comprehensive respiratory nursing* [p. 677]. Philadelphia: W. B. Saunders.)

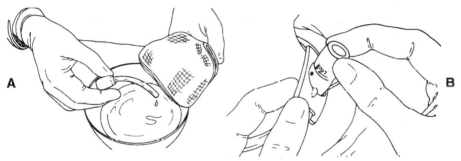

FIGURE 33-2. A, Rinse and shake dry. **B,** Reinsert cannula and turn clockwise to lock in place. (From Kersten, L. [1989]. *Comprehensive respiratory nursing* [p. 677]. Philadelphia: W. B. Saunders.)

7. Immerse the tip of the catheter into the saline and aspirate a small amount to lubricate the catheter.
8. For endotracheal suctioning, have your assistant stabilize the tube to prevent excessive movement or tube displacement.
9. Gently insert the catheter through the tube and advance the catheter until resistance is met. Pull the catheter back 1 cm. Do not apply suction during the introduction of the catheter.
10. Withdraw the catheter slowly while applying intermittent suction and rotating the catheter for no longer than 10 seconds (Chulay, 2001).
11. Use the ventilator to hyperventilate and hyperoxygenate the patient or have your assistant hyperventilate the patient with 100% oxygen via the bag-valve-mask. Postoxygenation should be given for 30 seconds (5-6 breaths) after suctioning or until the alert patient signals recovery (Chulay, 2001).
12. Reconnect the patient to the ventilator or T-piece.
13. Rinse the catheter and connecting tubing by aspirating sterile water or saline through the tubing.
14. Repeat steps 8-11 if excessive secretions exist. Allow the patient at least 1 minute to recover before repeating the procedure.
15. If necessary, suction the nares or the oropharynx before disposing of the catheter and gloves.
16. For a tracheostomy, dry and replace the clean inner cannula (Figure 33-2).

Alternative Technique: Closed-Suction System

1. The closed-suction system device is placed between the endotracheal or tracheostomy tube and the ventilator or T-piece to permit suctioning without interrupting oxygenation or ventilation. The attached sheathed suction catheter passes through a seal into the tracheal tube (Figure 33-3).
2. Attach the suction-connecting tubing to the open end of the closed-suction system near the lock.
3. Depress the suction-control valve and set the suction gauge between 100 and 120 mm Hg (Chulay, 2001). Keep the control valve depressed until the desired suction level is set.
4. Connect the T-piece of the suction system to the ventilator tubing and then attach the T-piece to the endotracheal or tracheostomy tube.
5. Use the ventilator to hyperventilate and hyperoxygenate the patient or have your assistant hyperventilate the patient with 100% oxygen via the bag-valve-mask for 30 seconds or at least 5-6 hyperinflations (Chulay, 2001).
6. Use your nondominant hand to stabilize the T-piece and gently advance the sleeved catheter through the tracheal tube with your dominant hand.
7. Use your dominant hand to grasp the suction-control valve. Depress the valve intermittently while withdrawing the suction catheter in a straight motion in 10 seconds or less (Chulay, 2001). Be sure to withdraw the suction catheter completely to prevent occlusion or irritation of the airway.
8. Use the ventilator to hyperventilate and hyperoxygenate the patient or have your assistant hyperventilate the patient with 100% oxygen via the bag-valve-mask. Postoxygenation should be given for 30 seconds (5-6 breaths) after suctioning or until the alert patient signals recovery (Chulay, 2001).
9. Repeat suctioning as needed. Flush the suction catheter by instilling sterile normal saline or water through the irrigation port until the catheter and connecting tubing are clear. A self-sealing system prevents the fluid from entering the tracheal tube.
10. After flushing, lock the catheter by turning the suction control valve to the lock position or following the manufacturer's instructions on the package insert.

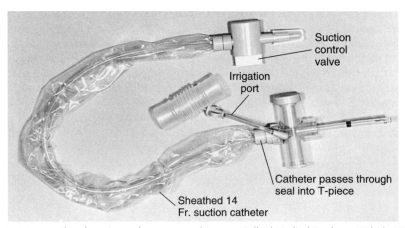

FIGURE 33-3 Closed-suction catheter system. (Courtesy Ballard Medical Products, Midvale, UT.)

11. Repeat steps 5-8 if additional suctioning is required. To provide adequate pre-oxygenation, allow the patient to rest at least 1 minute before repeating the procedure.
12. A 7.0 endotracheal tube is the smallest size that can be used with an adult closed-suction system. The 14 French catheter in the prepackaged suction kit will leave half the airway open in a 7.0 endotracheal tube, which prevents interruption of ventilation during the suctioning.

Sputum Trap for Specimen Collection

1. Connect the suction tubing to the open port of the sputum trap. Attach the suction catheter to the port of the sputum trap by means of the soft rubber extension tubing (Figure 33-4). Use the same setup as you would if you were preparing to suction.
2. Insert the suction catheter and use the suction technique as previously described.
3. Flush the suction catheter with approximately 10 ml of normal saline and remove the catheter and the tubing from the sputum trap.
4. As preparation for shipment to the laboratory, connect the rubber tubing port to the plastic port of the sputum trap.

AGE-SPECIFIC CONSIDERATIONS

1. Suction catheter insertion should stop short of the carina in infants and children. Using the endotracheal tube markings as a guide, insert the suction catheter only 1 cm beyond the tube (Curley & Thompson, 2001).
2. Hyperoxygenation and hyperventilation are often accompanied by hyperinflation in pediatric patients. Hyperinflation is accomplished by delivering breaths approximately 1.5 times the patient's usual tidal volume or increasing peak inspiratory pressure 10 cm H_2O above the patient's usual requirements. Hyperoxygenate pediatric patients for 60 seconds after suctioning (Curley & Thompson, 2001).

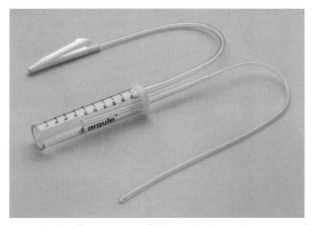

FIGURE 33-4 Sputum trap collection system. (From Argyle De Lee mucus trap with vacuum breaker [product information]. [1998]. Courtesy Sherwood Davis & Geck, St. Louis.)

3. To avoid hyperoxemia in children, consider using less than 100% oxygen. For preoxygenation, use 10%-20% more oxygen than baseline and titrate to maintain the oxygen saturation at 92%-94% (Curley & Thompson, 2001).
4. Monitor the heart rate in children during suctioning because vagal stimulation may cause bradycardia. Bradycardia is usually quickly reversed with the administration of supplemental oxygen and the cessation of suctioning.
5. Select the correct catheter size for effective suctioning. As general guidelines, use a 10-16 French suction catheter for an adult, an 8-10 French suction catheter for a child, and a 6-8 French for a small child. Neonatal and pediatric sizes of closed-suction catheters are available.

COMPLICATIONS

1. Prolonged suctioning may cause hypoxia or atelectasis.
2. Hypoxia, hypercarbia, or stimulation of the cough reflex during endotracheal or tracheostomy suctioning increases cerebral blood volume and intracranial pressure. Use caution when providing respiratory care to a patient with a head injury by limiting suctioning to duration and number of passes per suction event.
3. The procedure may create a feeling of suffocation in the patient and lead to excessive anxiety.
4. An improper suctioning technique may traumatize the tracheal mucosa.
5. A respiratory tract infection may result from colonization of the airway with bacteria.
6. Aspiration of vomit may occur if the tracheal cuff is faulty. Postintubation aspiration has been reduced with the advent of low-pressure, high-volume cuffs.
7. Suctioning may stimulate a vagal response that may result in hypotension or bradycardia.
8. Patients receiving anticoagulants or thrombolytics may have blood-tinged secretions. Suctioning should be limited in these patients.

PATIENT TEACHING

1. To decrease the incidence of mucosal damage at the point of entry (mouth or nose) and at the tracheal entry area, avoid touching or moving the endotracheal or tracheostomy tube.
2. Report any respiratory distress immediately.

REFERENCES

Chulay, M. (2001). Endotracheal or tracheostomy tube suctioning (pp. 41-48). In Lynn-McHale, D.J., & Carlson, K.K. (Eds.). *AACN procedure manual for critical care*, 4th ed. Philadelphia: W.B. Saunders.

Curley, M.A.Q., & Thompson, J.E. (2001). Oxygenation and ventilation (pp. 233-308). In Curley, M.A.Q., & Maloney-Harmon, P.A. (Eds.), *Critical care nursing of infants and children*, 2nd ed. Philadelphia: W.B. Saunders.

Kersten, L. (1989). *Comprehensive respiratory nursing*. Philadelphia: W.B. Saunders.

Ventilation

Mouth-to-Mask Ventilation

Ruth L. Schaffler, PhD(c), CEN, ARNP

Mouth-to-mask ventilation is also known as face-mask and face-shield ventilation.

INDICATION

To ventilate a patient who has ineffective or absent spontaneous respirations and to protect the rescuer from direct contact with the patient's mouth or secretions. Mouth-to-mask ventilation may provide a greater tidal volume than ventilation with a bag-valve-mask, especially if the rescuer is not highly skilled in the use of the bag-valve-mask.

CONTRAINDICATIONS AND CAUTIONS

1. Clear the airway of any obstruction before ventilating the patient.
2. Masks should be made of a transparent material so that lip color, vomit, blood, or other foreign material in the airway is visible. A mask with a one-way valve is preferred.
3. Both hands of the rescuer are needed to provide an adequate seal around the mask and to maintain an open airway. If cardiopulmonary resuscitation (CPR) is indicated, two rescuers are preferred because it is difficult for one person to simultaneously open the airway and quickly reestablish the mask seal with each return to the patient's head after performing chest compressions. Use of a face shield that drapes over the patient's face facilitates CPR by one rescuer.
4. The concentration of oxygen delivered in exhaled air is approximately 16%, but delivery to the patient can be enhanced by adding supplemental oxygen via a port (present on some masks).
5. Use of a face mask may not be appropriate for patients who have severe facial trauma, trismus, excessive oral bleeding, or vomiting.
6. Face masks are not used for patients who have a postlaryngectomy stoma.
7. Low tidal volumes without supplementary oxygen may be ineffective for maintaining adequate arterial oxygen saturation, resulting in hypercarbia and acidosis.

EQUIPMENT

Face mask (Figure 34-1) or face shield (flexible plastic sheet with filter or one-way valve)
Oropharyngeal or nasopharyngeal airway (if needed)
Oxygen tubing and source (optional, but preferred)
Suction equipment (if needed)

PATIENT PREPARATION

1. Place the patient in a supine position on a firm surface when possible. If necessary, ventilations can be delivered to persons who are seated or who are floating in water.

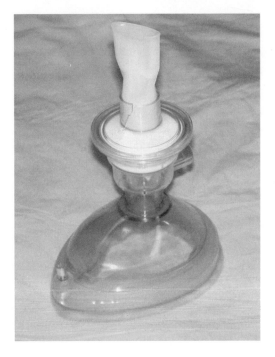

FIGURE 34-1 Example of a face mask with a one-way valve.

2. Open the airway by using the head-tilt, chin-lift, or jaw-thrust maneuver (see Procedure 3).
3. An oral or nasal airway may be used to maintain airway patency (see Procedures 5 and 6).
4. Assess airway patency and breathing status.
5. The rescuer should be positioned to use either a cephalic (above the patient's head) or a lateral (beside the victim's head) technique for rescue breathing.

PROCEDURAL STEPS
Mouth-to-Mask Ventilation

1. Place the mask over the patient's nose and mouth with the narrow end of the mask over the nose. A properly sized mask should extend from the bridge of the nose to the space between the lower lip and the chin and should provide an airtight seal on the face.
2. If you are using the cephalic technique, apply pressure to both sides of the mask by using the thumbs and thenar aspects of the palms to seal the cuff of the mask tightly against the face(Figure 34-2). If you are using the lateral technique, place the thumb and index finger of your hand closest to the top of the patient's head over the upper border of the mask and the thumb of your opposite hand (closes to the victim's chin) over the lower border of the mask. Use the remaining fingers to maintain the correct jaw position.
3. Lift upward on the patient's mandible, using the index, middle, and ring fingers of your hands to maintain a head tilt.
4. If an assistant is available, have him or her apply cricoid pressure. Cricoid pressure helps prevent gastric inflation and regurgitation. It is applied by

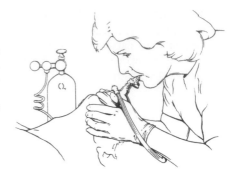

FIGURE 34-2 Mouth-to-mask ventilation. Place mask over mouth and nose and maintain a tight seal against the face by using both hands. Observe the rise and fall of the chest during the respiratory cycle. (From American Heart Association. [1997]. *Textbook of advanced cardiac life support* [pp. 2–8]. Dallas. Reproduced with permission. Copyright American Heart Association.)

pressing down on the cricoid cartilage to compress the esophagus against the cervical vertebrae (AHA, 2001).

5. Blow into the opening of the mask until you observe the chest rise. If oxygen is not available, the tidal volume should be approximately 100 ml/kg (700-1000 ml) in an adult. If oxygen is being provided, a lower tidal volume of 7 ml/kg (400-600 ml) is recommended. These volumes reduce the risk of gastric inflation (AHA, 2001).
6. For an adult, rescue breaths should be slow, at least 2 seconds each (AHA, 2001).
7. Remove your mouth from the opening to allow passive exhalation by the patient.
8. Ventilate the adult patient (a patient older than 8 years of age) 12 times per minute.
9. Connect oxygen tubing to the mask as soon as possible (if an inlet is present) and adjust the flow rate to 10-15 L/min (AHA, 2001).

Face Shield

1. Place the shield on the patient's face with the filter or one-way valve over the mouth. If the shield has a tube to fit in the mouth, insert the tube on the top of the tongue.
2. Position yourself to the side of the patient's head.
3. Pinch the patient's nose by using the thumb and index finger of one hand and maintain the head tilt with the other hand.
4. Take a deep breath and blow for at least 2 seconds through the one-way valve on the face shield as you watch for the chest to rise.
5. Lift your mouth off the shield to allow the patient to exhale passively. Expired air will flow out under the face shield. Leave the shield on the patient's face during resuscitation.
6. Rescue breathing should be performed 12 times per minute for an adult.
7. Every few minutes, reassess the need for continued assisted ventilation.
8. Oxygen delivery to the patient may be enhanced if the rescuer wears a nasal cannula dispensing oxygen at a flow rate of 6 L/min.
9. Face shields should be replaced by mouth-to-mask or bag-mask devices as soon as possible.

AGE-SPECIFIC CONSIDERATIONS

1. In children, respiratory problems are a more likely cause of cardiopulmonary arrest than cardiac problems (AHA, 2001). Rescue breathing should begin immediately in apneic patients. In the out-of-hospital setting, notify the emergency medical service (EMS) after the first minute of rescue efforts on a pediatric patient. Rescue efforts should begin on an adult after the EMS is activated.
2. For pediatric patients (birth to 8 years of age), the volume of ventilations should be sufficient to cause the chest to rise without causing gastric distention. Because of a wide variation in the compliance and size of children's lungs (AHA, 2001), no prescribed volume or pressure is offered.
3. Children's airways are small and are easily obstructed by mucus, edema, or both. Frequent suctioning may be required. The tongue is the most common cause of airway obstruction in a child (AHA, 2001).
4. Hyperextension of the neck should be avoided in an infant or a small child, because it may obstruct the narrow, pliable airway. Pushing on the soft tissues under the chin may also obstruct the airway.
5. Use appropriately sized infant and pediatric masks.
6. Rescue breaths for pediatric victims should be slow (1-1½ seconds), with only enough volume to cause the chest to rise. Gastric distention occurs easily in infants and children, generally as a result of overly rapid delivery or excessive volume of ventilations. Distention can be minimized by delivering rescue breaths slowly. In addition, cricoid pressure may decrease the amount of air reaching the stomach (AHA, 2001).
7. Geriatric patients may have decreased pulmonary function associated with aging or chronic diseases. Ventilation may be difficult because of decreased vital capacity, decreased lung compliance, and poor alveolar gas exchange.
8. Dentures may interfere with artificial ventilation efforts. If they are loose or ill fitting, they should be removed.

COMPLICATIONS

1. Loss of oxygen and tidal volume caused by an ineffective seal around the face mask
2. Insufficient airway patency as a result of improper chin-lift or head-tilt positions
3. Failure to recognize an obstruction caused by vomiting, excessive secretions, or bleeding in the upper airway
4. Gastric distention resulting from ventilations that are excessive in volume or are delivered too rapidly
5. Improperly assembled one-way valves that do not permit air to enter the patient's lungs

REFERENCE

American Heart Association. (2001). *BLS for healthcare providers*. Dallas: Author.

Bag-Valve-Mask Ventilation

Teresa L. Will, RN, MSN, CEN

The bag-valve-mask is also known as BVM, Ambu bag, self-inflating bag, or manual resuscitator.

INDICATION

To provide positive-pressure ventilatory support manually in the presence of inadequate spontaneous ventilation or apnea

CONTRAINDICATIONS AND CAUTIONS

1. Excessive airway pressure or tidal volume can cause gastric distention and pneumothorax.
2. Care should be taken to ensure a properly fitted mask and provide a good seal. Frequently, two people are required to provide adequate ventilation to a non-intubated patient. One member of the team maintains the airway positioning and the mask seal while the other delivers the volume of air via the bag. Mouth-to-mask ventilation (see Procedure 34) may be more effective in some situations. One rescuer can provide adequate ventilation using a bag-valve-mask device if the rescuer has some experience and practice with this device.

EQUIPMENT

Oral or nasal airway
Masks of various sizes
Pharyngeal suctioning equipment
Self-inflating bag with oxygen reservoir and attached oxygen-connecting tubing

PATIENT PREPARATION

1. Secure an open airway and position the patient's head and neck properly. Methods of establishing an airway include:
   Procedure 3–Airway Positioning
   Procedure 4–Airway Foreign Object Removal
   Procedure 5–Oral Airway Insertion
   Procedure 6–Nasal Airway Insertion
   Procedure 7–Laryngeal Mask Airway
   Procedure 8–Esophageal Obturator Airway and Esophageal Gastric Tube Airway
   Procedures 9-13–Endotracheal Intubation
   Procedure 15–Pharyngeal Tracheal Lumen Airway
   Procedure 16–Combitube Airway
   Procedure 17–Cricothyrotomy
   Procedure 19–Tracheostomy
2. Suction any foreign matter out of the airway (see Procedure 31).

PROCEDURAL STEPS

1. Connect the oxygen tubing to the oxygen flowmeter and set at 10-15 L/min. Using a bag-valve-mask with a reservoir significantly increases the oxygen concentration that is administered. If no oxygen is readily available, the bag-valve-mask device can be used on room air until oxygen becomes available.

2. For the nonintubated patient, choose the appropriate size of mask and secure it to the bag. The mask should be large enough to seal around the mouth and nose without covering the eyes. Ensure that the equipment is functioning by placing the mask against your hand and noting the gas flow through the mask. Stand behind the patient's head. Seat the mask on the face by covering the nose, the mouth, and the tip of the chin. The narrow end of the mask goes over the nose. Hold the mask firmly with your thumb over the patient's nose and your fingers grasping the bony edge of the mandible (Figure 35-1). A two-person technique may be used with one team member maintaining the airway and mask seal while the other delivers the air from the bag (Figure 35-2).

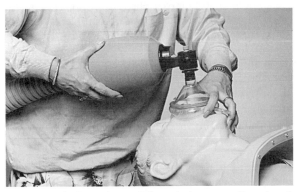

FIGURE 35-1 Application of a bag-valve-mask by a single rescuer. (From Jesudian, M.C., Harrison, R.R., & Keenan, R.L., et al. [1985]. Bag-valve-mask ventilation: two rescuers are better than one: preliminary report. *Critical Care Medicine, 13*[2], p. 122.)

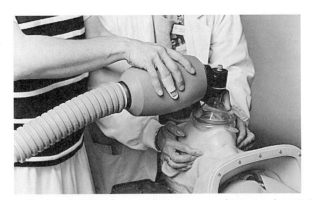

FIGURE 35-2 Application of a bag-valve-mask by two rescuers. (From Jesudian, M.C., Harrison, R.R., & Keenan, R.L., et al. [1985]. Bag-valve-mask ventilation: two rescuers are better than one: preliminary report. *Critical Care Medicine, 13*[2], p. 122.)

3. To help minimize gastric inflation and passive regurgitation in the unconscious patient, consider the application of cricoid pressure (the Sellick maneuver) to minimize the passage of air into the esophagus. Using the fingers and thumb of one hand on either side of the trachea, gently compress the cricoid ring posteriorly (toward the cervical spine). This technique occludes the esophagus (Figure 35-3).

4. For the intubated patient, attach the bag to the connector or adapter of the endotracheal tube. When one hand is needed to maintain the tube position, the free hand can compress the bag and thus inflate the lungs.

5. If two hands are not available to squeeze the bag, compress the bag against your thigh or chest or the stretcher to assist in decompressing the bag and generating additional tidal volume.

6. The gentle symmetrical rise and fall of the chest signals an adequate tidal volume and mask seal or endotracheal tube to bag seal. A tidal volume of 6-7 ml/kg or 400-600 ml over 1-2 seconds is recommended for bag-mask ventilation with oxygen. When no oxygen is connected to the bag-valve-mask ventilation system, a slightly larger chest rise should be seen, with a slightly longer inspiratory time. A tidal volume of 10 ml/kg or 700-1000 ml given over 2 seconds is recommended with room air (AHA, 2001).

7. While ventilations continue, auscultate breath sounds bilaterally to assess adequacy of air flow.

AGE-SPECIFIC CONSIDERATIONS

1. Children have fewer and smaller alveoli, which predisposes them to alveolar collapse because of their lower elastic recoil. To prevent barotrauma, look for a gentle rise and fall of the chest rather than an exaggerated or pronounced expansion.

2. Bag-valve devices are generally made with pop-off valves set at 30-35 cm H_2O pressure to prevent overinflation of the lungs. In children with poor compliance or high resistance during lung insufflation, you may not get chest rise before the valve "pops." In this instance, the pop-off valve may have to be occluded or you may have to switch to a bag without a pop-off valve for the delivery of higher pressure gradients.

3. The tidal volume to be delivered for either adults or children is 6-10 ml/kg of body weight (AHA/ILCOR, 2000). Higher tidal volumes have been associated with increased risk of barotrauma, gastric inflation, and longer hospital stays (ARDS Network, 2000). To help minimize the risk of overinflation, inadver-

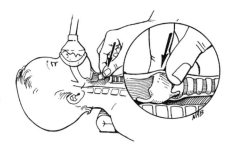

FIGURE 35-3 Gentle pressure on the cricothyroid membrane occludes the esophagus and helps prevent gastric distention during positive pressure ventilation. (From Walsh-Sukys, M.C. [1997]. Orotracheal intubation [pp. 36-41]. In Walsh-Sukys, M.C. & Krug, S.E. [Eds.], *Procedures in infants and children*. Philadelphia: W.B. Saunders.)

tent gastric inflation, or barotrauma, choose the appropriate bag size. The bag size recommended for infants and children is 450-500 ml and for adults is 1600 ml (AHA/ILCOR, 2000). Inadequate tidal volumes may result in hypoxia and hypercarbia. Supplementary oxygen will ensure the maintenance of oxygen saturation at these smaller tidal volumes (AHA/ILCOR, 2000).

4. When applying cricoid pressure in children, gentle pressure is sufficient to occlude the esophagus effectively. You may use fewer than three fingers for compression, and a fingertip may be all that is required for the infant. In children of all ages, care should be taken to avoid excessive pressures that may compress the trachea and cause inadvertent obstruction (AHA/ILCOR, 2000).

5. If the mask used is too large, pressure may be placed on the eyes. This can cause vagal stimulation, especially in children.

COMPLICATIONS

1. Excessive tidal volumes cause gastric distention, leading to vomiting and aspiration or pulmonary impingement. Insert a gastric tube as soon as possible if prolonged bag-valve-mask ventilation is necessary (see Procedure 101). Children are highly susceptible to gastric distention.

2. Excessive airway pressures can result in pneumothorax or other barotrauma.

3. An inadequate seal of the face mask can cause an air leak that may result in inadequate ventilation.

4. Ophthalmic damage can occur if the mask is too large because pressure is exerted on the eyes during ventilation.

REFERENCES

Acute Respiratory Distress Syndrome (ARDS) Network. (2000). Ventilation with lower tidal volumes as compared with traditional tidal volumes for acute lung injury and the acute respiratory distress syndrome. *New England Journal of Medicine, 342*(18), 1301-1308.

American Heart Association (AHA). (2001). *Advanced cardiac life support provider manual.* Dallas: Author.

American Heart Association & International Liaison Committee on Resuscitation (AHA/ILCOR). (2000). Guidelines 2000 for cardiopulmonary resuscitation and emergency cardiovascular care: international consensus on science. *Circulation, 102* (Suppl): I1-I384.

Walsh-Sukys, M.C. (1997). Orotracheal intubation (pp. 36-41). In Walsh-Sukys, M.C., & Krug, S.E. (Eds.), *Procedures in infants and children.* Philadelphia: W.B. Saunders.

Anesthesia Bag Ventilation

Teresa L. Will, RN, MSN, CEN

Anesthesia bags are also known as flow inflating bags, Ayre's bag, A-bag. Jackson-Rees circuit, Mapleson-F circuit, bellows, manual resuscitators, or balloon bags. This type of resuscitation bag relies on a continuous source of compressed oxygen or mixed gases to deliver ventilations. Anesthesia bags cannot be operated on room air; thus, a self-filling bag-valve-mask device should also be available.

INDICATIONS

1. To provide manual ventilation in the event of apnea, when there is a continuous source of compressed gases
2. To assist respiration in the event of an ineffective respiratory pattern
3. To deliver a specifically blended concentration of oxygen (up to 100%) via a compressed gas system

CONTRAINDICATIONS AND CAUTIONS

1. Anesthesia bags are difficult to use in nonintubated patients, and, frequently, two people are needed to ventilate the nonintubated patient effectively via an anesthesia bag. For this reason, a self-filling bag-valve-mask is preferable (see Procedure 35).
2. Overinflation of the lungs may result in gastric distention or pneumothorax.
3. Barotrauma can result from an inability to control gas flow. Balancing inflow, controlling leaks, and allowing sufficient outflow or exhaust are essential to prevent over-inflation or underinflation.
4. If the minute volume of gas is two to three times the minute tidal volume delivered, a nonrebreathing condition occurs. One must provide an outflow leak to permit exhalation.

EQUIPMENT

Anesthesia bag
Oxygen or air flowmeter
Oxygen-connecting tubing
Suction equipment
Mask (if patient is not intubated)
Pressure gauge (if the anesthesia bag has a pressure gauge port)
Compressed oxygen continuous flow or compressed room air continuous flow

PATIENT PREPARATION

1. Secure an open airway and position the patient's head and neck properly. Methods of establishing an airway include:
Procedure 3 Airway Positioning
Procedure 4 Airway Foreign Object Removal

2. Suction any foreign matter out of the airway (see Procedure 31).

PROCEDURAL STEPS

1. Connect the oxygen tubing to the oxygen flowmeter and the gas inlet on the anesthesia bag. If less than 100% oxygen is indicated, an air or oxygen blender is needed.
2. Turn on the oxygen flowmeter to allow the bag to fill halfway. Adjust the flow-control valve to keep the bag approximately half full. This allows ease in compression of the bag and usually delivers adequate tidal volumes (6-10 L/min) (AHA/ILCOR, 2000).
3. If the patient is not intubated, choose a mask that covers the patient's, nose, mouth, and tip of the chin. Attach the mask or the endotracheal tube to the anesthesia bag.
4. Test the unit by placing the mask against your hand and squeezing the bag to feel the flow. Observe the cycle of inflation, gas delivery, and re-inflation.
5. A pressure gauge is optional. If there is a pressure port, attach the pressure gauge to the bag. Pressure measurement is not a primary concern in the adult patient, but the gauge must be attached for the bag to inflate properly (Figure 36-1).
6. If you are using a mask, stand behind the patient's head and seat the mask on the face by covering the nose, mouth, and tip of the chin. Hold the mask firmly in place by using your thumb and forefinger of one hand and allowing your remaining fingers to grasp the bony edge of the mandible (see Procedure 34 and Figure 35-1).
7. For the intubated patient, attach the bag to the connector or adapter of the endotracheal tube.
8. With your free hand, squeeze the bag to force air into the lungs. If the anesthesia bag does not have a flow-control valve, you need to occlude the distal opening of the bag as you squeeze. If two people are available for airway management, one person can maintain the airway and mask seal while the other

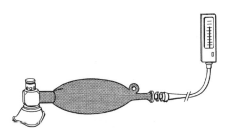

FIGURE 36-1 An anesthesia bag requires a constant gas flow to inflate. (From Walsh-Sukys, M.C. [1997]. Bag and mask ventilation [p. 29]. In Walsh-Sukys, M.C. & Krug, S.E. (Eds.), *Procedures in infants and children*. Philadelphia: W.B. Saunders.)

ventilates (see Procedure 35 and Figure 35-2). Anesthesia bags are less fatiguing to the hands in prolonged use. Watch for rise and fall of the chest and feel for lung compliance and increasing pressure when you are squeezing the bag.

9. To help minimize gastric inflation and passive regurgitation in the unconscious, nonintubated patient, consider the application of cricoid pressure (the Sellick maneuver) to minimize the passage of air into the esophagus. Using the fingers and thumb of one hand on either side of the trachea, gently compress the cricoid ring posteriorly (toward the cervical spine). This occludes the esophagus (see Procedure 35 and Figure 35-3).
10. Symmetrical rise and fall of the chest and good breath sounds bilaterally indicate adequate tidal volume and mask seal.

AGE-SPECIFIC CONSIDERATIONS
1. Children have fewer and smaller alveoli, which are more susceptible to collapse because of lower elastic recoil; therefore airway pressures need to be monitored carefully to prevent barotrauma.
2. The tidal volume delivered for both the child and the adult is 6-10 ml/kg. The size of the anesthesia bag should be chosen on the basis of volume: for neonates, 450 ml; for children, 750 ml; and for adults, 1600 ml (AHA/ILCOR, 2000).
3. When applying cricoid pressure in children, gentle pressure effectively occludes the esophagus. You may use two fingers for compression, and a fingertip may be all that is required for the infant. Care should be taken in children of all ages to avoid excessive pressures that may produce tracheal compression and inadvertent obstruction.
4. If a mask that it too large is used, pressure may be placed on the eyes. This can cause vagal stimulation, especially in children.

COMPLICATIONS
Via Bag-Mask
1. Overinflation can result in gastric distention that may lead to vomiting and aspiration or limited lung expansion. Insert a gastric tube as soon as possible to decompress the stomach (see Procedure 101).
2. Inadequate pressure on the bag leads to low delivered volume and inadequate ventilation.
3. Inadequate seal of the face mask resulting in an inadvertent air leak may cause inadequate ventilation.
4. Damage to the eyes can occur if the mask is too large and pressure is exerted during the bag-mask ventilation.

Via Bag-Endotracheal Tube
1. Delivery of excessive volume can result in barotrauma, such as a pneumothorax.
2. Inadequate pressure can result in inadequate ventilation.

REFERENCE
American Heart Association & International Liaison Committee on Resuscitation (AHA/ILCOR). (2000). Guidelines 2000 for cardiopulmonary resuscitation and emergency cardiovascular care: international consensus on science. *Circulation, 102* (Suppl), I1-I384.

Mechanical Ventilators

Reneé Semonin Holleran, RN, PhD, CEN, CCRN, CFRN, SANE
and Michael Rouse, MSN, CRNA

Mechanical ventilators are also known as ventilators, vents, and respirators; they may also be known by a specific brand name.

INDICATIONS
1. The primary purpose of mechanical ventilation is to maintain alveolar ventilations or the exchange of fresh gas between the lungs and the ambient air by causing air to flow in and out of the lungs via changing airway pressures.
2. To deliver a specific and reliable concentration of oxygen to an ill or injured patient who is hypoxic or in danger of becoming hypoxic because of illness or injury. A partial pressure of arterial oxygen of less than or equal to 50 mm Hg indicates a critical level of oxygen, which requires intervention.
3. To assist or provide mechanical ventilation for the patient who is experiencing respiratory distress or impending respiratory arrest.
4. To decrease the work of breathing for the ill or injured patient and prevent respiratory muscle fatigue. Respiratory muscle fatigue results from depletion of energy stores because of an increased ventilatory workload. Disease states such as weakness, chronic obstructive pulmonary disease, and shock may lead to respiratory muscle fatigue (Burns, 2001).
5. To avoid prolonged use of a manual bag-valve device, which could cause hypocapnia or hypercapnia, during transport of patients who require ventilatory support.

CONTRAINDICATIONS AND CAUTIONS
1. There are no specific contraindications for the use of mechanical ventilation other than it must be initiated and monitored by skilled personnel who understand not only the physiologic aspects of mechanical ventilation but also how to perform a patient-ventilator systems check. However, mechanical ventilation can cause pulmonary injury as well as leave the patient at risk for respiratory infections and generalized sepsis.
2. The safety and effectiveness of positive-pressure mechanical ventilation is dependent on the proper placement of the endotracheal, tracheostomy, or cricothyrotomy tube. Assess proper tube placement before connecting the patient to the ventilator and periodically while the patient remains on the ventilator. At the first change in the patient's condition, you must confirm proper tube placement before considering other causes (see Procedure 9). *If the cause of the problem cannot be determined, remove the patient from the ventilator and provide manual ventilation with a bag-valve device until the source of the alarm can be identified.*

3. During positive-pressure ventilation, the rate, tidal volume, oxygen concentration, and airway pressures must be appropriate for the patient's age, lung compliance, and airway resistance.

4. Mechanical ventilation may cause further damage to an injured lung or may injure remaining healthy lung tissue (Burns, 2001; Sherwood & Hartsock, 2002). Patients with a chest injury or a pulmonary disease, such as asthma and emphysema, should be monitored carefully when they undergo mechanical ventilation. Increased airway pressures may lead to the development of a pneumothorax or a tension pneumothorax. In some cases, prophylactic chest tubes may be inserted to prevent the development of a tension pneumothorax.

5. Anxiety can interfere with mechanical ventilation. Sedation may be required to decrease anxiety, which in turn decreases the work of breathing and decreases oxygen consumption, allowing the patient to breathe with the ventilator. Narcotics cause respiratory depression; therefore, they may be particularly beneficial in patients who have uncontrolled tachypnea and resist or "buck" the ventilator. Some patients may require neuromuscular blocking agents (NMBs) to facilitate mechanical ventilation. It is important to confirm that the patient is receiving adequate sedation and analgesia when NMBs are used. A potentially fatal situation exists if a patient receiving NMBs inadvertently becomes disconnected from the ventilator; therefore appropriate safeguards, alarms, and monitors should be in place.

6. The patient-ventilator system should be assessed every hour. This check should include airway pressures (peak inspiratory pressure and peak end-expiratory pressure), fraction of inspired oxygen (FIO_2), tidal volume, and verification that alarms are set properly.

EQUIPMENT

Intubation equipment (see Procedure 9)
Bag-valve-mask with oxygen reservoir connected to an oxygen source and appropriately fitting mask in case intubation fails
Suction setup
Mechanical ventilator (see following discussion) (Figure 37-1)
Oxygen source for ventilator
Compressed air source
Humidifier
Ventilator circuit to supply gas to the patient
Cardiac monitor
Pulse oximeter
End tidal CO_2 monitor

Ventilators

Ventilators fall into two general categories: negative-pressure and positive-pressure ventilators.

Negative-Pressure Ventilators: These ventilators work by applying subatmospheric pressure at a prescribed rate per minute to the thorax of a patient enclosed in an airtight body suit. The ventilator creates a pressure gradient that causes air to move passively into the lungs. The old iron lung is an example of a negative-pressure ventilator, although

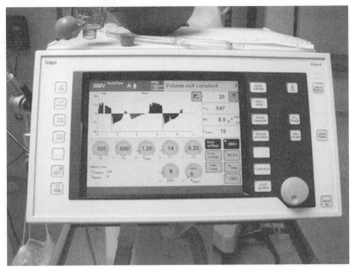

FIGURE 37-1 Example of a ventilator that may be used in an emergency department. (Courtesy Rose DeJarnette.)

today's models in no way resemble their historic counterpart. Negative-pressure ventilation provides the advantage of not requiring an artificial airway, thus allowing the patient to communicate and eat normally. Today, negative-pressure ventilators are used in a home-care setting for patients who have normal lung function and who suffer from neuromuscular diseases, or who require ventilatory support during sleep (Nettina, 2001).

Positive-Pressure Ventilators: These ventilators employ an artificial airway that forces air into the lungs. Expiration during positive-pressure ventilation occurs passively as a result of the elastic recoil of the lungs and the chest wall. Positive-pressure ventilators are classified according to the cycling mechanism or the method by which inspiration is terminated and expiration is initiated.

Volume-Cycled Ventilators: These are the ventilators used most often in the emergency department. Inspiration ends when a preselected volume of gas has been delivered. One of the advantages of volume-cycled ventilators is that they can be programmed to overcome changes in lung compliance and airway resistance.

Pressure-Cycled Ventilators: In these ventilators, inspiration ends when a preset driving pressure is attained. The pressure is constant, so that tidal volume is dependent on lung compliance and airway resistance. These ventilators are used mainly for patients who require short-term ventilation, such as those who have undergone surgery.

Flow-Cycled Ventilators: In these ventilators, inspiration ends when the flow rate of gas delivered drops below a preset level. As lung volume increases and lung compliance decreases, the flow rate of gas decreases progressively and is sensed by the ventilator, which then interrupts gas flow, allowing exhalation.

Time-Cycled Ventilators: These ventilators are used primarily for neonates and incorporate a timing mechanism that controls the inspiratory phase. The ventilator delivers a determined flow, for a given time, which determines tidal volume.

Ventilator Settings (Figure 37-2)

Tidal Volume: The amount of air that moves in and out of the lungs in one breath. Normally calculated at 10-15 ml/kg of body weight.

Rate: The number of breaths delivered per minute.

FIO_2: The fraction of inspired oxygen is discussed as a percentage, although it is often expressed as a decimal. Room air is 21% (or 0.21) oxygen. Typically, the FIO_2 used in an emergency situation is 100% (or 1.0).

Peak Inspiratory Pressure (PIP): The highest pressure generated by the ventilator to deliver the preset tidal volume, PIP varies depending on airway resistance and lung compliance. In adults, PIP is optimally less than 40 cm H_2O. A pressure alarm should be set at 5-10 cm H_2O above the PIP. An alarm may indicate kinked ventilator tubing, the patient's biting the tube or coughing, or water in the circuit. A low-pressure alarm usually signals that the patient has been disconnected from the ventilator.

Positive End-Expiratory Pressure (PEEP): Resistance is applied to the expiratory phase of ventilation, so that positive airway pressure is maintained throughout exhalation. The primary use of PEEP is to improve oxygenation in patients who do not respond to increases in FIO_2. PEEP also aids in preventing collapsed alveoli and in opening already collapsed alveoli to prevent atelectasis. Usually, PEEP begins at 3-5 cm H_2O. Low levels of PEEP may be set just to help overcome the effects of the dead space in the ventilator circuit. Severe lung disease may require a PEEP level of at least 30 cm H_2O. Patients receiving PEEP need to be monitored closely for barotrauma.

Continuous Positive-Airway Pressure (CPAP): Essentially the same as PEEP, except that the patient has spontaneous respirations and is unaided by mechanical positive-pressure breaths. The positive pressure is usually delivered by mask.

Ventilation Modes

Ventilators have the capacity to operate in different ventilatory modes.

Assist Mode: When the patient begins to inhale, the ventilator senses the negative pressure created by the patient's effort and delivers a ventilator breath at the prescribed tidal-volume setting. This mode allows the patient some control over ventilation; however, if the patient becomes apneic, the machine does not deliver a breath.

Control Mode: The ventilator is not sensitive to the patient's ventilatory efforts, and it delivers a prescribed rate of ventilation per minute.

Assist/Control Mode: This mode is used most often in the setting of acute respiratory failure and is tolerated well by the awake patient. The ventilator senses the patient's effort and delivers a ventilator breath, allowing

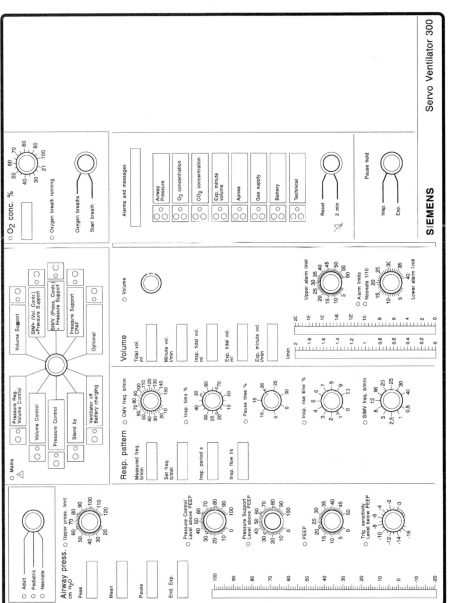

FIGURE 37-2 Ventilator control panel (Servo Ventilator 300). (Courtesy Siemens Life Support Systems, Danvers, MA.)

for a rate faster than the set rate on the ventilator. If the patient's inspiratory effort ceases, however, the ventilator continues to deliver mechanical breaths at the prescribed rate.

Intermittent Mandatory Ventilation (IMV): Often this mode is used to wean patients off the ventilator. The patient on IMV breathes spontaneously between mechanical breaths delivered by the ventilator. The spontaneous breaths vary in tidal volume based on the patient's effort, but the ventilator ensures that the patient receives a prescribed number of breaths per minute.

Pressure Support Ventilation (PSV): This mode is used when the patient is spontaneously breathing. When using pressure support ventilation, inspiratory pressure, PEEP amount, and sensitivity are selected. During patient inspiration, a high flow of gas is delivered to the preselected inspiratory pressure, and this pressure is then maintained throughout inspiration.

Synchronous Intermittent Mandatory Ventilation (SIMV): The ventilator senses the patient's spontaneous breath and does not deliver a ventilator breath until the patient has completely exhaled. This avoids hyperinflation caused by the delivery of a mechanical breath during the inspiratory phase of a spontaneous, patient-initiated breath, referred to as "breath stacking."

PATIENT PREPARATION

Intubate the patient or obtain airway access surgically or percutaneously (see Procedures 9-13, 17, 19).

PROCEDURAL STEPS

1. Plug the ventilator into an oxygen source. Turn the machine on and check that the equipment is functioning properly according to the equipment manual.
2. Set the FIO_2. In the emergency department, it is usually set at 100% initially. The oxygen setting should be manipulated based on the clinical and physiologic assessment of the patient, including arterial blood gases.
3. Set the tidal volume based on the patient's weight (10-15 ml/kg; it is sometimes set as low as 5-8 ml/kg, depending on the cause of the patient's hypoxia).
4. Set the respiratory rate based on the patient's age and clinical condition (adult, 10-12; child, 14-24; and infant, 20-40).
5. Set the ventilator mode (CMV, AC, IMV, PSV, SIMV).
6. Ensure that all of the alarms are turned on and functioning. Common alarms include disconnect alarms (low-pressure or low-volume alarms) and pressure alarms (high-pressure alarms, low-pressure alarms) minute ventilation alarms, FIO_2 alarms, silence or pause alarms.
7. Connect the endotracheal tube (or tracheostomy/cricothyrotomy tube) to the ventilator.
8. Research has demonstrated that barotrauma causes serious injury and may lead to additional respiratory problems. A respiratory therapist or intensivist should be consulted when applying pressure to the airway. If respiratory care personnel are not available, PEEP should start at 5 cm H_2O or less, and the maximum airway pressure at 6-10 cm H_2O (Burns, 2001).
9. To evaluate the patient's clinical condition, arterial blood gases should be drawn 15-30 minutes after the patient has been connected to the ventilator. The ventilator should be adjusted as indicated.

10. The patient should be placed on a cardiac monitor, a pulse oximeter, and when available, an end-tidal CO_2 monitor to continuously monitor tube placement and ventilations.
11. Check that the humidifier has adequate distilled water and that the thermostat is adjusted to the manufacture's recommended temperature. Drain ventilator tube as needed to prevent condensation and aerolization of bacteria into the patient's lungs.
12. Patients who remain in the emergency department for extended periods of time should be periodically repositioned. Repositioning has been shown to improve oxygenation (Vollman, 2001).

AGE-SPECIFIC CONSIDERATIONS

1. Infants' and young children's chests are more compliant, which results in a greater change in volume when there is a change in pressure.
2. The pediatric patient's alveoli fill and empty more quickly than the adult's.
3. Tidal volume for the pediatric patient is generally calculated at 10-15 ml/kg.
4. Infants' and young children's respiratory rates are faster than those of adults, and the ventilator rate should be set appropriately.
5. Infants are ventilated with pressure-cycled machines that leave them at risk for barotrauma, and they must be monitored closely for complications.
6. An uncuffed endotracheal tube may cause an increase in PIP without an increase in ventilation. The child should be monitored closely for this, and an assessment should include periodic blood gas analysis and continuous pulse oximetry.
7. Owing to the short length of infant endotracheal tubes, a change of the head position may dislodge the tube. Small-diameter pediatric tubes may also become plugged and nonfunctional easily, causing deterioration in ventilation.
8. The geriatric patient who requires mechanical ventilation may have preexisting diseases that may lead to more complications with mechanical ventilation, such as emphysema or congestive heart failure.
9. Aging leads to reduction in lung mass, decreased expansion of the rib cage, and decreased vital capacity (Atwell, 2002).

COMPLICATIONS

1. Whenever there is a complication related to mechanical ventilation that is serious enough to cause patient compromise, the patient should be disconnected from the ventilator and manual bag-valve ventilation should be initiated until the problem is identified and corrected.
2. Increased intrathoracic pressure from mechanical ventilation may cause decreased venous return to the heart and hypotension. The emergency care provider should first determine whether medication or the patient's clinical condition (e.g., shock) is the cause of hypotension. This effect is exacerbated by PEEP.
3. Mechanical ventilation causes barotrauma and acute lung injury. Monitor the patient for the development of a pneumothorax or a tension pneumothorax.
4. The awake patient may "fight" the ventilator. Patients may require sedation and analgesia as well as neuromuscular blocking agents. Once these medications are given, spontaneous ventilatory efforts are impaired, and if the ventilator fails, the patient requires assistance with a bag-valve device until the

ventilator is functioning again. Inadequate sedation and analgesia when NMBs are being used can cause physiologic and psychological complications, such as hypertension and release of stress hormones.

5. Other complications that may occur with mechanical ventilation include cuff leak, mucus plugs in the tube, displaced tube (e.g., right main stem), tear in the ventilator tubing, malfunctioning alarms, pulmonary infections, sepsis, and lack of humidification.

PATIENT TEACHING

1. Explain the need for mechanical ventilation and the importance of not touching the ventilator or any other equipment surrounding the patient.
2. Notify the nurse of system disconnections or if anything does not appear or "feel" right when the patient is being ventilated.
3. While the patient is on the ventilator, encourage family members to provide support and reassurance to the patient by means of conversation and touch.

REFERENCES

Atwell, S.L. (2002). Trauma in the elderly (pp. 772-787). In McQuillan, K., Von Rueden, K., Hartsock, R., Flynn, M., & Whalen, E. (Eds.). *Trauma nursing: from resuscitation through rehabilitation*. 3rd ed. Philadelphia: W. B. Saunders.

Burns, S. (2001). Ventilatory management: volume and pressure modes (pp. 178-195). In Lynn-McHale, D.J., & Carlson, K.K. (Eds.). *AACN procedure manual for critical care*, 4th ed. Philadelphia: W.B. Saunders.

Nettina, S.M. (Ed.) (2001). Lippincott manual of nursing practice. Philadelphia: J.B. Lippincott.

Sherwood, S.F. & Hartsock, R.L. (2002). Thoracic injuries (pp. 543-590). In McQuillan, K., Von Rueden, K., Hartsock, R.L., Flynn, M., et al. (Eds.). *Trauma nursing: from resuscitation through rehabilitation*, 3rd ed. Philadelphia: W.B. Saunders.

Vollman, K. M. (2001). Manual pronation therapy (pp. 83-94). In Lynn-McHale, D.J. & Carlson, K.K. (Eds.). *AACN procedure manual for critical care*, 4th ed. Philadelphia: W. B. Saunders.

Inhalation Therapy

Nebulizer Therapy

*Margo E. Layman, MSN, RN, RNC, CN-A
and Jean A. Proehl, RN, MN, CEN, CCRN*

Nebulizer therapy is also known as "neb," updraft, SVN (small-volume nebulizer), or "acorn neb."

INDICATIONS
To deliver medications directly to the respiratory tract for the treatment of the following:
1. Acute bronchospasm due to reactive airway disease (asthma) and other causes
2. Excessive mucus buildup
3. Croup
4. Epiglottitis

Nebulizers use baffles to break down particles to a size small enough to be inhaled into more distal parts of the tracheobronchial tree (Curley & Thompson, 2001). There are several advantages of nebulized medications. The medication is delivered directly to the site of action (the lungs); therefore a low dose may be used (Witek, 2000). The low dose decreases systemic absorption and side effects. Moreover, delivery of nebulized medications to the lungs is very rapid, so the onset of action is faster than with subcutaneous or oral routes. The delivery of nebulized medications also humidifies inspired air, which helps loosen bronchial secretions.

CONTRAINDICATION AND CAUTIONS
1. An unconscious or confused patient who cannot cooperate with the procedure may require a mask; but the mask lessens effectiveness significantly.
2. Chronic obstructive pulmonary disease patients should generally receive nebulizer treatments with compressed air instead of oxygen.
3. Nebulized medications are contraindicated in the presence of absent or severely diminished breath sounds unless the nebulized medication is delivered through an endotracheal tube that uses positive pressure. A patient with decreased air exchange may not be able to move the medication adequately into the respiratory tract.
4. Use catecholamines with caution in patients with cardiac irritability. When inhaled, catecholamines increase the cardiac rate and may precipitate dysrhythmias.

EQUIPMENT
Nebulizer and connecting tubing (Figure 38-1)
Short, corrugated tubing
Oxygen cannula
Compressed gas source (oxygen or air) or air compressor
Medication to be administered by nebulizer (Table 38-1)

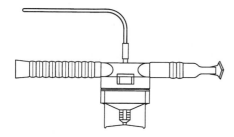

FIGURE 38-1 Nebulizer assembled to allow corrugated tubing to function as a reservoir.

TABLE 38-1

MEDICATIONS COMMONLY ADMINISTERED BY NEBULIZER

Generic name	Type of Medication	Trade name
Isoproterenol hydrochloride, isoproterenol sulfate	Bronchodilator	Isuprel
Metaproterenol	Bronchodilator	Alupent
Albuterol	Bronchodilator	Ventolin, Proventil
Cromolyn sodium	Mast cell stabilizer, antiasthmatic	Intal
Ipratropium bromide	Anticholinergic bronchodilator	Atrovent

PATIENT PREPARATION

1. Place the patient in an upright position (40-90 degrees), which allows deep ventilation and maximal diaphragmatic movement (see Procedure 20).
2. Assess the breath sounds, pulse rate, respiratory status, oxygen saturation (see Procedure 23), and peak flow (see Procedure 25), if possible, before administering the medication.
3. Assess the heart rate during the treatment. If the heart rate increases by 20 beats per minute, stop the nebulizer treatment. In pregnant patients, the fetal heart rate should also be assessed (see Procedure 112).
4. Instruct the patient take slow deep breaths through the mouth and hold at end inspiration (Curley & Thompson, 2001).

PROCEDURAL STEPS

1. Place the patent on supplemental oxygen, with the flow rate determined by the patient's condition, pulse oximetry, and/or arterial blood gases. The inhalation of a catecholamine alters pulmonary ventilation-perfusion ratios and may exacerbate hypoxemia for a short period (Anderson, 1989).
2. Assemble the nebulizer and the tubing and instill the medication into the nebulizer.
3. Add the amount of sterile normal saline to the nebulizer as prescribed; 2.5 ml is a common amount of diluent. Some medications come prediluted with saline.

4. Attach the nebulizer to a source of compressed gas. Oxygen (rate of 6-8 L/min) can be used, but room air via an air compressor increases the humidity of the inhaled gas because of the water vapor content in room air. Adjust the flow rate until a light mist is created. If too forceful a stream is generated, the medication may be wasted.

5. Attach the corrugated tubing to the nebulizer. Some references place the tubing between the nebulizer and the mouthpiece to allow large droplets to "rain out" into the tubing; this decreases deposition of these droplets on the tongue and may reduce side effects. Other sources place the tubing on the opposite side of the nebulizer to serve as a reservoir.

6. Give the patient the mouthpiece or place the mask on the patient.

7. Coach the patient in the correct breathing technique.

8. Tap the sides of the nebulizer occasionally to decrease dead volume in the container.

9. Continue treatment until nebulizer starts sputtering.

10. Reassess breath sounds, pulse rate, oxygen saturation, respiratory rate, and peak flow.

11. Medications may be combined in the nebulizer.

AGE-SPECIFIC CONSIDERATIONS

1. Use of a mask guarantees better compliance for the elderly patient as well as the pediatric patient who is unable to cooperate by holding a nebulizer mouthpiece and inhaling appropriately. Never administer nebulizer treatments to a crying child; crying completely prevents absorption of nebulized medications (Fink, 2000).

2. If a child resists wearing a mask, the medication stream can be directed into the face in a blow-by fashion.

COMPLICATIONS

Nausea, vomiting, tremors, bronchospasm, headache, and tachycardia are common medication-related side effects.

PATIENT TEACHING

If the nebulizer is sent home with the patient, instruct him or her to wash the nebulizer in soapy water, rinse, and air dry daily. Additional cleansing should be performed according to manufacturer's recommendations.

REFERENCES

Anderson, M.R. (1989). The pharmacology of intervention for respiratory emergencies. *Emergency Care Quarterly, 5,* 23-26.

Curley, M.A.Q., & Thompson, J.E. (2001). Oxygenation and ventilation (pp. 233-308). In Curley, M.A.Q., & Moloney-Harmon, P.A. *critical care nursing of infants and children,* 2nd ed. Philadelphia: W.B. Saunders.

Fink, J.B. (2000). Aerosol device selection: evidence to practice. *Respiratory Care, 45,* 874-884.

Witek, T.J. (2000). The fate of inhaled drugs: the pharmacodynamics of drugs administered by aerosol. *Respiratory Care, 45,* 826-830.

Metered-Dose Inhaler

Margo E. Layman, MSN, RN, RNC, CN-A

Metered-dose inhalers are also known as MDIs or "puffers." They disperse medication into the lungs through aerosol spray, mist, or fine powder.

INDICATIONS

To administer medications directly to pulmonary structures and to assist in the relief of bronchospasm in reversible obstructive airway disease, or to prevent exercise-induced bronchospasm. Advantages of medication delivery via MDIs include a decreased likelihood of systemic side effects and an immediate relief of symptoms. The types of medications used with metered-dose inhalers include the following:

1. Bronchodilators: Relax the muscles around the bronchial tubes
2. Corticosteroids: Decrease inflammation and swelling in the airways
3. Cromolyn: Reduces the reactions of antigens in the airways

CONTRAINDICATIONS AND CAUTIONS

1. Improper technique results in medication not reaching the bronchial tubes or air passages.
2. Remember to remove the mouthpiece cap and shake the canister to mix the medication properly.
3. The patient may be unable to use an MDI because of altered mental status or deterioration of the clinical condition.

EQUIPMENT

Metered-dose inhaler with prescribed medication
Spacer (e.g., AeroChamber) (optional)
Facial tissues (optional)
Wash basin or sink with warm water
Paper towel

PATIENT PREPARATION

1. Assess breath sounds, heart rate, and respiratory rate.
2. Assess peak flow if indicated (see Procedure 25).
3. Assist the patient to an upright sitting position.

PROCEDURAL STEPS

1. Warm by rolling in hands and shake the inhaler canister immediately before using. Remove the protective cap and make sure the metal canister is firmly seated in the plastic case.
2. Hold the mouthpiece 2.5-5.0 cm (1-2 inches) from the mouth, keeping the canister in an upright position (Fink, 2000).

3. At the end of expiration, depress the metal canister (with two of your fingers on top of the canister and your thumb on the bottom of the plastic metered-dose inhaler) while the patient inhales deeply and slowly through the mouth (Fink, 2000).
4. Have the patient hold the breath as long as possible, at least 4-10 seconds (Fink, 2000).
5. Wait 30-60 seconds and then repeat steps 2-4.
6. To use a spacer, insert the canister into the spacer and put the mouthpiece into the patient's mouth before activating the MDI (Figure 39-1). The spacer traps the medication mist inside the chamber, allowing the patient to inhale and exhale slowly several times without removing the mouth from the spacer. This ensures maximal medication delivery.

AGE-SPECIFIC CONSIDERATIONS
1. Hand strength diminishes with age and may cause difficulty in ensuring enough pressure on the canister for the patient to receive a proper dose of medication.
2. A child may need the nose plugged during inhalation.
3. Spacers can be used with a mask attachment for infants and small children; this allows the child 5-6 breaths to inhale medication. Children are not able to use a metered-dose inhaler without a spacer until they are old enough to understand and perform the technique. A mask can be used and a nurse, parent, or caretaker can depress the metered-dose inhaler with the child's inspiration.

COMPLICATIONS
1. Cardiac dysrhythmias (tachycardia)
2. Hyperventilation with dizziness, lightheadedness, tingling, and palpitations
3. Paroxysmal bronchospasm
4. Thrush in patients receiving corticosteroid inhalations. Use of a spacer and a thorough mouth rinse after each application helps prevent thrush.

PATIENT TEACHING
1. Do not attempt to instruct the patient on using the metered-dose inhaler during an episode of shortness of breath.
2. Use a placebo metered-dose inhaler to teach patient the appropriate breathing technique. Placebo MDIs are available from pharmaceutical company representatives (Togger & Brenner, 2001).
3. Clean the MDI plastic canister after each use and dry it thoroughly. This prevents clogging of the valve in the mouthpiece.
4. Observe the MDI to make sure it is dispensing medication.

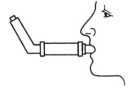

FIGURE 39-1 Metered-dose inhaler attached to a spacer. (From Proehl, J.A., & Jones, L.M. [1998]. *Mosby's emergency department patient teaching guides.* St. Louis: Mosby.)

5. Notify a physician if shortness of breath or difficulty in breathing persists after the metered-dose inhaler is used as prescribed.

REFERENCES

Fink, J.B. (2000). Aerosol device selection: evidence to practice. *Respiratory Care, 45,* 874-885.

Togger, D.A., & Brenner, P.S. (2001). Metered dose inhalers. *American Journal of Nursing, 101,* 26-32.

Pleural Decompression

Emergency Needle Thoracentesis

Deborah A. Upton, RN, BSN, CEN

Emergency needle thoracentesis is also known as needling a chest.

INDICATIONS

To provide immediate decompression of a tension pneumothorax with respiratory or cardiovascular compromise or both. Tension pneumothorax is suspected in the presence of the following:

Respiratory distress
Unilateral decreased or absent breath sounds
Signs of hypoxemia
Jugular venous distention (indicates elevated central venous pressure)
Hypotension
Unilateral hyperresonance
Tracheal deviation
Pulseless electrical activity, especially when preceded by trauma

Performance of needle thoracentesis converts a tension pneumothorax to a simple pneumothorax.

CONTRAINDICATIONS AND CAUTIONS

1. If this procedure is used in the absence of a tension pneumothorax, there is a risk of producing a pneumothorax, causing damage to the lung or blood vessels (Sullivan, 2001).

2. Needle thoracentesis is performed as an interim procedure until tube thoracostomy (chest tube placement) can be carried out. Anticipate thoracostomy as a follow-up procedure.

3. Initial presentation of a traumatic ruptured diaphragm with herniation of abdominal contents into a hemithorax can mimic a tension pneumothorax. Placement of a needle in this instance can result in bacterial contamination of the pleural cavity. Suspect a ruptured diaphragm in a patient with a history of application of sudden, compressive forces to the abdomen.

4. Owing to the urgent nature of a tension pneumothorax, consideration should be given to training nursing and ancillary personnel in this procedure in areas in which there is no immediate access to a physician. The patient may suffer cardiac arrest without immediate intervention.

5. Research demonstrates that in some adults, the standard 3-cm, over-the-needle catheter may not reach the pleural cavity at the second intercostal space. Insufficient cannula length may contribute to the failure of the procedure. A minimum length of 4.5 cm (1.77 inches) is recommended (Britten et al., 1996).

EQUIPMENT

Antiseptic solution
Local anesthetic
Syringe and needles for local anesthesia
10- to 18-G over-the-needle catheter (4.5-6.0 cm in length)
3-inch collapsible tubing for flutter valve (Penrose drain or Heimlich valve)
   or sterile rubber glove
Suture ties or small rubber band

PATIENT PREPARATION

1. Chest radiographs may be deferred initially, depending on the patient's presentation. Consider obtaining films before performing needle thoracentesis if a ruptured diaphragm is suspected.
2. If time allows, cleanse the chest with an antiseptic solution on the side of the tension pneumothorax. The usual site for needle insertion is the second intercostal space at the midclavicular line (Figure 40-1). The fifth intercostal space, midaxillary line can also be used (Wolfe & Smith-Coggins, 2001).
3. Place the patient in an upright position if cervical spine pathology is ruled out and the patient's condition permits.
4. Administer high-flow oxygen.

PROCEDURAL STEPS

1. *Infiltrate the area with local anesthetic if the patient is conscious and the patient's condition permits.
2. *Insert the needle through the skin and direct it toward the top of the second rib. Then, direct the needle over the top of the rib (intercostal nerves and arteries run inferior to the rib) and into the pleural space.

Site for chest decompression

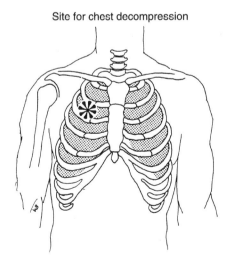

FIGURE 40-1 The usual site for needle thoracostomy. (From Caroline, N.L. [1983]. *Emergency care in the streets,* 2nd ed. [p. 226]. Boston: Little, Brown.)

---

*Indicates portions of the procedure usually performed by a physician or an advanced practice nurse.

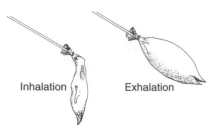

FIGURE 40-2 Flutter valve made from the finger of a rubber glove. (From Caroline, N.L. [1983]. *Emergency care in the streets,* 2nd ed. [p. 226]. Boston: Little, Brown.)

Inhalation   Exhalation

3. *Egress of air confirms the diagnosis of tension pneumothorax. If no air is released or if signs and symptoms do not improve, consider the presence of pericardial tamponade, myocardial contusion, or air embolism.
4. *Remove the needle and leave the catheter in place. The catheter may now be secured with tape and left open to the air. A simple pneumothorax now exists.
5. Assemble the equipment and prepare for subsequent chest tube placement (see Procedure 41). If there is a delay in chest tube placement (e.g., during transport), a flutter valve can be placed over the hub of the catheter. A simple form of flutter valve could be a ¼-inch sterile rubber drain or a finger of a sterile glove with the tip removed. The flutter valve can then be secured to the hub of the catheter with tape or a suture (Figure 40-2).

    Intubated patients receiving positive-pressure ventilation do not require a flutter valve.
6. After chest tube placement is carried out, remove the catheter. Apply antibiotic ointment and a sterile dressing over the puncture site.
7. Obtain a chest x-ray film after the procedure.

AGE-SPECIFIC CONSIDERATIONS
1. The use of accessory muscles and nasal flaring may also be indicators of tension pneumothorax in children.
2. Landmarks and insertion techniques are the same in children and adults. A relatively smaller needle/catheter is used for children.

COMPLICATIONS
1. Creation of a pneumothorax if a tension pneumothorax did not exist before procedure was performed.
2. Hematoma at insertion site.
3. Perforation of abdominal viscera if ruptured diaphragm or herniation of abdominal contents is present.
4. Placement of the needle close to the sternum may result in a laceration of the internal mammary artery with significant blood loss and resultant hemothorax.
5. Failure to decompress a tension pneumothorax (Sullivan, 2001).
6. Infection of puncture site (late).

---

*Indicates portions of the procedure usually performed by a physician or an advanced practice nurse.

REFERENCES

Britten, S., Palmer, S.H., & Snow, T.M. (1996). Needle thoracocentesis in tension pneumothorax: insufficient cannula length and potential failure. *Injury, 27*, 321-322.

Sullivan, D.M. (2001). Myths in trauma (pp. 702-709). In Ferrera, P.C., Colucciello, S.A., Marx, J.A., Verdile, V.P., & Gibbs, M.A. (Eds.), *Trauma management: an emergency medicine approach.* St. Louis: Mosby.

Wolfe, M.B., & Smith-Coggins, R. (2001). Needle thoracostomy (pp. 38-39). From Rosen, P., Chan, T.C., Vilke, G.M., & Sternbach, G. (Eds.), *Atlas of emergency procedures.* St. Louis: Mosby.

PROCEDURE 41

Chest-Tube Insertion

Deborah A. Upton, RN, BSN, CEN

Chest-tube insertion is also known as tube thoracostomy.

INDICATIONS

1. To remove air, blood, or both from the pleural cavity in the presence of a pneumothorax (free air in the pleural space), hemothorax (free blood in the pleural space), or hemopneumothorax (combination of air and blood).
2. To remove fluid from the pleural cavity in the presence of a large pleural effusion, empyema, or chylothorax. Iatrogenic pleural collections are most commonly seen after central venous access procedures.
3. To provide prophylactic chest drainage in patients with severe blunt chest trauma (flail chest or pulmonary contusions) who will require positive-pressure ventilatory support. Prophylactic chest tubes may also be inserted in patients with penetrating thoracic injuries, even in the absence of evidence of pneumothorax.

CONTRAINDICATIONS AND CAUTIONS

1. A patient's hemodynamic status may deteriorate rapidly after the evacuation of a massive hemothorax (larger than 1000-2000 ml). Initiate fluid resuscitation before performing chest decompression and anticipate the need for high-volume resuscitation. Autotransfusion may be indicated if available. A large left hemothorax may signal an aortic or great vessel injury.
2. The use of trocar chest tubes is controversial and is not recommended by most authors, because trocar use has been associated with damage to the thoracic structures. If a trocar is used, it should be used only to guide the

tube through an opening already created by blunt dissection, rather than to enter the chest forcibly (Kirsch & Mulligan, 2004).
3. A patient with a previous thoracostomy may have scar tissue and adhesions, making chest-tube placement difficult.
4. Consideration should be given to decompression of a pneumothoraces before attempting air transport, because the size of the pneumothorax may increase with altitude.
5. Chest-tube insertion is not indicated if an emergency thoracotomy is imminent.

EQUIPMENT
Antiseptic solution
Local anesthetic
Syringes and needles for local anesthesia
No. 10 scalpel
Large, curved hemostat
Suture scissors
Needle holder
Sterile towels or drapes
Chest tube
36-40 French for blood or viscous fluid
12-22 French for air only
Large silk suture (0-0 to 2-0)
3-inch tape
Occlusive dressing (gauze impregnated with petroleum jelly) (optional)
Gauze dressings (4 × 4, split drain sponges)
Chest-drainage device
Autotransfusion equipment if indicated or available
NOTE: Most institutions have preassembled trays containing much of this equipment.

PATIENT PREPARATION
1. Obtain a chest x-ray film unless the patient's condition mandates immediate chest tube placement.
2. If time allows, cleanse the insertion site with antiseptic solution. The usual site for chest tube placement is the fourth or fifth intercostal space in the anterior or midaxillary line (Figure 41-1). Alternatively, the level of the nipple line can be used as a marker, especially in the unstable patient who requires immediate tube placement. In women with pendulous breasts, the lateral crease of the breast is a more stable landmark. Insertion through a lower site risks subdiaphragmatic placement, possibly into the liver or spleen.
3. Place the patient in a supine position with the arm over the head on the involved side. If the patient's injuries permit, elevate the trunk to a 30- to 60-degree angle.
4. Administer sedation and analgesia as prescribed. This is an extremely uncomfortable and painful procedure.
5. Prepare the chest-drainage device (see Procedures 42-49).
6. Prepare autotransfusion equipment if indicated (see Procedures 79-83).

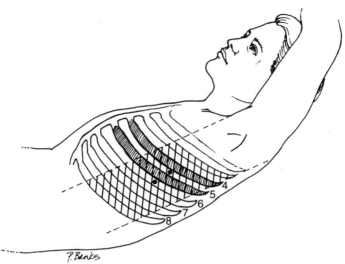

FIGURE 41-1 Acceptable and preferred locations for chest-tube placement. (From Dalbec, D., & Krome, R.L. |1986|. Thoracostomy. *Emergency Medical Clinics of North America, 4,* 449.)

PROCEDURAL STEPS

1. *Cleanse the insertion site with an antiseptic solution.
2. *Drape the chest with sterile drapes.
3. *Infiltrate the area with a local anesthetic if the patient is conscious and if the patient's condition permits.
4. *Using the chest tube, measure the distance from the insertion site to the apex of the lung and note the distance on the tube.
5. *Make a 2- to 4-cm incision through the chest wall parallel to the ribs. The incision is made one interspace below the desired interspace. Making an incision below the pleural cavity entry site permits blunt dissection over the superior surface of the rib and creates a tunnel that allows later removal of the tube without an air leak.
6. *Bluntly dissect over the superior surface of the rib with the curved hemostat (nerves and arteries run inferior to the ribs). Enter the pleural cavity with the hemostat. The patient will experience pain as the pleural cavity is entered (Figure 41-2).
7. *Widen the pleural opening and the skin incision by pulling the opened hemostat back out of the chest wall.
8. *With a gloved finger, palpate through the incision to verify entry into the pleural space and to check for adhesions of the pleura and for intrathoracic or intraabdominal organs (Figure 41-3).
9. *Direct the chest tube upward through the incision. Use a large hemostat to introduce the tube. Advance the tube to the premeasured distance. The

---

*Indicates portions of the procedure usually performed by a physician or an advanced practice nurse.

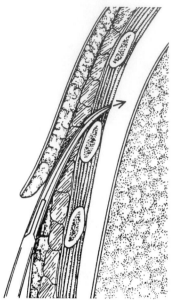

FIGURE 41-2 Enter the pleural space with a Kelly clamp. (From Yeston, N., & Neihoff, J. [1989]. Important procedures in the intensive care unit [p. 249]. In Civetta, J.M., Taylor, R., & Kirley, R. et al. [Eds.], *Critical care*. Philadelphia: J.B. Lippincott.)

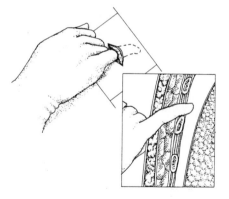

FIGURE 41-3 Place a gloved finger into the incision to confirm pleural penetration and assess for the presence of adhesions. (From Yeston, N. & Neihoff, J. [1989]. Important procedures in the intensive care unit [p. 249]. In Civetta, J.M., Taylor, R., & Kirley, R. et al. [Eds.], *Critical care*. Philadelphia: J.B. Lippincott.)

immediate return of blood, air, or both confirms the appropriate placement.

10. *Connect the chest tube to the chest-drainage device.
11. Tape all connections in the chest drainage system. One inch of tape is placed horizontally, extending over connections. Reinforce this with tape placed vertically so that it encircles both ends of the connector (Figure 41-4).
12. *Suture the chest tube in place with silk suture.
13. Place an occlusive dressing. Petroleum-impregnated gauze may be wrapped around the tube close to the insertion site if the air leak is large. However,

---

*Indicates portions of the procedure usually performed by a physician or an advanced practice nurse.

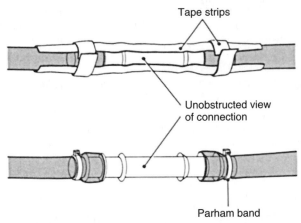

FIGURE 41-4 Securing of connection points. (From Kersten, L.D. [1989]. Comprehensive respiratory nursing. In Gordon, P., Norton J., & Merrell, R [Eds], *Dimensions of Critical Care Nursing,* 14, 6-13. Philadelphia: W.B. Saunders.)

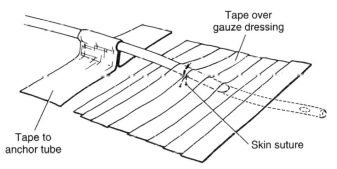

FIGURE 41-5 Occlusive chest tube dressing. (From Kersten, L.D. [1989]. Comprehensive respiratory nursing. In Gordon, P., Norton, J., & Merrell, R. [Eds.], *Dimensions* of *Critical Care Nursing,* 14, 6-13. Philadelphia: W.B. Saunders.)

this may cause maceration of the skin and is not routinely necessary (Barefoot, 2001) (Figure 41-5).

14. Apply split drain sponges around the chest tube, one over the top and one underneath the tube.
15. Apply two or three gauze pads (4 × 4) on top of the split sponges.
16. Tape the dressing to the skin.
17. Tape the chest tube to the skin.
18. Obtain a chest x-ray film to confirm the correct tube placement (the last hole on the tube should be inside the pleural space) and to assess the status of the pneumothorax or hemothorax.
19. Monitor the chest-drainage device for the presence of large, continuous air leaks (may signal esophageal or large airway damage) or excessive blood

loss. Indications for surgical intervention include massive blood loss (>1000-1500 ml initially or 300 ml in the first hour), massive or persistent air leaks (Kirsch & Mulligan, 2004).

AGE-SPECIFIC CONSIDERATIONS

1. Usual tube sizes for pediatric patients are 16-, 20-, and 24-French tubes. Small infants may require 8- to 12-French tubes.
2. For newborn infants the tube is placed in the fifth intercostal space of the anterior axillary line and directed onteriorly (Kirsch & Mulligan, 2004).
3. In a small infant, be sure that the dressing is not so large as to splint a large part of the chest wall and interfere with effective ventilation (Walsh-Sukys, 1997).

COMPLICATIONS

1. A malpositioned, nonfunctioning tube (with the last hole in the tube outside of the pleural space or the tube malpositioned in the subcutaneous space)
2. Bleeding from the skin incision, from intercostal arteries or veins, or from a pulmonary artery or vein (risk is increased if chest tube with trocar is used)
3. Organ or structure injury (diaphragm, liver, spleen, stomach, or colon)
4. Vasovagal response
5. Dyspnea
6. Hypovolemia secondary to rapid fluid loss with a hemothorax
7. Hemothorax
8. Re-expansion pulmonary edema
9. Occlusion or kinking of the tube (which may result in the formation of a tension pneumothorax)
10. Pain with re-expansion of the lung
11. Local hematoma
12. Local cellulitis (late)
13. Atelectasis or pneumonia due to splinting by the patient
14. Reoccurrence of pathology after removal of the tube

PATIENT TEACHING

1. Request assistance when moving or turning in bed or when getting out of bed.
2. Immediately report any shortness of breath, chest pain, or disconnections in the system.
3. Do not lie on the tubing or allow it to be kinked.

REFERENCES

Barefoot, W. (2001). Thoracentesis (pp. 145-150). In Lynn-McHale, D., & Carlson, K. (Eds.), *AACN procedure manual for critical care*, 4th ed. Philadelphia: W.B. Saunders.

Walsh-Sukys, M.C. (1997). Thoracostomy (pp. 160-165). In Walsh-Sukys, M.C., & Krug, S.E. (Eds.), *Procedures in infants and children*. Philadelphia: W.B. Saunders.

Kirsch, T.D., & Mulligan, J.P. (2004). Tube thoracostomy (pp. 187-209). In Roberts, J.R., & Hedges, J.R. (Eds.), *Clinical procedures in emergency medicine*, 4th ed. Philadelphia: W.B. Saunders.

Management of Chest-Drainage Systems

Deborah A. Upton, RN, BSN, CEN and
Jean A. Proehl, RN, MN, CEN, CCRN

The information contained in this procedure should be used in conjunction with that in the procedures pertaining to specific chest-drainage systems (see Procedures 43-49).

INDICATION

To evacuate air, fluid, or both from the pleural space and re-expand the lung by restoring negative intrapleural pressure.

CONTRAINDICATIONS AND CAUTIONS

1. Water-seal devices must be kept upright; otherwise, intrapleural negativity may be lost with air entry into the pleural space.
2. Do not clamp the tube unless it is absolutely necessary (to change the chest drainage device or to check for air leaks), because a tension pneumothorax may develop.
3. Do not raise the device above the patient's chest level, because fluid may re-enter the chest and increase the probability of infection (applies to water-seal systems only).
4. Do not allow the tubing to coil below the top of the device or lie on the floor, because dependent fluid-filled loops require increased intrathoracic pressure to continue the emptying of the pleural space.
5. "Milking," or stripping, chest tubes can result in more than 400 cm H_2O of negative pressure within the pleural space (Duncan & Erickson, 1982). This negative pressure may damage the lung tissue, and therefore, stripping of chest tubes should not be performed routinely. Milking may be necessary when a clot is suspected of obstructing the tube, as is the case when the flow of sanguinous drainage suddenly slows or stops. To milk the tube, fold the tubing over on itself three times. Each fold should be approximately three inches long. Squeeze the folded tubing 3-4 times and release.

GENERAL INFORMATION

1. The fluid level in the water-seal tube should rise with inspiration and fall with expiration. If fluctuations are not present, the lung is either fully re-expanded or there is an obstruction. Check the tubing for kinks or occlusions. The most common cause is the patient lying on the tubing. Positive-pressure ventilation dampens these fluctuations.
2. For water-seal units, the water in the water-seal chamber should bubble during expiration. If it bubbles constantly, check for an air leak.

187

a. Clamp the chest tube near the insertion site. If the bubbling stops, the leak is from either the insertion site or the patient's lung.

b. Reinforce the occlusive dressing over the chest-tube insertion site. If the bubbling continues, the air leak is coming from the patient's lung. If this is a new finding, report the observation to the physician immediately.

c. If the bubbling continues after clamping at the insertion site, then the air leak is located either in the tubing or in the equipment. Check the integrity of the unit and all its connections. If a prefabricated, disposable unit is in use (Emerson, Pleur-Evac, Thora-Klex, Atrium, or Argyle), replace the entire unit.

AGE-SPECIFIC CONSIDERATIONS

1. Adult chest-drainage units may be used for children; however, pediatric chest-drainage devices are available from most manufacturers. The pediatric collection chamber is smaller than its adult counterpart and has smaller incremental markings for accurate measurement of small volumes. Autotransfusion is not usually available on pediatric units, but adult autotransfusion units may be used instead.

2. Negative 10-20 cm H_2O is the suction level usually recommended for pediatric patients.

3. Milking or stripping of chest tubes is contraindicated in children.

COMPLICATIONS

1. A tension pneumothorax may develop if there are obstructions in the system. Kinked or clamped tubing is the most likely source of obstruction.

2. If the device breaks or the system becomes disconnected, a loss of intrapleural negativity may result, and an open pneumothorax may develop. If the tubing becomes disconnected from the patient or the device breaks, place the end of the drainage tubing (approximately 2.5 cm) in a container of sterile water until another chest drainage device can be prepared.

3. Accidental dislodgement of the chest tube: If this happens, have the patient cough or exhale forcibly. Apply an occlusive dressing to the area and tape it on three sides. Notify the physician immediately. Check the oxygen saturation as measured by pulse oximetry (SpO_2) and administer oxygen. Monitor the patient closely for development of a tension pneumothorax until another chest tube can be inserted.

PATIENT TEACHING

1. Request assistance when moving or turning in bed or when getting out of bed.

2. Report any shortness of breath, chest pain, or disconnections in the system immediately.

3. Do not lie on the tubing or allow it to be kinked.

REFERENCE

Duncan, C., & Erickson, R. (1982). Pressures associated with chest tube stripping. *Heart and Lung, 11*, 166-171.

One-Way Valve

Deborah A. Upton, RN, BSN, CEN

A one-way valve is also known as a Heimlich valve or a flap valve.

INDICATION
To allow air and fluid to drain from the pleural cavity and simultaneously prevent re-entry of air into the pleural space. Patients who have chronic pneumothorax or pleural effusion can benefit from a one-way valve because no other chest drainage device is required. Using the one-way valve, these patients can ambulate and, in some cases, can be discharged from the hospital. The valve can also be employed during interhospital transport instead of, or in addition to, a chest-drainage unit.

CONTRAINDICATIONS AND CAUTIONS
If a hemothorax or pleural effusion is present, it may be necessary to replace the valve or add a regular chest-drainage unit for fluid collection.

EQUIPMENT
    One-way valve
    Adhesive tape
    Padded hemostat
    Urinary catheter drainage collection bag or sterile glove (if necessary for fluid collection)
    Sutures ties or small rubber band

PATIENT PREPARATION
1. Insert a chest tube or chest-drainage catheter (see Procedure 41).
2. Instruct the patient to rest during the procedure and report pain or shortness of breath.
3. If possible, have the patient sit at a 45- to 90-degree angle.

PROCEDURAL STEPS
1. If the chest tube is connected to a chest-drainage unit, untape the connection.
2. If drainage of blood or other fluid is anticipated, attach a urinary catheter collection bag to the distal end of the valve. A sterile glove can be used if only a small amount of drainage is present.
3. Disconnect the chest tube from the chest-drainage unit and immediately connect to the blue end of the one-way valve. The "collapsed end" of the valve is the distal end, which allows the fluid or air to drain out of the pleural space but does not allow the air to re-enter (Figure 43-1). If fluid is draining actively, the chest tube may be clamped briefly during this step. Do not clamp the chest tube until you are ready to place the valve, and remove the clamp as soon as the valve is in place.

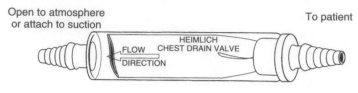

Open to atmosphere   To patient
or attach to suction

One-way air flow

FIGURE 43-1 Heimlich or one-way valve. The "collapsed end" is placed distally to allow drainage out of the chest. (From Kirsch, T.D., & Mulligan, J.P. [2004] Tube thoracostomy [p. 201]. In Roberts, J.R. & Hedges, J.R. (Eds.), *Clinical procedures in emergency medicine*, 4th ed. Philadelphia: W.B. Saunders.)

4. Ask the patient to cough or exhale forcibly.
5. Tape the connections securely and anchor the chest tube and valve to the patient's chest.
6. If using a flutter valve, no dressing is necessary.
7. Intubated patients receiving positive pressure ventilation do not necessarily need a flutter valve.
8. Obtain a chest x-ray film to determine whether air has re-entered the pleural cavity.

COMPLICATIONS
1. Infection resulting from a break in aseptic technique
2. Tension pneumothorax if the chest tube is clamped, kinked, or occluded

PATIENT TEACHING
1. Report chest pain, shortness of breath, or any disconnection in the system immediately.
2. Do not attempt to reposition the chest tube or valve.

PROCEDURE 44

Chest-Drainage Bottles

Deborah Upton, RN, BSN, CEN

The information in this procedure should be used in conjunction with that in Procedure 42.

INDICATION
See Procedure 42.

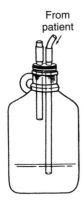

From
patient

FIGURE 44-1 One-bottle chest-drainage system. (From Wieck, L., King, E.M., & Dyer, M. [1986]. *Illustrated manual of nursing techniques,* 3rd ed. [p. 285]. Philadelphia: J.B. Lippincott.)

CONTRAINDICATIONS AND CAUTIONS

1. See Procedure 42.
2. The one-bottle system can be used for removing fluid; however, a two- or three-bottle system is preferred because it reduces the need for frequent readjustment of the water-seal tube to maintain appropriate submersion (the same bottle is used as a water-seal and as a collection chamber). Also, suction cannot be used with a one-bottle system.
3. The bottle system is rarely used now because most facilities have replaced it with prefabricated, disposable chest-drainage systems. The prefabricated systems can be used either as gravity or suction-drainage systems. They are easier to set up and maintain, and their components are less fragile than glass bottles.

PATIENT PREPARATION
Insert a chest tube (see Procedure 41).

ONE-BOTTLE SYSTEM: GRAVITY DRAINAGE
Equipment
Sterile water-seal device or collection bottle (Figure 44-1)
Sterile water or saline
Holder for bottle
3-4 ft of sterile tubing
Tubing connectors, ¼-inch internal diameter
Adhesive tape

Procedural Steps
1. Add enough sterile water or saline solution to the bottle to submerge the end of the water-seal tube 2.5 cm below the water level. The water-seal tube is attached to the tubing that exits the patient. This provides the water-seal necessary for preventing back flow. The short, rigid tube is the vent tube (see Figure 44-1).
2. Attach the chest tube to the drainage tubing with a connector.
3. Connect the drainage tubing to the water-seal tube.
4. Secure the connection sites with adhesive tape.

TWO-BOTTLE SYSTEM: GRAVITY DRAINAGE
Equipment
Sterile collection and water-seal bottles (Figure 44-2)
Sterile water or saline solution
Holder for bottles
3-4 ft of sterile tubing
Tubing connectors, 1/4-inch internal diameter
Adhesive tape

Procedural Steps
1. Add enough sterile water or saline solution to the water-seal bottle to submerge the end of the water-seal tube 2.5 cm below the water level. This provides the water seal necessary for preventing back flow. The short, rigid tube is the vent tube.
2. Attach the drainage bottle to the water-seal bottle via the short length of sterile tubing that is attached to the water-seal tube.
3. Attach the chest tube to the drainage tubing via a connector.
4. Connect the drainage tubing to the other short, rigid tube in the drainage bottle (see Figure 44-2).
5. Secure the connections with adhesive tape.

TWO-BOTTLE SYSTEM: SUCTION DRAINAGE
Equipment
Sterile water-seal/collection bottle and suction-control bottle (Figure 44-3)
Sterile water or saline solution
Holder for bottles
3-4 ft of sterile tubing
Tubing connectors, 1/4-inch internal diameter
Suction setup
Adhesive tape

Procedural Steps
1. Add enough sterile water or saline solution to the water-seal/collection bottle to submerge the end of the water-seal tube 2.5 cm below the water level. This provides a water seal necessary for preventing back flow.

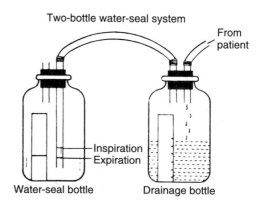

FIGURE 44-2 Two-bottle gravity-drainage system. (From Brunner, L.S., & Suddarth, D.S. [1988]. *Textbook of medical-surgical nursing,* 6th ed. [p. 151]. Philadelphia: J.B. Lippincott.)

Two-bottle water-seal system

From patient

Inspiration
Expiration

Water-seal bottle   Drainage bottle

2. The suction-control bottle has three openings in the cap. The long, rigid tube in the center works as the manometer tube. Fill the suction-control bottle with enough sterile water or saline to submerge the manometer tube in about 10 cm of water. Connect the suction-control bottle to the water-seal/collection bottle with a short length of sterile tube. Connect the other short, rigid tube in the suction-control bottle to the continuous-suction device. The level of submersion of the manometer tube, rather than the suction regulator device, determines how much suction is applied (Brunner & Suddarth, 1988):

> 1 cm manometer of submersion = 1 cm of negative water pressure

3. Attach the chest tube to the drainage tubing with a connector.
4. Attach the drainage tube to the water-seal tube of the collection bottle (see Figure 44-3).
5. Secure the connections with adhesive tape.

THREE-BOTTLE SYSTEM
Equipment
Sterile collection, suction, and water-seal (overflow) bottles (Figure 44-4)
Sterile water or saline
Holder for bottles
4-5 ft of sterile tubing
Tubing connectors, ¼-inch internal diameter
Adhesive tape
Suction setup

Procedural Steps
1. Add enough sterile water or saline solution to one of the bottles with two openings in the cap to submerge the end of the long, rigid tube 2.5 cm below the water level. This provides the water seal necessary for preventing back flow. This is the water-seal and collection overflow bottle.

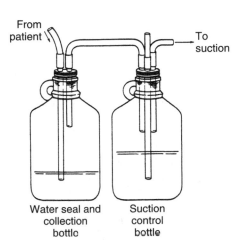

From patient

To suction

Water seal and collection bottle

Suction control bottle

FIGURE 44-3 Two-bottle chest-drainage with suction. (From Wieck, L., King, E.M., & Dyer, M. [1986]. *Illustrated manual of nursing techniques,* 3rd ed. [p. 287]. Philadelphia: J.B. Lippincott.)

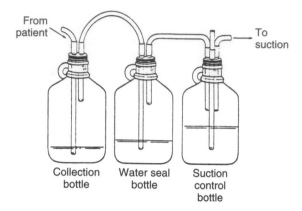

FIGURE 44-4 Three-bottle chest-drainage system. (From Wieck, L., King, E.M., & Dyer, M. [1986]. *Illustrated manual of nursing techniques,* 3rd ed. [p. 287]. Philadelphia: J.B. Lippincott.)

2. The other bottle with two openings in the cap is the collection bottle. One of the short, rigid tubes is connected to the drainage tubing, and the other is connected to the water-seal tube via a short length of sterile tubing.
3. The suction bottle has three openings in the cap. The long, rigid tube in the center is the manometer tube. Fill the suction bottle with enough sterile water to submerge the manometer tube in about 10 cm of water. Connect one of the short, rigid tubes of the suction bottle to the water-seal bottle via a short length of sterile tubing. Connect the other short rigid tube in the suction bottle to the suction device. The depth the manometer tube is submerged in the water, rather than the suction regulator device, determines the amount of suction that is applied (Brunner & Suddarth, 1988).

   1 cm manometer of submersion = 1 cm of negative water pressure

4. Attach the chest tube to the drainage tube via a connector.
5. Attach the drainage tube to the other short, rigid tube of the collection bottle (see Figure 44-4).
6. Secure the connection sites with adhesive tape.

COMPLICATIONS
1. See Procedure 42.
2. When the suction source is functioning, there is continuous bubbling from the manometer tube in the suction bottle. If the bubbling stops, check the suction source. If the suction source is malfunctioning, disconnect the manometer tube from the suction bottle to provide an air vent for gravity drainage.

PATIENT TEACHING
See Procedure 42.

REFERENCE
Brunner, L.S., & Suddarth, D.S. (1988). *Textbook of medical-surgical nursing,* 6th ed. Philadelphia: J.B. Lippincott.

Chest-Drainage Devices: Emerson

Deborah Upton, RN, BSN, CEN, and
Jean A. Proehl, RN, MN, CEN, CCRN

The information in this procedure should be used in conjunction with that in Procedure 42.

INDICATION
See Procedure 42.

CONTRAINDICATIONS AND CAUTIONS
1. See Procedure 42.
2. The Emerson pump is a high-pressure, high-flow system capable of generating pressures of 60 cm H_2O. Bottles are used infrequently because most facilities now use low-pressure, prefabricated, disposable chest-drainage systems.

EQUIPMENT
Emerson pump-bottle set (connectors, drainage tubes, bottles, bottle cap assemblies, bottle tubes, large tubing, pump, mobile stand with a triangular tray)
or
Disposable Emerson chest-drainage unit for Emerson pump or wall-suction setup (for disposable unit with manometer only)
Sterile water or saline solution
Tape

PATIENT PREPARATION
Insert a chest tube (see Procedure 41).

PROCEDURAL STEPS
Bottle System for Emerson Pump (Emerson, 1989c) (Figure 45-1)
1. Add enough sterile water or saline solution to the water-seal collection bottle to fill it up to the water line. Write the time and date on the bottle. Attach the two, short, rigid, narrow tubes to the underside of the cap via three connectors. These tubes should be submerged in 1-2 cm of sterile water in the bottle. This provides the water seal necessary for preventing back flow.
2. If the patient has only one chest tube, cover one of the openings in the bottle cap with the plastic adapter.
3. Attach the water-seal bottle and the fluid-trap bottle via the short, wide connection tube.

195

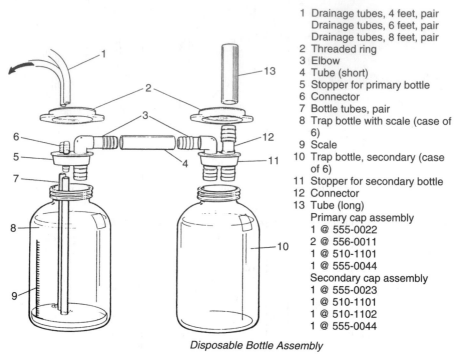

1 Drainage tubes, 4 feet, pair
   Drainage tubes, 6 feet, pair
   Drainage tubes, 8 feet, pair
2 Threaded ring
3 Elbow
4 Tube (short)
5 Stopper for primary bottle
6 Connector
7 Bottle tubes, pair
8 Trap bottle with scale (case of 6)
9 Scale
10 Trap bottle, secondary (case of 6)
11 Stopper for secondary bottle
12 Connector
13 Tube (long)
   Primary cap assembly
   1 @ 555-0022
   2 @ 556-0011
   1 @ 510-1101
   1 @ 555-0044
   Secondary cap assembly
   1 @ 555-0023
   1 @ 510-1101
   1 @ 510-1102
   1 @ 555-0044

Disposable Bottle Assembly

FIGURE 45-1 Emerson bottle setup. (Courtesy J.H. Emerson Co., Cambridge, MA.)

4. Attach the fluid-trap bottle to the pump via the large, wide connection tube.
5. Plug in the machine and make sure that the red indicator light goes on.
6. Plug in the two small connectors on the primary bottle cap and adjust the speed of the motor until the desired suction is attained (–20 to –30 cm H_2O).
7. Remove the cap(s) and connect the long tube(s) (if there are two chest tubes) to the cap of the water-seal collection bottle.
8. Connect the drainage tube(s) to the chest tube(s).
9. Tape all the connections and make sure the caps are tight.
10. Turn on the machine and adjust the pressure to the prescribed level.
11. To determine the negative pressure in the patient's pleural space, subtract the depth of submersion of the tube tips in the water-seal collection bottle from the pressure on the machine. For example, if the pressure on the machine is set at –30 cm of water and the tubes in the water-seal collection bottle are submerged to 20 cm of water, then the pressure in the patient's pleural space is –10 cm of water. Therefore, to maintain the desired pressure, it is necessary to increase the pressure setting on the machine as fluid accumulates in the water-seal collection bottle. Fluid should not be allowed to fill more than one quarter of the bottle (the machine capacity is –60 cm H_2O; higher fluid levels require increased pressure settings on the machine to maintain the desired pressure level).

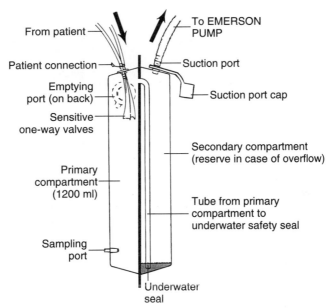

FIGURE 45-2 Emerson disposable thoracic drainage set for use with the Emerson suction regulator or the Emerson pump. (Courtesy J.H. Emerson Co., Cambridge, MA.)

Disposable System for Emerson Pump (Emerson, 1989a) (Figure 45-2)

1. Add water through the suction port up to the water-seal mark.
2. Place the disposable unit in the stand (Figure 45-3) or suspend it from the bed by using ties or accessory metal hangers.
3. Connect the patient tube(s) to the patient fittings on the disposable unit.
4. Connect the flexible corrugated tube to the suction port on the disposable unit and the fitting on the bottom of the Emerson pump.
5. Turn on the pump. The level of accumulated fluid in the disposable unit does not affect the vacuum level applied to the patient, because there is no underwater seal in the primary collecting compartment.

Disposable System for Wall Suction (Emerson, 1989b) (Figure 45-4)

1. Add water through the suction port up to the water-seal mark.
2. Add water through the manometer air intake to the desired level of suction. The air intake port must be left uncapped to allow air to enter and relieve excess negativity.
3. Connect the patient tube(s) to the patient fittings on the disposable unit.
4. Connect the reducing adapter to the suction port and attach it to the wall-suction device. Adjust the wall-suction device until bubbles appear in the bottom of the manometer column.

AGE-SPECIFIC CONSIDERATION

There are no pediatric versions of the bottle or disposable units, but the adult units can be used for infants and children.

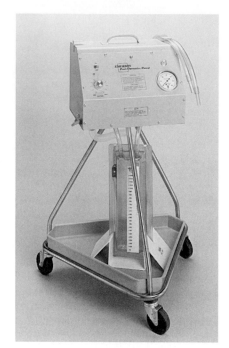

FIGURE 45-3 Emerson pump with disposable chest drainage unit. (Courtesy J.H. Emerson Co., Cambridge, MA.)

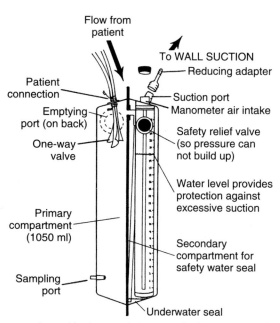

FIGURE 45-4 Emerson disposable thoracic drainage set (with manometer) for use with any regulated suction source. (Courtesy J.H. Emerson Co., Cambridge, MA.)

COMPLICATIONS

1. See Procedure 42.
2. If there is a loss of electrical power or if the Emerson pump malfunctions, the internal vacuum blower has an air vent to the atmosphere, so there is no danger of pressure accumulation (R. Felt, personal communication, February 1998).

PATIENT TEACHING

See Procedure 42.

REFERENCES

J.H. Emerson Co. (1989a). *Emerson disposable thoracic drainage set: instructions for use.* Form 903-6001-2. Cambridge, MA: Author.

J.H. Emerson Co. (1989b). *Emerson disposable thoracic drainage set: instructions for use with wall suction.* Form 902-4001. Cambridge, MA: Author.

J.H. Emerson Co. (1989c). *Emerson post-operative pumps: operation and maintenance.* Cambridge, MA: Author.

PROCEDURE 46

Chest-Drainage Devices: Pleur-Evac

Deborah A. Upton, RN, BSN, CEN

Pleur-Evac and Sahara chest-drainage units are products of the Deknatel Product Group, Genzyme Surgical Products (Fall River, MA).

The information in this procedure should be used in conjunction with the information in Procedure 42.

INDICATIONS

1. See Procedure 42.
2. The Sahara units are totally dry and, thus, quick and easy to set up.
3. All Sahara units have 100% latex free pathway and tubing.
4. The Sahara and dry suction-control units can achieve greater levels of suction (as much as -40 cm H_2O) than the wet suction-control units.

CONTRAINDICATIONS AND CAUTIONS

See Procedure 42.

EQUIPMENT

Pleur-Evac (wet or dry suction control) water-seal unit or Sahara (dry)
    chest-drainage unit
Sterile water
Adhesive tape
Suction setup
Needle and a 30-ml syringe (to fill the air-leak chamber of the Sahara unit)

PATIENT PREPARATION

Insert a chest tube (see Procedure 41).

PROCEDURAL STEPS

Pleur-Evac: Wet Suction Control (Deknatel, 1997a) (Figure 46-1)

1. Attach a funnel to the suction-tubing connector and fill it to the 2-cm level
   with sterile water (approximately 70 ml). Use the "Fill to Here" mark as a
   guide. The water turns blue for enhanced visibility. Disconnect the funnel. If
   necessary, the unit can now be attached to the patient.
2. Remove the atmospheric vent cover (muffler) and fill the suction-control
   chamber with enough sterile water to achieve the desired level of suction;
   -20 cm H_2O is the standard setting. Replace the muffler, making sure that you
   do not occlude the atmospheric vent.
3. Attach the long tube from the collection chamber to the patient's chest tube
   and tape all the connections securely.
4. Attach the tubing from the suction-control chamber to a suction source.
   Adjust the suction until gentle, continuous bubbling occurs in the suction-
   control chamber. Increasing the suction from the suction source increases
   bubbling and air flow through the system but does not increase the suction
   delivered to the pleural cavity; additional water must be added to the chamber to accomplish this.
5. If gravity drainage is desired, omit step 4 and leave the suction tubing open
   and unclamped to prevent positive pressure buildup.

Pleur-Evac: Dry-Suction Control (Deknatel, 1997b) (Figure 46-2)

1. Attach a funnel to the suction-tube connector and fill it to the 2-cm level ("Fill
   to Here" mark) with sterile water (approximately 70 ml). The water turns
   blue for enhanced visibility. Disconnect the funnel.
2. Attach the long tube from the collection chamber to the patient's chest tube
   and tape all connections securely.
3. Attach the tubing from the suction-control chamber to a suction source. The suction is controlled by a dial that is preset at -20 cm H_2O. Turn on the suction and
   increase it until the orange float is visible in the suction-control indicator
   window. Increasing the suction from the source increases the air flow through
   the system without increasing the negativity delivered to the patient; if more negativity is desired, change the suction-control dial. If the suction level is decreased
   after the initial setup, the negativity delivered to the patient may not change
   unless the excess negativity is vented with the high-negativity relief valve.
4. If gravity drainage is desired, omit step 3 and leave the suction tubing open
   and unclamped to prevent positive pressure buildup.

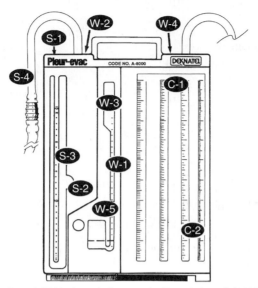

FIGURE 46-1 Pleur-Evac A-8000 chest-drainage unit. (From Deknatel. [1989]. *Pleur-Evac: instructions for use.* Fall River, MA: Pfizer Hospital Products Group, Inc. Copyright 1989 by Pfizer Hospital Products Group.)

S-1: Atmospheric vent: Fill the suction control chamber through this opening. Do not cover the vent with anything other than the muffler provided. The muffler allows air to enter the suction control chamber, but it decreases evaporation and noise.

S-2: Self-sealing diaphragm to inject or withdraw fluid to adjust the water level in the suction-control chamber.

S-3: Suction-control pressure scale.

S-4: Suction tubing.

W-1: Water-seal pressure scale: Oscillations (tidaling) occur in this chamber with respirations, but they may not be present when the suction is on, the lung is fully expanded, or the tubing is obstructed or kinked.

W-2: Positive-pressure relief valve: Opens to vent increased positive pressure within the system and prevent pressure accumulation (tension pneumothorax).

W-3: High-negativity float valve: Preserves the water seal in the presence of high negativity. The high-negativity relief valve may be used to reduce negativity.

W-4: Filtered high-negativity relief valve: Depress this button to relieve excess negativity within the system (i.e., after "milking" or stripping the tube to clear clots). If this button is depressed in the absence of suction, negative pressure may be lost and atmospheric pressure may be attained.

W-5: Self-sealing diaphragm: Injects or withdraws fluid to adjust the water level in the water-seal chamber.

C-1: Collection chamber: 2500-ml capacity with overflow from one compartment to the next.

C-2: Self-sealing diaphragm on the back of the collection chamber: Obtains laboratory samples of drainage.

Sahara (Deknatel, 1997) (Figure 46-3)

    1. Attach the long tube from the collection chamber to the patient's chest tube and tape all connections securely (Figure 46-4). No fluid needs to be added to the system before it is connected to the patient, because there is a one-way valve, not a water seal, which prevents air from re-entering the thoracic cavity.

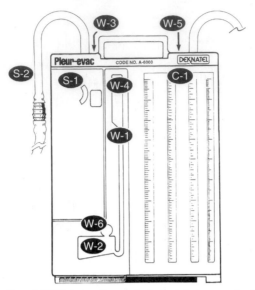

FIGURE 46-2 Pleur-Evac A-6000 dry-suction control chest-drainage unit. (From Deknatel. *Pleur-Evac: instructions for use.* [1989]. Fall River, MA: Pfizer Hospital Products Group, Inc. Copyright 1989 by Pfizer Hospital Products Group.)

S-1: Suction-control dial and indicator: When the orange float appears in this window, the suction is operating at the level indicated by the dial.

S-2: Suction tubing: Connects to the suction source.

W-1: Water-seal pressure scale: Oscillations (tidaling) occur in this chamber with respirations, but they may not be present when the suction is on, the lung is fully expanded, or the tubing is obstructed or kinked.

W-2: Patient air-leak meter. The higher the number of the column in which bubbles are seen, the larger the air leak.

W-3: Positive-pressure relief valve: Opens to vent increased positive pressure within the system and prevent pressure accumulation (tension pneumothorax).

W-4: High-negativity float valve: Preserves the water seal in the presence of high negativity. The high-negativity relief valve may be used to reduce negativity.

W-5: Filtered high-negativity relief valve: Depress this button to relieve excess negativity within the system (i.e., after "milking" or stripping the tube to clear clots). If this button is depressed in the absence of suction, negative pressure may be lost and atmospheric pressure may be attained.

W-6: Self-sealing diaphragm: Injects or withdraws fluid to adjust the water level in the water-seal chamber.

C-1: Collection chamber, 2500-ml capacity with overflow from one compartment to the next.

2. Use an 18-G or smaller needle and a 30-ml syringe to inject 30 ml of sterile water or saline through the injection port on of the unit into the patient air-leak meter.

3. Connect the suction source to the suction port. The suction-control dial is preset at –20 cm H_2O; if a different level of suction is prescribed, turn the dial until it clicks into place. Increase the suction from the suction source until

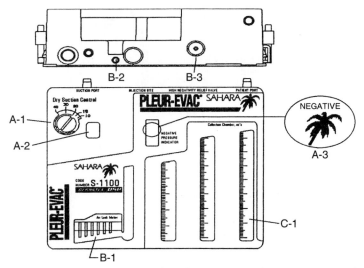

FIGURE 46-3 Pleur-Evac S-1100 Sahara chest-drainage system. (From Deknatel DSP. [1996]. Fall River, MA: Author. Copyright 1996 by DSP Worldwide, Inc.)

A-1: Suction dial: Preset to −20 cm H_2O.

A-2: Suction indicator: When the orange float appears in this window, the suction is operating at the level indicated by the dial.

A-3: Negative-pressure indicator: If a palm tree can be seen in this window, negative pressure exists within the collection chamber. The palm tree should be continuously visible when suction is in use. During gravity drainage, the palm tree may be visible intermittently.

B-1: Air-leak meter: When filled with fluid, this chamber indicates the degree of air leak from the chest cavity. The higher the number of the column in which bubbles are seen, the larger the air leak.

B-2: Positive-pressure relief valve: Opens to vent increased positive pressure within the system and prevent pressure accumulation (tension pneumothorax).

B-3: Filtered high-negativity relief valve: Depress this button to relieve excess negativity within the system (i.e., after "milking" or stripping the tube to clear clots). If this button is depressed in the absence of suction, negative pressure may be lost and atmospheric pressure attained. There is an automatic high-negative, pressure-relief valve that limits negative pressure to approximately −50 cm H_2O.

C-1: Collection chamber: 2000-ml capacity with overflow from one compartment to the next.

the orange float appears in the suction-control indicator window (Figure 46–5). Increasing the suction from the source increases the air flow through the system without increasing the negativity delivered to the patient; if more negativity is desired, change the suction-control dial. If the suction level is decreased after the initial setup, the negativity delivered to the patient may not change unless the excess negativity is relieved by use of the high-negativity relief valve.

4. If gravity drainage is desired, omit step 3 and leave the suction port open to prevent positive pressure buildup.

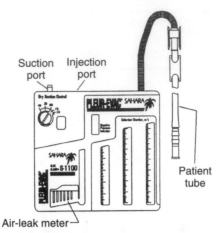

Suction   Injection
port   port

Patient
tube

Air-leak meter

FIGURE 46-4 Pleur-Evac S-1100 Sahara chest-drainage system components for basic setup. (From Deknatel DSP. [1996]. Fall River, MA: Author. Copyright 1996 by DSP Worldwide, Inc.)

FIGURE 46-5 Pleur-Evac S-1100 Sahara chest-drainage system suction indicator window. (From Deknatel DSP. [1996]. Fall River, MA. Copyright 1996 by DSP Worldwide, Inc.)

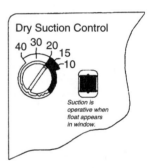

Dry Suction Control

40 30 20
          15
         10

Suction is
operative when
float appears
in window.

AGE-SPECIFIC CONSIDERATIONS

1. All these devices may be used for children. Infant versions are available for both the wet and the dry water-seal devices; the most significant differences in the infant versions are that the drainage chamber is smaller than its adult counterpart, with finer gradations for accurate measurement of drainage and no autotransfusion capability. There is no infant version of the Sahara drainage device.
2. See Procedure 42.

COMPLICATIONS
See Procedure 42.

PATIENT TEACHING
See Procedure 42.

REFERENCES
Deknatel Product Group, Genzyme Surgical Products. (1997). *Pleur-Evac Sahara* (product insert). Fall River, MA: Author.

Deknatel Product Group, Genzyme Surgical Products. (1997a). *Pleur-Evac adult/pediatric single-use chest drainage unit: A-8000* (product insert). Fall River, MA: Author.

Deknatel Product Group, Genzyme Surgical Products. (1997b). *Pleur-Evac adult/pediatric single-use chest drainage unit: Dry suction control A-6000* (product insert). Fall River, MA: Author.

PROCEDURE 47

Chest-Drainage Devices: Thora-Klex

Deborah A. Upton, RN, BSN, CEN

Thora-Klex is a registered trademark of Genzyme Surgical Products.

The information in this procedure should be used in conjunction with that in Procedure 42.

INDICATIONS

1. See Procedure 42.
2. To ensure maintenance of the one-way seal, regardless of the position of the chest-drainage unit in relation to the patient (i.e., tipping or horizontal placement does not result in loss of the one-way seal with this unit).

CONTRAINDICATIONS AND CAUTIONS

1. See Procedure 42.
2. For patients who have a significant change in air leak or an inconsistent suction source, the unit requires frequent manual adjustments.

EQUIPMENT

Thora-Klex chest-drainage unit (Figure 47-1)
  15 ml sterile water
  20-ml syringe and needle
  1- or 2-inch tape
  High-flow, continuous-suction device with a regulator, such as wall suction or an Emerson pump. Some portable suction pumps cannot generate sufficient air flow capacity (20 L/min desired).

PATIENT PREPARATION

Insert a chest tube (see Procedure 11).

PROCEDURAL STEPS (Genzyme Corporation, 1997)

1. The chest-drainage unit is ready to use directly from the package. Instructions are on a pull-out card attached to the front of the unit.
2. Attach the long tube from the collection chamber to the chest tube and tape it securely.
3. The unit must be kept at least 30 cm below the patient's chest level (Elliot, 1990). Secure it to the bed rail or beside the floor stand with the attached hooks.
4. There is no true water seal in the Thora-Klex device, because it is a dry system. The seal is maintained by a one-way vacuum seal valve that is preset at 1.5-2.0 cm H_2O. The one-way valve maintains a closed system and allows air to flow in only one direction, away from the patient. The effective seal is not lost when the unit is tipped in any direction.
5. To maximize air flow, push and turn the suction control dial counterclockwise until it is fully open (Figure 47-2). Do not use the manual vent when the device is set on gravity drainage.

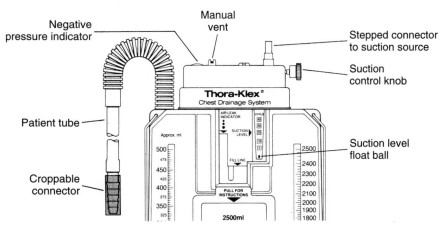

FIGURE 47-1 Thora-Klex chest-drainage unit. (From Davol [1990]. *Thora-Klex 2500/4000 mL chest-drainage system: quick reference guide.* Cranston, RI: Genzyme Corporation. Copyright 1997 by Genzyme Corporation.)

FIGURE 47-2 Top of Thora-Klex chest-drainage unit. (From Davol [1990]. *Thora-Klex 2500/4000 mL chest-drainage system: quick reference guide.* Cranston, RI: Genzyme Corporation. Copyright 1997 by Genzyme Corporation.)

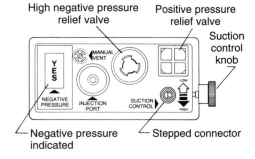

6. Attach the tubing from the suction source to the suction connector on top of the control mode (see Figure 47-2).

7. Adjust the suction control on the chest-device unit by pushing and turning the suction control knob clockwise until it is closed.

8. Adjust the suction pressure at the suction source: -80 to -120 mm Hg on wall suction; -40 to -60 cm H_2O on the portable suction pump. Higher vacuum is used for large air leaks. Adding suction to the system improves the evacuation of gas from the pleural space by creating a lower pressure within the unit than within the patient.

9. Push in the suction-control knob and turn until the float ball sits at the desired level in the suction-level chamber (Figure 47-3). Settings range from -10 to -40 cm H_2O; -20 cm H_2O is the usual setting.

10. If the minimal desired suction level is not attained when the control knob is fully open (counterclockwise), the suction source must be increased. Clockwise movement of the control knob decreases suction; counterclockwise movement increases suction.

11. As an air leak develops or suction pressure varies, the suction level to the patient changes. Therefore, to detect changes, observe the position of the float ball frequently. This requires manual resetting of the control knob.

12. The collection chambers hold up to 2500 ml and are calibrated for easy measurement. Recognize that the two collection columns have different total volumes (500 vs. 2000). Assess and record the type and volume of drainage. If blood in large quantities is evacuated, add an autotransfusion system (ATS). All Thora-Klex units are compatible with ATS units (see Procedure 81).

13. Avoid dependent loops in the patient's tubing, because this generates the same effect as a higher water-seal level and requires more effort to evacuate fluid and air.

14. To create a fluid-filled chamber for detecting air leaks, inject 15 ml of sterile water into the air-leak indicator chamber via the injection port on the top of the unit. The fluid turns blue for enhanced visibility.

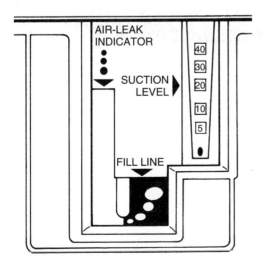

FIGURE 47-3 Suction control meter and air-leak indicator of Thora-Klex chest-drainage unit. (From Davol [1990]. *Thora-Klex 2500/4000 mL chest-drainage system: quick reference guide.* Cranston, RI: Genzyme Corporation. Copyright 1997 by Genzyme Corporation.)

15. In the air-leak indicator, the fluid rocks gently or tidals in response to respirations. The fluid rises with spontaneous inspiration (more negative) and falls (more positive) with expiration; however, the opposite occurs with positive-pressure ventilation. Oscillation is less evident when suction is applied. Rocking decreases or stops if the patient's tubing is kinked, obstructed, or disconnected, or if the lung has re-expanded.

16. A pleural or system air leak is detectable by bubbles passing from left to right in the air-leak indicator (see Figure 47-3). Air leaks do not always occur with each breath, so careful observation is necessary. Pleural air evacuation can be seen on exhalation; if it occurs on inspiration as well (constant bubbling), a significant pulmonary air leak may be present or there may be a leak within the system.

17. If there is a large pleural leak, the suction control knob should be turned counterclockwise as far as possible to increase air flow capacity. To do this, however, a physician's order may be necessary, because the suction level is changing in the suction chamber as it is in the water-seal systems.

18. The presence of negativity within the unit is displayed on the top of the unit by a "Yes" indicator. In gravity systems, the "Yes" displays intermittently with the respiratory pattern; but in suction systems, the "Yes" indicator should be constant. The unit must remain negative to continue to evacuate fluid and air from the chest.

19. Negativity within the system arises from the suction level setting (cm H_2O); from maneuvers to clear the drainage tubing by "milking," or stripping; and from the patient during increased inspiratory efforts. The degree of negativity is reflected by the suction-level float ball with a range of -0 to -40 cm H_2O.

20. Excess negativity (≥ 50 cm H_2O) is automatically reduced to a relatively safe level of approximately -35 cm H_2O by a high-negative pressure-relief valve (see Figure 47-2). The manual vent on top of the unit lowers the negative pressure further to return to the desired level. The manual vent is activated by the use of a coin or a pen; it cannot be adjusted accidentally. To confirm that suction control is restored to the desired level after decreasing negativity within the system (i.e., stripping the chest tube), and after any change from a higher to a lower suction setting, adjust the suction control (float ball) to the desired setting and depress the manual vent until a bubble that passes from left to right is released. If the system negativity exceeds that of the suction control, fluid rises up the left side of the air-leak indicator, and bubbling may occur from right to left. The manual vent procedure should be followed. A similar phenomenon occurs when the lung re-expands, but there is a concurrent lack of rocking or tidaling and no bubbling. Do not activate the manual vent button during gravity drainage.

21. Excess positive pressure (>2 cm H_2O) is automatically relieved.

22. The best fluid samples are taken from the self-sealing rubber tubing, although a port is available on the back of the first collection chamber.

AGE-SPECIFIC CONSIDERATION

A pediatric unit is available, but adult units can also be used for infants and children.

COMPLICATIONS

See Procedure 42.

PATIENT TEACHING
See Procedure 42.

REFERENCES
Genzyme Corporation. (1997). *Thora-Klex 2500-ml chest-drainage and autotransfusion system*. Fall River, MA: Author.
Elliot, D. (1990). *Why waterless chest drainage?* Report No. 118910M. Cranston, RI: C.R. Bard.

PROCEDURE 48

Chest-Drainage Devices: Argyle

Deborah A. Upton, RN, BSN, CEN

The information in the procedure should be used in conjunction with the information in Procedure 42.

INDICATION
See Procedure 42.

CONTRAINDICATIONS AND CAUTIONS
See Procedure 42.

EQUIPMENT
Chest-drainage unit (Aqua-Seal, Thora-Seal III, or Sentinel Seal)
Sterile water
1- or 2-inch tape
Suction setup

PATIENT PREPARATION
Insert a chest tube (see Procedure 41).

PROCEDURAL STEPS
Aqua-Seal (Figure 48-1)
1. Fill the water-seal chamber. Lower the preattached syringe and fill it to the top with approximately 45 ml of sterile fluid (Figure 48-2). Raise the syringe and

allow the fluid to flow into the water-seal chamber up to the 2-cm line. The water turns blue for enhanced visibility. Remove the tubing and the syringe from the water-seal chamber and discard them. If necessary, the unit can be connected to the patient now. If the water-seal level needs to be adjusted later, use the needleless access port on the back of the water-seal chamber.

2. Fill the suction-control chamber. Pour sterile fluid directly into the "suction-control fill opening" to the prescribed level; -20 cm H_2O is the usual setting for patients who are older than 6 months of age. Close the suction control chamber with the attached cap; make sure that the cap snaps into place (suction greater than -25 cm H_2O can be achieved with the suction-control

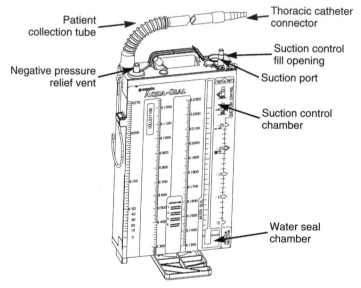

FIGURE 48-1 Aqua-Seal chest-drainage unit. (Courtesy Tyco Healthcare, Mansfield, Ma.)

FIGURE 48-2 Filling the water seal chamber of the Aqua-Seal. (Courtesy Tyco Healthcare, Mansfield, Ma.)

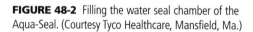
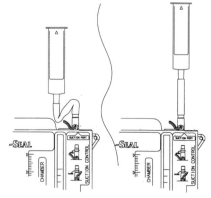

bypass adaptor on the back of the unit; see the package insert for more information).

3. Attach the chest tube to the thoracic catheter connector (if not done in step 1). Tape the connection securely.
4. Turn the black valve on the suction port clockwise to the closed position (Figure 48-3). Connect a regulated suction source to the suction port. Turn the vacuum on and open the black suction valve until a gentle bubbling is achieved in the suction-control chamber.
5. Excess negative pressure can be relieved with the negative-pressure relief vent on the top of the unit. Excess positive pressure is automatically relieved by a valve on top of the unit.

Thora-Seal III (Figure 48-4)

1. Fill the water-seal bottle. Remove the water-seal cap from the top of the unit (middle bottle). Pour approximately 120 ml of sterile fluid directly into the

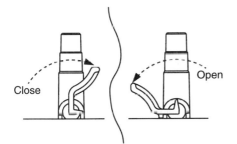

FIGURE 48-3 Aqua-Seal suction-control valve. (Courtesy Tyco, Healthcare, Mansfield, Ma.)

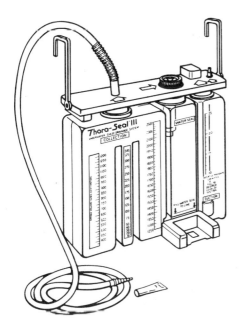

FIGURE 48-4 Thora-Seal III underwater chest drainage system. (Courtesy Tyco, Healthcare, Mansfield, Ma.)

opening to the line indicated on the water-seal bottle. Replace the cap. If necessary, the unit can be connected to the patient now.

2. Fill the suction-control bottle. Pour sterile fluid into the opening on the top of the suction-control bottle to the prescribed level; -20 cm H_2O is the usual setting for patients who are older than 6 months of age.

3. Attach the chest tube to the thoracic catheter connector (if this did not occur in step 1). Tape the connection securely.

4. Attach the suction tubing to the connection port on top of the suction bottle, turn on the vacuum, and adjust until a gentle bubbling is achieved in the suction-control bottle.

5. To change the collection bottle, remove the floor stand. With the physician's approval, clamp the patient's connecting tubing *for a brief time*. Rotate the collection bottle clockwise and pull it down. Insert a new bottle into the manifold and rotate until the bottle neck snaps into a locked position. *Remove the clamp from the patient's connecting tubing*. Replace the floor stand.

Sentinel Seal (Figure 48-5)

1. Fill the underwater-seal chamber. Remove the "suction regulator" from the top of the unit by twisting it at the base. Pour approximately 90 ml of sterile fluid through the opening and fill to the red "-2-" line on the suction control chamber. Replace the suction regulator and twist it into place. Remove the red protector ring from the suction regulator and discard it.

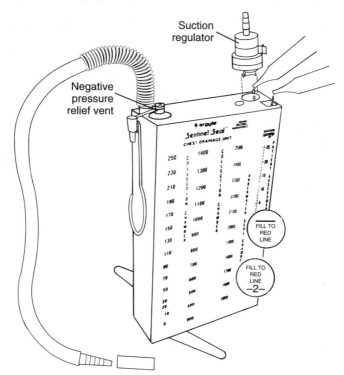

FIGURE 48-5 Sentinel-Seal chest drainage unit. (Courtesy Tyco, Healthcare, Mansfield, Ma.)

2. Fill the patient assessment chamber. Remove the instruction tape from the top of the unit and fill the chamber to the red line with approximately 30 ml of sterile fluid. The fluid turns blue for enhanced visibility.
3. Attach the chest tube to the thoracic catheter connector. Tape the connection securely.
4. Connect the suction source to the suction regulator. Set the wall suction source to at least 160 mm Hg (set a portable suction source to at least 50 cm H_2O). Watch the patient assessment chamber while turning the suction regulator until the fluid reaches the prescribed suction level; −20 cm H_2O is the usual setting for patients who are older than 6 months of age. Turn the suction regulator clockwise to increase the negative pressure. To release excess negative pressure, remove the red cap and depress the negative-pressure relief vent. To decrease the vacuum, depress the negative-pressure relief vent while turning the suction regulator counterclockwise. Do not depress the negative-pressure relief vent unless the unit is connected to the suction source or the intrapleural negativity may be lost.
5. For gravity drainage, disconnect the suction tubing from the suction regulator.

AGE-SPECIFIC CONSIDERATION
Argyle does not make a pediatric chest-drainage unit, but all units can be used for pediatric patients.

COMPLICATIONS
1. See Procedure 42.
2. Tipping the units may result in mixing of fluid from some chambers or loss of the water seal.

PATIENT TEACHING
See Procedure 42.

PROCEDURE 49

Chest-Drainage Devices: Atrium

Deborah A. Upton, RN, BSN, CEN

The information in this procedure should be used in conjunction with the information in Procedure 42.

INDICATIONS
1. See Procedure 42.
2. The dry-suction system has the advantages of quick setup, quiet operation, and the ability to use high levels of controlled suction.

CONTRAINDICATIONS AND CAUTIONS
See Procedure 42.

EQUIPMENT
Atrium chest-drainage unit (wet- or dry-suction control)
Sterile water or saline
Tape
Suction setup

PATIENT PREPARATION
Insert a chest tube (see Procedure 41).

PROCEDURAL STEPS
Wet-Suction Control (Figure 49-1) (Atrium, 1996a)
1. Turn the suction-control stopcock to the on position. Fill the water-seal chamber with sterile water by holding the preattached funnel level with the unit. Add water to the top of the funnel. Raise the funnel and empty the water into the water-seal chamber up to the 2-cm line. The water turns blue to assist in air-leak detection. If too much water is added, the excess can be removed by inserting a needle and syringe through the face grommet. When the water has passed to the chamber, the suction-control stopcock must be returned to the off position before it is connected to the unregulated suction device. Discard the funnel after use or use it to fill the suction-control chamber.
2. To fill the suction-control chamber, remove the suction-control vent plug and pour into the chamber the amount of sterile water or saline needed to achieve the desired suction pressure (Table 49-1). The water turns blue when the chamber is filled. The usual pressure setting for adults is −20 cm H_2O.
3. Replace the suction-control vent plug.
4. Remove the cap from the patient-tube connector and attach it to the chest tube.
5. Position the unit below the patient's chest level and keep it upright by using either the bed attachment hooks or the floor stand.
6. Connect the suction source to the suction-control stopcock. Tape all the connections to prevent accidental disconnections.
7. Turn on the suction-control stopcock and increase the suction pressure slowly until constant gentle bubbling occurs in the suction-control chamber. To increase or decrease the suction pressure delivered to the patient, adjust the fluid level in the suction-control chamber by injecting or withdrawing water via the face grommet.
8. Observe the water seal for air leaks and changes in pressure. Absence of bubbling with minimal float-ball oscillation indicates that there is no air leak. Constant or intermittent bubbling, with air bubbles going from right to left in the air-leak zone, indicates a leak in either the chest-drainage system or the thoracic cavity (Figure 49-2).

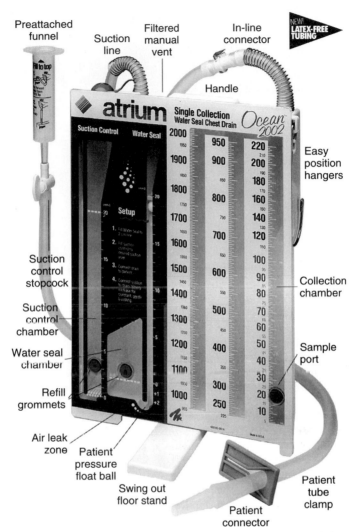

FIGURE 49-1 Atrium water seal chest-drainage unit with wet-suction control. (Courtesy Atrium Medical Corporation, Hudson, NH.)

TABLE 49-1

WATER NEEDED FOR VARIOUS SUCTION LEVELS

Suction pressure	Water/saline volume needed
-20 cm H_2O	320 ml
-15 cm H_2O	190 ml
-10 cm H_2O	80 ml

From Weimer, C. (1998) Personal communication. Atrium.

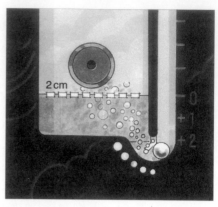

FIGURE 49-2 Atrium water seal with float ball in the air-leak zone. (Courtesy Atrium Medical Corporation, Hudson, NH.)

9. Changes in patient pressure are detected by observing the float ball in the calibrated water-seal column. When the chest tube is connected to the suction chamber, the patient's pressure is equal to the suction-control setting plus the float-ball level. Accumulated positive pressure is automatically released by the in-line positive-pressure valve.

Dry-Suction Control (Figure 49-3) (Atrium, 1996b)

1. Turn the suction-control stopcock to the on position. Fill the water-seal chamber with sterile water by holding the preattached funnel level with the unit. Add water to the top of the funnel. Raise the funnel and empty the water into the water-seal chamber up to the 2-cm line. The water turns blue to assist in air-leak detection. If too much water is added, the excess can be removed by inserting a needle and syringe through the face grommet.
2. Remove the cap from the patient-tube connector and attach it to the chest tube.
3. Connect the chest-drain suction line to the suction source. The suction-control regulator is preset to −20 cm H_2O. Increase the suction source to −80 mm Hg or higher. The suction-monitor bellows must be expanded to the mark or beyond it for a −20 cm H_2O or higher setting. The monitor bellows does not expand when suction is not operating or is disconnected. The regulator-control dial on the side of the drain can be set between −10 and −40 cm H_2O (Figure 49-4). To change the suction pressure, dial down to lower the suction pressure and up to increase it.
4. Observe the calibrated water-seal column for changes in patient pressure. When the suction is operating, the patient pressure equals the suction-control setting plus the water-seal column level. For gravity drainage, the patient pressure equals the calibrated water-seal column level only.
5. Observe the water seal for air leaks. Absence of bubbling with minimal float-ball oscillation indicates that there is no air leak. Constant or intermittent bubbling indicates a leak in either the chest-drainage system or the thoracic cavity (see Figure 49-2).

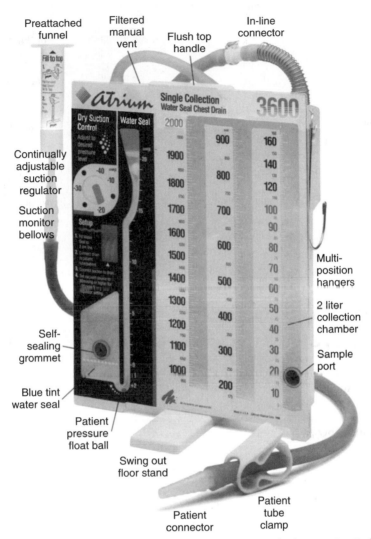

FIGURE 49-3 Atrium dry-suction collection unit. (Courtesy Atrium Medical Corporation, Hudson, NH.)

AGE-SPECIFIC CONSIDERATION

Infant or pediatric collection units are available in either wet- or dry-suction control models. The drainage chamber is smaller than the adult counterpart, and it has large, easy-to-read drainage gradations.

COMPLICATIONS

See Procedure 42.

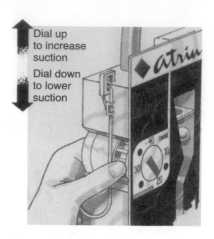

Dial up
to increase
suction

Dial down
to lower
suction

FIGURE 49-4 Dry-suction control regulator.
(Courtesy Atrium Medical Corporation, Hudson, NH.)

PATIENT TEACHING

See Procedure 42.

REFERENCES

Atrium. (1996a). *Atrium 2002 single collection water seal drainage unit instruction sheet.* Hudson, NH: Author.

Atrium. (1996b). *Atrium 3600 single collection dry suction chest drainage manual.* Hudson, NH: Author.

PROCEDURE 50

Thoracentesis

Deborah A. Upton, RN, BSN, CEN

INDICATION

Thoracentesis removes fluid (pleural effusion) from the pleural cavity for diagnostic or therapeutic purposes. Air or fluid in the pleural space may affect ventilatory mechanisms. Emergency needle thoracentesis for tension pneumothorax is discussed in Procedure 40.

CONTRAINDICATIONS AND CAUTIONS

1. An absolute contraindication for thoracentesis is needle insertion into an area of infection.

2. Relative contraindications include bleeding dyscrasias and anticoagulant therapy.
3. Caution should be used in the presence of a compromised respiratory status (e.g., a ventilator dependency, ruptured diaphragm, emphysema) or pleural adhesions, because of a higher incidence of pneumothorax secondary to lung perforation.

EQUIPMENT

Antiseptic solution
Sterile towels
Local anesthetic
Gauze dressings
Tape
Syringes and needles for local anesthesia
For aspiration:
    18- to 22-G needle, 3.75-5 cm long or
    16- to 20-G over-the-needle catheter or
    14- to 16-G through-the-needle catheter with plastic sleeve
    50- to 60-ml syringe
Three-way stopcock
Two curved hemostats
Intravenous (IV) extension tubing
18-G needle
Sterile basin (if vacuum bottle is not used)
500- to 1000-ml vacuum bottle(s) (optional)
NOTE: Preassembled kits containing some of this equipment are available.

PATIENT PREPARATION

1. Place the patient in a sitting position, leaning forward on a bedside table with arms crossed. If the patient cannot tolerate a sitting position, place him or her in a supine position.
2. Cleanse the site with an antiseptic solution. For the patient in a supine position, drape the area with a sterile towel. For the removal of pleural fluid, the insertion site is the posterior axillary line one intercostal space below the top of the fluid (Barefoot, 2001).
3. Administer atropine, if prescribed, to prevent a vasovagal response.
4. Instruct the patient to refrain from coughing during the procedure to prevent trauma to the lung.

PROCEDURAL STEPS

1. *Infiltrate the area with a local anesthetic directly inferior to the selected site. The needle-insertion site is directly over the top of the rib. Change to the 22-G needle and continue the anesthetic infiltration to the periosteum. If a rigid needle is used to withdraw fluid, advance the anesthetic needle until the pleural space is entered and fluid can be withdrawn. Note the depth of penetration at which fluid is aspirated by clamping a hemostat at the skin line of the anesthetic needle.

---

*Indicates portions of the procedure usually performed by a physician or an advanced practice nurse.

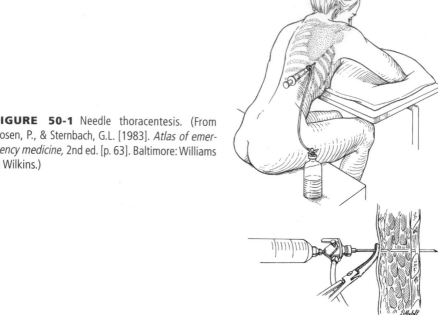

FIGURE 50-1 Needle thoracentesis. (From Rosen, P., & Sternbach, G.L. [1983]. *Atlas of emergency medicine,* 2nd ed. [p. 63]. Baltimore: Williams & Wilkins.)

2. *Insert the needle or catheter into the pleural space. The needle should be inserted directly over the top of a rib. A pop may be felt as the pleural space is entered.
   a. Rigid needle: Attach a 50- to 60-ml syringe to the needle via a three-way stopcock. Place a hemostat on the needle at the same depth as the hemostat on the anesthetic needle. Insert the needle to the depth of the hemostat (Figure 50-1).
   b. Over-the-needle catheter: Attach a 14- to 18-G over-the-needle catheter to a 50- to 60-ml syringe. Aspirate as the needle is advanced. After entering the pleural space, advance the catheter off the needle and withdraw the needle. Cover the open end of the catheter with a sterile, gloved finger when the needle is withdrawn.
   c. Through-the-needle catheter: Attach a three-way stopcock to the catheter and then turn it to the off position. Insert the needle into the pleural space. Guide the catheter, within the plastic sleeve, through the needle. Discard the plastic sleeve. Withdraw the needle, leaving the catheter in the pleural space (Figure 50-2). Cover the needle with the plastic needle guard.
3. *Withdraw fluid via a syringe and stopcock or a vacuum bottle.
   a. Syringe and stopcock: Attach the 50- to 60-ml syringe to the needle or catheter via a three-way stopcock. Withdraw the fluid and then turn the

---

*Indicates portions of the procedure usually performed by a physician or an advanced practice nurse.

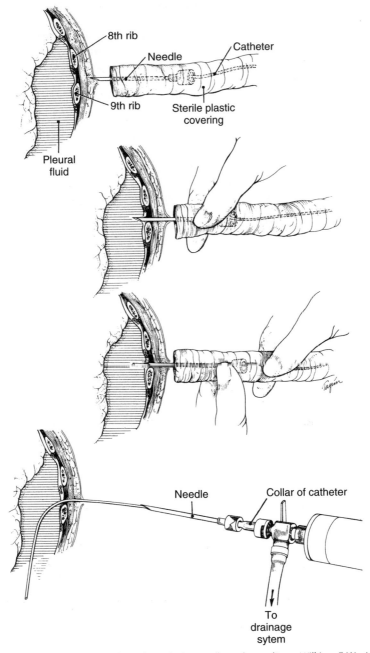

FIGURE 50-2 Thoracentesis with a through-the-needle catheter. (From Wilkins, E.W., Jr. [1989]. Thoracentesis [p. 1022]. In Wilkins, E.W. et al. [Eds.], *Emergency medicine: scientific foundations and current practice,* 3rd. ed. Baltimore: Williams & Wilkins.)

stopcock off to the patient to empty the syringe into a basin. Repeat until the desired amount of fluid is withdrawn.

   b. Vacuum bottle: Attach one end of the IV extension tubing to the catheter via a three-way stopcock, and the other end to an 18-G needle. Insert the needle into the top of the vacuum bottle and open the stopcock between the bottle and the patient.

4. *Withdraw the desired amount of fluid; 50-100 ml of fluid is required for laboratory diagnosis. For therapeutic drainage, fluid is removed in 50-ml increments until respiratory distress is relieved. It is recommended that no more than 1000-1500 ml of fluid be removed at a time owing to the risk of postprocedure pulmonary edema, hypovolemia, or hypoxemia (Barefoot, 2001). Turn the stopcock off to the tubing and withdraw the needle from the patient.

5. Apply a sterile dressing and obtain a chest x-ray film.

6. Fluid from the syringe or the bottle may be sent to the laboratory for analysis. Analyses that are performed frequently include Gram's stain, culture and sensitivity, acid-fast staining and culture, differential cell count, cytology, pH, specific gravity, total protein, glucose, and lactate dehydrogenase.

AGE-SPECIFIC CONSIDERATION

Landmarks and insertion techniques are the same for both pediatric and adult patients. A smaller needle or catheter is used for pediatric patients.

COMPLICATIONS

1. Pulmonary edema can result from removal of a large quantity of fluid. Do not remove more than 1000-1500 ml of fluid at one time.

2. Shearing of the plastic catheter may occur if the catheter is withdrawn through the needle.

3. Hypoxia may develop in patients with underlying respiratory pathology.

4. A hemothorax can result from laceration of the lung, diaphragm, or intercostal vessels.

5. Lung perforation can create a pneumothorax. Other internal organs, such as the spleen and liver, may also be perforated.

6. A hematoma may appear at the insertion site.

7. Vasovagal response.

PATIENT TEACHING

1. Immediately report any shortness of breath, faintness, bloody sputum, or chest pain.

2. Remain in a position of comfort for 1 hour after the procedure.

REFERENCE

Barefoot, W. (2001). Performing thoracentesis (pp. 145-150). In Lynn-McHale, D.J., & Carlson, K.K. (Eds), *AACN procedure manual for critical care*, 4th ed. Philadelphia: W.B. Saunders.

*Indicates portions of the procedure usually performed by a physician or an advanced practice nurse.

Circulation Procedures

Positioning the Hypotensive Patient

Maureen T. Quigley, MS, ARNP, CEN

INDICATION
Symptomatic hypotension caused by hypovolemia, vasovagal reaction, or medication.

CONTRAINDICATIONS AND CAUTIONS
1. Ensure the adequacy of airway, breathing, and circulation before initiating treatment.
2. The Trendelenburg position should be avoided in the presence of potential head or spinal cord injuries.
3. Patients who are in cardiogenic or anaphylactic shock may not be able to tolerate a supine or modified Trendelenburg position.
4. There is no measurable improvement of cardiopulmonary performance with the Trendelenburg position as compared with the supine position (Rivers et al., 2000).
5. Pulmonary gas exchange may decline, and the likelihood of aspiration of emesis may be increased in the Trendelenburg position (Rivers et al., 2000).
6. The Trendelenburg position is no longer a recommended treatment because of the potential for respiratory compromise due to the pressure on abdominal organs (Nettina, 2001).

PROCEDURAL STEPS
1. Place the patient in a supine position.
2. Raise the lower extremities to a maximum elevation of 45 degrees. This is known as the modified Trendelenburg position (Figure 51-1).

FIGURE 51-1 Modified Trendelenburg position. (From Finis, N.M. [1995]. Abdominal trauma [p. 241]. In Kitt S., Selfridge-Thomas J., Proehl J.A., & Kaiser J. [Eds.], *Emergency nursing: a physiologic and clinical perspective,* 2nd ed. Philadelphia: W.B. Saunders.)

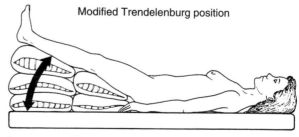

Modified Trendelenburg position

Lower extremities elevated   Patient flat

3. Do not lower the patient's head below the level of the body, because this places pressure on the diaphragm that may result in respiratory distress. It also increases intracranial pressure, potentially harming a patient with a neurologic deficit.

PATIENT TEACHING
1. Explain that the position is temporary.
2. Immediately report any difficulty in breathing.

REFERENCES
Nettina, S.M. (2001). *Lippincott manual of nursing practice*, 7th ed. Philadelphia: Lippincott Williams & Wilkins.

Rivers, E.P., Rady, M.Y. & Bilkovski, R. (2000). Approach to the patient in shock (pp. 215-228). In Tintinalli, J., Kelen, G., & Stapczynski, J.S. Hill (Eds.), *Emergency medicine: a comprehensive study guide*, 5th ed. New York: McGraw-Hill.

PROCEDURE 52

Doppler Ultrasound for Assessment of Blood Pressure and Peripheral Pulses

Maureen T. Quigley, MS, ARNP, CEN

INDICATIONS
1. To measure the blood pressure, pulse, or both, when auscultation by stethoscope is unsuccessful (i.e., in the presence of hypotension, faint Korotkoff sounds, or a noisy environment)
2. To assess peripheral blood flow when circulatory impairment or vascular trauma is suspected

CONTRAINDICATIONS AND CAUTIONS
1. Use of an ultrasonic transmission gel assists in optimal sound transmission and protects the crystals, which are found in the probe. The crystals transmit and receive signals. In emergency situations, a water-soluble gel, such as Surgilube, may be substituted for a conductive gel (Gorgas, 2004).

2. The probe should be checked regularly for damage to the electrode and integrity of the crystals.
3. Improper probe placement may lead to erroneous interpretations. Care should be taken to verify that the signal is coming from the intended vessel and not a collateral vessel. This can be determined by assessing the quality of the sound, as described in the Complications section of this procedure.
4. Excess pressure on the probe may compress the artery and abolish the signal.
5. Verify sensitivity when signals are absent from a position where they would normally be expected. Sensitivity may be verified by checking one's own pulses with the Doppler device.
6. The presence of a signal does not always indicate that circulation and perfusion are adequate to maintain viable tissue, just as absence of a signal does not always indicate that there is no blood flow through the vessel.
7. Tissue penetration varies, depending on which Doppler instrument is used. The higher-frequency sound waves yield better resolution for superficial vessels, and the lower-frequency sound waves allow penetration of deeper tissues with less scatter. Most Doppler instruments are supplied with a fixed frequency. The frequency required for the assessment of blood pressure and superficial peripheral blood flow is 2-10 MHz.
8. Falsely elevated pressures may be observed in patients with diabetes, obesity, or calcified vessels (Gorgas, 2004).

EQUIPMENT

Doppler probe with a frequency of 5-10 MHz (for limb arteries and veins)
    and an amplifier (Figure 52-1)
Ultrasonic transmission gel
Blood pressure cuff
Wet towel or tissue

PROCEDURAL STEPS
Blood Pressure Measurement

1. Place the blood pressure cuff on the upper arm, the thigh, or the ankle and apply a transmission gel to the skin over the brachial/popliteal artery or the

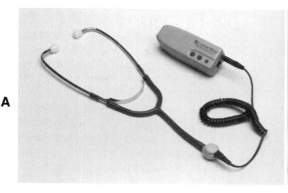
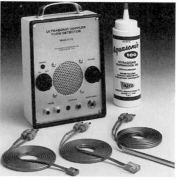

A   B

FIGURE 52-1 Examples of two commercially available Doppler devices. (Courtesy Medasonics, Newark, CA, and Parks Medical Electronics, Aloha, OR.)

posterior-tibial artery. Be sure the cuff is high enough on the limb that the Doppler probe can access the area with the strongest pulse.

2. Turn on the Doppler instrument and turn down the volume. Insert the stethoscope earpieces, if applicable.

3. Adjust the volume control as necessary.

4. Identify the brachial/popliteal pulse or the posterior-tibial pulse with the Doppler instrument.

5. Position the probe over the artery and tilt it so that it is at a 45-degree angle along the length of the vessel to optimize frequency shifts and signal amplitude (Figure 52-2).

6. Inflate the blood pressure cuff until the arterial sounds are no longer audible.

7. Deflate the cuff slowly, listening for the first sound, which reflects the systolic pressure. Diastolic pressure is recorded at the point at which there is a decrease in arterial wall motion (Pickering, 2002).

8. Clean the gel from the patient's skin with a wet towel or tissue.

9. Clean the face of the Doppler probe with a damp towel or tissue. Do not use alcohol or other organic solvents to clean the probe. The probe may be gas sterilized, but it should not be autoclaved or immersed in liquid.

Assessment of Peripheral Blood Flow

1. Apply a transmission gel to the skin over the vessel.

2. Turn on the Doppler instrument and turn down the volume. Insert the stethoscope earpieces, if applicable.

3. Place the probe over the vessel to be assessed and tilt the probe so that it is at a 45-degree angle to the vessel. Standard arterial locations include the brachial, radial, femoral, popliteal, dorsalis pedis, and posterior tibial pulses.

4. Adjust the volume control as necessary.

5. Mark the pulse location with a waterproof marker. Compare the blood flow bilaterally. Begin assessment of the extremity at its most distal aspect. If you do not find a pulse with the Doppler instrument, move to a more proximal site. Continue to move more proximally until you are able to identify the

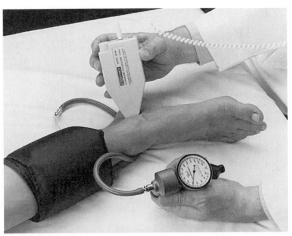

FIGURE 52-2 Measurement of systolic blood pressure in the ankle. (Courtesy Medasonics, Newark, CA.)

blood flow. The findings may then be recorded by describing the pulses at each location as absent, present, or diminished.

AGE-SPECIFIC CONSIDERATION

In infants, auscultation or Korotkoff sound techniques may underestimate true systolic pressure, and ultrasonic flow detectors are recommended (Pickering, 2002).

COMPLICATIONS

1. Absence of a Doppler signal may be due to any of the following:
   a. Blood flow at a speed less than the Doppler instrument can detect
   b. Excess pressure on the probe, causing occlusion of the vessel
   c. Too low volume setting
   d. Insufficient transmission gel
   e. Dead battery
   f. Damaged equipment
2. The signal may also be misinterpreted. Arterial sounds are loud, pulsatile, pumping sounds that are repeated with each cardiac cycle. Venous sounds are normally cyclic. They occur with respirations and on expiration; they produce a high-pitched sound that resembles a rushing wind.
3. The output of ultrasonic signals from diagnostic Doppler applications is very low; nevertheless, prolonged, unnecessary exposure to ultrasonic signals should be avoided to prevent tissue damage (Medasonics, 1985).

REFERENCES

Gorgas, D.L. (2004). Vital sign measurement (pp. 3-28). In Roberts, J.R., & Hedges, J.R. (Eds.), *Clinical procedures in emergency medicine*, 4th ed. Philadelphia: W.B. Saunders.

Medasonics (1985). *A Doppler instrument for the detection of blood flow: Ultrasound stethoscope, model BF4A*. Newark, CA: Author.

Pickering, T.G. (2002). Principles and techniques of blood pressure measurement. *Cardiology Clinics*, 20(2), 207-223.

Measuring Postural Vital Signs

*Margo E. Layman, MSN, RN, RNC, CN-A
and Maureen T. Quigley, MS, ARNP, CEN*

Postural vital signs are also known as orthostatic vital signs, tilt test.

INDICATIONS
1. To safely and noninvasively evaluate a patient's fluid status
2. To assess response to fluid therapy
3. To evaluate a patient with a history of known or suspected fluid loss secondary to vomiting, diarrhea, diaphoresis, bleeding, blunt abdominal or chest trauma, abdominal pain, unexplained syncope, weakness or dizziness, or autonomic dysfunction.

CONTRAINDICATIONS AND CAUTIONS
1. An assistant may be necessary because a patient with hypovolemia may experience dizziness, lightheadedness, or syncope when moving from a lying to a standing position for postural vital sign measurement. Do not leave the patient alone during this procedure.
2. Checking orthostatic vital signs is contraindicated in patients with supine hypotension, shock, or severe alteration in mental status, as well as in those who may have spinal, pelvic, or lower-extremity injuries (Gorgas, 2004).
3. Certain medications, such as sympatholytic drugs, diuretics, nitrates, narcotics, antihistamines, psychotropic agents, barbiturates, antihypertensives, and anticholergenics, can predispose a patient to orthostatic hypotension in the absence of hypovolemia. Studies have demonstrated a significant incidence of orthostatic hypotension, even in euvolemic patients.
4. Paradoxical bradycardia may be observed in hypovolemic patients who have rapid and massive bleeding; this may be interpreted as orthostasis (Gorgas, 2004).
5. Prevent unreliable results by avoiding invasive or painful procedures during the measurement of postural vital signs.

PATIENT PREPARATION
Have the patient lie in a supine position for 2-5 minutes before taking the initial measurements.

PROCEDURAL STEPS
1. Measure the blood pressure and heart rate measurements after the patient has been in supine position for 2-3 minutes. Taking two sets of measurements

and using the second set as baseline helps prevent false-positive results that are based on patient's sympathetic response (Roper, 1996).

2. Have the patient move from the supine to the sitting position (if three measurements are taken) or from supine to standing. If the patient is unable to stand for blood pressure measurement, try the high Fowler's position, although the results may be less credible. A supine-to-standing measurement is more accurate than a supine-to-sitting measurement (Gorgas, 2004).

3. Question the patient about weakness, dizziness, or visual dimming associated with a change of position. Note any pallor or diaphoresis. These symptoms are as important as the measurement of vital signs. If the patient becomes extremely dizzy and needs to lie down or becomes syncopal, the measurement should be terminated.

4. Take the standing or sitting blood pressure (in the same arm as the initial readings) and the heart-rate measurement within 1 minute. Support the patient's forearm at heart level when taking the blood pressure to prevent an inaccurate measurement.

5. If an intermediate sitting measurement was taken, have the patient move into the standing position and repeat steps 3 and 4.

6. Return patient to supine or sitting position.

7. Note all measurements on the patient record, including the position in which they were taken (i.e., with the patient lying, sitting, or standing). Positive findings are considered to be heart rate increase of 30 beats/min in adults and any postural fall in blood pressure that results in symptoms of cerebral hypofusion, such as dizziness and syncope (Gorgas, 2004). There may be accompanying changes in blood pressure; these changes are too variable to be considered a reliable indicator of blood loss (Gorgas, 2004).

AGE-SPECIFIC CONSIDERATIONS

1. The usefulness of orthostatic vital signs in children is not clear. Postural near-syncope or an increase in heart rate of 25 beats or more may be a predictor of dehydration in children (Gorgas, 2004).

2. Patients with nondemand pacemakers or those taking beta-blocking medications may not have significant changes in heart rate.

COMPLICATIONS

Weakness, dizziness, syncope, and falls

PATIENT TEACHING

Educate elderly patients or patients with postural symptoms about the importance of sitting for 5 minutes before getting out of bed, or standing after sitting for an extended length of time.

REFERENCES

Gorgas (2004). Vital-sign measurement procedures (pp. 3-28). In Roberts J.R., & Hedges J.R. (Eds.), *Clinical procedures in emergency medicine*, 4th ed. Philadelphia: W.B. Saunders.

Roper, M. (1996). Back to basic assessing orthostatic vital signs. *American Journal of Nursing*, 96(8), 43-46.

Pneumatic Antishock Garment

Reneé Semonin Holleran, RN, PhD, CEN, CCRN, CFRN, SANE

Also known as PASG, military antishock garment (MAST), or shock pants

INDICATIONS

Indications, contraindications, and cautions remain controversial and depend on local protocols. PASG use should be considered a short-term intervention until definitive care can be initiated. Indications for the use of PASG include the following:

1. Hypovolemic shock
2. Relative hypovolemia and hypotension:
   Neurogenic shock
   Drug overdose
   Septic shock
   Anaphylaxis
3. Stabilization of pelvic fractures with hypotension (American College of Surgeons, 2002; McSwain et al., 2003)
4. Significant trauma (see 1-3 above) followed by prolonged transport times (i.e., longer than 1 hour) (American College of Surgeons, 2002)

CONTRAINDICATIONS AND CAUTIONS

1. Absolute contraindications to the application of a PASG include the following:
   Pulmonary edema
   Congestive heart failure
   Penetrating thoracic injuries
2. Relative contraindications to the use of a PASG include the following:
   Cautious use during pregnancy (attempt to stabilize the patient by using the proper position [left lateral recumbent, tilted 15 degrees to the left] and inflation of the leg compartments only)
   Abdominal evisceration
   Impaled foreign body
3. The application of MAST or PASG for isolated lower-extremity fractures is not recommended because of the risk of the development of compartment syndrome (McSwain et al., 2003). A traction splint provides a better method of stabilizing isolated lower-extremity fractures.
4. During long transports (>1 hour), significant alterations in fluid and electrolyte balance may occur and may complicate management and recovery. The patient is also at great risk of developing pressure sores as well as compartment syndrome the longer the pants remain inflated.

5. The PASG application should always be used in combination with oxygen administration and intravenous (IV) fluid resuscitation.
6. If the patient is transported to a higher altitude (air transport or over mountain passes), the air in the PASG expands and the pressure inside the garment increases. Monitor the PASG pressures carefully in these situations.

EQUIPMENT

Pneumatic antishock garment (Figure 54-1)
Long spine board or scoop stretcher

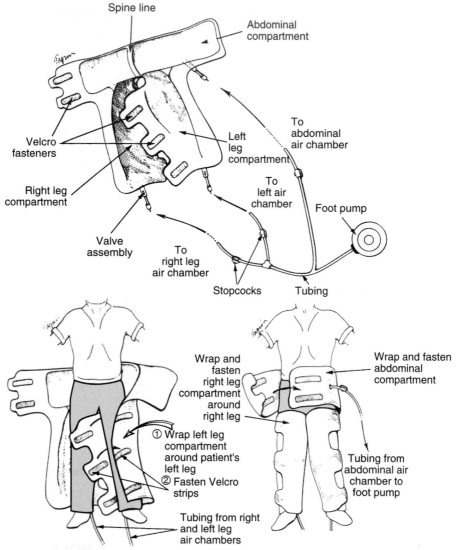

FIGURE 54-1 The pneumatic antishock garment (PASG). (From Wilkins, E.W., Jr. [Ed.] [1989]. *Emergency medicine: scientific foundations and current practice* [p. 23]. Baltimore: Williams & Wilkins.)

Foot pump or inflation device that comes with the pants
Board straps or cravats

PATIENT PREPARATION

1. If the mechanism of injury warrants immobilization, place the patient on a long spine board or a scoop stretcher (see Procedure 115). Position the garment on the board or the scoop stretcher before the patient. The patient may be log rolled onto the garment and the garment slid up under the patient (technique A), or, alternatively, the garment may be placed on the patient like trousers (technique B).
2. Remove all clothing and anything else below the waist to prevent compression injuries from objects such as belts when the pants are inflated.

PROCEDURAL STEPS (INFLATION)

1. Place the garment on the patient by using one of the following techniques:

Technique A

a. Release the leg and abdominal Velcro closures. Lay the garment out flat. Maintain in-line spinal immobilization if indicated (Figure 54-2).
b. One or more persons may then slide the garment underneath the patient. Raise the feet and slide the PASG under the buttocks. Elevate the buttocks slightly to place the pants properly.
c. Match the Velcro straps on the leg compartments and secure them (some models color code the Velcro closures). Fasten the Velcro straps on the abdominal compartment.

Technique B

(This method is contraindicated in persons with suspected or confirmed spinal fractures.)

a. Lay the garment out flat near the patient. Match the Velcro closures. Close the Velcro straps loosely on all three compartments.
b. Maintain in-line spinal immobilization, if appropriate. Position at least one person on each side of the patient near the patient's hips. If additional people are available, they may help elevate the hips or feet. Simultaneously, elevate the feet carefully while sliding the trousers over the feet and up the legs. Elevate the hips to allow the proper placement of the garment.
c. Readjust the Velcro straps to ensure a snug fit.

2. The abdominal compartment should be placed just below the rib cage so as not to reduce vital capacity and impair respiration.
3. Close the stopcock to the abdominal compartment and open the stopcocks to the leg compartments.
4. Attach the tubing from the foot pump to the three compartments. Some models have color-coded tubing for the different compartments.
5. Inflate the leg compartments with the pump until the pressure gauge (if present) indicates the appropriate amount of pressure. Some pants have a pop-off valve that limits the inflation pressure to 104 mm Hg. Crackling of the Velcro closures also indicates sufficient inflation. The goal is to achieve a systolic pressure of 100 mm Hg while using the lowest inflation pressure possible (<40 mm Hg). Patients in extremis may need rapid, simultaneous inflation of

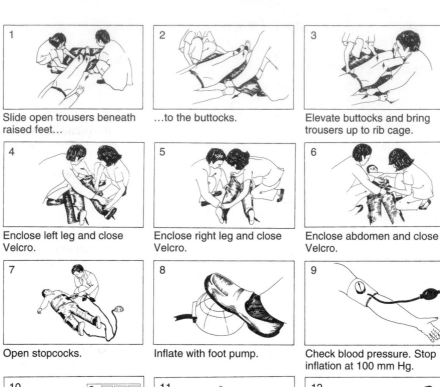

1 Slide open trousers beneath raised feet...	2 ...to the buttocks.	3 Elevate buttocks and bring trousers up to rib cage.
4 Enclose left leg and close Velcro.	5 Enclose right leg and close Velcro.	6 Enclose abdomen and close Velcro.
7 Open stopcocks.	8 Inflate with foot pump.	9 Check blood pressure. Stop inflation at 100 mm Hg.
10 Velcro straps, pop-off valves, or gauges prevent overinflation.	11 Close stopcocks.	12 The device can be left in place fully inflated for two hours if necessary.

FIGURE 54-2 Application of the pneumatic antishock garment. (Courtesy the American College of Surgeons, Committee on Trauma, with permission)

all three compartments to 100 mm Hg immediately on application of the garment. If the foot pump is not available, sufficient pressures may be obtained by manually inflating the compartments.

6. Recheck the patient's vital signs. Inflation should be stopped when the systolic pressure reaches 100 mm Hg.
7. If the systolic pressure has not increased to more than 100 mm Hg, inflate the abdominal compartment. (NOTE: This is a relative contraindication in pregnancy.)
8. Assess vital signs and respiratory effort frequently.
9. Secure the patient to the long board or scoop stretcher as necessary.

PROCEDURAL STEPS (DEFLATION)

1. Any patient who has had the PASG applied and inflated must be stabilized before the garment is deflated. Stabilization may be accomplished via intravenous fluids, hemorrhagic control, vasopressors, or surgical intervention. Deflation of the garment must be done slowly. Remind all providers that this device should never be cut off!
2. Assess vital signs while the garment is inflated.
3. Gradually release air from the abdominal compartment and recheck the vital signs. If the blood pressure has dropped more than 5 mm Hg, deflation should be stopped and more fluids administered (if necessary) to restore pressure. In addition to the drop in pressure, some protocols suggest stopping deflation if the heart rate increases by 10 beats per minute after deflation. If pressure is not restored, reinflate the abdominal compartment.
4. Continue to release air from the abdomen, assessing the patient's vital signs each time. Some protocols suggest waiting 5 minutes between each step of deflation, although this has not been fully researched or documented.
5. Release air from one leg of the PASG at a time, following the same procedure as above. If one leg is injured, release the pressure from the uninjured leg first.
6. Reassess the patient's condition frequently after deflation.
7. Do not remove the deflated garment from the patient, in the event that rapid reapplication is necessary.

AGE-SPECIFIC CONSIDERATIONS

1. Use of the PASG for children is not recommended in the prehospital setting (NIITSA, 1990).
2. Pediatric and toddler-sized PASGs are available.
3. If an adult-sized PASG must be used for a child, inflate the leg compartments only (Eichelberger et al., 1998).

COMPLICATIONS

1. Sudden and severe hypotension may ensue after sudden removal of the garment.
2. Metabolic acidosis may develop after prolonged use of the garment as a result of a release of lactic acid from peripheral tissues.
3. Respiratory compromise may occur as a result of decreased vital capacity or pulmonary congestion (see Contraindications and Cautions).
4. Decreases in renal blood flow may result in a decline in renal perfusion, glomerular filtration rate, and urine output.
5. Inflation of the abdominal compartment may aggravate lumbar instability because of the circumferential compartment expansion.
6. Bleeding from lower-extremity wounds may increase with increased blood pressure.
7. Skin breakdown and decubitus ulcer formation may occur.
8. Compartmental syndrome may develop in the lower extremities.

PATIENT TEACHING

1. The PASG is a temporary measure to help increase blood pressure or splint pelvic fractures.
2. Report any increases in pain in areas under the PASG.

REFERENCES

American College of Surgeons, Committee on Trauma. (2002). *Advanced trauma life support manual*. Chicago: Author.

Eichelberger, M.R., Partsch, G.S., Ball, J.W., Clark, J.R. et al. (1998). *Pediatric emergencies: a manual for prehospital care providers*, 2nd ed. Upper Saddle River, NJ: Brady Communications, Prentice-Hall.

McSwain, N., Frame, S., & Salomone J. (2003). *Basic and advanced prehospital trauma life support*. St. Louis: Mosby.

National Highway Transportation and Safety Administration (NHTSA). (1998). *Emergency medical technician: national standard curriculum*. Washington, DC: Author.

PROCEDURE 55

Therapeutic Phlebotomy

Maureen T. Quigley, MS, ARNP, CEN

Therapeutic phlebotomy (TP) is also known as blood letting. It is a simple and easy method to remove red blood cell mass and blood volume. For every 500 ml of blood withdrawn, 200-250 ml of iron is removed (Means, 1999). Iron is mobilized from tissue stores by the bone marrow as it replaces the lost hemoglobin.

INDICATIONS

1. To decrease blood volume in the presence of high blood viscosity (e.g., polycythemia vera). In patients with severe polycythemia (hematocrit >55%), phlebotomy enables a decrease in mean pulmonary artery pressure and pulmonary vascular resistance and improves exercise performance (Means, 1999).
2. To decrease iron stores in iron overload syndromes, such as hemochromatosis and both sporadic and familial porphyria cutanea tarda.
3. Rarely, therapeutic phlebotomy is advised in the patient with acute decompensation of cor pulmonale with marked polycythemia or for the rare patient who remains significantly polycythemic despite appropriate long-term oxygen therapy (Wiedemann, 2002).

CONTRAINDICATIONS AND CAUTIONS

1. A physician from the blood bank should be involved in the decision to perform therapeutic phlebotomy (American Association of Blood Banks, 2001).
2. A written order, including medical record number, date of birth, or social security number must be obtained before therapeutic phlebotomy. Also included should be the diagnosis, most recent hemoglobin or hematocrit

value, and the amount of blood to be removed. One unit is considered to be 450 ml (American Association of Blood Banks, 2001).

3. Patients who have bleeding disorders and those who are taking anticoagulant medications should be monitored closely.

4. Generally, less than 500 ml of blood is slowly removed, and the volume can be replaced with normal saline (Hamilton & Janz, 2002).

5. For patients with known atherosclerotic symptoms, such as angina or transient ischemic attacks, care should be given to prevent a large reduction in blood volume at one time (Bottomley & Lee, 1999).

EQUIPMENT

500- to 1000-ml vacuum bottle (a 1000-ml bottle may create too much negative pressure and collapse the vein)

Phlebotomy tubing with needles on both ends

or

Saf-T donor set (36-inch tubing with a 17-G needle on one end and a 15-G stopper-piercing needle on the other end) (anticoagulant is not required)

Blood pressure cuff or tourniquet

Antiseptic solution

Local anesthesia (optional)

Occlusive dressing (e g , Op-Site)

Gauze dressing

Hemostat

PROCEDURAL STEPS

1. Apply the tourniquet or blood pressure cuff and locate the most suitable antecubital vein.

2. Remove the tourniquet or deflate the blood pressure cuff.

3. Cleanse the site with antiseptic solution.

4. Clamp the tubing with the hemostat at the patient's end and insert the other end into the vacuum bottle. If using the Saf-T donor set, clamp the tubing to maintain the vacuum in the bottle and connect the 15-G stopper-piercing needle to the bottle.

5. Reapply the tourniquet or inflate the blood pressure cuff to a pressure between the patient's systolic and diastolic readings.

6. Inject 1-2 ml of local anesthetic intradermally at the venipuncture site or spray the site with ethyl chloride (optional).

7. Perform the venipuncture with the needle on the proximal end of the tubing.

8. Tape the needle in place and cover the site with an occlusive dressing.

9. Unclamp the hemostat and collect the desired amount of blood, usually 250 ml, in the collection bottle.

   a. If the blood return is slow, have the patient pump his or her hand. Reapply the tourniquet or blood pressure cuff. Increase the distance between the patient and the collection bottle. Check the position of the needle.

   b. When the blood collection takes longer than 10-15 minutes, a blood pressure cuff is more comfortable than a tourniquet. Release the cuff every 10-15 minutes.

10. Reclamp the tubing with the hemostat.

11. Release the tourniquet or deflate the cuff.

12. Withdraw the needle and apply pressure with a gauze dressing until the bleeding stops.
13. Assess and document the patient's vital signs.

AGE-SPECIFIC CONSIDERATION

Removal of smaller volumes of blood during therapeutic phlebotomy is recommended in the elderly.

COMPLICATIONS

Adverse effects include fainting, nausea, vomiting, and muscular twitching. If adverse effects occur, clamp the tubing and notify the physician.

PATIENT TEACHING

1. Rest for 15 minutes before moving to a sitting or standing position.
2. Eat and drink before the procedure, and drink after the procedure if not contraindicated.
3. Avoid vigorous exercise within 24 hours of therapeutic phlebotomy.
4. For patients with iron overload problems, iron supplements should not be used.
5. Patients with porphyria cutanea should avoid alcohol to prevent relapse.
6. Contact the American Porphyria Foundation (P.O. Box 22712, Houston, TX 77227; [713] 266-9617) for additional patient information.

REFERENCES

American Association of Blood Banks (AABB), (2001). *Standards for blood banks and transfusion services: technical manual*, 21st ed. Bethesda, MD: Author.

Bottomey, S.S., & Lee, G.R. (1999). Porphyria (pp. 1071-1102). In Lee (Ed.), *Wintrobe's clinical hematology*, 10th ed. Baltimore: Williams & Wilkins.

Hamilton, G.G., & Janz, T.G. (2002). Anemia, polycythemia and white blood cell disorders (pp. 1665-1687). In Marx, J.A, et al. (Eds.), *Rosen's emergency medicine: concepts and clinical practice*, 5th ed. St. Louis: Mosby.

Means, R. (1999). Polycythemia: erythrocytosis (pp. 1538-1554). In Lee G.R., Hockberger, R.S., & Walls, R.M., (Ed.), *Wintrobe's clinical hematology*, 10th ed. Baltimore: Williams & Wilkins.

Wiedemann, H.L. (2002). *Cor pulmonale.* UpToDate, version 10.2. Uptodate.com

Pericardiocentesis

Jean A. Proehl, RN, MN, CEN, CCRN
and Daun A. Smith, RN, MS, CEN

Pericardiocentesis is also known as pericardial "tap."

INDICATIONS

1. To assist in the diagnosis of pericardial tamponade in patients with decreased cardiac output, elevated central venous pressure with jugular vein distention, muffled heart tones, and hypotension (also known as Beck's triad) who have sustained blunt or penetrating trauma to the chest
2. To relieve pericardial tamponade secondary to infection, tumor, bleeding diathesis, or recent intracardiac instrumentation, such as pacemaker insertion
3. To assist in the diagnosis and treatment of patients in pulseless electrical activity
4. Computed tomography (CT)-guided pericardiocentesis is used in some situations (Duvernoy & Magnusson, 1996).

CONTRAINDICATIONS AND CAUTIONS

1. Extreme caution is necessary when performing pericardiocentesis on patients who are taking anticoagulant medication.
2. All equipment must be secured and properly grounded to prevent the delivery of current to the myocardium, which could cause ventricular fibrillation.
3. In CT-guided pericardiocentesis, impaired imaging can result in accidental cardiac or blood vessel perforation (Duvernoy & Magnusson, 1996).
4. Pericardiocentesis may be inadequate for traumatic pericardiocentesis; a pericardial window or other operative intervention may be necessary.

EQUIPMENT

16- or 18-G cardiac or spinal needle or 6-inch over-the-needle catheter
60-ml syringe
3-way stopcock
Alligator clamps/cable
Kelly clamp
Tape
12-lead electrocardiography (ECG) machine or 5-lead ECG monitor
Antiseptic solution
Gauze dressings
Local anesthetic (optional)
Syringe and needles for local anesthetic (optional)
Sterile gloves

Gown and mask

Cardiac resuscitation equipment at the bedside

Specimen containers for requested diagnostic tests (e.g., culture, cytology)

PATIENT PREPARATION

1. If possible, obtain a chest x-ray film and a 12-lead ECG before starting the procedure (see Procedure 59). Initiate pulse oximetry and ECG monitoring (Procedures 23 and 58).
2. If the patient is stable and able to tolerate sitting, place the patient in the semi-Fowler's position to facilitate the pooling of blood in the apex of the heart and to lower the diaphragm and abdominal organs.
3. Insert a nasogastric tube to decompress the stomach (see Procedure 101).
4. Connect the ECG limb leads to the patient.

PROCEDURAL STEPS

Standard Pericardiocentesis

1. Cleanse the chest from the left costal margin to the xiphoid process with an antiseptic solution.
2. *Infiltrate the area with a local anesthetic (if indicated).
3. *Nick the skin with the No. 11 blade (optional).
4. Attach the alligator clamp to the metal hub of the needle and to any anterior chest V ECG lead or the chest lead of a five-lead system. A rhythm strip of the V lead is then recorded to monitor for contact with the ventricle. If the patient does not have an organized electrical rhythm with an obvious ST segment, ECG monitoring via the alligator clamp is not indicated.
5. *Palpate the junction of the xiphoid process and the left costal arch. Insert the needle with obturator below the xiphoid process at a 30- to 45-degree angle and direct it toward the left shoulder (Figure 56-1). As soon as the needle punctures the skin, remove the obturator and attach a 60-ml syringe with a 3-way stopcock (Harper, 2004).
6. *Aspirate the plunger of the syringe gently as the needle is advanced. If the needle is inserted under electrocardiographic guidance, observed the V lead for a significant elevation of the ST segment or premature ventricular contractions (see Procedure 89: Temporary Transvenous Pacemaker Insertion, Figure 89-2, for an illustration of ST segment elevation).
7. *After a blood flash is seen, the following may occur:
   a. If blood is obtained and the monitor does not show ST-segment or T-wave changes; large, widened QRS complexes; or premature ventricular contractions, then as much blood or fluid as possible is withdrawn.
   b. Should any of the above ECG changes occur (indicating that the needle is in the epicardium or the myocardium), the needle is withdrawn slowly until the patient's baseline rhythm returns. It is important to note that myocardial scarring due to an infarction or disease may prevent an injury pattern from occurring (Harper, 2004).

---

*Indicates portions of the procedure usually performed by a physician or an advanced practice nurse.

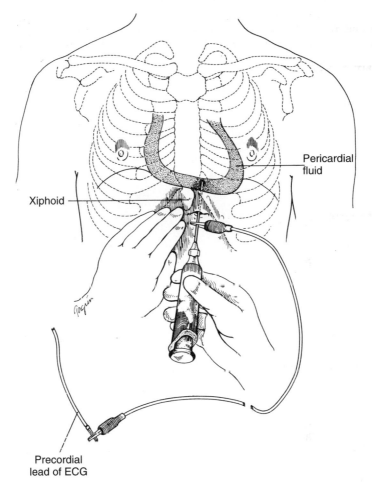

FIGURE 56-1 Pericardiocentesis guided by ECG. (From Wilkins, E.W., Jr. [Ed.] [1989]. *Emergency medicine: scientific foundations & current practice* [p. 1017]. Baltimore: Williams & Wilkins.)

8. *If the syringe becomes full during the aspiration of blood, use the stopcock to expel the blood from the syringe into an emesis basin instead of disconnecting the needle. After as much blood as possible is aspirated (anywhere from 10-150 ml), the syringe is removed, the three-way stopcock closed, and the needle is taped securely to the chest or sutured in place, or the Kelly clamp is attached at the level of the skin and secured to prevent advancement or displacement of the needle. Blood removed from the pericardial sac generally does not clot; however, brisk bleeding may result in blood being withdrawn from the ventricle before defibrination occurs and, therefore, the blood may clot (Harper, 2004).

9. Monitor the patient closely for recurring symptoms of cardiac tamponade.

---

*Indicates portions of the procedure usually performed by a physician or an advanced practice nurse.

CT-Guided Pericardiocentesis

1. Place the patient in a supine position on the movable CT tabletop.
2. *Determine the entry site based on contiguous slices of the heart and the pericardium.

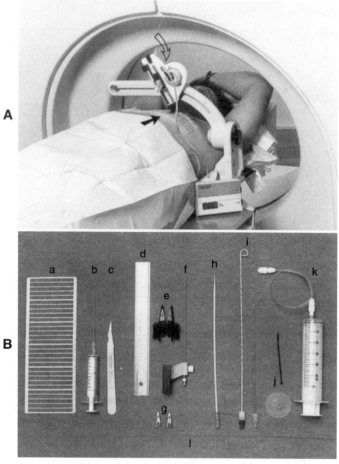

FIGURE 56-2 A, CT-guided pericardiocentesis. The CT guide (*open arrow*) is positioned at the level of the entry site. After the skin is disinfected, a sterile radiopaque grid (*solid arrow*) is placed over the entry area. **B,** Equipment includes *(a)* radiopaque grid, *(b)* 20-ml syringes, *(c)* scalpel, *(d)* ruler, *(e)* needle guide, *(f)* needle holder with 0.9-mm needle, *(g)* alligator cable, *(h)* 3.3-mm dilator, *(i)* 2.3-mm drainage catheter with stiffening cannula, *(j)* retention disk, *(k)* 60-ml syringe with connecting tubing, *(l)* 0.46-mm guide wire. (From Duvernoy, O., & Magnusson, A. [1996]. CT-guided pericardiocentesis [p. 776]. *Acta Radiologica, 37,* 775-778.)

---

*Indicates portions of the procedure usually performed by a physician or an advanced practice nurse.

3. The base of the guidance device is placed under the patient at the level of the entry site.
4. *Disinfect the skin site and place a sterile, radiopaque grid over the entry area (Figure 56-2).
5. *The needle path, direction, and depth is determined by the radiologist, and the puncture is performed when the needle tip reaches the determined site.
6. *The needle placement is confirmed and the fluid is drained.
7. The patient is monitored as noted earlier.

Echocardiographic-Guided Pericardiocentesis
1. *The skin is anesthetized and the probe is positioned on the skin.
2. *The needle is set at an unchangeable angle to the probe (Suehiro et al., 1996).
3. *The puncture is made, and after the tip of the needle enters the pericardial space, as seen on the monitor, a J wire is inserted through the needle until its tip enters the pericardial space.
4. *The needle is removed and an angiographic catheter is inserted.
5. *The effusion is drained and the catheter is connected to the extension tubing for continuous drainage.
6. The patient is monitored as noted above.

COMPLICATIONS
1. Laceration of the ventricle or a coronary vessel, which may result in tamponade or myocardial infarction
2. Puncture of the lung resulting in a pneumothorax
3. Cardiac dysrhythmia, including cardiac arrest
4. Puncture of the aorta, inferior vena cava, esophagus, stomach, liver, or peritoneum
5. Decreased cardiac output caused by continued leakage into the pericardial sac
6. Venous air embolism
7. Sudden ventricular dilatation and pulmonary edema (Simon & Brenner, 2002)
8. Pericarditis (late)

REFERENCES
Duvernoy, O., & Magnusson, A. (1996). CT-guided pericardiocentesis. *Acta Radiologica, 37,* 775-778.
Harper, R.J. (2004). Pericardiocentesis (pp. 305-322). In Roberts, J.R., & Hedges, J.R. (2004). *Clinical procedures in emergency medicine,* 4th ed. Philadelphia: W.B. Saunders.
Suehiro, S., Hattori, K., Shibata, T., et al. (1996). Echocardiography-guided pericardiocentesis with a needle attached to a probe. *Annals of Thoracic Surgery, 61,* 741-742.
Simon, R.R., & Brenner, B.E. (2002). *Emergency procedures & techniques,* 4th ed. Philadelphia: Lippincott Williams & Wilkins.

*Indicates portions of the procedure usually performed by a physician or an advanced practice nurse.

Emergency Thoracotomy and Internal Defibrillation

Jean A. Proehl, RN, MN, CEN, CCRN
and Daun A. Smith, RN, MS, CEN

Emergency thoracotomy is also known as open or resuscitative thoracotomy, "cracking the chest."

INDICATIONS

To maximize resuscitative efforts for penetrating trauma patients in the face of actual or impending cardiac arrest.

The specific goals of emergency thoracotomy are the following (Boczar & Rivers, 2004):

1. To relieve cardiac tamponade
2. To support cardiac function via direct cardiac compression, cross-clamping of the aorta, and internal defibrillation
3. To control hemorrhage from the heart or great vessels

CONTRAINDICATIONS AND CAUTIONS

1. The health-care team's risk of exposure to blood and body fluids is high, especially if internal massage is performed on a patient who has fractured ribs.
2. Emergency thoracotomy is not indicated for patients who have massive central nervous system injuries, blunt trauma, or other injuries that are incompatible with life.
3. The ideal location for a thoracotomy is the operating room. A thoracotomy should be performed in the emergency department only when the patient is too unstable to be transported to the operating room. If no operating room or surgeon is available to assume the patient's care after initial management in the emergency department, this procedure should not be performed.
4. In the patient who has intra-abdominal bleeding, a major risk associated with thoracotomy is release of abdominal tamponade before aortic control can be achieved. This results in rapid exsanguination and death.
5. If the patient is presumed or known to have been in cardiac arrest for a prolonged period of time, the chance for survival after emergency thoracotomy is small. Indicators of poor prognosis include multiple major injuries; blunt trauma to the thorax, abdomen, or both; absent pupillary reflexes; no respiratory effort; and no palpable pulse. Patients with the best prognosis for survival after an emergency thoracotomy are those who have suffered a single penetrating injury to the left side of the chest and who have had vital signs and pupillary response within the 5 minutes before the thoracotomy is performed (Aihara et al., 2001; Coats et al., 2001; Miglietta et al., 2001; Clemence, 2000).

6. On rare occasions, patients regain consciousness during thoracotomy. In this event, chemical and physical restraint are required immediately to prevent the patient from causing further injury by pulling on clamps, tubes, and so forth. If chemical paralytics are used, analgesics and sedatives should also be given to any patient who demonstrates viable perfusion during resuscitation.

EQUIPMENT

Antiseptic solution
Gown, gloves, mask, and protective eyewear for all team members
Suction setup with long extension tubing and a Yankauer tip
Sterile thoracotomy tray consisting minimally of the following:
    Knife handles (2 long and 2 short)
    No. 11 blade
    Rib cutter
    Rib spreaders
    Long scissors (Mayo), curved and straight
    Vascular clamps (Mixter), extra long, medium long, and regular Satinsky clamp
    Needle holders, regular and 9-inch vascular
    Tissue forceps (Russian, DeBakey, and thoracic DeBakey)
    Toothed forceps (Brown, 8-inch Peons)
    Noncrushing clamps (bronchial)
    Lebsche knife and mallet (optional)
    Lap pads (sterile gauze sponges in packages of five, each marked with a blue tab for ease in counting, which are used to absorb blood)
Cardiac monitor and defibrillator
Internal defibrillator paddles and cable
Pledgets
Nonabsorbable suture (e.g., 3-0 silk)
Skin stapler with 6-mm staples (optional)
Sterile saline solution
Gauze dressings

PATIENT PREPARATION

1. If time allows, prepare the patient's chest by scrubbing it with an antiseptic solution, wiping it with a sterile towel, and applying antiseptic as a paint solution. In most situations, time does not permit thorough skin cleansing, and in these situations, pouring full-strength antiseptic solution on the patient's chest before making the incision is acceptable.
2. Mechanical ventilation via an endotracheal tube must be in progress.
3. Establish large-bore intravenous (IV) access and request blood for transfusion immediately.
4. For patients in cardiac arrest, continue external cardiac massage until the thoracic incision is made.
5. Attach the electrocardiograph leads to the patient's limbs (see Procedure 58).

PROCEDURAL STEPS

1. Turn on full-strength suction and attach it to a sterile Yankauer tip via the extension tubing. Assemble the internal paddles.

2. *Make an anterolateral incision in the fourth or fifth intercostal space (Figure 57-1).
3. *Incise the skin and subcutaneous tissue until the intercostal muscles are exposed (Figure 57-2).
4. *Enter the pleural space by pushing your index finger through the intercostal space near the sternal border, and then, posteriorly, running along the superior border of the rib (Figure 57-3). Ventilations should be interrupted until the incision is complete.
5. *Insert the rib spreaders and expose the pleural cavity. Pick up the pericardium with the toothed forceps and open it with scissors, taking care not to sever the phrenic nerve (Figure 57-4).

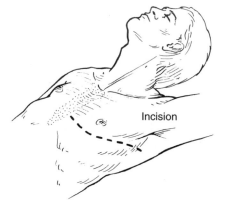

FIGURE 57-1 Anterolateral incision for thoracotomy. (From Rosen, P., & Sternbach, G.L. [1983]. *Atlas of emergency medicine,* 2nd ed. [p. 51]. Baltimore: Williams & Wilkins.)

Incision

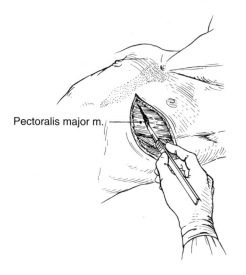

FIGURE 57-2 Intercostal muscle dissection. (From Rosen, P., & Sternbach, G.L. [1983]. *Atlas of emergency medicine,* 2nd ed. [p. 51]. Baltimore: Williams & Wilkins.)

Pectoralis major m.

*Indicates portions of the procedure usually performed by a physician or an advanced practice nurse.

6. *Inspect the heart. If there is a penetrating injury, it can be occluded temporarily with direct pressure by placing a finger into the hole (Figure 57-5). Alternatively, a large Foley catheter (e.g., 28 French) can be inserted, and the inflated balloon can be used to occlude the hole. Be sure to inflate the balloon with sterile fluid. Also, blood and IV fluid can be infused directly into the heart via the catheter. The defect is then sutured with a nonabsorbable suture and pledgets. Pledgets are used to help hold the sutures in the friable myocardial muscle (Figure 57-6). The defect may also be stapled shut with a skin stapler for temporary control of hemorrhage (Boczar & Rivers, 2004).

7. *Cardiac massage may be performed with either one or two hands by compressing the heart against the sternum. Compress in a superior-to-inferior direction to mimic the normal blood flow from the atria to the ventricles.

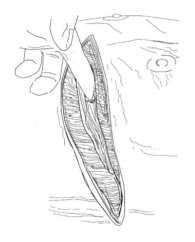

FIGURE 57-3 The fastest way to enter the pleural space without risking injury to the underlying lung is to push the index finger through the intercostal space near the sternal border and then forcefully push it posteriorly, running it along the superior border of the rib. (From Wahlstrom, H.E., Carroll, B.J., & Phillips, E.H. [1986]. Emergency thoracotomy: indications and technique. *Surgical Rounds, 9,* 25.)

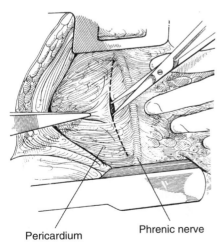

Pericardium   Phrenic nerve

FIGURE 57-4 Release of pericardial tamponade. (From Wilkins, E.W., Jr. [Ed.]. [1989]. *Emergency medicine: scientific foundations and current practice,* 3rd ed. [p. 1019]. Baltimore: Williams & Wilkins.)

---

*Indicates portions of the procedure usually performed by a physician or an advanced practice nurse.

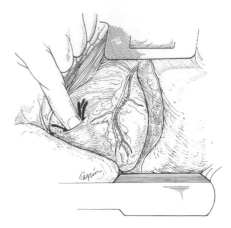

FIGURE 57-5 Occlusion of bleeding after a penetrating injury to the myocardium. (From Wilkins, E.W., Jr. [Ed.]. [1989]. *Emergency medicine: scientific foundations and current practice,* 3rd ed. [p. 1019]. Baltimore: Williams & Wilkins.)

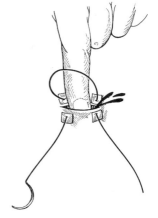

FIGURE 57-6 Use of Teflon pledgets to close a myocardial defect. (From Wilkins, E.W., Jr. [Ed.]. [1989]. *Emergency medicine: scientific foundations and current practice,* 3rd ed. [p. 1020]. Baltimore: Williams & Wilkins.)

8. *Retract the lung and inspect the descending aorta. The descending aorta may be occluded until the intravascular volume is restored and the blood pressure returns to normal. This is accomplished by compressing the aorta against the spine or by cross-clamping (Figure 57-7).
9. Document the time that the aorta is clamped.
10. *Pulmonary injuries may be controlled by clamping across the parenchyma proximal to the injury or across the hilum of the lung (Figure 57-8), or by wrapping the hilum with a Penrose drain and then providing traction to occlude the vessels and control hemorrhage.
11. To perform internal defibrillation:
    a. Place the sterile paddles on the sterile field and have the physician hand you the connector end of the cable to plug into the monitor or defibrillator, or pick up the connector without contaminating the field.
    b. Turn on the defibrillator and charge the paddles (usually 30 joules for adults). Internal paddles are programmed to deliver no more than 50 joules.

---

*Indicates portions of the procedure usually performed by a physician or an advanced practice nurse.

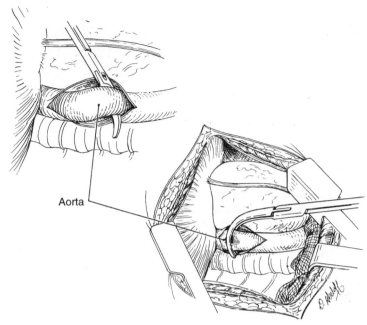

FIGURE 57-7 Cross-clamping the aorta. (From Rosen, P., & Sternbach, G.L. [1983]. *Atlas of emergency medicine,* 2nd ed. [p. 56]. Baltimore: Williams & Wilkins.)

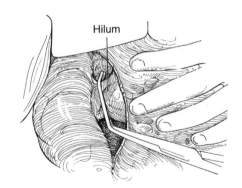

FIGURE 57-8 Clamping the hilum of the lung with an appropriate vascular clamp. A Satinsky clamp is shown. (From Wilkins, E.W., Jr. [Ed.]. [1989]. *Emergency medicine: scientific foundations and current practice,* 3rd ed. [p. 1020]. Baltimore: Williams & Wilkins.)

   c. *Place the paddles on opposite sides of the myocardium. A saline-soaked gauze dressing between the paddles and the myocardium may be used to improve conduction and decrease myocardial injury (Figure 57-9). Make sure all personnel clear the stretcher; state, "All clear"; and discharge the current into the paddles. (NOTE: Some monitors or defibrillators require a second person to discharge the paddles from the defibrillator. In this instance, the physician holding the paddles should say "All clear" before the paddles are discharged.)

---

*Indicates portions of the procedure usually performed by a physician or an advanced practice nurse.

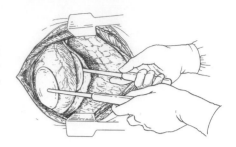

FIGURE 57-9 Internal defibrillation. (From Rosen, P., & Sternbach, G.L. [1983]. *Atlas of emergency medicine,* 2nd ed. [p. 55]. Baltimore: Williams & Wilkins.)

    d. Monitor the electrocardiograph for improvement in rhythm and repeat these steps as necessary.

12. If the patient appears to be salvageable, plan an immediate transport to the operating room. In anticipation of the transfer, notify the operating room and prepare the patient (e.g., move all IV fluids, the portable oxygen tank, the cardiac monitor, and so forth, to the stretcher). If necessary, have the security personnel or other staff members clear the corridors and secure an elevator to expedite the transfer.

AGE-SPECIFIC CONSIDERATIONS

1. Small-scale equipment is needed for pediatric patients, including rib spreaders, vascular clamps, and internal paddles for defibrillation. Four-cm paddles are used for large children, whereas 2-cm paddles are used for infants and toddlers (Clemence, 2000).
2. Only 5-20 joules are used for pediatric patients, compared with 30-50 joules for adults (Clemence, 2000).

COMPLICATIONS

1. Accidental lung injury occurring during incision leading to the pleural space
2. Phrenic nerve transection causing diaphragmatic paralysis
3. Injury to coronary arteries while suturing lacerations or attempting to relieve a pericardial tamponade
4. Injury to the heart while performing compressions against a fractured sternum or rib
5. Hemorrhage from internal mammary arteries
6. Organ and tissue ischemia from aortic clamping (If the systolic blood pressure cannot be raised above 70 mm Hg after 30 minutes of cross-clamping the aorta, resuscitative efforts should be discontinued [Boczar & Rivers, 2004].)

REFERENCES

Aihara, R., Millham, F.H., Blansfield, J., & Hirsch, E.F. (2001). Emergency room thoracotomy for penetrating chest injury: effect of an institutional protocol. *Journal of Trauma, 50,* 1027-1030.

Boczar, M.E., & Rivers, E. (2004). Resuscitative thoracotomy (pp. 336-353). In Roberts J.R. & Hedges J.R. (Eds.), *Clinical procedures in emergency medicine,* 4th ed. Philadelphia: W.B. Saunders.

Clemence, B. (2000). Emergency department thoracotomy: nursing implications for pediatric cases. *International Journal of Trauma Nursing, 6*(4), 123-127.

Coats, T.J., Keogh, S., Clark, H., & Neal, M. (2001). Prehospital resuscitative thoracotomy for cardiac arrest after penetrating trauma: rationale and case scenarios. *Journal of Trauma, 50,* 670-673.

Miglietta, M.A., Robb, T.V., Eachempati, S.R., et al. (2001). Current opinion regarding indications for emergency department thoracotomy. *Journal of Trauma, 51,* 67—6.

PROCEDURE 58

Electrocardiographic Monitoring

Mike D. McMahon, RN, BSN

Electrocardiographic monitoring is also known as ECG or EKG monitoring or cardiac monitoring. EKG monitoring is from the term "Elektrokardiogramme" used by Einthoven over 100 years ago.

INDICATION
To continuously monitor cardiac rate and rhythm.

CONTRAINDICATIONS AND CAUTIONS
1. All equipment should be well grounded to prevent electrical shock and electrical interference on the ECG tracing.
2. Always remember to treat the patient and not the monitor because the patient's clinical condition is more important than the rhythm.
3. Monitors and printers may be capable of displaying heart rhythms at different frequency ranges. Diagnostic frequency (0.05-150 Hz) should be used for interpreting such points as waveform duration and ST changes. If the monitor and the printer are at different frequencies, subtle changes may be seen in the ECG between the two sources. Twelve-lead ECGs are interpreted at the frequency range of 0.05 to 150 Hz.
4. Standard calibration is 1 mV = 10 mm, and standard speed is 25 mm/sec. Changes in either parameter should be documented in the patient's record.
5. Changes in body position may cause changes in the patient's rhythm, the same as changing electrode positions.

EQUIPMENT
Cardiac monitor
ECG cable (3 or 5 lead system)

Pregelled disposable electrodes (3-5)
Razor (optional)
Alcohol wipes (optional)
Dry gauze dressings (optional)

PROCEDURAL STEPS

1. Turn on the monitor.
2. Select the desired lead (Figures 58-1 through 58-4). Lead II is the most commonly used monitoring lead. Marriott's modified chest lead 1 (MCL_1) aids in QRS morphology differentiation, as does Marriott's MCL_6 (Wagner, 2001).
3. Connect the electrodes to the lead wires and place electrodes on clean, dry skin at the appropriate sites, per Figures 58-1 to 58-4. Avoid placing the electrodes over large muscle masses and bony structures.
4. Observe the ECG tracing. Ideally, the tracing should be free of excessive artifact and should have an R wave that is adequate to allow for accurate heart-rate determinations.
5. Set the heart-rate alarm limits (based on institutional or unit policy/standards) and turn on the alarms.

TROUBLESHOOTING ECG TECHNICAL PROBLEMS

1. Alternating current interference (also known as 60-cycle interference) (Figure 58-5).
   Possible causes
   a. Nearby electrical equipment, power cords, electrical wiring in room walls and floors

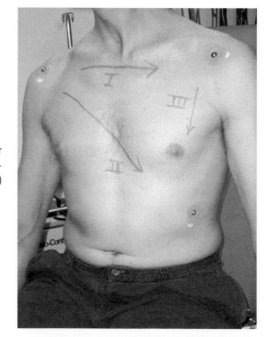

FIGURE 58-1 Electrode placement for leads I, II, and III. The arrows point to the positive electrode. (Courtesy Mike D. Mc Mahon.)

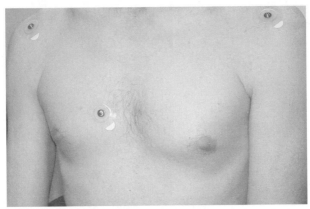

FIGURE 58-2 Marriott's MCL$_1$ using a 3-wire cable. The right and left arm leads remain in the standard position. The left leg lead is placed at the V$_1$ position, and the monitor is set to display lead III. (Courtesy Mike D. Mc Mahon.)

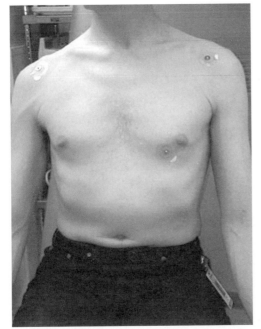

FIGURE 58-3 Marriott's MCL$_6$ using a 3-wire cable. The right and left arm leads remain in the standard position. The left leg lead is placed at the V$_6$ position, and the monitor is set to display lead III. (Courtesy Mike D. Mc Mahon.)

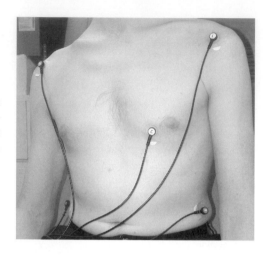

FIGURE 58-4 Five-wire placement. The limb leads are placed in the standard positions, and the chest lead can be placed across the chest. V$_3$ lead placement is shown here. (Courtesy Mike D. Mc Mahon.)

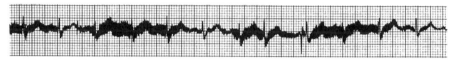

FIGURE 58-5 Common ECG problem patterns: alternating-current electrical interference (60 cycles per second).

    b. Improper grounding of electrical equipment in the area
    c. Unshielded lead wires or patient cable
    d. Loose connections in the system (e.g., electrodes, lead wires, cable)
    e. Inadequate skin preparation
    f. Dry electrodes
    g. Stress on patient cables
  Solutions
    a. Ground equipment in patient area properly.
    b. Verify connections of electrodes, leads, and cable.
    c. Prepare the skin by performing the following procedure:
       Clip hair as necessary
       Cleanse the skin with an alcohol wipe
       Abrade the skin with a dry gauze pad
       Apply new electrodes
2. Low voltage (Figure 58-6)
  Possible causes
    a. Low-gain setting on the ECG monitor
    b. Poor electrode contact or disconnected electrode
    c. Broken or disconnected lead wire
    d. Loose cable connection
    e. Low amplitude of QRS signal due to changing the patient's position

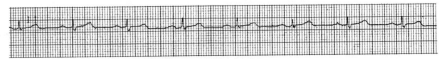

FIGURE 58-6 Common ECG problem patterns: low voltage.

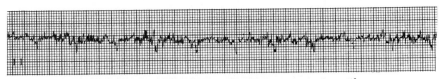

FIGURE 58-7 Common ECG problem patterns: excessive artifact.

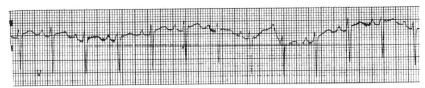

FIGURE 58-8 Common ECG problem patterns: wandering baseline.

Solutions
a. Increase the gain on the monitor.
b. Verify that all the connections are intact.
c. Change the electrodes.
d. Select another lead to monitor.

3. Excessive artifact (Figure 58-7)
   Possible causes
   a. Patient movement
   b. Loose electrode, lead, or cable connections
   c. Intermittent electrical interference
   Solutions
   a. Verify the placement of the electrodes, or move the electrodes to new locations, where there is less skeletal muscle.
   b. Replace any loose electrodes.
   c. Check the connections.
   d. Support the lead wires and the cable to prevent tension on the cable-lead system caused by patient movement.

4. Wandering baseline (Figure 58-8)
   Possible causes
   a. Cable movement with respirations or patient movement
   b. Poor electrode contact or location
   c. Excess tension on the cable-lead system

Solutions
a. Reposition the cable to a place where there is less movement.
b. If necessary, change the electrodes and select a new location.
c. Secure the cable-lead system to reduce tension.

PATIENT TEACHING
1. Report any chest discomfort, palpitations, shortness of breath, or related symptoms immediately.
2. Report any disconnections in the system.

REFERENCE

Wagner, G.S. (2001). *Marriott's practical electrocardiography*, 10th ed. Philadelphia: J.B. Lippincott.

PROCEDURE 59

12-, 15-, and 18-Lead Electrocardiograms

Mike D. McMahon, RN, BSN

The 12-lead electrocardiogram is also known as a 12-lead ECG. The 15-lead ECG involves using right-sided chest wall lead placements of V_{4R}, V_{5R}, and V_{6R} in the ECG. The 18-lead ECG includes the left posterior leads, V_7, V_8, and V_9.

INDICATIONS
1. To aid in the diagnosis of acute myocardial ischemia, injury, or infarction (MI)
   a. 12-lead ECG is an American Heart Association class I recommendation for prehospital advanced life support units when presented with a patient suspected of having an acute MI.
   b. A 15-lead ECG is used to determine right ventricular myocardial infarction. A 15-lead ECG is indicated when an inferior wall MI is suspected. Patients who present with a right ventricular infarct associated with an inferior wall MI tend to have a worse cardiac output (Fijewski et al., 2002).
   c. An 18-lead ECG is used to determine posterior wall myocardial infarction. An 18-lead ECG is indicated when there is ST-segment depression in the precordial leads (V_{1-3}) of the 12-lead ECG (Wung & Drew, 2001).

2. To diagnose and differentiate cardiac dysrhythmias and conduction defects
3. Patients who present to the emergency department after injuries that cause blunt chest trauma (Walsh et al., 2001).

CONTRAINDICATIONS AND CAUTIONS

1. The sensitivity of a 12-lead ECG in the diagnosis of acute MI is approximately 50% on initial presentation to the emergency department. Serial ECGs or ST-segment trending (Procedure 60) should be performed to observe for changes in the patient's ECG (Green & Hill, 2000).
2. All electrical equipment, including the ECG machine, should be well grounded to prevent electrical shock and electrical interference on the ECG tracing.
3. Do not touch the ECG machine, the patient cable, or the patient during cardioversion or defibrillation.
4. When collecting ECGs with placements other than the standard lead placements, the lead placements that were used should be labeled on the printout.

EQUIPMENT

Multiple-lead ECG machine, including cable and leads
Electrodes (pregelled disposable electrodes, suction cups, or plates)
Electrical conductive gel (if suction cups or plates are used)

PATIENT PREPARATION

1. Center the patient on the bed so that no part of the body touches the side rails, the head, or the foot of the bed
2. To obtain a good tracing, place the head of the bed as flat as the patient can tolerate.

PROCEDURAL STEPS

1. Connect the power cord to a grounded electrical outlet and turn on the ECG machine.
2. Enter the patient demographic information necessary for your equipment.
3. Apply limb leads. If plates or suction cups are used, a conductive gel must be used. Limb leads are placed on the medial aspect of each lower leg. Plates and suction cups are placed on the medial aspect of each forearm, and pregelled electrodes are placed on the outer aspect of each upper arm.
4. Apply the precordial leads. For a 12-lead ECG, lead V_1 is located in the fourth intercostal space (ICS) along the right sternal border. Lead V_2 is located in the fourth ICS along the left sternal border. Lead V_4 is located in the fifth ICS at the midclavicular line. Lead V_3 is located midway between V_2 and V_4 in the fifth ICS. Lead V_6 is located at the midaxillary line. Lead V_5 is located midway between V_4 and V_6. Leads V_{4-6} share the horizontal axis (Figure 59-1).
5. Connect the electrodes to the appropriate lead wires. Lead wires are labeled for each location.
6. Instruct the patient to relax and lie as still as possible. Assure the patient that this procedure takes only 10-15 seconds.
7. Press the appropriate button to record the ECG.
8. Precordial lead placement for the 15-lead ECG (right-sided) is as follows (Figure 59-2). V_{1R} is at the fourth ICS along the left sternal border (same as

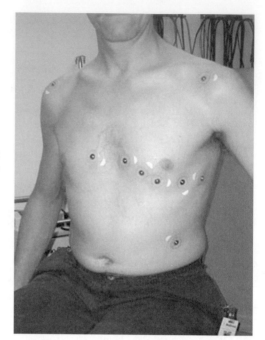

FIGURE 59-1 Standard precordial chest lead placement for a 12-lead ECG. (Courtesy Mike D. Mc Mahon.)

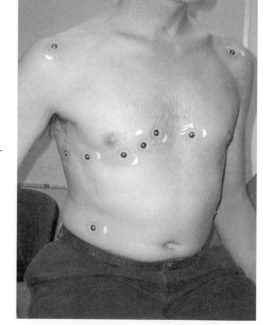

FIGURE 59-2 Precordial leads for right-sided ECG. (Courtesy Mike D. Mc Mahon.)

V_2). V_{2R} is at the fourth ICS along the right sternal border (same as V_1). V_{4R} is at the fifth ICS at the right midclavicular line. V_{3R} is placed between leads V_{2R} and V_{4R}. V_{6R} is at the right midaxillary line, and V_{5R} is placed between V_{4R} and V_{6R}. V_{4-6R} all share the same horizontal axis.

9. For the 18-lead ECG (posterior) placement, lead V_7 is placed on the posterior axillary line, lead V_8 is placed on the posterior midclavicular line, and lead V_9 is placed on the left paraspinal border. Leads V_{7-9} share the same horizontal axis as leads V_{4-6}.
10. Repeat steps 5-7 to record the additional leads, and mark the printed ECG to show the changed lead positions.
11. Remove the cables from the electrodes. If the patient is likely to undergo a repeat ECG, you may leave the pregelled electrodes in place; otherwise, remove the electrodes and cleanse the skin as needed.

AGE-SPECIFIC CONSIDERATIONS
1. Pediatric patients should have an ECG that includes leads V_{3-4R} to evaluate the possibility of right ventricular hypertrophy.
2. Leads V_{1R-4R} display a prominent R wave up to age 8 years.
3. Flat or inverted T waves may be a sign of hypothyroidism.
4. T waves in lead V_1 should never be positive before age 6; this may continue into adolescence (Bernstein, 2000).

COMPLICATIONS
1. Equipment malfunction
2. Electric microshock

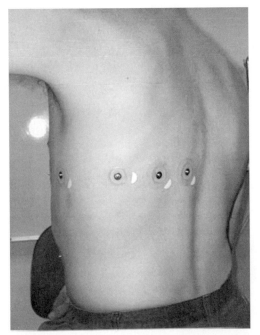

FIGURE 59-3 Precordial lead positions for posterior-view ECG. (Courtesy Mike D. Mc Mahon.)

TROUBLESHOOTING ECG TECHNICAL PROBLEMS
1. Alternating current interference (see Procedure 58)
2. Wandering baseline (see Procedure 58)
3. Tremor
Possible causes
a. Patient is tense or uncomfortable.
b. If electrode plates are used, the straps may be too tight.
Solutions
a. Help the patient to find a comfortable position and encourage the patient to relax.
b. Loosen the electrode straps.
4. Intermittent or jittery waveforms
Possible causes
a. Loose connections
b. Broken lead wires
c. Poor skin preparation
d. Contaminated conductive gel
e. Patient movement and tension
Solutions
a. Check all the connections.
b. Test the lead wires for breaks by wiggling them and watching for the effect on the recording.
c. Reapply the electrodes with proper skin-preparation technique and with fresh electrode-conductive gel.

PATIENT TEACHING
Lie as still as possible with your muscles relaxed. Do not talk during the recording.

REFERENCES
Bernstein, D. (2000). Electrocardiography (pp. 1351-1355). In Behrman R.E., Kliegman R.M., & Jenson H.B. (Eds.), *Textbook of pediatrics*. Philadelphia: W.B. Saunders.

Fijewski, T.R., Pollack, M.L., Chan, T.C., Brady, W.J., et al. (2002). Electrocardiographic manifestations: right ventricular infarction. *Journal of Emergency Medicine, 2*, 189-194.

Green, B.B., & Hill P.M. (2000). Approach to chest pain and possible myocardial ischemia (pp. 341-352). In Tintinalli, J.E., Kelen, G.D., & Stapszynski, J.S. (Eds.), *Emergency medicine*. New York: McGraw-Hill.

Walsh, P., Marks, G., Arangun, C. et al. (2001). Use of V_{4R} in patients who sustain blunt chest trauma. *Journal of Trauma, 51*, 60-63.

Wung, S., & Drew, B. (2001). Extra electrocardiographic leads: right precordial and left posterior leads (pp. 271-277). In Lynn-McHale, D.J., & Carlson, K.K. (Eds.), *AACN procedure manual for critical care*. Philadelphia: W.B. Saunders.

Continuous ST-Segment Monitoring

Mike D. McMahon, RN, BSN

INDICATIONS

1. To assist with the early detection and identification of myocardial ischemia or myocardial infarction (MI) before other symptoms (Herren et al., 2001), or, in situations such as general anesthesia, in which the patient is unable to communicate with the staff (Landesberg et al., 2002).
2. To facilitate the ruling out of myocardial infarction in low- to moderate-risk outpatients who do not have active chest pain, laboratory changes, or ischemic electrocardiogram (ECG) changes.
3. To monitor patients with asymptomatic forms of ischemia and unstable angina.
4. To monitor patients for reperfusion during thrombolytic therapy (Kucia & Zeitz, 2002).
5. To follow the clinical progress of an MI (Schröder et al., 2001).

CONTRAINDICATIONS AND CAUTIONS

The following are clinical conditions that may alter ST-segment findings:
1. Acute pericarditis (Wagner, 2001)
2. Acute cor pulmonale
3. Pulmonary emphysema
4. Hypokalemia
5. Digitalis
6. Balloon inflation during percutaneous transluminal coronary angioplasty
7. Pericardial tamponade
8. Intracranial hemorrhage (related to T-wave changes)
9. Hypothermia
10. Bundle branch blocks
11. Body position changes (Pelter & Adams, 2001)
12. Paced beats
13. Changes in cardiac rhythm
14. Noisy signals
15. Misplacement of leads
16. Elevation just before reperfusion (Kucia & Zeitz, 2002)
17. Left ventricular hypertrophy (Brady et al., 2001)
18. Benign early repolarization
19. Ventricular aneurysm
20. ST-segment changes have been documented during exercise ECG testing. Rapid up-sloping of the ST segment is a normal finding during exercise

(Chaitman, 2001). ST-segment changes in three or more consecutive leads may be considered abnormal.
21. Valsalva maneuver (Mirvis & Goldberger, 2001)
22. Hyperventilation
23. Drinking cold water

Situations that may invalidate ST-segment findings include the following:
1. Low-frequency filters on the cardiac monitors. Some new monitors have software that is activated to adjust to ST-segment monitoring automatically.
2. Poor electrode contact. Reduce the resistance across the skin to allow for a clean ECG tracing.
3. Poor patient positioning. The precordial leads are especially susceptible to shifts.
4. Improper electrode placement

EQUIPMENT
ST-segment ECG monitor
ECG cable: three-, five-, or 12-lead
Electrodes
Alcohol sponges
Gauze sponges
Razor (optional)
Scissors

PATIENT PREPARATION
1. If possible, choose flat, nonmuscular areas for electrode placement (see Procedure 59).
2. Good skin preparation and electrode placement are essential to perform the sensitive analysis of an ECG signal, to detect ST-segment changes, and to reduce artifact and false alarms. Clip or shave the chest hair as necessary. Cleanse the electrode placement sites with a mild soap and water to remove all oily residue and dead skin.
3. Allow the skin to dry and then apply the electrodes.

PROCEDURAL STEPS
1. Follow the manufacturer's instructions for setting up your monitoring system. Equipment that is currently available can analyze two, three, four, and 12 leads, depending on the model. Some systems have stand-alone ST-segment trending and can trend ST, T waves, QRS fractionation, and QRS difference in all leads.
2. If the patient's condition allows, obtain 12-lead ECGs while the patient is lying on the right and on the left sides. This may help if ST-segment changes occur as a result of patient movement (Pelter & Adams, 2001).
3. Choose the appropriate grouping of leads for ST-segment monitoring. Determine the patient's ischemic "fingerprint" from a 12-lead ECG, noting which leads show the most ST-segment displacement. Use the lead or leads with the most ST-segment displacement as the bedside ST-segment monitoring leads. If no ischemic fingerprint is available, consider the following recommendations (Table 60-1). Landesberg et al. (2002) found that V_4 is the most sensitive precordial lead for ischemia and infarction while undergoing sur-

gery. If you are unsure about where the occlusion is located, or the patient has no ECG changes, leads II, III, and V_1 usually provide good data regarding all three vessels.

4. A dominant rhythm is identified, from which the monitor creates a template. The template develops a median beat from each monitored lead. The ST segment is isoelectric (a flat line). The amplitude of the ST segment is determined from the J point (junction point, at the end of the S wave) to the beginning of the T wave (Figure 60-1).

TABLE 60-1

MONITORING LEADS FOR DIFFERENT AREAS OF THE MYOCARDIUM

Infarct Location	Primary Leads	Reciprocal Leads	Artery Involved
Anterior wall	V_2, V_3, V_4,	II, III, aV_F	Left coronary artery
Lateral wall	I, aV_L, V_5, V_6	II, III, aV_F	Circumflex branch of left anterior descending artery (LAD)
Posterior wall	V_1, V_2, V_3		Right coronary artery (RCA), circumflex branch of LAD
Inferior wall	II, III, aV_F	I, aV_L	RCA

Marquette Electronics, Inc., 1995. From *The golden minutes and ST segment monitoring.* Milwaukee, WI: Author, with permission.

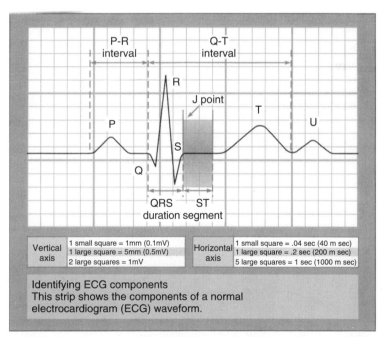

FIGURE 60-1 ECG wave form with J point. (From 12 lead ECG Monitoring. [1996]. (poster). Milwaukee, WI: Author. Courtesy Marquette Medical Systems Worldwide, Milwaukee, WI.)

5. When the ST-segment baseline analysis is complete, the monitor continuously updates changes in specific time intervals. A change of the ST segment off the baseline represents myocardial ischemia.
6. If changes in ST-segment amplitude exceed the parameters set in the alarm for more than the set duration, an alarm sounds. A 12-lead ECG should verify these changes in case the alarm has been triggered by artifact. Assess the patient to determine the cause of the changes (e.g., hypothermia, hyperventilation, or suctioning vs. myocardial ischemia).
7. After detecting a change in the ST segment, the system automatically resets the template based on the new ST-segment level. After treating the patient (for a non–MI-related cause of the alarm), you may need to reset the parameters of the monitor to create a new template.

TROUBLESHOOTING
See Procedure 58.

PATIENT TEACHING
1. Report any chest pain, palpitations, shortness of breath, or related symptoms immediately. Any unusual signs and symptoms should also be reported, taking into account that ischemic presentations in women differ from those in men (Douglas, 2001).
2. Report any disconnections in the system.
3. If the patient is discharged to home, aftercare instructions should include the following:
   a. Signs and symptoms that indicate myocardial ischemia (pain in the chest, jaw, epigastrium, or shoulder; sweating; shortness of breath; a feeling of impending doom; nausea; palpitations)
   b. How to access the emergency medical services system; stress the importance of accessing emergency care quickly if symptoms of myocardial ischemia occur
   c. Risk factors for coronary artery disease and follow-up with a primary care provider to develop a plan to decrease risks (e.g., smoking cessation, diet modification, exercise, medications)
   d. A copy of the resting 12-lead ECG, which the patient can bring to future visits in the emergency department or to the primary care provider

REFERENCES
Brady, W.J., Perron, A.D., Ullman, E.A. et al. (2001). Cause of ST segment abnormality in ED chest pain patients. *American Journal of Emergency Medicine*, *19*, 25-28.
Chaitman, B.R. (2001). Exercise stress testing (pp. 129-159). In Braunwald W., Zipes D.P., & Libby P. (Eds.), *Heart disease*, 6th ed. Philadelphia: W.B. Saunders Company.
Douglas, P.S. (2001). Coronary artery disease in women (pp. 129-159). In Braunwald, W., Zipes, D.P., & Libby, P. (Eds.), *Heart disease*, 6th ed. Philadelphia: W.B. Saunders.
Herren, K.R., Mackway-Jones, K., Richards, C.R. et al. (2001). Is it possible to exclude a diagnosis of myocardial damage within six hours of admission to an emergency department? Diagnostic cohort study. *British Medical Journal*, *323*, 1-4.
Kucia, A.M., & Zeitz, C.J. (2002). Failed reperfusion after thrombolytic therapy: recognition and management. *Heart & Lung*, *31*, 113-121.

Landesberg, G., Mosseri, M., Wolf, Y., Vesselov, Y., & Weissman, C. (2002). Perioperative myocardial ischemia and infarction. *Anesthesiology, 96*, 264-270.

Mirvis, D.M., & Goldberger, A.L. (2001). Electrocardiography (pp. 82-128). In Braunwald, W., Zipes, D.P., & Libby, P. (Eds.), *Heart disease*, 6th ed. Philadelphia: W.B. Saunders Company.

Pelter, M.M., & Adams, M.G. (2001). ST segment monitoring (pp. 349-353). In Lynn-McHale, D.J., & Carlson, K.K. (Eds.), *AACN procedure manual for critical care*. Philadelphia: W.B. Saunders.

Schröder, K., Wegscheider, K., Zeymer, U. et al. (2001). Extent of ST-segment deviation in the single ECG lead of maximum deviation present 90 or 180 minutes after start of thrombolytic therapy best predicts outcome in acute myocardial infarction. *Z Kardiol, 90*, 557-567.

Wagner, G.S. (2001). *Marriott's practical electrocardiography*, 10th ed. Philadelphia: Lippincott Williams & Wilkins.

PROCEDURE 61

Phlebotomy for Laboratory Specimens

Jean A. Proehl, RN, MN, CEN, CCRN

Phlebotomy for laboratory specimens is also known as blood draw, blood collection, blood tests, or venipuncture.

INDICATION
To obtain blood for laboratory studies.

CONTRAINDICATIONS AND CAUTIONS
1. Patients undergoing thrombolytic therapy should have as few punctures as possible. If venipuncture is absolutely necessary, use the smallest possible needle (i.e., a 23-G needle).
2. Whenever possible, patients should have blood specimens drawn when the intravenous (IV) line is started; this limits the number of punctures. This increases the likelihood of hemolysis (Grant, 2003). However, it results in only 4%-8% hemolysis, and thus 92%-96% of patients can benefit from this technique by only having one puncture (Proehl, 2003).
3. Blood should never be drawn close to a running IV line. It is preferable to draw from the other arm, but if this is not possible, turn off the fluids before drawing blood.

4. Because of the risk of syncope, never perform a venipuncture on a standing patient.
5. Avoid venipuncture in an arm that has an arteriovenous shunt or fistula or on the same side as a radical mastectomy.
6. Label all tubes immediately after blood collection. Do not allow unlabeled tubes to leave the patient's bedside or the phlebotomist's possession.
7. Patients from whom it is very difficult to draw blood or those who should not have large volumes of blood drawn, such as patients who are receiving hemodialysis or who have blood dyscrasias, may benefit from the use of neonatal or pediatric blood-sample tubes.
8. Informed consent may be required before you perform testing for the human immunodeficiency virus. Refer to your institution's policy for more information.

EQUIPMENT

Tourniquet or blood pressure cuff
Antiseptic solution or preparation pads
Blood-sampling options:
  Needles (21 G or 23 G) and syringe
  21-G or 23-G butterfly needle and syringe or vacuum-tube adapter
  Tube holder and needle or vacuum-tube adapter (Figure 61-1)
Cotton balls or 2- × 2-inch gauze dressings
Tape
Patient labels
Evacuated tubes (Check with your laboratory for specific requirements. Common color codes include a purple top for hematology; a red, gold, green, or speckled top for chemistry; a blue top for coagulation; and a yellow top [sterile] for blood cultures.)

PATIENT PREPARATION

1. Make a positive identification of the patient.
2. Check for restrictions, such as IV, shunts, thrombolytic therapy, or an uncooperative patient.
3. Place the patient in a sitting position with the arm extended and supported comfortably or in a supine position with the arm extended at the side.
4. To prevent aspiration in the event of syncope, be sure the patient does not have gum or candy or any other substance in his or her mouth.

PROCEDURAL STEPS

1. Assemble equipment (with extra tubes, needles, and syringes) within easy reach.

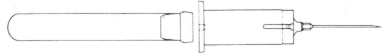

FIGURE 61-1 Vacutainer blood collection set. (Courtesy Becton Dickinson Vacutainer Systems, Franklin Lakes, NJ.)

2. Select a site. The most common sites are the veins in the antecubital fossa—the cephalic, basilic, and median cubital (also known as the median basilic) veins—but any vein may be used. The median cubital is a good choice because it is fairly stationary and close to the surface, and nerves and tendons are farther away than they are from some other veins.
3. Apply the tourniquet or cuff within 3-4 inches of the puncture site.
4. Have the patient make a fist and hold it.
5. Palpate to locate the vein. Even if the vein is visible, palpation is necessary to confirm location, direction, and suitability. A vessel that pulsates is an artery, whereas a vein feels like an elastic tube. Thrombosed veins roll and feel hard or rigid. Tendons may feel like veins. If in doubt, release the tourniquet while palpating; fullness should disappear if the structure is a vein.
6. Find the best vein, but do not leave the tourniquet on for more than 1 minute (NCCLS, 1998), because it may alter some laboratory values.
7. If you are having difficulty finding a vein, try the following:
   a. Be sure the arm is in a dependent position.
   b. Switch to the other arm.
   c. Gently massage the arm from wrist to elbow.
   d. Flick over the vein site with your finger.
   e. Apply a warm compress.
   f. Use a blood pressure cuff instead of a tourniquet.
8. Cleanse the site according to institutional policy and anchor the selected vein by placing your nondominant thumb 1-2 inches below the intended venipuncture site. If blood is being drawn for blood alcohol determination, use a non-alcohol cleaning solution, such as povidone-iodine or saline.
9. Perform the venipuncture with the bevel of the needle up and inserted at approximately a 15-degree angle in line with the vein. The needle may be inserted directly over the vein or off to the side and then directed into the vein.
10. If no blood is obtained, try the following:
   a. Reposition the needle by withdrawing, advancing, or rotating it slightly. Do not probe, because it is painful to the patient.
   b. Loosen the tourniquet; if it is too tight, it may be obstructing blood flow.
   c. Select a different tube, because some tubes lack an adequate vacuum.
   d. Choose another venipuncture site.
11. Withdraw the blood.
   a. *Using a syringe:* With one hand, pull the plunger gently while stabilizing the syringe and needle with the other hand. Aspirating too forcefully may collapse the vein or hemolyze the specimen. The syringe method is often used when the veins are small, such as those in the hand or those in elderly or chronically ill patients, because a vacuum tube may provide too much suction. After the blood is drawn, remove the stopper from the tube and the needle from the syringe and expel the blood gently into the tube. (Blood that is injected through the stopper with a needle has a higher risk of hemolysis.) Replace the stopper and vent with a needle puncture. Devices to facilitate blood transfer from syringe to evacuated tube are available.
   b. *Vacuum-tube method:* The first tube may be placed in the holder and pushed to the line without loss of vacuum before you perform the

venipuncture. One hand stabilizes the holder while the other presses the tube onto the needle. The tube fills and automatically stops when the vacuum is exhausted. If multiple samples are drawn, keep the holder and the needle stable as the tubes are exchanged. Be sure to use a multiple-sample needle to prevent blood from leaking as the tubes are changed. If no blood enters the tube and the needle is thought to be in the vein, change the tube before withdrawing the needle to ensure that the tube does have a vacuum.

   c. *Butterfly method:* A winged collection set may be used with either a syringe or a tube holder and an adapter for difficult veins. This method allows you to withdraw blood with very little manipulation of the needle within the vein.

   d. *Intravenous catheter:* Adapters are available to facilitate drawing directly from IV catheters into vacuum tubes during the placement of an IV line. This method increases the likelihood of hemolysis (Grant, 2003).

12. To prevent contamination of samples with bacteria (in the case of cultures) or tube additives, blood samples should be collected (or specimen tubes filled) in the following order (NCCLS, 1998):

   a. Blood cultures (see the special procedural steps that follow)

   b. Red-top tubes (contain no anticoagulant or clot activator; used to obtain serum)

   c. Blue-top tubes (contain sodium citrate; used to obtain plasma samples for coagulation studies). There are two common sizes of blue-top tubes for coagulation studies. The half-draw tube requires 2.7 ml, and for accurate test results, it must be allowed to fill completely to the line indicated on the label. If there is no line on the label, the tube is a full-draw tube and should be filled to the top of the label (4.5 ml).

   d. Gold-top tubes, tiger-top tubes, serum separator tubes, or red-and-black-top tubes (contain no anticoagulant; contain clot activator and/or silicon gel for cell/serum separation)

   e. Green-top tubes (contain heparin; used to obtain plasma)

   f. Lavender-top tubes (contain the anticoagulant ethylene diamine tetraacetic acid [EDTA]; used to obtain whole blood or plasma samples)

   g. Gray-top tubes (contain sodium fluoride oxalate for plasma samples)

13. Have the patient open the hand as soon as the blood flow is established.

14. To properly mix samples, invert the collection tubes gently five to eight times as soon as they are filled. Do not shake the tubes.

15. The tourniquet may be released as soon as blood enters the collection system, or it may be left on throughout the procedure.

16. On completion of the blood collection, release the tourniquet (if not previously released). Activate needle blunting device (if used).

17. Apply a gauze dressing over the site and gently withdraw the needle. Activate the needle shielding device (if used). Apply pressure until the bleeding has stopped.

18. Tape the gauze dressing firmly in place.

19. Label the blood samples per the policy of the institution.

20. Place specimens on ice if necessary. Specimens that commonly require cooling include ammonia, lactic acid, gastrin, catecholamines, and parathyroid hormone. Check with your laboratory for specific requirements.

Blood Cultures

Cultures are performed in an effort to evaluate bacteremia, which may be intermittent, transient, or continuous. The ideal time to obtain cultures is 1 hour before the onset of fever or chills because there is usually a delay between the influx of bacteria and a fever spike or chill. However, this is rarely possible in the emergency department setting. Two blood cultures from two separate sites may be obtained before antimicrobial therapy is initiated. Multiple bottles from the same site should be considered a single sample. For confirmation of bacteremia and to rule out contamination or a lapse in skin-cleaning technique, both cultures must be positive.

1. Remove the covers from the blood culture bottles and cleanse the bottle tops with 70% isopropyl alcohol and allow them to air dry.
2. Cleanse the venipuncture site vigorously with 70% isopropyl alcohol and allow it to air dry for 1-2 minutes. Apply 2% tincture of iodine to the site, starting in the center and moving outward in a circular pattern. Allow the site to air dry for 1-2 minutes. A double application of alcohol may be used for patients who are allergic to iodine.
3. Apply the tourniquet and perform the venipuncture. Obtain 20-30 ml of blood by following procedural steps 13-19 above. Sterile gloves may be worn to avoid contaminating the prepared skin. Holders that allow direct collection into the blood-culture bottle are available. These holders are bulky and should be used in conjunction with a butterfly needle, which minimizes difficulty in positioning during venipuncture.
4. If a syringe is used, it is preferable to draw two syringes in order to inoculate each bottle with a different syringe and reduce the risk of aerosolization of blood during inoculation. Change to a sterile needle before inoculating the culture bottle. Inject at least 10 ml of blood into each culture bottle.
5. Swab the bottle tops with 70% isopropyl alcohol and allow them to air dry.
6. On the laboratory slip, note the time, site, and any previous administration of antibiotics.

AGE-SPECIFIC CONSIDERATIONS

1. Consult your laboratory regarding the minimal sample volume and the appropriate collection tubes for blood studies in infants and small children.
2. Small blood-collection tubes, which allow the collection of capillary blood from a heel stick, are available. See Procedure 22 for capillary blood collection technique.
3. A butterfly needle facilitates venipuncture in small children because it is easier to obtain samples without moving the needle.
4. Use of a tight tourniquet on elderly patients with friable veins may cause the vein to rupture if it is punctured. Use a loose tourniquet or no tourniquet at all.

COMPLICATIONS

1. Vasovagal syncope
2. Failure to obtain blood, usually due to incorrect needle positioning or a tube without a vacuum
3. Hematoma formation at the puncture site
4. Hemolysis of the sample. Hemolysis is more likely to occur when blood is drawn through IV catheters, especially when an adaptor is used to draw

directly into vacuum tubes (Grant, 2003). Tips to help prevent hemolysis include:

   a. Allow the site to air dry before venipuncture.

   b. Make sure the needle is tight on the syringe to prevent frothing during collection.

   c. Angle the tube so that the blood runs down the side during collection.

   d. Aspirate gently when using a syringe. Hemolysis can be associated with either large- or small-gauge needles if excessive force is applied via syringe or evacuated tube.

   e. Gently invert the tube to mix additives; do not shake.

   f. Fill tubes completely. Partially filled tubes are more prone to hemolysis when they are transported via a pneumatic tube system.

   g. Avoid injecting blood from a syringe through a needle via the stopper of the tube. Use a blood transfer device or remove the needle from the syringe and the stopper from the tube and gently fill the tube.

5. Clotted sample that was not mixed properly when drawn. Gently invert each tube several times to ensure mixing.

6. Local reaction to skin-cleansing agent. Remove any residual iodine solutions after venipuncture and before dressing application.

PATIENT TEACHING

Report ongoing bleeding or pain at the venipuncture site.

REFERENCES

Grant, M.S. (2003). The effect of blood drawing techniques and equipment on hemolysis of ED laboratory blood samples. *Journal of Emergency Nursing, 29*, 116-121.

National Committee for Clinical Laboratory Standards (NCCLS). (1998). *Procedures for the collection of diagnostic blood specimens by venipuncture*, 4th ed; approved standard, 18 (7). Wayne, PA: Author.

Proehl, J.A. (2003). *ED hemolysis rates in laboratory specimens*. Unpublished data, Dartmouth-Hitchcock Medical Center, Lebanon, NH.

Blood Glucose Monitoring

Daun A. Smith, RN, MS, CEN
and Mary E. Wood, RN, MS, CDE, BC-ADM

INDICATION
To measure whole blood glucose levels at the bedside.

CONTRAINDICATIONS AND CAUTIONS
1. Do not obtain blood from a site that is vascularly compromised (cold, mottled, cyanotic); the sample may not produce an accurate result.
2. Severely decreased peripheral blood flow, such as occurs in the presence of hypotension, shock, peripheral vascular disease, or the severe dehydration of diabetic ketoacidosis or hyperglycemic hyperosmolar nonketotic syndrome, may lead to inaccurate results. An initial serum glucose determination performed simultaneously with a bedside blood glucose test determines concordance (Ray, et al., 2001).
3. There are many types of blood glucose meter, and each uses its own specific test strips. The user must be familiar with the test strips that must be used for the model he or she operates. Some meters test only capillary whole blood. Others can also accommodate venous, arterial, neonatal, or capillary blood.
4. An accurate result depends on a competent operator, properly stored supplies, and clean, functional equipment that is calibrated correctly and tested routinely for quality control.
5. If the results are inconsistent with the patient's clinical picture or otherwise appear inaccurate, validate the result with a serum glucose test, recheck the blood glucose meter manufacturer's instructions, review the test procedure, verify that the quality control results are in the desired range, check the expiration date of the test strips, and repeat the test.
6. For results that are critically high or low (hospital policy may dictate these values) or for other questionable results, validate the result with a serum glucose test.
7. Limitations of the procedure may include a very high or low hematocrit or elevated uric acid, oxygen, or ascorbic acid levels (Louie et al., 2000). Falsely high glucose results may occur in patients who use EXTRANEAL (icodextrin) peritoneal dialysis solution (Baxter Healthcare Corporation, 2001). See the blood glucose test strip package insert for specific limitations.
8. A complete bedside blood glucose monitoring program includes administrative responsibility for the program, a written policy or procedure, training for personnel who perform the test, quality control standards, and a program of equipment maintenance (American Diabetes Association, 2003; The National Committee for Clinical Laboratory Standards, 1994).

EQUIPMENT
Lancet or lancet device
Alcohol swab
Gloves
Cotton balls or gauze pad
Blood glucose meter
Blood glucose test strip

PATIENT PREPARATION
1. Select a puncture site. The fingertip or earlobe is acceptable for adults.
2. Cleanse the site with alcohol. Allow to dry. If the site is cold, warm it with a hot pack to increase vasodilatation.

PROCEDURAL STEPS
NOTE: Each blood glucose meter or system has specific procedural steps. Consult the meter manual for the specific system to be used.
1. Prepare the meter by turning it on and making sure that the calibration code on the meter matches the code on the package of test strips. If indicated, enter operator and patient identification.
2. Ensure that the meter and strip are ready to accept the drop of blood.
3. Prepare the lancet or lancet device.
4. Hold the lancet firmly to the site and perform the puncture.
5. Gently squeeze the finger and release to allow blood to flow. Obtain a drop of blood that is adequate to fill the test area of the strip.
6. Lightly touch the reagent area of the strip to the drop of blood, filling the entire area. Avoid smearing the blood. (Some meters allow the addition of a second drop if the first is insufficient. Check the meter manual.) When applying blood to the test strip from a syringe, obtain a drop at the tip of the syringe and allow the capillary action of the strip to draw the blood.
7. Read the value at the conclusion of the test.

AGE-SPECIFIC CONSIDERATION
The heel may be used as a puncture site in neonates; toes should not be used.

COMPLICATIONS
1. Discomfort at the puncture site
2. Infection (rare)
3. Inaccurate blood glucose result

PATIENT TEACHING
1. Review home blood glucose monitoring procedure and interpretation of the results.
2. Watch for signs and symptoms of infection.
3. Alternate sites, such as the forearm, should not be used if hypoglycemia is suspected or within 1 hour of a meal or insulin injection (Jungheim & Koschinsky, 2002).

REFERENCES

American Diabetes Association. (2003). Position statement: bedside blood glucose monitoring in hospitals. *Diabetes Care, 26* (Suppl. 1), S119.

Baxter Healthcare Corporation. (2001). *EXTRANEAL product insert.* McGaw Park, IL: Author.

Jungheim, K., & Koschinsky, T. (2002). Glucose monitoring at the arm: risky delays of hypoglycemia and hyperglycemia detection. *Diabetes Care, 25,* 956-960.

Louie, R.F., Tang, Z., Sutton, D.V. et al. (2000). Point-of-care glucose testing: effects of critical care variables, influence of reference instruments, and a modular glucose meter design. *Archives of Pathology and Laboratory Medicine, 124,* 257-266.

Ray, J., Hamielec, C., & Mastracci, T. (2001). Pilot study of the accuracy of bedside glucometry in the intensive care unit. *Critical Care Medicine, 29,* 2205-2207.

The National Committee for Clinical Laboratory Standards (1994). *Ancillary blood glucose testing in acute and chronic care facilities: approved guideline.* Villanova, PA: Author.

Vascular Access

Peripheral Intravenous Cannulation

Jean A. Proehl, RN, MN, CEN, CCRN
and Margo E. Layman, MSN, RN, RNC, CN-A

INDICATION

To establish venous access for the administration of fluids, electrolytes, intravenous (IV) medications, blood components, or total parenteral nutrition.

CONTRAINDICATIONS AND CAUTIONS

1. If the patient has a coagulation disorder, care should be taken to prevent bleeding from unsuccessful venipuncture sites.
2. A hematoma may form if the needle punctures both the anterior and the posterior walls of the vein.
3. Attempt to draw any necessary blood specimens through the IV catheter to decrease the number of venipunctures the patient has to undergo (see Procedure 61).
4. Avoid placing IV lines over joints because the movement of the joint may cause infiltration.
5. Rotate IV sites in adult patients every 72-96 hours to help prevent the development of phlebitis and infection (O'Grady et al., 2002).
6. Remove IV catheters inserted under emergency conditions and restart at a new site within 48 hours (O'Grady et al., 2002).
7. Remove IV catheters promptly on evidence of edema, redness, phlebitis, pain, or subcutaneous infiltration.
8. Do not apply antibiotic ointment or creams to insertion sites, because they may promote fungal infections and antibiotic resistance (O'Grady et al., 2002).
9. Shaving the site for intravenous cannulation may promote bacterial growth; if hair removal is necessary, clipping is preferred.
10. Never withdraw the catheter over the needle; this could shear off the catheter inside the vein.
11. Embolisms occur rarely from IV sites in patients with poor venous return. In adults, the feet and ankles are poor sites for IV cannulation because venous return may be sluggish.

EQUIPMENT

IV solution and tubing
or
IV lock and saline flush
Over-the-needle IV catheter

T-piece or short extension set
Tourniquet
Gauze dressings
Transparent dressing (optional)
Tape
Vacuum tubes, syringe, or adapter for blood sampling (optional)
Local anesthetic or saline, tuberculin syringe (optional)
Arm board (optional)

PATIENT PREPARATION

Assemble IV fluid and tubing or a saline lock. A T-piece or short extension set is recommended on all IV sites to facilitate tubing changes with minimal catheter hub manipulation and dressing changes.

PROCEDURAL STEPS

1. Apply a tourniquet above the intended site of cannulation. Tuck the tail of the tourniquet under the tourniquet to permit one-handed release as soon as the vein is cannulated.
2. Identify a vein. If the vein is not distended and is easily palpable, lightly pat the area. Have the patient open and close the fist and lower the extremity below the level of the heart. An alternative is to apply a warm pack to help distend a vein. Make the initial venipuncture in the distal extremity to preserve proximal sites for potential later use. Bifurcations are good sites for venipuncture because they are stable and are not prone to roll.
3. Cleanse the skin with an antiseptic solution by using a firm, circular swabbing motion outward from the center of the site. Allow the skin to air dry for 30 seconds (povidone-iodine should be allowed to dry for at least 2 minutes). Acceptable skin cleansing solutions include 2% chlorhexidine, tincture of iodine, an iodophor, or 70% alcohol (O'Grady et al., 2002).
4. Inject an intradermal wheal of local anesthetic or saline solution at the intended puncture site (optional). This is not recommended when the vein is difficult to see, because the skin wheal may obscure the site.
5. Using the thumb of your nondominant hand, apply slight traction to the distal vein to help stabilize the vein during venipuncture. Insert the needle through the skin at a 10- to 30-degree angle with the bevel up, in line with and alongside the vein. Alternatively, you may insert the needle directly over the vein, but there is an increased risk of posterior wall puncture with this technique (Figure 63-1).
6. When the vein is punctured, a flash of blood appears in the hub of the catheter. Advance the needle and stylet another $1/8$ inch into the vein (adult patient).
7. Advance the catheter over the needle and into the vein. If any resistance is met on advancement of the catheter, stop immediately, remove the needle and catheter, and apply pressure to the site. Activate any needle shield or safety device as indicated.
8. If blood specimens are to be drawn through the IV catheter, attach the syringe or vacuum-tube adapter to the needle hub and withdraw the required samples (see Procedure 61).
9. Release the tourniquet.
10. Connect the IV tubing and open the roller clamp or attach the saline lock.

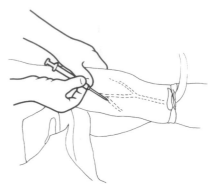

FIGURE 63-1 Insert the intravenous catheter along the vein while stabilizing the vein with your other thumb. (From Simon, R.R., & Brenner, B.E. [2002]. *Emergency procedures and techniques,* 4th ed. [p. 450]. Baltimore: Williams & Wilkins.)

11. Apply ¼-inch tape across the hub of the catheter to secure it. Do not place the tape over the insertion site or at the junction of the needle and tubing. Place a small sterile dressing over the insertion site. Alternatively, apply a transparent dressing over the site and needle hub.
12. Tape the IV tubing or saline lock securely.
13. Tape a label to the IV site with the date, the time, the size of the catheter, and your initials.
14. Adjust the drip rate as ordered or flush the saline lock. Assess the site for infiltration.
15. Before injecting medication through an injection port, clean the port with 70% alcohol or an iodophor (O'Grady et al., 2002).

AGE-SPECIFIC CONSIDERATIONS
1. Pediatric patients should not have routine rotation of IV sites; replace peripheral catheters only when clinically indicated (O'Grady et al., 2002).
2. Pediatric or elderly patients may require an arm board to protect the IV site. Wrapping the extremity with gauze can help prevent the patient from manipulating the catheter.
3. It may be helpful to secure the hand of a small child to an IV board before the venipuncture.
4. In infants and small children, advance the catheter off of the needle as soon as you see the blood flashback. This helps avoid puncture of the posterior wall of the vein. In adults with large, rope-like veins, advance the needle and stylet together approximately ¼ inch to prevent the catheter tip from catching on the thick wall of the vein.
5. Scalp veins can be used for IV access in infants, although they are inadequate for large volumes of fluids or medications that must be administered quickly. A rubber band can be used as a tourniquet to distend the veins (Figure 63-2). Determine which direction the blood is flowing by occluding the vein with your finger and "milking" it. The IV catheter should be inserted in the same direction the blood is flowing. The rubber band has to be cut away carefully after the IV catheter is in place. A plastic medicine cup can be used to protect the IV line (Figure 63-3).
6. A T-piece or a short extension set should be used on all pediatric IV lines to facilitate the injection of medications near the site and to avoid flushing long lengths of tubing to ensure that the medication has been infused.

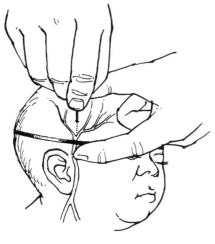

FIGURE 63-2 Use a rubber band as a tourniquet for scalp veins. (From Lozon, M.M. [2004]. Pediatric vascular access and blood sampling techniques [p. 367]. In Roberts J.R., & Hedges, J.R. [Eds.], *Clinical procedures in emergency medicine*, 4th ed. Philadelphia: W.B. Saunders.)

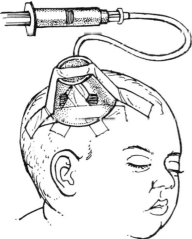

FIGURE 63-3 A plastic medicine cup can be used to protect a scalp intravenous line. (From Lozon, M.M. [2004]. Pediatric vascular access and blood sampling techniques [p. 367]. In Roberts J.R., & Hedges, J.R. [Eds.], *Clinical procedures in emergency medicine*, 4th ed. Philadelphia: W.B. Saunders.)

7. A local anesthetic may not be the best option in children, who approach any puncture with fear. An anesthetic cream (eutectic mixture of local anesthetics, EMLA) may be used to anesthetize the site, but this takes 20-60 minutes to be effective. School-aged children may be able to decide whether they want intradermal local anesthesia, which can be described as "a sting that makes the skin go to sleep so the needle doesn't hurt so much."

8. Avoid using a tourniquet in elderly patients who have fragile veins to decrease the risk of blowing the vein.

9. Using vacuum tubes to draw blood directly from the IV catheter increases the risk of blowing the vein in elderly patients.

COMPLICATIONS

1. Hematomas may form at unsuccessfully cannulated sites.

2. Inadequate cleansing of the skin at the cannulation site may result in the introduction of bacteria into the vein, which can lead to local infection or bacteremia.

3. Phlebitis may develop.
4. Catheter embolism may occur if the catheter shears off as it is withdrawn over the stylet.
5. Infiltration of the surrounding tissue can occur because of a displaced catheter. Some medications can cause serious tissue damage if they infiltrate the tissue.

PATIENT TEACHING
1. Do not bend, pinch, or adjust the flow rate of the tubing.
2. Report any sensations of swelling, heat, pain, or drainage at the puncture site.

REFERENCE
O'Grady, N.P., Alexander, M., Dellinger, E.P. et al. (2002). Guidelines for prevention of intravascular catheter–related infections. *Morbidity and Mortality Weekly Report, 51,* 1-28.

PROCEDURE 64

Rapid-Infusion Catheter Exchange

Reneé Semonin Holleran, RN, PhD, CEN, CCRN, CFRN, SANE

Rapid-infusion catheter exchange is also known as RIC.

INDICATIONS
1. To increase the size of a functioning peripheral intravenous (IV) line
2. To provide access for volume resuscitation of the patient in shock
3. To provide percutaneous access for the introduction of invasive monitoring lines, diagnostic catheters, or temporary pacing wires

CONTRAINDICATIONS AND CAUTIONS
1. These catheters are for peripheral IV use only.
2. A 20-G or larger catheter must be established before this device can be used.
3. Patency of the established catheter must be ensured through an adequate blood return.

EQUIPMENT

Antiseptic solution
Local anesthetic
Rapid-infusion catheter exchange set (guide wire, sheath or dilator combination, No. 11 scalpel, 7.0- or 8.5-French catheter)
IV dressing supplies

PATIENT PREPARATION

1. Place the patient in a supine position.
2. Remove the IV dressing over the established catheter.
3. Ensure that the existing peripheral IV catheter is 20 G or larger.

PROCEDURAL STEPS

1. *Infiltrate the area around the catheter with a local anesthetic.
2. Cleanse the entire area, including the puncture site and indwelling catheter, with an antiseptic solution.
3. *Disconnect the IV tubing from the catheter and insert the guide wire through the indwelling catheter and into the vein (Figure 64-1, *A*). If resistance is met, withdraw the guide wire and reinsert. If resistance persists, the procedure must be stopped.
4. *When the guide wire has been inserted into the indwelling catheter, remove the existing catheter.
5. *Pass the sheath or dilator over the guide wire (Figure 64-1, *B*).
6. *Nick the skin with the scalpel blade at the insertion site (approximately 5 mm) (Figure 64-1, *C*).
7. *Thread the tapered tip of the dilator over the guide wire and advance the dilator and sheath into the vessel, using a slight twisting motion (Figure 64-1, *D*).
8. *Advance the sheath over the dilator by grasping the skin and using a slight twisting motion.
9. *Make sure the sheath is held in place and then remove the dilator and guide wire. The free flow of blood demonstrates that the catheter is in place (Figure 64-1, *E*).
10. Connect the catheter to the IV tubing. Blood tubing or large-bore tubing should be used if fluid resuscitation is indicated.
11. Secure the catheter with tape or a suture. Apply a dressing.

AGE-SPECIFIC CONSIDERATION

This procedure is not recommended for infants and small children because of the size of the peripheral catheter. All patients receiving fluids through this catheter must be closely monitored because excessive amounts of fluid may be delivered, which can be deleterious to the patient (Clark, 2002).

COMPLICATIONS

1. Rupture of the vein and hematoma formation may occur when the catheter being inserted is larger than the vessel.

---

*Indicates portions of the procedure usually performed by a physician or an advanced practice nurse.

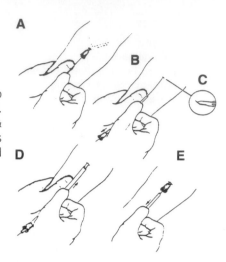

FIGURE 64-1 Percutaneous insertion of a 7.0- to 8.5-French introducer (see text for explanation). (Reproduced From Herron, H., Falcone, R., Dean, B., & Werman, H. [1997]. 8.5 French peripheral intravenous access during air medical transport of the injured patient. *Air Medical Journal, 16*[1], 8.)

2. Leaving the vessel dilator in place after catheter insertion may lead to limited function as well as the potential for the dilator to dislodge from the vessel and enter the systemic circulation.
3. Infiltration and infusion of fluids, blood, or medications into surrounding tissues may occur with this procedure.

PATIENT TEACHING

1. Keep the limb where the catheter is inserted immobilized to prevent dislodgement of the catheter.
2. Report immediately dampness, pain, or swelling at the IV site, or any disconnection in the equipment.

REFERENCE

Clark, D.Y. (2002). Prehospital care of the trauma patient. In McQuillan, K., Von Rueden, K., Hartsock, R., Flynn, M., & Whalen, E. (Eds.), *Trauma nursing: from resuscitation through rehabilitation*, 3rd ed. (pp. 94-106). Philadelphia: W.B. Saunders.

External Jugular Venous Access

Reneé Semonin Holleran, RN, PhD, CEN, CCRN, CFRN, SANE

INDICATIONS

NOTE: Although the external jugular vein is usually considered a peripheral intravenous (IV) site, some institutions consider the external jugular site to be central line access instead of peripheral line access. Consult your institution's policies and procedures for clarification on whether registered nurses may insert external jugular catheters.

1. To obtain peripheral venous access for fluid resuscitation, blood products, or medication administration
2. To obtain peripheral venous access when no sites are available on the extremities
3. To obtain peripheral venous access to draw blood for laboratory evaluation

CONTRAINDICATIONS AND CAUTIONS

1. If the head must be moved for catheter insertion, external jugular venous access is contraindicated in the patient who has a suspected cervical spine injury.
2. Use of the external jugular vein is contraindicated in a patient who has a penetrating injury to the neck, and it should be avoided when there is significant blunt trauma and soft tissue injury to the face, neck, and upper chest.
3. External jugular venous access should be used with caution in patients who cannot tolerate a supine or head-down position.
4. External jugular venous access should be used with caution when the anatomy of the external jugular vein is not clearly discernible.
5. Securing an external jugular venous line can be difficult, and this increases the potential for accidental dislodgement.

EQUIPMENT

Antiseptic solution
Caps, masks, and sterile gloves
IV solution and tubing
IV needle and catheter (size and length are dependent on the need for the line)
Dressing supplies
5-ml syringe; 18-G, 25-G, or 27-G needles for local anesthesia
Local anesthetic
20- to 30-ml syringes to obtain blood samples
Assorted blood collection tubes

PATIENT PREPARATION

1. Place the patient in a supine, head-down position, with the head turned away from the side where the catheter is to be inserted. Please note that external jugular vein access may be obtained in the trauma patient, but the patient's head cannot be moved or lowered.
2. Cleanse the area overlying the external jugular vein with antiseptic solution. The external jugular vein runs downward and backward obliquely behind the angle of the mandible and across the sternomastoid muscle. It then courses deeply into the neck just above the midclavicular area. The external jugular vein enters the subclavian vein (Figure 65-1).

PROCEDURAL STEPS

1. *If the patient is conscious, anesthetize the insertion site with a local anesthetic.
2. *Attach the IV catheter to a syringe and align the needle with the external jugular vein, directing the needle tip toward the ipsilateral shoulder.
3. *Lightly "tourniquet" the distal end of the external jugular vein (just above the clavicle) with the opposite index finger. The opposite thumb can also be used on the proximal portion of the vein to assist in anchoring it for puncture (Figure 65-2).
4. *Perform the venipuncture midway between the angle of the jaw and the clavicle.

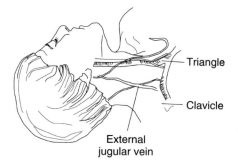

FIGURE 65-1 Anatomy of the external jugular vein. (From American Heart Association. [1997]. *Textbook for advanced cardiac life support* [p. 6-4]. Dallas: Author. Reproduced with permission. Copyright American Heart Association.)

Triangle

Clavicle

External jugular vein

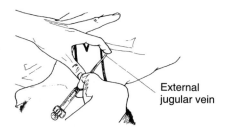

FIGURE 65-2 External jugular venipuncture. (From American Heart Association. [1997]. *Textbook for advanced cardiac life support* [p. 6-5]. Dallas: Author. Reproduced with permission. Copyright American Heart Association.)

External jugular vein

---

*Indicates portions of the procedure usually performed by a physician or an advanced practice nurse.

5. *When a blood return is noted in the syringe, advance the catheter off the needle to the hub. If you are using another type of device (i.e., a triple-lumen catheter), advance according to the package instructions.
6. *If blood is to be obtained, withdraw the desired amount. Detach the syringe and place a gloved finger over the hub to prevent the introduction of air.
7. Connect the IV tubing and initiate the flow of the fluid. Monitor for signs of infiltration.
8. Apply a dressing over the area. Secure the catheter with tape. Looping the IV tubing around the ear may add additional security. Sedation may be required to help keep the patient from moving and dislodging the catheter (Fleck, 2001).

AGE-SPECIFIC CONSIDERATIONS
1. For the pediatric patient, the external jugular vein is a relatively safe place to gain venous access, because it is superficial and visible (Markenson, 2002).
2. The pediatric airway may be compromised when the child's head is turned for placement.
3. Any patient taking anticoagulants has an increased the risk of bleeding around the catheter, which may result in the development of an airway compromise from an expanding hematoma.

COMPLICATIONS
1. Infection and phlebitis. Risk factors associated with the development of infection and phlebitis include type of catheter, frequency of catheter manipulation, and patient-related factors (O'Grady et al., 2002).
2. Turning a patient's head for better visualization of the external jugular vein may cause airway compromise.
3. Hematoma formation at the site of the insertion may cause airway compromise.
4. Inadvertent puncture of the carotid artery may occur.
5. The catheter may shear and an embolus may form.
6. An air embolus can result from the insertion.

PATIENT TEACHING
1. Avoid excessive head movement.
2. Report any pain, shortness of breath, bleeding, or dampness at the site immediately.

REFERENCES
Fleck, D. (2001). Central line insertion (perform). In Lynn-McHale, D.J., Carlson, D.J., & Carlson, K.K. (Eds.), *AACN procedure manual for critical care*, 4th ed. (pp. 503-521). Philadelphia: W.B. Saunders.
Markenson, D.S. (2002). *Pediatric prehospital care*. Upper Saddle River, NJ: Prentice Hall.
O'Grady, N.P., Alexander, M., Dellinger, E.P. et al. (2002). Guidelines for prevention of intravascular catheter-related infections. *Morbidity and Mortality Weekly Report, 51*, 1-28.

---

*Indicates portions of the procedure usually performed by a physician or an advanced practice nurse.

Subclavian Venous Access

Reneé Semonin Holleran, RN, PhD, CEN, CCRN, CFRN, SANE

INDICATIONS

1. To obtain central venous access through the subclavian vein when peripheral access is unobtainable, such as occurs in a patient who is in profound shock or cardiac arrest, or in a patient with peripheral vascular access limitations, such as an intravenous substance abuser or one with severe peripheral vascular disease
2. To monitor the patient's central venous pressure (CVP)
3. To administer intravenous fluids, blood products, or medications, especially those likely to cause complications if administered via a smaller peripheral vein
4. To administer long-term parenteral nutrition
5. To provide a site for the insertion of a transvenous pacemaker or a pulmonary-artery catheter.

CONTRAINDICATIONS AND CAUTIONS

1. The only contraindication to subclavian venous access is a lack of skill on the part of the emergency-care provider who is inserting the line.
2. A patient who has a coagulopathy from either a disease process or a medication must be monitored carefully for bleeding. A femoral site is preferred because the vessel can be compressed if bleeding should occur.
3. Fibrinolytic therapy must be administered with extreme caution when any central line is in place.
4. A patient who is agitated or uncooperative is at risk for injury during the procedure.
5. A femoral vein should be used in a patient with a chest injury, and a subclavian or internal jugular vein should be used in a patient with a pelvic injury (Markenson, 2002).
6. Special care must be taken when inserting a central line into a patient with distorted landmarks caused by obesity, deformity of the chest wall, previous subclavian insertion, clavicle fracture, or radiation therapy to the area of insertion (Simon & Brenner, 2002).
7. Cannulization of the subclavian vein should be avoided in patients on positive end-expiratory pressure or continuous positive-airway pressure or in patients with pulmonary emphysema because of the increased risk of causing a pneumothorax.

EQUIPMENT

Antiseptic solution
Local anesthetic
5-ml syringe; 18-G, 25-G, or 27-G needles for local anesthesia

Central venous access kit (Most kits contain an 8.5-French introducer, which can be used for large fluid-volume resuscitation or for the introduction of a transvenous pacemaker or a pulmonary artery catheter.)
or
Multiple lumen catheter (used for fluid administration and allows insertion of invasive lines, transvenous pacemakers as well as ports for medication administration and obtaining blood)
or
16-G, 8-inch, single-lumen catheter
No. 11 scalpel
IV solution and tubing
Flushing solution (heparinized solution or 0.9% saline solution per institutional policy)
Silk suture (2-0 or 3-0) with a needle holder
Sterile towels
Masks, caps, goggles, sterile gloves, and gowns
Dressing supplies (gauze or a transparent dressing) NOTE: When the patient is diaphoretic or the site is oozing, it should be covered with gauze instead of a transparent dressing (O'Grady et al, 2002).

PATIENT PREPARATION

1. Place the patient on a cardiac monitor and pulse oximeter (See Procedures 23 and 25).
2. Place the patient in a supine, 20-degree Trendelenburg position with a small, rolled towel placed between the shoulder blades to improve access. If the patient cannot tolerate the Trendelenburg position, elevate the legs for a modified Trendelenburg position (Procedure 51). Turn the patient's head to the side opposite the insertion.
3. *Cleanse the chest with an antiseptic solution. The subclavian vein rises as a continuation of the axillary vein, with its origin near the lateral portion of the first rib. The vein runs medially, passing under the middle third of the clavicle, and unites with the internal jugular vein near the sternum to form the brachiocephalic (innominate) vein.
4. *Drape the patient, using a sterile technique. In addition to gloves, masks and goggles should be worn for this procedure.
5. If a multiple lumen catheter is being used, be sure that the ports have been flushed using the solution recommended by the hospital's policies and procedures.
6. The right subclavian is the preferred site because the vein is shorter and provides a more direct route (Fleck, 2001).

PROCEDURAL STEPS

1. *Locate the landmarks for the subclavian vein and anesthetize the insertion site.
2. *Place the middle finger of your nondominant hand in the suprasternal notch.
3. *Locate the tubercle, which is approximately one third of the distance along the sternum from the clavicle.
4. *With the middle finger still in the suprasternal notch and the thumb on the inferior tubercle of the clavicle, insert the needle attached to the syringe

---

*Indicates portions of the procedure usually performed by a physician or an advanced practice nurse.

under the tubercle along the undersurface of the clavicle, directing it toward the suprasternal notch (Figure 66-1). If the patient is awake and cooperative, have him or her take a deep breath and hold it during needle insertion.

5. *While aspirating, advance the needle approximately 3-5 cm.

6. *When the vein has been located, detach the needle from the syringe and place a gloved finger over the hub to prevent the introduction of air.

7. *Gently insert the guide wire through the needle hub (Figure 66-1).

8. *After the guide wire is in place, remove the needle and allow the wire to remain in the vein.

9. *Use the No. 11 blade to make a small nick in the skin where the wire enters (see Figure 66-1).

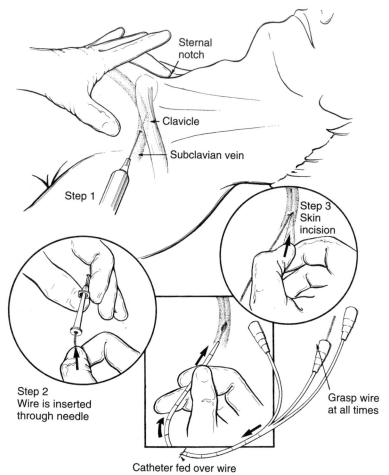

FIGURE 66-1 Subclavian vein cannulation. (From Dunmire, S., & Paris, P. [1994]. *Atlas of emergency procedures* [p. 199]. Philadelphia: W.B. Saunders.)

---

*Indicates portions of the procedure usually performed by a physician or an advanced practice nurse.

10. *Some kits contain a separate dilator, whereas others have the catheter and dilator joined together. If the dilator is separate, insert it into the hub and leave the wire in place.
11. *Insert the catheter over the wire, making sure to maintain control of the wire at all times.
12. *Once the catheter has been inserted, remove the wire and the dilator (if it is joined to the catheter).
13. *Aspirate and ascertain that there is good blood flow.
14. Draw the blood as needed for the laboratory evaluation.
15. Attach the catheter to the IV solution.
16. *Suture the catheter in place.
17. Apply a sterile gauze or transparent dressing and tape it to secure the catheter and the tubing (O'Grady et al., 2002).
18. Obtain a chest x-ray film to verify the catheter placement and to rule out any postprocedural complications, such as a pneumothorax.
19. Attach the catheter to the monitoring device, that is, the CVP monitor (if indicated).
20. CVP monitoring may be altered by dysrhythmias (Fleck, 2001).

AGE-SPECIFIC CONSIDERATIONS

1. For a young child, an infraclavicular approach may be a good route because it allows the catheter to be secured comfortably to the chest wall (Buntain, 1995; Fernandez et al., 1997). The landmarks for the infraclavicular approach are the bend of the clavicle and the suprasternal notch. The needle is inserted a few millimeters caudally and a few millimeters medially to the bend of the clavicle. The needle should be "walked" along the clavicle and kept parallel to the chest. The needle is advanced toward the suprasternal notch. When a blood return has been obtained, the procedure should be continued as previously described (Buntain, 1995).
2. Complications related to central venous cannulation are more common in children than in adults; therefore, it is recommended that the procedure be performed or supervised by an experienced practitioner.
3. The femoral vein is the area of choice for placement of a central line in the pediatric patient (Fernandez et al., 1997).
4. The size of the catheter is based on the child's age and weight (Evans & Bishop-Kurylo, 1996):
   <1 yr and <10 kg   =   3-French catheter
   1-12 yr and 10-40 kg   =   4-French catheter
   >12 yr and >40 kg   =   5- to 6-French catheter

COMPLICATIONS

1. Pneumothorax resulting from an overly acute angle of insertion
2. Insertion in the subclavian artery. (The needle should be removed immediately and direct pressure applied.)

---

*Indicates portions of the procedure usually performed by a physician or an advanced practice nurse.

3. Ventricular dysrhythmia as the result of insertion of the guide wire into the right ventricle
4. Air embolism as the result of not keeping the hub of the needle covered at all times (unless connected to the IV solution)
5. Guide wire embolism if the guide wire is not controlled during insertion
6. Hematoma formation from multiple attempts
7. Infection and phlebitis. Risk factors associated with the development of phlebitis include type of catheter, frequency of catheter manipulation, and patient-related factors (O'Grady et al., 2002).

PATIENT TEACHING

1. Report any chest pain or shortness of breath, as well as any disconnections or dampness around the dressing site.
2. Do not touch the area where the catheter has been inserted.

REFERENCES

Buntain, W. (1995). *Management of pediatric trauma.* Philadelphia: W.B. Saunders.

Evans, T., & Bishop-Kurylo, D. (1996). Pediatric procedures. *Topics in Emergency Medicine, 18,* 30-45.

Fernandez, E., Sweeney, M., & Green, T. (1997). Central venous catheters (pp. 196-202). In Dieckmann R., Fiser, D., & Selbst, S. (Eds.), *Pediatric emergency and critical care procedures.* St. Louis: Mosby.

Fleck, D. (2001). Central venous catheter insertion (perform) (pp. 503-521). In Lynn-McHale, D.J., & Carlson, K.K. (Eds.), *AACN Procedure Manual for Critical Care,* 4th ed. Philadelphia: W.B. Saunders.

Markenson, D.S. (2002). *Pediatric prehospital care.* Upper Saddle River, NJ: Prentice Hall.

O'Grady, N.P., Alexander, N.P., Dellinger, E.P. et al. (2002). Guidelines for prevention of intravascular catheter-related infections. *Morbidity and Mortality Weekly Report, 51,* 1-28.

Simon, R., & Brenner, B. (2002). *Emergency procedures and techniques,* 4th ed. Baltimore: Williams & Wilkins.

Internal Jugular Venous Access

Reneé Semonin Holleran, RN, PhD, CEN, CCRN, CFRN, SANE

INDICATIONS

1. To obtain central venous access when peripheral access is unattainable, such as occurs in a patient who is in profound shock or cardiac arrest or in a patient who is an intravenous (IV) drug abuser. There is a lower risk of pleural puncture when using the internal jugular (IJ) vein than when using the subclavian vein. In the obese or elderly patient, the IJ vein may afford easier access than the subclavian vein (Simon & Brenner, 2002)
2. To place a catheter to monitor central venous pressure
3. To provide a site for insertion of a transvenous pacemaker or a pulmonary artery catheter
4. To administer large amounts of fluid, blood products, or medications, especially those likely to cause complications if they are administered via a smaller peripheral vein

CONTRAINDICATIONS AND CAUTIONS

1. This procedure is contraindicated in any patient with a potential cervical spine injury because positioning the patient for this procedure requires movement of the head.
2. Proceed with caution in the presence of an anatomic distortion (e.g., massive soft tissue injury) or patient habitus (obese, short neck) that interferes with the location of the anatomic landmarks.
3. A patient with a coagulopathy, either from a disease process or from medication, must be monitored carefully for bleeding at the insertion site.
4. An infection in the area of the insertion precludes the use of that site.
5. Fibrinolytic therapy must be given with extreme caution to the patient with a central line in place.
6. If a hematoma develops on one side of the neck, insertion on the other side should be avoided or should be accomplished with extreme caution because of the potential for airway compromise if hematomas form bilaterally.
7. When selecting a site to insert a central line, several things should be considered, including selecting a site that with the lowest risk of complications, such as infection; anticipated duration of catheter placement; and type of fluids or medications that are to be administered through the device (O'Grady et al, 2002).

EQUIPMENT

Antiseptic solution

Local anesthetic

5-ml syringe; 18-G, 25-G, or 27-G needles for local anesthesia administration

Central venous kit (Most kits contain an 8.5-French introducer, which can be used for fluid-volume resuscitation or for the introduction of a trans-venous pacemaker or a pulmonary-artery catheter.)

or

Multilumen catheter (used for fluid administration and allows insertion of invasive lines, transvenous pacemakers, as well as ports for administering medication and obtaining blood)

or

16-G, 8-inch single-lumen catheter

No. 11 scalpel

Intravenous solution and tubing

Normal saline flush

Silk suture (2-0 or 3-0) with a needle holder

Masks, caps, goggles, sterile gloves, and gowns

Dressing supplies (gauze or a transparent dressing). NOTE: When the patient is diaphoretic or the site is oozing, it should be covered with gauze instead of a transparent dressing (O'Grady et al, 2002).

PATIENT PREPARATION

1. Place the patient on a cardiac monitor and pulse oximeter.
2. Place the patient in a Trendelenburg position and turn the head away from the site of insertion. Placing a pillow or towel roll under the patient's shoulder can facilitate patient positioning (American Heart Association [AHA], 2002). If the patient cannot tolerate the Trendelenburg position, elevate the legs for a modified Trendelenburg position (Procedure 51). Turn the patient's head to the side opposite the insertion.
3. *Cleanse the area of insertion with an antiseptic solution. The IJ vein runs posteriorly and laterally to the internal and common carotid artery. As the vein nears the thoracic area, it becomes more lateral and more anterior to the common carotid artery. Another landmark used for accessing the IJ vein is the sternocleidomastoid muscle. The IJ vein runs medially to this muscle in its upper part and then passes posteriorly to the inferior heads of the muscle in its midportion. Landmarks for the IJ vein are the angle of the mandible, the clavicle, the suprasternal notch, the external jugular vein and the carotid pulsation, the two heads of the sternocleidomastoid muscle, and the triangle formed by the two heads and the clavicle (Figure 67-1).
4. *Drape the patient's head with sterile towels.

PROCEDURAL STEPS

1. *Locate the landmarks of the IJ vein and infiltrate the area of insertion with a local anesthetic.
2. The three approaches to accessing the IJ vein are the middle, the anterior, and the posterior approaches. The posterior and middle approaches are the most commonly used and are described as follows (see Figure 67-1):

---

*Indicates portions of the procedure usually performed by a physician or an advanced practice nurse.

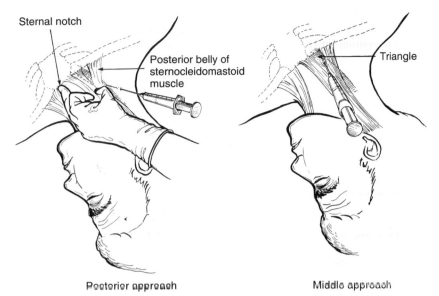

FIGURE 67-1 Internal jugular vein cannulation. (From Dunmire, S., & Paris, P. [1994]. *Atlas of emergency procedures* [p. 201]. Philadelphia: W.B. Saunders.)

a. *Middle approach: Locate the triangle formed by the bifurcation of the sternocleidomastoid muscle and the clavicle. Attach the needle to a syringe and insert it at the apex of the triangle at a 30- to 45-degree angle to the skin. During insertion, the needle should be directed at the ipsilateral nipple. The needle should not be inserted farther than 5 cm. If the vein cannot be located immediately, the needle should be withdrawn and redirected just lateral to the ipsilateral nipple.

b. *Posterior approach: Locate the posterior border of the sternocleidomastoid muscle and insert the needle attached to a syringe under the posterior border, directing the needle toward the sternal notch. If the vein is not located after 4-6 cm of insertion, remove the needle and redirect it toward the contralateral nipple.

3. *Once the vein has been located, detach the syringe and place a gloved finger over the hub. Gently thread the guide wire through the hub of the needle. When the wire has been inserted 8-20 cm, remove the needle and leave the guide wire in place. Using the No. 11 blade, make a nick in the skin where the wire enters the skin. If there is a vein dilator, thread it over the wire to the hub and then remove the dilator, leaving the wire in place. Sometimes, the catheter and the dilator are inserted together over the wire. During insertion, always maintain control of the wire. Once the catheter is inserted, remove the wire and the dilator, if it is present. When the catheter is in place, confirm its location again by withdrawing some blood. Blood may also be drawn for a

---

*Indicates portions of the procedure usually performed by a physician or an advanced practice nurse.

laboratory evaluation. If the catheter has been found to be patent, connect it to the intravenous solution. Secure the catheter with a suture and apply a transparent, sterile dressing.
4. *Suture the catheter in place.
5. Apply a dressing and secure the catheter and the tubing with tape.
6. Obtain a chest x-ray film to check the line placement and to rule out complications, such as a pneumothorax.

AGE-SPECIFIC CONSIDERATIONS

1. Only skilled personnel (or less experienced providers under the direct supervision of a skilled clinician) can safely access the IJ vein in the infant and young child (AHA, 2002).
2. The right IJ vein is the preferred site for the pediatric patient because it has a lower risk of causing a pneumothorax or possible damage to the thoracic duct than does the left IJ vein. Accessing the right IJ vein in the pediatric patient increases the likelihood that the catheter may pass into the superior vena cava instead of the right subclavian vein (AHA, 2002).

COMPLICATIONS

1. Pneumothorax
2. Hematoma formation from either a venous or an arterial bleed. If the carotid artery is nicked, apply direct pressure to control bleeding.
3. Air embolism resulting from an introduction of air into the catheter
4. Thoracic duct injury because of a perforation of the thoracic duct
5. Infection and phlebitis. Risk factors associated with the development of infection and phlebitis include type of catheter, frequency of catheter manipulation, and patient-related factors (O'Grady, et al., 2002).

PATIENT TEACHING

1. Report any chest pain or shortness of breath or any disconnections or dampness around the dressing site immediately.
2. Do not touch the area where the catheter is inserted.

REFERENCES

American Heart Association (AHA). (2002). *Textbook of pediatric advanced life support*. Dallas: Author.

O'Grady, N.P., Alexander, M., Dellinger, E.P. et al. (2002). Guidelines for prevention of intravascular catheter–related infections. *Morbidity and Mortality Weekly Report, 51*, 1-28.

Simon, R.R., & Brenner, B.E. (2002). *Emergency procedures & techniques*, 4th ed. Baltimore: Williams & Wilkins.

---

*Indicates portions of the procedure usually performed by a physician or an advanced practice nurse.

Femoral Venous Access

Reneé Semonin Holleran, RN, PhD, CEN, CCRN, CFRN, SANE

INDICATIONS

1. To place a large (i.e., 6-9 French) vascular access device for the administration of medications, intravenous (IV) fluids, and blood products
2. To gain central-venous access during cardiopulmonary resuscitation (CPR) for rapid distribution of medications and/or fluids.

NOTE: During CPR, venous return from below the diaphragm is diminished. For this reason, if the femoral site is used for access, the catheter should be long enough to pass above the level of the diaphragm, and large quantities of flush solution are recommended after IV medication.

3. To provide access for insertion of invasive devices, such as pulmonary catheters, transvenous pacemakers, hemodialysis catheters, and cardiac catheters.

CONTRAINDICATIONS AND CAUTIONS

1. Relative contraindications for femoral access devices include an abnormal vascular status of the lower extremities, congenital malformation of the lower extremity, femoral hernia, abdominal or pelvic tumor or trauma, abdominal ascites, and infection of the tissue overlying the puncture site (Lavelle & Costarino, 1997).
2. Caution should be exercised if a patient is receiving an anticoagulant or fibrinolytic therapy. In such a patient, femoral vein cannulation should be performed by using the single-wall puncture technique (Grossman & Baim, 1991). The patient should be monitored continuously for excessive bleeding.

EQUIPMENT

Commercially available central line kit or assemble the following:
Polyurethane, radiopaque, indwelling catheter
6- to 9-French catheter or a 10-cm length catheter with or without side ports for infusions while monitoring central venous pressure
14- to 18-G or 20-cm, single- or multiple-lumen catheters
Vessel dilator
J-tip spring-wire guide
Percutaneous entry needle (18 G, 7 cm)
10-ml syringe
Local anesthetic (e.g., lidocaine 1%)
Syringe and needles for local administration of anesthesia
Scalpel (No. 11 blade)
Needle holder
Suture scissors

Suture (2-0 silk or nylon)
Sterile gloves
Antiseptic solution
Saline flush
Dressing supplies (gauze or a transparent dressing) NOTE: When the patient
   is diaphoretic or the site is oozing, it should be covered with gauze
   instead of a transparent dressing (O'Grady et al., 2002).
Tape
IV solution and tubing
Blood-collection tubes

PATIENT PREPARATION

1. Place the patient in a flat, supine position with the legs fully extended.
2. Shave or clip the hair around the insertion site as needed and cleanse the area
   with an antiseptic solution.

PROCEDURAL STEPS

1. *Locate the femoral artery (Figure 68-1) by palpating the pulsation 1-3 cm
   below the inguinal ligament, which runs from the anterosuperior iliac spine

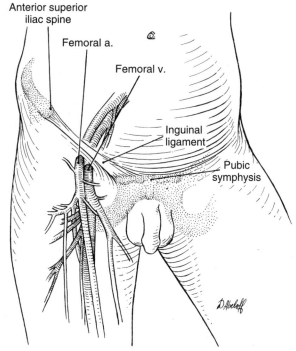

FIGURE 68-1 Anatomy of the femoral vein. (From Rosen, P., & Sternbach, G.L. [1983]. *Atlas of emergency medicine,* 2nd ed. [p. 83]. Baltimore: Williams & Wilkins, with permission.)

---

*Indicates portions of the procedure usually performed by a physician or an advanced practice nurse.

to the pubic tubercle. The femoral vein lies approximately 1-2 cm medial to the artery, along a parallel course. Easy location of the vein depends on the presence of a pulse in the femoral artery. During CPR, the arterial pulse may be weak or absent, but it may also be present in the femoral vein because of venous backflow during CPR. Therefore, unsuccessful attempts to cannulate the vein medial to the pulsations should lead to a more lateral approach.

2. *Infiltrate the insertion site with a local anesthetic by creating a linear intradermal wheal with a short needle. Once the dermal layer is anesthetized, make a small transverse skin puncture with a No. 11 scalpel. Replace the needle with a longer needle and continue to infiltrate the tissue with lidocaine to the periosteum.

3. *Attach a 10-ml syringe to the 18-G, 7-cm percutaneous entry needle and enter the insertion site at the transverse skin puncture (Figure 68-2, *A*). Approach the femoral vein at a 45- to 90-degree angle cephalad, and aspirate gently with the syringe while advancing. Once the wall of the vein is penetrated, blood should be aspirated freely.

NOTE: After any unsuccessful attempts at venous wall puncture, apply pressure at the site for 5 minutes.

4. *If only blood samples are desired, aspirate the quantity needed and withdraw the needle. Apply pressure to the site for 5 minutes. Monitor the site frequently for continued bleeding.

5. *As soon as the blood is aspirated freely from the femoral vein, remove the syringe and place the J-tip spring wire through the needle into the vein (Figure 68-2, *B*).

6. *Withdraw the needle while holding the J-wire firmly with the left hand to ensure that it remains in the vein (Figure 68-2, *C*). After the needle is removed, wipe the protruding wire with a moistened gauze pad to remove clotted blood and facilitate the advancement of the dilator or catheter.

7. *Thread the catheter or the dilator-catheter over the J-wire into the vein. Advance the dilator-catheter until it is seated at the hub (Figure 68-2, *D*). Remove the J-wire and then the dilator, if used. Aspirate the blood via the catheter to remove any air bubbles. Attach the primed IV tubing and the solution to the catheter.

8. The IV fluid should flow freely. The catheter position in the vein can be verified by withdrawing the blood or lowering the IV bag below the level of the entrance site and noting the blood reflux into the IV tubing.

9. *Secure the catheter to the skin. This is generally accomplished by suturing the catheter hub to the patient's skin.

10. Apply a dressing to the site.

AGE-SPECIFIC CONSIDERATIONS

1. For pediatric patients, slightly rotate the leg externally (Spivey & Hodge, 1996).

2. For children, the femoral site is the first choice for emergency placement of a central venous catheter because the anatomic landmarks are easily identifiable, hemostatic pressure can be applied easily in the event of bleeding at

---

*Indicates portions of the procedure usually performed by a physician or an advanced practice nurse.

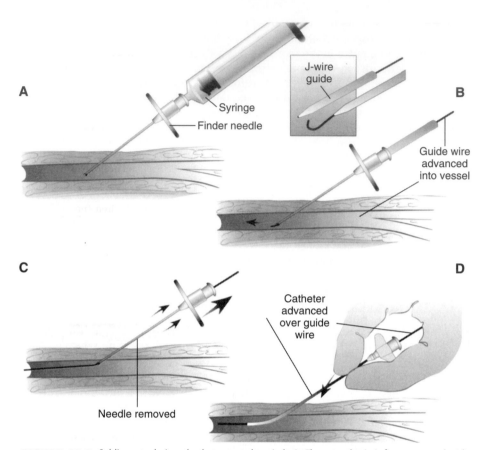

FIGURE 68-2 Seldinger technique (catheter over the wire). **A,** The central vein is first punctured with a percutaneous needle. **B,** The syringe is removed, and the guide wire is inserted through the needle into the vein. **C,** The needle is removed, and the wire is left in place. **D,** The dilator or catheter is inserted over the guide wire, and the wire is removed. (From Lavelle, J., & Costarino, A., Jr. [1997]. Central venous access [p. 259]. In Henretig, F.M., & King, C.G. [Eds.], *Textbook of pediatric emergency procedures*. Baltimore: Williams & Wilkins.)

the site, and there is no interference with airway management or chest compressions (Lavelle & Costarino, 1997).

COMPLICATIONS

1. Hematoma at the puncture site of the vein or femoral artery
2. Arteriovenous fistula
3. Inadvertent cannulation of the femoral artery
4. Infection and phlebitis. Risk factors associated with the development of infection and phlebitis include type of catheter, frequency of catheter manipulation, and patient-related factors (O'Grady et al., 2002).
5. Thrombosis
6. Injury to the femoral nerve

PATIENT TEACHING

1. Avoid flexion of the affected leg.
2. Report any wetness felt at the site or any blood on the dressing.
3. Report any pain, numbness, or tingling in the leg.

REFERENCES

Grossman, W., Baim, D.S. (1991). Cardiac Catheterization, angiography, and intervention, 4th ed. Philadelphia: Lea & Febiger.

Lavelle, J., & Costarino, A., Jr. (1997). Central venous access (pp. 251–277). In Henretig, F.M. & King, C. *Textbook of pediatric emergency procedures*. Baltimore: Williams & Wilkins.

O'Grady, N.P., Alexander, M., Dellinger, E.P. et al. (2002). Guidelines for prevention of intravascular catheter–related infections. *Morbidity and Mortality Weekly Report, 51*, 1-28.

Spivey, W.H., & Hodge, D., III (1996). Vascular access in infants and children (pp. 88-92). In Tintinalli, J.E. et al. (Eds.), *Emergency medicine: a comprehensive study guide*, 4th ed. New York: McGraw-Hill.

PROCEDURE 69

Venous Cutdown

Reneé Semonin Holleran, RN, PhD, CEN, CCRN, CFRN, SANE and Jean A. Proehl, RN, MN, CEN, CCRN

INDICATION

To provide venous access when peripheral sites are either unavailable or inadequate

CONTRAINDICATIONS AND CAUTIONS

1. Venous access via cutdown may be more time consuming than percutaneous central venous access; other types of venous access should be considered before a venous cutdown is performed.
2. This procedure is contraindicated in patients who have injury proximal to the cutdown site (Krug, 1997).
3. The presence of a coagulopathy is a relative contraindication (Krug, 1997).

EQUIPMENT

Intravenous (IV) setup (fluid and tubing)
1-piece or short extension set

Large-bore IV catheter (Infant feeding tubes or an IV extension set with the distal end cut at a bevel can also be used.)
Antiseptic solution
Tourniquet (optional)
Local anesthetic (optional)
Syringe and needles for local anesthetic administration
No. 11 and No. 15 blade scalpels
Tissue scissors (iris or Metzenbaum)
Tissue forceps
Vein retractor
Hemostats
Needle holder
Catheter introducer (optional)
Silk suture 1-0 to 4-0
Dressing supplies (gauze or transparent)
NOTE: Most facilities have prepackaged venous cutdown trays with much of this equipment already assembled.

PATIENT PREPARATION

1. Assemble the IV solution and tubing. Prime the T-piece with the saline solution and leave a syringe of the saline solution attached.
2. Place the chosen extremity in an extended position. The sites most commonly used are the saphenous vein (just anterior and superior to the medial malleolus of the tibia or superficial and medial to the femoral artery and vein in the groin) or the basilic vein (medial aspect of antecubital fossa). The cephalic vein (lateral aspect of the antecubital fossa) can also be used, but passing a catheter through the sharp angulation where the vein enters the axillary vein makes this route difficult if central access is desired (Simon & Brenner, 2002).
3. Place a venous tourniquet proximally if a distal extremity site is chosen (optional).

PROCEDURAL STEPS

1. Cleanse the site with an antiseptic solution and then drape it.
2. *Infiltrate the area over the vein with a local anesthetic if the patient is conscious and time permits.
3. *Make a transverse skin incision over the vein (Figure 69-1).
4. *Dissect bluntly down to the vein.
5. *Isolate the vein with silk ligatures proximally and distally.
6. *Tie the distal ligature.
7. *Make a small incision into the vein between the ligatures and insert the catheter toward the heart. A catheter introducer may facilitate this procedure. Alternatively, cannulate the vein with an over-the-needle or through-the-needle catheter (Krug, 1997).
8. Remove the tourniquet (if used).

---

*Indicates portions of the procedure usually performed by a physician or an advanced practice nurse.

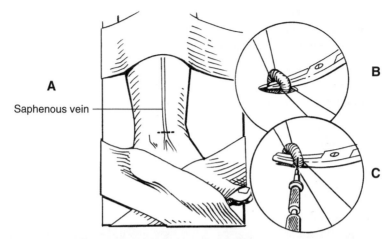

FIGURE 69-1 A, Make transverse incision over the distal saphenous vein. **B,** Use silk ligatures to isolate and expose the vein. **C,** Cannulate the exposed vein. (From Krug, S. [1997]. Venous cutdown [p. 96] In Walsh-Sukys, M.C., & Krug, S.E. [Eds.], *Procedures in infants and children.* Philadelphia: W.B. Saunders.)

9. Connect the primed T-piece and syringe assembly to the catheter and aspirate to confirm the placement. Flush the tubing with a saline solution from the syringe, disconnect the syringe, and connect the IV tubing to the T-piece.
10. *Tie the proximal ligature to secure the catheter in place.
11. *Suture the skin around the catheter and suture the catheter in place.
12. Apply a dressing.
13. Tape the tubing securely.
14. Observe the patient closely for signs of swelling from a hematoma formation or a fluid infiltration.

AGE-SPECIFIC CONSIDERATION

For children, the saphenous vein at the ankle is the preferred peripheral cutdown site, and the saphenous vein at the groin is the preferred central cutdown site (Krug, 1997).

COMPLICATIONS

1. Blood loss
2. Inadvertent "cannulation" of a tendon or an artery, or false passage of the catheter between layers of the vessel wall
3. Loosening of ligatures with resultant bleeding and hematoma formation
4. Embolization
5. Infiltration of IV fluid
6. Thrombophlebitis
7. Infection and sepsis
8. Injury to adjacent nerves and arteries

---

*Indicates portions of the procedure usually performed by a physician or an advanced practice nurse.

PATIENT TEACHING

1. Do not manipulate or move the catheter.
2. Report any disconnections or dampness at the site immediately.

REFERENCES

Krug, S. (1997). Venous cutdown (pp. 94–97). In Walsh-Sukys, M.C. & Krug, S.E. (Eds.), *Procedures in infants and children*. Philadelphia: W.B. Saunders.

Simon, R.R., & Brenner, B.E. (2002). *Emergency procedures and techniques*, 4th ed. Baltimore: Williams & Wilkins.

PROCEDURE 70

Intraosseous Access

Reneé Semonin Holleran, RN, PhD, CEN, CCRN, CFRN, SANE

INDICATIONS

Intraosseous (IO) infusion is indicated when rapid access to the circulation for the administration of fluids or medications is needed. IO infusion should be given any time intravenous (IV) cannulation is either too difficult or too time consuming to accomplish. IO needles are recommended for resuscitation in any age group (American Heart Association [AHA], 2001). Some specific indications include the following:

1. Administration of crystalloids, colloids, or blood for resuscitation of patients in shock states. However, flow rates may not be sufficient to fully treat severe hypovolemia or hemorrhagic shock.
2. Administration of medications
3. Diagnostic studies, such as electrolytes, blood cultures, blood gases, and hemoglobin, may be obtained through the IO route, although these studies are not primary indications for this procedure.

CONTRAINDICATIONS AND CAUTIONS

1. An IO infusion is not recommended in any fractured extremities because of the risk of fluid and medication infiltration into the surrounding tissue.
2. To decrease the risk of infection, avoid placing the IO line through burned or infected tissue.
3. General contraindications may include patients who have bone disorders, such as osteoporosis and osteogenesis imperfecta.

4. Avoid placing the needle in a site where there is obvious soft tissue infection.

5. Do not infuse marrow-toxic medications (e.g., certain antibiotics) via the IO route.

EQUIPMENT

Antiseptic solution

Local anesthetic (optional, but should be used if the patient is conscious)

Several large-bore (18 G or larger) IO needles (Figures 70-1 and 70-2); products that are commonly available include the following:

Jamshidi Illinois sternal (Baxter Healthcare): 15-18 G, adjustable plastic sleeve to control depth of penetration

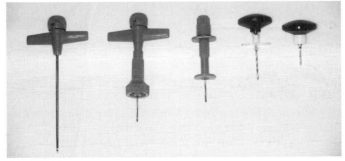

FIGURE 70-1 Types of intraosseous needles. (From Stanley, R. [2004]. Intraosseous infusion [p. 478]. In Roberts, J.R. & Hedges, J.R. (Eds.), *Clinical procedures in emergency medicine,* 4th ed. Philadelphia: W.B. Saunders, with permission.)

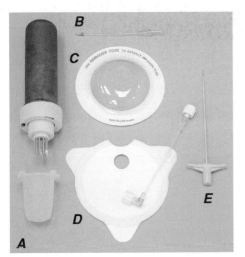

FIGURE 70-2 The F.A.S.T. intraosseous infusion system. *A,* Introducer with depth control. *B,* Infusion tube. *C,* Protector dome. *D,* Target/strain-relief patch. *E,* Remover. (Courtesy the Pyng Medical Corp., Richmond, BC.)

Cook IO needle (Cook Critical Care): 16-18 G, relatively large, round, detachable handles; various tips include bevel, pencil-point tip, and 45-degree trocar

Sur-Fast (Cook Critical Care): Has a threaded shaft to assist in more secure needle placement

B.I.G. bone injection gun (WaisMed, Ltd.): Available in two sizes: a blue case for the 15-G needle (adults and children older than 12 years of age) and a red case for the 18-G needle (children 0-12 years of age). This device is a triggered mechanism, which inserts a trocar needle into the bone.

F.A.S.T. IO infusion system (Pyng Medical Corp.): An adult IO needle that is inserted in the sternum. Each kit contains a 16-G introducer with depth control, an infusion tube, a protector dome, target strain-relief patch, and a remover.

Syringe for aspiration

Normal saline solution for irrigation

Tape, an arm or leg board, or hemostats, for stabilization of the needle

Dressing supplies

IV tubing and a fluid bag or bottle

Pressure infusion bag

PROCEDURAL STEPS

1. Select the potential site for the infusion. Consider the patient's age, size, site accessibility, and any other procedures that may be needed. The tibial plateau (approximately 1 cm below the tibial tuberosity and medially on the tibial plateau) is the most popular and common site for insertion of the needle (AHA, 2002) (Figure 70-3). This location is preferred because it is a relatively flat surface and there is very little overlying soft tissue, which facilitates stabilizing the needle. The medial malleolus site (approximately 2 cm proximal to the tip of the medial malleolus) may also be used, although it may be more difficult to stabilize the needle over the rounded bony prominences. The distal femur and the iliac crest are occasionally used, but they may be more difficult to access because of greater amounts of overlying tissue and rounded bone. The needle should be inserted 2-3 cm above the femoral condyles at an angle of 10-15 degrees from the vertical position (Stanley, 2004). In the adult patient, the manubrium on the midline and 1.5 cm (⅝ inch) below the sternal notch can be accessed for IO insertion. Two other additional access sites include the posterior-distal metaphysis of the radius opposite the radial pulse and the anterior head of the humerus.

2. Position the patient (depending on the site of the insertion) and stabilize the area for insertion.

3. Cleanse the area with an antiseptic solution.

4. Anesthetize the area (this is not necessary in moribund or obtunded patients).

5. Insert the needle.

   a. Manual insertion: With the needle pointed slightly away from the joint or at a 90-degree angle (AHA, 2002; Stanley, 2004), puncture the skin, and use a rotary motion to push the needle into the bony cortex. Feel for a "pop." The needle should feel firm in the bone, but not stable.

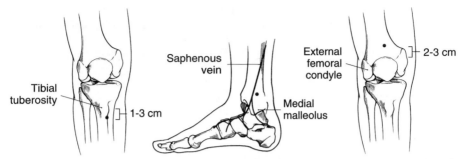

FIGURE 70-3 Examples of insertion sites for intraosseous needles. (From Stanley, R. [2004]. Intraosseous infusion [p. 479]. In Roberts, J.R., & Hedges, J.R. (Eds.), *Clinical procedures in emergency medicine,* 4th ed. Philadelphia: W.B. Saunders.)

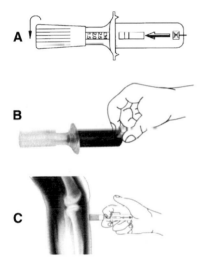

FIGURE 70-4 Insertion of the B.I.G. **A,** Adjust the depth of penetration. **B,** Pull out the safety latch. **C,** trigger the device by pressing the rear part against the shoulder of the housing. (Courtesy Wais Med Ltd., Kress USA Corporation, Overland Park, KS.)

b. Bone injection gun (B.I.G.) (WaisMed, Ltd., 2000) (Figure 70-4): Adjust the depth of penetration by unscrewing the sleeve from the cylindrical housing. Squeeze the sides of the safety latch together and remove it. Place the device against the insertion site and hold it firmly against the extremity while triggering it. The kickback of the device can push your hand back and prevent the needle from entering the bone if you do not hold it firmly enough. Trigger the device by pushing the rear part against the two shoulders of the housing. Remove the B.I.G. and separate the trocar needle from its housing.

c. F.A.S.T.: (Pyng Medical Corp., 2001) (Figure 70-5): Locate the patient's manubrium and place the target patch (See Figure 70-5, *A*). Place the introducer in the target zone on the patch, perpendicular to the skin (See Figure 70-5, *B*). Push on the introducer and then pull it straight back. This will

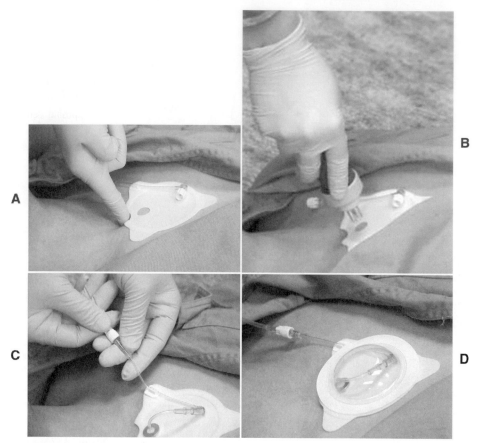

FIGURE 70-5 Insertion of the F.A.S.T. intraosseous infusion system. (Courtesy Pyng Medical Corp., Richmond, BC.)

expose the infusion tube and a two-part support sleeve (See Figure 70-5, *C*), which will fall away. Correct placement is verified by observation of marrow entering the infusion tube. Connect the IV to the infusion tube. place the protective dome over the site and press down firmly over the target patch to engage the Velcro fastening. This prevents the needle from moving. This device must be removed using the remover to disengage the infusion tube from the bone.

6. Remove the stylet and confirm the placement by aspirating the blood or the marrow contents or irrigating with a normal saline solution. In addition, the IV fluid should run steadily. Remember that laboratory tests can be obtained from the bone marrow, if needed. X-ray films may also be used to confirm placement.

7. Connect the syringe or the IV tubing.

8. Apply a sterile dressing and stabilize the needle and the tubing. Stabilize site with tape and dressings or hemostats (Figure 70-6). If the B.I.G. is used, the

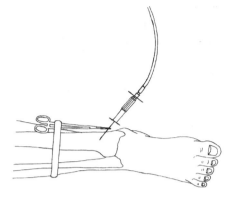

FIGURE 70-6 A hemostat may be placed on the shaft or hub of the needle and then taped to the ankle or leg to stabilize the needle. Be careful not to clamp the needle too tightly. Opposing hemostats further increase the stability of the needle.

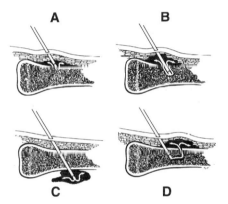

FIGURE 70-7 Placement should be carefully assessed to avoid leakage of fluid around the insertion site. **A,** Incomplete penetration of the bony cortex. **B,** Penetration of the posterior cortex. **C,** Fluid escaping around the needle through the puncture site. **D,** Fluid leaking through a nearby previous puncture site. (From Stanley, R. [2004]. Intraosseous infusion [p. 483]. In Roberts J.R. & Hedges, J.R. (Eds.), *Clinical procedures in emergency medicine,* 4th ed. Philadelphia: W.B. Saunders.)

safety latch can be placed around the needle to provide additional stabilization. If the F.A.S.T. is used, a protector dome is supplied for stability. A small plastic cup can be placed over the needle to provide further protection against dislodgment.

9. Reassess the patency of the site.

AGE-SPECIFIC CONSIDERATIONS

1. IO access is widely recommended for use in the pediatric population (AHA, 2002), and it is now recommended in the management of adult patients who are critically ill (Waisman & Waisman, 1997; Frascone et al., 2001).
2. The F.A.S.T. (sternal site) is contraindicated in the pediatric patient.
3. The lower femur can be used safely only in small infants (Krug, 1997).
4. Adult patients with sternal trauma or chest deformities should not have a sternal IO placed.
5. IO placement in adult patients may be difficult because of the thickness of the bony cortex.

COMPLICATIONS

1. Unsuccessfully attempting to penetrate the bony cortex or bending the needle by use of excessive force delays vascular access (Figure 70-7).

2. Puncture of the posterior cortex as a result of excessive pressure during the insertion of the needle (see Figure 70-7)
3. Fluid leakage from the infusion site. Fluid extravasation may occur, especially if the insertion was difficult or both cortices were penetrated (see Figure 70-7). This fluid extravasation may lead to compartmental syndrome.
4. Fat embolism resulting from use of high-pressure volume infusions (Iserson & Criss, 1986; O'Neill, 1945)
5. Potential osteomyelitis, which appears to be associated with prolonged continuous infusions (Heinild et al., 1947)
6. Clot formation within the bone marrow needle, causing slowing of the rate of infusion. The use of a pressure bag often alleviates this problem.
7. Tibial fractures

REFERENCES

American Heart Association. (AHA). (2002). *Pediatric advanced life support manual*. Dallas: Author.

American Heart Association (AHA). (2001). *Advanced cardiac life support manual*. Dallas: Author.

Frascone, R., Dries, D., Gisch, T., Kaye, K., & Jensen, J. (2001). Obtaining vascular access: is there a place for the sternal IO? *Air Medical Journal, 20*(6), 20-22.

Heinild, S., Sondergaard, T., & Tudvad, F. (1947). Bone marrow infusion in childhood. *Journal of Pediatrics, 30*, 400-412.

Iserson, K.V., & Criss, E. (1986). Intraosseous infusions: a usable technique. *American Journal of Emergency Medicine, 4*, 540.

Krug, S. (1997). Intraosseous infusion (pp. 134-139). In Walsh-Sukys, M.C., & Krug, S. (Eds.), *Procedures in infants and children*. Philadelphia: W.B. Saunders.

O'Neill, J.F. (1945). Complications of intraosseous therapy. *Annals of Surgery, 2*, 266.

Pyng Medical Corp. (2001). *F.A.S.T.™ intraosseous infusion system with depth control* (product brochure). Richmond, BC: Author. Available at http://www.pyng.com/.

Stanley, R. [2004]. Intraosseous infusion (pp. 475-485). In Roberts J.R., & Hedges, J.R. (Eds.), *Clinical procedures in emergency medicine*, 4th ed. Philadelphia: W.B. Saunders.

Waisman, M., & Waisman, D. (1997). Bone marrow infusion in adults. *Journal of Trauma, 42*, 288-293.

WaisMed, Ltd. (2000). *Bone injection gun (B.I.G.™) instructions*. Caesarea, Israel. Retrieved 5/16/2003 from http://www.waismed.com/.

Accessing Preexisting Central Venous Catheters

Reneé Semonin Holleran, RN, PhD, CEN, CCRN, CFRN, SANE

There are many types of preexisting central venous catheters, including the Hickman-Broviac right atrial catheter, the Groshong catheter, the peripherally inserted central catheter (PICC), and the hemodialysis catheter. Most are available in single- or multilumen configurations (Table 71-1). Most patients carry an identification card that displays the manufacturer's name, model, and instructions. For the latest information, contact the manufacturer of the specific catheter.

INDICATIONS
To gain venous access in patients with preexisting central venous catheters to:
1. Administer intravenous (IV) fluids, medications, and blood products
2. Obtain venous blood samples
3. Administer parenteral nutrition

CONTRAINDICATIONS AND CAUTIONS
1. Use only a clamp without teeth or a padded clamp on central venous catheters. Other clamps may damage the catheter. Bulldog clamps are safe and convenient (Figure 71-1).
2. To prevent an air embolism in the event that the catheter is disconnected or damaged, clamp the catheter or place the patient in a supine position and ask the patient to perform the Valsalva maneuver (take a deep breath and bear down).
3. Use needles of 1 inch or smaller when inserting a needle into the male adapter plug of a central venous catheter because longer needles may puncture the catheter. When available, needleless systems are recommended.
4. Tape all connections to prevent inadvertent disconnection or air embolism.
5. When whole blood or packed red blood cells are administered through a PICC line, it may be necessary to use a pressure infusor (Procedure 78). Adding 50 ml of normal saline solution to the blood bag or running a normal saline solution concomitantly with the blood reduces viscosity and improves flow rates.
6. When performing central venous pressure monitoring via a Groshong catheter, subtract the "valve-closing pressure" from the manometer reading (5.44 H_2O or 4 mm Hg) to give the true central venous pressure reading (Davol, 1994a).
7. If administration of chemotherapy or other vesicant agents is anticipated, ensure patency of the catheter by aspirating blood before infusion. If there is any question of patency, evaluation of the catheter by dye studies is recommended before infusion.
8. Rapid or forceful flushing may dislodge a clot into the central circulation.

TABLE 71-1

SELECTED CENTRAL VENOUS CATHETERS

Catheter Type/Name	Description of Catheter	Recommended Flush Protocol	Comments
Right atrial catheter (Hickman, Broviac)	Tunneled, cuffed silicone catheter (see Figure 71-2) surgically inserted, usually in subclavian vein, but may also use femoral access. Available in single-, double-, or triple-lumen configuration.	Heparin, 10-100 units/ml, 2.5-5 ml every 12-24 hr, or after each use. Flush each lumen separately.	Check for closed clamp. *Do not flush vigorously or against resistance—catheter may rupture.*
Groshong	Tunneled, cuffed silicone catheter, surgically inserted, usually in subclavian vein. Available in single-, double-, and triple-lumen configurations. A three-way slit valve helps prevent air intake or bleeding if catheter comes apart (see Figure 71-3).	Heparin is not necessary. Flush after each use, or once per week with 5 ml of normal saline (use 20 ml after blood draw). Flush each lumen separately.	Need to flush with enough turbulence to clear blood from closed-tip catheter. No clamp necessary, owing to the three-way valve.
PICC (peripherally inserted central catheter)	Silicone or polyurethane catheter with insertion site near antecubital fossa and catheter tip threaded into central vein. Some catheters may not have tip placed in central vein (this is known as a midline catheter). Available in single- or double-lumen configurations.	Heparin 10-100 units/ml, 1-2.5 ml every 12 hr, or after each use. Flush each lumen separately. No heparin needed for Groshong PICC; use normal saline solution as described above.	*Avoid vigorous flushing.* Do not flush against resistance—catheter may rupture. Use 10-ml or larger syringe. Do not use affected arm for venipuncture or blood pressures.
Hemodialysis catheter (Quinton, HEMED, Vas-Cath)	Silicone or polyurethane, usually subclavian or femoral access. Catheters maintained by dialysis personnel and not routinely used for IV therapy.	Heparin flush dose and strength should be by specific physician order only. Typical dose is heparin 1000-5000 units/ml, 1.5 ml instilled into each lumen after flushing with 20 ml of normal saline.	Aspirate heparin before use to avoid heparin-induced coagulopathy. Most hemodialysis catheters tolerate very high flow rates and pressures and provide good access for resuscitation efforts.

Data from Clemence, M. A., Walker, D., & Farr, B. M. (1995). Central venous catheter practices: results of a survey. *Journal of Vascular Access Devices, 1,* 30-38; Davol (1994a). *Nursing procedure manual, Groshong C. V. catheter.* Cranston, R. I.: Author; Davol. (1994b). Hickman subcutaneous ports and Hickman/Broviac catheters wall poster. Cranston, R. I.: Author; Mayo D. J., Dimond, E. P., Kramer, W., & Horne, M. K. (1996). Discard volumes necessary for clinically useful coagulation studies from heparinized Hickman catheters. *Oncology Nursing Forum, 23,* 671-675, with permission; Terry, J., Baranowski, L., Lonsway, R. A., & Hedrick, C. (1995). *Intravenous-therapy: clinical principles and practice.* Philadelphia: W. B. Saunders, with permission; Weinstein, S. M. (1993). *Plumer's principles and practice of intravenous therapy,* 5th ed. Philadelphia: J. B. Lippincott.

IV, Intravenous; PICC, peripherally inserted central catheter.

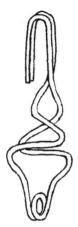

FIGURE 71-1 Bulldog catheter clamp.

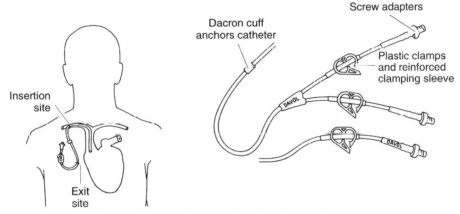

FIGURE 71-2 Schematic of tunneled catheter. (Courtesy Davol. [1994b]. Hickman subcutaneous ports and Hickman/Broviac catheters wall poster. Cranston, RI: Author.)

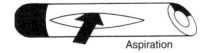

Aspiration

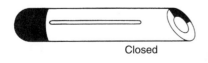

Closed

FIGURE 71-3 The Groshong three-position valve. (Courtesy Davol. [1994b]. Hickman subcutaneous ports and Hickman/Broviac catheters wall poster. Cranston, RI: Author.)

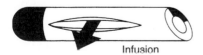

Infusion

EQUIPMENT
Bulldog or padded clamp
Nonsterile gloves
10-ml syringe to withdraw blood for discard, or an extra blood-specimen
    collection tube if you are using a vacuum tube
Sampling syringes for blood specimens
Blood-specimen tubes
Antiseptic swabs
Normal saline solution for injection
Heparin or saline flush, as needed (see Table 71-1 for recommended flush
    protocols)

PATIENT PREPARATION
Place the patient in a supine position or make sure that the catheter is clamped.
For a PICC line, place the patient in any comfortable position.

PROCEDURAL STEPS
Fluid Administration
1. Prepare the appropriate fluids and prime the tubing.
2. Clamp the catheter and remove the male adapter plug from the hub of the
    catheter if a continuous IV infusion is to be administered.
3. Attach the primary tubing to the hub of the catheter.
4. Unclamp the catheter and adjust the IV flow to the prescribed rate.

Medication Administration
NOTE: For administration of IV push medications or flush solutions, care must be
taken to avoid excessive pressure on the syringe, which could rupture the
catheter. Smaller syringes create higher pressures. Therefore a syringe no smaller
than 10 ml should be used for an IV push administration through any silicone elas-
tomer catheter. Table 71-2 lists recommended flow rates.
1. Check the compatibility of the prescribed medication with heparin. If the
    medication is potentially or actually incompatible with heparin, flush the
    catheter with 5 ml of normal saline solution for injection before administer-
    ing the medication.
2. Flush the catheter with 5 ml of normal saline solution after the administra-
    tion of the medication and before administering the heparin flush.

Additional Interventions (Smith et al., 2000)
1. If blood cannot be aspirated from the catheter:
    Use less negative pressure
    Have the patient change position
    Ask the patient to hold his/her breath or "bear down"
2. If air enters the catheter:
    Clamp the catheter
    Turn the patient onto the left side
    Administer oxygen
    Notify physician immediately

TABLE 71-2

MAXIMUM FLOW RATES FOR SELECTED CATHETERS AS RECOMMENDED BY THE MANUFACTURER

Catheter Type/Name	Maximum Flow Rate
Hickman 9.6 Fr (1.6 mm)	0.5 ml/sec (30 ml/min)
Hickman 1.3 mm	0.5 ml/sec (30 ml/min)
Broviac 6.6 Fr (1.0 mm)	0.5 ml/sec (30 ml/min)
Broviac 4.2 Fr (0.7 mm)	205 ml/hr (3 ml/min)
Broviac 2.7 Fr (0.5 mm)	49 ml/hr (0.8 ml/min)
Groshong 4 Fr (18 G)	500 ml/hr (PICC or tunneled)
Per-Q-Cath PICC 1.9 Fr (23 G)	125 ml/hr (2 ml/min)
Per-Q-Cath PICC 2.8 Fr (20 G)	250 ml/hr (4 ml/min)
Per-Q-Cath PICC 3.8 Fr (18 G)	350 ml/hr (6 ml/min)
Per-Q-Cath PICC 4.8 Fr (16 G)	450 ml/hr (7 ml/min)
Clinicath PICC 4 or 5 Fr (16 or 18 G)	>999 ml/hr (16 ml/min)
Clinicath PICC 3 Fr (20 G)	453 ml/hr (7.5 ml/min)

Data modified from SIMS Deltec. (1996). Clinicath peripherally inserted catheters wall poster. St. Paul, MN: Author; Gesco (1990). Gesco Per-Q-Cath package Insert. San Antonio, TX: Author; and Bard (1992). *How to care for your Hickman or Broviac catheter.* Salt Lake City, UT: Author.

Blood Sampling

NOTE: Using a heparinized catheter to collect blood samples for coagulation studies is not recommended if results are intended to monitor anticoagulant therapy or evaluate coagulopathy, because this technique yields falsely elevated levels (Mayo et al., 1996). If coagulation studies are necessary for such an evaluation, use a separate peripheral site for venipuncture. Blood samples from a heparinized catheter may be used to determine whether coagulation study results are normal (Mayo et al., 1996).

Blood Sampling Using a Syringe

1. If a continuous IV infusion is running, stop the infusion for 1 minute before drawing the blood specimens.
2. Clamp the catheter and remove the IV tubing or the male adapter plug.
3. Attach an empty 10-ml syringe to the hub of the catheter, unclamp the catheter, withdraw 5-10 ml of blood, and discard it (Terry et al., 1995).
4. Aspirate gently, because forceful aspiration may collapse the catheter. To facilitate blood return, have the patient raise both arms, cough, perform the Valsalva maneuver, or change position (Terry et al., 1995).
5. Withdraw the amount of blood needed, transfer blood to the tubes with a transfer device or remove the stopper(s) from the blood tube(s) and gently inject the blood along the side of the tube(s).
6. After the blood is drawn, flush the catheter with 10 ml of normal saline solution (20 ml for the Groshong catheter).
7. Reestablish the IV fluids or administer an appropriate heparin flush through a new male adapter plug.

Blood Sampling Using a Vacuum Tube

NOTE: Vacuum tubes may collapse the catheter. If this occurs, use the syringe method as described earlier.

1. When drawing blood specimens through a multilumen catheter, use the largest lumen if it is known, or use the distal lumen. Avoid the lumen that is used for nutritional solutions (total parenteral nutrition).
2. Turn off all the running infusions for 1 minute before withdrawing blood specimens.
3. Leave the male adapter plug on the catheter. Clean the catheter injection port with an antiseptic solution.
4. Place the vacuum tube in the tube holder and insert the adapter or needle into the injection port of the catheter.
5. Withdraw 5-10 ml of blood into an extra tube and discard it.
6. Draw the appropriate number and types of tubes needed (see Procedure 61).
7. After the blood is drawn, flush the catheter with 10 ml of normal saline solution (20 ml for the Groshong catheter).
8. Reestablish IV fluids or administer an appropriate saline or heparin flush through the male adapter plug.

AGE-SPECIFIC CONSIDERATIONS

1. For neonatal and pediatric patients, withdraw two to three times the volume of the catheter for discard before drawing blood samples. If the catheter volume is unknown, check the information on Figure 71-4 or contact the IV team, central supply services, operating room, or intensive care nursery for package insert information.
2. Blood discard may be avoided by first flushing the catheter with normal saline solution for injection, and then alternately aspirating the blood and reinjecting it several times to clear the line of any IV fluid or medication. Finally, proceed with the blood draw.

COMPLICATIONS

Table 71-3 lists complications of this procedure.

PATIENT TEACHING

These are preexisting central catheters, so most patients should be familiar with self-care measures. Patient teaching should be focused on handling catheter-related complications pertinent to the patient's presenting problem. If it is determined that the patient requires further training for home management of the catheter, a referral to a home health service or to the primary provider should be considered.

GUIDE TO COMMON CATHETER VOLUMES

Arrow International / Arrow PICC

Single Lumen Catheter
PK01451		0.45mL

Dual Lumen Catheter
PK01552		0.48mL/0.52mL

BARD ACCESS SYSTEMS

Broviac®
Single Lumen Vascular Access Catheter
60004	2.7 FR	0.15mL
60006	4.2 FR	0.3mL
60010	6.6 FR	0.7mL
60012	6.6 FR (short sheath)	0.7mL

Groshong™
Single Lumen Catheter with Vitacuff®
3.5 FR		0.13mL
5.5 FR		0.4mL
7.0 FR		0.7mL
8.0 FR		0.9mL
8.0 FR (Extra-Long Length)		1.2mL

Dual Lumen Catheter with Vitacuff®
9.5 FR Red	1.33mm	0.83mL
9.5 FR White	1.10mm	0.52mL
9.5 FR Red	1.33mm (Extra-Long Length)	0.94mL
9.5 FR White	1.10mm (Extra-Long Length)	0.57mL

GISH BIOMEDICAL, INC.
Hemed Catheter Sys.

Single Lumen Catheter
CVAC 1200	4.0 FR	0.4mL
CVAC 1221	4.0 FR	0.4mL
CVAC 1231	4.0 FR	0.4mL
CVAC 2200	6.6 FR	0.8mL
CVAC 2231	6.6 FR	0.8mL
CVAC 2221	6.6 FR	0.8mL
CVAC 3200	9.5 FR	1.8mL
CVAC 3221	9.5 FR	1.8mL
CVAC 3231	9.5 FR	1.8mL

Double Lumen Catheter
CVAC 4200	14.0 FR	1.9mL/1.9mL
CVAC 4221	14.0 FR	1.9mL/1.9mL
CVAC 4231	14.0 FR	1.9mL/1.9mL
CVAC 5200	11.0 FR	1.1mL/2.3mL
CVAC 5221	11.0 FR	1.1mL/2.3mL
CVAC 5231	11.0 FR	1.1mL/2.3mL
CVAC 6200	7.0 FR	0.7mL/1.1mL
CVAC 6221	7.0 FR	0.7mL/1.1mL
CVAC 6231	7.0 FR	0.7mL/1.1mL
CVAC 7200	9.0 FR	1.2mL/1.2mL
CVAC 7231	9.0 FR	1.2mL/1.2mL

Triple Lumen Catheter
CVAC 9200	12.0 FR	0.8mL/0.8mL/1.8mL
CVAC 9231	12.5 FR	0.8mL/0.8mL/1.8mL

Hickman®

Single Lumen Catheter
60016	9.6 FR	1.3mL
60018	9.6 FR	1.3mL
60020	9.6 FR	1.3mL
60028	10.8 FR	0.9mL
60030	14.4 FR	1.4mL

Dual Lumen Catheter
60031	7.0 FR (C.8mm/1.0mm)	0.6mL/0.3mL
60032	9.0 FR (C.7mm/1.3mm)	0.5mL/1.3mL
60033	9.0 FR (C.7mm/1.3mm)	0.6mL/1.3mL
60049	13.5 FR (2.0mm/2.0mm)	1.4mL/1.3mL
	28cm	1.23mL/1.28mL
	36cm	1.47mL/1.51mm
	40cm	1.60mL/1.51mm
60066-2 (Proximal/Distal)		1.47mL/1.51mm
60068-2 (Proximal/Distal)		1.23mL/1.28mm
60069-6 (Proximal/Distal)		1.60mL/1.51mm
60368-2 (Proximal/Distal)		1.23mL/1.28mm
60069-2 (Proximal/Distal)		1.60mL/1.51mm
60370-2 (Proximal/Distal)		1.47mL/1.51mm

Triple Lumen Catheter
60036	1.0mm,1.5mm,1.0mm	0.7mL/1.6mL/0.7mL

Leonard®
Dual Lumen Catheter
60034	10.3 FR	1.3mL/1.3mL

MENLO CARE, INC.
Centermark™ P ICC
Single Lumen Tray/Guidewire
C2-181-58G	18 guage	0.53mL
C2-201-58G	20 guage	0.23mL

Landmark®
Single Lumen Tray/Guidewire — Hydrated Volume
P2E20S	18 guage	0.55mL
P2E22S	20 guage	0.17mL
P2E24S	22 guage	0.94mL

STRATO MEDICAL CORP.
Infuse-a-Cath™
CVC 100-65	9.0 FR (single)	1.3mL
CVC 100-50	9.0 FR (single)	1.0mL
CVC 200-68	10.0 FR (dual)	1.0mL
CVC 200-60	10.0 FR (dual)	0.9mL

Groshong® PICC
Single Lumen Catheter
7715300	3.0 FR	0.31mL
7715305	3.0 FR	0.31mL
7715307	3.0 FR	0.31mL
7715400	4.0 FR	0.49mL
7715405	4.0 FR	0.49mL
7715407	4.0 FR	0.49mL

Dual Lumen Catheter
7725500	5.0 FR	0.62/0.48mL
7725505	5.0 FR	0.62/0.48mL
7725507	5.0 FR	0.62/0.48mL

Hohn®
Central Venous Catheter
60070	4F	0.2mL
60071	5F	0.3mL
60071-2	5F	0.3mL
60072-2	5F	0.3mL
60073	7F (0.8mm/1.1mm)	0.3mL/0.2mL

GESCO INTERNATIONAL, INC.
Per-Q-Cath PICC
Single Lumen Tray
P2	2.0 FR	0.04mL
P3	3.0 FR	0.11mL
P4	4.0 FR	0.25mL

QUINTON
Mahurkar
Double Lumen Catheter
10 FR	(9.5 cm)	1.0mL/1.1mL
10 FR	(5.0 cm)	0.9mL/1.0mL
10 FR	(12.0 cm)	0.8mL/0.9mL
11.5 FR	(24.0 cm)	1.4mL/1.5mL
11.5 FR	(9.5 cm)	1.2mL/1.3mL
11.5 FR	(16.0 cm)	1.1mL/1.2mL
11.5 FR	(13.5 cm)	1.0mL/1.1mL

VAS-CATH
Flexxicon® II
Double Lumen Catheter
CXC-4000	(6"-5 cm)	1.2mL/1.2mL
CXC-4400	(8"-20 cm)	1.4mL/1.4mL
CXC-4424	(9.5/2.6 cm)	1.6mL/1.6mL
CXC-3500-PC	(5"-2.5 cm)	1.5mL/1.2mL
CXC-3800-PC	(6"-15 cm)	1.6mL/1.3mL
CXC-3800-PC	(8"-20 cm)	1.7mL/1.4mL

Soft-Cell™
Double Lumen Catheter
PDLC-5512PC/PDLC-5512	12 cm	1.3mL/1.4mL
PDLC-5519PC/PDLC-5519	19 cm	1.5mL/1.6mL
PDLC-5523PC/PDLC-5523	23 cm	1.7mL/1.8mL

Per-Q-Cath PICC (cont.)
Single Lumen Tray/Guidewire
PSG	3.0 FR	0.34mL

Dual Lumen/Tray
PAD	4.0 FR	0.06mL/0.13mL
PSD	5.0 FR	0.27mL/0.27mL
PBD	6.0 FR	0.27mL/0.27mL

HDC
Chemo-Cath®
Single Lumen Catheter
330-04	4.0 FR	0.4mL
330-06	6.6 FR	0.7mL
330-09	9.6 FR	1.8mL
330-08	9.6 FR	1.8mL

Double Lumen Catheter
330-07	7.0 FR	0.55mL/1.0mL
330-10	9.6 FR	0.6mL/1.3mL
330-12	12.0 FR	1.8mL/1.8mL

V-Cath PICC®
Single Lumen Catheter
350-00	2.0 FR	0.08mL
360-00	3.0 FR	0.15mL
380-00	4.0 FR	0.4mL

Dual Lumen Catheter
395-60	4.5 FR	0.35mL/0.35mL

VYGON
Lifevac PICC
Single Lumen Catheter
2190.10 CN	3 FR	0.3mL
2190.20 CN	4 FR	0.4mL
1262.30	2 FR	0.16mL

Abbott Laboratories
North Chicago, IL 60064
410-081-3896 R1 • October 1995 • Printed in U.S.A.

FIGURE 71-4 Selected catheter volumes. (Modified from *Guide to common catheter volumes*. Publication No. 410-081-3896 RI [1995]. Courtesy of Abbott Laboratories, North Chicago, North Chicago: Author.)

TABLE 71-3

IDENTIFICATION AND MANAGEMENT OF CENTRAL LINE COMPLICATIONS

Complication	Signs and Symptoms	Management
Infection	Redness, tenderness at site; may be pus or induration. May have fever, chills, or signs of sepsis.	Culture site (semiquantitative method). Blood culture through catheter and separate venipuncture. Antibiotics through catheter may resolve catheter-related bloodstream infections, but catheter may need to be removed to resolve infection. Do not remove except by physician order.
Infiltration or extravasation	Pain and/or swelling of the neck, shoulder, arm, and/or chest. Fluid may be visible at insertion site. Rate may slow or stop.	Note that blood return may still be present if fibrin sheath has formed. Stop IV or slow rate until patency is confirmed. Venography is diagnostic. Remove catheter only by physician order. If fibrin sheath is confirmed, thrombolytic therapy may be considered with or without catheter removal.
Central vein thrombosis	No blood return; slow flow rate; pain; redness, induration, or edema of shoulder; arm or neck on affected side. Development of collateral circulation in chest, decreased venous emptying time on affected side.	Stop or slow rate. Watch for infiltration. Venography is diagnostic. If thrombosis is confirmed, thrombolytic therapy may be considered with or without catheter removal.
Pinch-off syndrome	Intermittent inability to aspirate blood return or infuse that is affected by a change in position of the arm or shoulder, caused by pinching of the catheter between the first rib and the clavicle.	Most common with silicone catheters. To confirm, order upright chest x-ray film and ask radiologist to check for pinch-off. If no blood return, venography will identify transection. If catheter is intact, may be used with caution. External rotation of shoulder may facilitate blood return. Do not irrigate against resistance. Catheter may need to be replaced; if it is nonfunctioning, contact the surgeon.
Damaged catheter	Catheter body or hub broken, cracked, or contaminated.	Immediately clamp catheter between break and body with a bulldog or other suitable clamp. Obtain repair kit (available from manufacturer). Repair according to repair-kit instructions. Ensure sterile technique. May be necessary to declot catheter following repair (see following text on "Occlusion").

TABLE 71-3

IDENTIFICATION AND MANAGEMENT OF CENTRAL LINE COMPLICATIONS

Complication	Signs and Symptoms	Management
Occlusion	Inability to aspirate or infuse caused by occlusion by blood or precipitate. NOTE: Management of occlusion by precipitate other than blood is mostly anecdotal. Check with pharmacy for most current literature.	By history, confirm occlusion by blood, then declot per Procedure 73. No blood work is necessary before declotting procedure. Recent ocular or cerebral bleed is a relative contraindication—check with physician first.
Air embolism	Hypotension, pulse rapid and weak, cyanosis, change in level of consciousness, shock, auscultation of coarse machinery noise over the precordium.	Place patient in left Trendelenburg position, administer oxygen, and provide life support as needed. To avoid air embolism, place patient in Trendelenburg position for central line insertion or whenever line is disconnected.

IV, Intravenous line.

REFERENCES

Bard. (1992). *How to care for your Hickman or Broviac catheter.* Salt Lake City, UT: Author.

Davol. (1994a). *Nursing procedure manual, Groshong C.V. catheter.* Cranston, RI: Author.

Davol. (1994b). Hickman subcutaneous ports and Hickman/Broviac catheters wall poster. Cranston, RI: Author.

Gesco. (1990). *Gesco Per-Q-Cath package insert.* San Antonio, TX: Author.

Mayo, D.J., Dimond, E.P., Kramer, W., & Horne, M.K. (1996). Discard volumes necessary for clinically useful coagulation studies from heparinized Hickman catheters. *Oncology Nursing Forum, 23,* 671-675.

SIMS Deltec. (1996). Clinicath peripherally inserted catheters wall poster. St. Paul, MN: Author.

Smith, S., Duell, D., & Martin, B. (2000). *Clinical nursing skills: basic to advanced.* Upper Saddle River, NJ: Prentice Hall Health.

Terry, J., Baronowski, L., Lonsway, R.A., & Hedrick, C. (1995). *Intravenous therapy: clinical principles and practice.* Philadelphia: W.B. Saunders.

Accessing Implanted Venous Port Devices

Reneé Semonin Holleran, RN, PhD, CEN, CCRN, CFRN, SANE

An implanted port consists of a tunneled catheter attached to an injection port with a self-sealing septum (Figure 72-1). The device is implanted under the skin and must be accessed through the skin. Although most frequently used for venous access, implanted ports may also be placed intra-arterially, epidurally, or intraperitoneally. Venous ports are usually located in the chest; however, some ports are located in the upper extremity, with the catheter insertion site in the basilic or cephalic vein and the tip threaded into a central vein, similar to a peripherally inserted central catheter (PICC). Catheter tip placement must be confirmed by aspiration of blood before the port is used. There are many brands of implanted ports, including one with the Groshong catheter attached. Many ports are available in single- or double-port or lumen configuration. Most septa are located on the top of the port. Patients may carry written information about their port.

INDICATIONS

To gain venous access in patients who have implanted venous port to:
1. Administer intravenous (IV) fluids, medications, blood, or blood products
2. Obtain samples of venous blood
3. Perform routine heparin flushes to maintain catheter patency

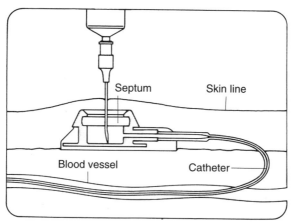

FIGURE 72-1 Implantable port configuration. (Courtesy Davol. *Davol implanted ports: Patient information.* Publication No. 99020 M [p. 4]. Cranston, RI: Author.)

CONTRAINDICATIONS AND CAUTIONS

1. Use strict sterile technique to avoid infection because the patient would require a surgical procedure to have the device removed.

2. Use only noncoring or Huber point needles to access an implanted port because other needles may damage the port septum, leading to extravasation of fluids or medications (Smith et al., 2000; Nettina, 2001). Noncoring needles are available in 19-, 20-, or 22-G sizes and either in a straight configuration for one-time access, or at a 90-degree angle with or without an attached extension set for continuous infusion (Figure 72-2). If blood samples are desired, use a 19-G noncoring needle.

3. Although the port is sutured in place, it is possible for it to flip over. Palpate the septum of the port to ensure that it is right side up before attempting needle insertion.

4. If the patient feels pain or an abnormal sensation at the port site during infusion, it may indicate that the medication has extravasated. The infusion should be stopped immediately until the port patency has been determined. A chest radiograph helps verify catheter placement if no blood return is obtained when the port is accessed. When port patency is uncertain, the only conclusive way to determine patency is to perform a cathetergram by injecting contrast dye into the port.

5. To administer whole blood or packed red blood cells, use a 19-G noncoring needle to access the port. It is usually necessary to use an infusion pump or add 50 ml of normal saline solution to the blood bag, or run a normal saline solution concomitantly with the blood to maintain adequate flow rates.

6. For a routine heparin flush of the port, use 5 ml of heparin (100 units/ml). Other concentrations of heparinized saline solution (10-1000 units/ml) may

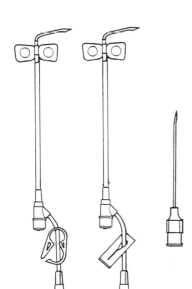

FIGURE 72-2 Noncoring (Huber) needle configuration. (Courtesy Pharmacia Deltec.)

be used, depending on the patient's medical condition, laboratory tests, and home care or physician protocols.

7. To avoid an air embolism, the patient should be supine and should perform the Valsalva maneuver, or the extension set should be clamped any time the IV line is disconnected.

8. The needle should be changed every 7 days or sooner if the flow rates decrease or blood return is absent (Intravenous Nurses Society, 2000; Nettina, 2001).

9. When not accessed, the port should be flushed once per month with 5 ml of heparin, 100 units/ml (Weinstein, 1993). Ports placed in the hepatic artery are flushed weekly.

EQUIPMENT

Two pairs of sterile gloves
Three antiseptic swab sticks (povidone-iodine preferred)
Sterile fenestrated drape
Noncoring or Huber needle
Luer-locking T extension set or short extension set if this is not already attached to the needle
Bulldog or padded clamp if not provided on the extension set
Sterile normal saline for injection
Two 10-ml syringes with needles
Dressing materials (if the port is to remain accessed), skin tapes, 4- to 5-cm transparent dressing, 2×2 sterile gauze dressings, tape
IV solution as precribed or a male adapter plug
Blood specimen tubes, if needed
5 ml of heparin (100 units/ml) if heparin lock is needed

PROCEDURAL STEPS
Port Access

1. Prepare all supplies on a sterile field.
2. Expose the chest and identify the septum by palpating the outer perimeter of the port. The septum is located in the middle of the port.
3. Using sterile gloves, clean the skin over the port with an antiseptic swab stick, working outward in a spiral motion to cover an area 4 inches in diameter (Terry et al., 1995). Clean with the second and third swab sticks in the same manner. Allow to air dry.
4. Apply the sterile fenestrated drape, leaving only the area over the port exposed.
5. Change gloves.
6. Fill the 5-ml syringes with normal saline solution. Attach the extension set to the noncoring needle, if necessary, and prime the needle or extension setup with the normal saline solution to purge all air. Leave the syringe attached to the needle or extension set.
7. Stabilize the port with the forefinger and thumb (one on each side of the port). Insert the noncoring needle through the skin and into the middle of the septum. Hold the needle perpendicular to the port and apply only downward pressure. Do not twist, rock, or manipulate the needle sideways during or after the needle insertion, because this may core the septum and cause leak-

ing from the port. Continue downward pressure on the needle until it hits the back of the septum and can go no farther (Figure 72-3).

8. Aspirate 5 ml of blood to confirm port patency. To facilitate blood return, have the patient raise his or her arms, cough, perform the Valsalva maneuver, or change position.

9. If no blood return is obtained, the needle may be located at the side of the septum over the outer periphery of the port. If you are unable to achieve a blood return, remove the needle and try again with a new needle. If there is visual confirmation that the new needle is in the port, attempt to irrigate the port with 10 ml of normal saline solution. If there is no resistance when irrigating, proceed with the infusion (the IV fluid should drip freely by gravity if the needle is in the port) while monitoring the patient for signs of extravasation. To assess for extravasation, place the patient on his or her back and compare the breasts and both sides of the chest and neck. Observe for asymmetry, swelling, redness, or the patient's complaint of tenderness. A chest radiograph helps confirm the catheter placement and rule out a catheter pinch-off or transection. The only definitive diagnostic study is a cathetergram with contrast into the port. If there is resistance to irrigation, a cathetergram is strongly recommended to determine catheter placement. Fibrinolytic therapy may be required to restore patency to a clotted catheter (see Procedure 73).

10. After port patency is confirmed and blood specimens are obtained, if necessary, flush the port with 10 ml of normal saline solution.

11. If the port is to remain accessed, apply a dressing as follows:
    a. Tape all connections that will be under the dressing with sterile tape.
    b. Place a 2 × 2 sterile gauze pad under the angled needle to provide support as needed.
    c. Place skin tapes over the needle to secure it in place. To facilitate patient assessment, do not obscure the needle insertion site.
    d. Cover the entire setup with a transparent dressing, leaving only the end of the extension set with the clamp exposed.
    e. Label the dressing with the date of the insertion and the needle size.

Blood Sampling

NOTE: The use of a heparinized catheter for blood sampling for coagulation studies is not recommended if results are to be used to monitor anticoagulant therapy

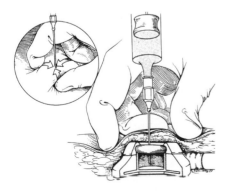

FIGURE 72-3 Accessing an implanted port. (Courtesy Davol. *Hickman subcutaneous port: use and maintenance.* Publication No. 11905 M [p. 6]. Cranston, RI: Author.)

or to evaluate coagulopathy, because they show be falsely elevated levels (Mayo et al., 1996). If coagulation studies are necessary for such an evaluation, use a separate peripheral site for the venipuncture. Blood samples from a heparinized catheter may be used to determine whether the coagulation studies are normal (Mayo et al., 1996). If the catheter must be used for coagulation studies, note this on the laboratory request form.

1. If a continuous IV is running, stop the infusion for 1 minute.
2. Aspirate and discard 10 ml of blood from the port (Weinstein, 1993).
3. Attach the sampling syringe, withdraw the amount of blood needed, and place it in appropriate specimen tubes.

Removing the Needle From the Port

1. Flush the port with 10 ml of normal saline solution for injection.
2. Flush the port with 5 ml of heparin (100 units/ml).
3. Stabilize the port with the thumb and forefinger of one hand while removing the needle with the other hand.
4. Clean the injection site and apply a bandage or small dressing.

AGE-SPECIFIC CONSIDERATION

A smaller port and a shorter catheter are used for infants and children; therefore there are lower blood discard volumes for laboratory draws and flushing volumes. Volumes should equal approximately two to three times the catheter or port volume, which can be found on the package insert. If the catheter volume is unknown, it is generally adequate to withdraw 5 ml of blood before the blood draw.

COMPLICATIONS

See Table 71-3 in Procedure 71.

1. Infection
2. Medication or fluid extravasation
3. Catheter pinch-off syndrome and transection
4. Catheter occlusion
5. Air embolism
6. Central venous thrombosis
7. Catheter rupture
8. Hematoma
9. Pneumothorax

PATIENT TEACHING

Ports are preexisting central catheters, so most patients should be familiar with self-care measures. Patients should be reminded to have the catheter flushed at monthly intervals when not in use. If it is determined that the patient requires further training for home management of the catheter, a referral to the home health service or the primary provider should be considered.

REFERENCES

Intravenous Nurses Society. (2000). Intravenous nursing standards of practice. *Journal of Intravenous Nursing*, Supplement, 2000.

Mayo, D.J., Dimond, E.P., Kramer, W., & Horne, M.K. (1996). Discard volumes necessary for clinically useful coagulation studies from heparinized Hickman catheters. *Oncology Nursing Forum, 23,* 671-675.

Nettina, S. (2001). *The Lippincott manual of nursing practice,* 7th ed. Philadelphia: Lippincott.

Smith, S., Duell, D., & Martin, B. (2000). *Clinical nursing skills,* 5th ed. Upper Saddle River, NJ: Prentice Hall Health.

Terry, J., Baronowski, L., Lonsway, R.A., & Hedrick, C. (1995). *Intravenous therapy: clinical principles and practice.* Philadelphia: W.B. Saunders.

Weinstein, S.M. (1993). *Plumer's principles and practice of intravenous therapy.* Philadelphia: J.B. Lippincott.

PROCEDURE 73

Declotting Central Venous Access Devices

Ruth Altherr Rench, MS, RN and Teresa L. Will, MSN, RN, CEN

Tissue plasminogen activator is also known as tPA, TPA, r-tPA, alteplase, Cathflo Activase.

INDICATION

TPA is indicated for the restoration of function to central venous access devices, as assessed by the ability to withdraw blood.

CONTRAINDICATIONS AND CAUTIONS

1. Known hypersensitivity to TPA or any component of the formulation is a contraindication.
2. Catheter dysfunction may be caused by many conditions other than thrombus formation, such as catheter malposition, mechanical failure, constriction of a suture, and lipid deposits or drug precipitates within the catheter lumen. These conditions should be ruled out before treatment with TPA is considered.
3. Avoid vigorous suction during attempts to determine catheter occlusion in order to avoid damage to the vessel wall or collapse of the catheter walls.
4. To prevent rupture of the catheter or expulsion of the clot into the systemic circulation, avoid excessive pressure when instilling TPA.
5. Bleeding is the most frequent adverse reaction associated with all thrombolytics in all approved indications. TPA use in this situation has not been studied in patients who are known to be at risk for bleeding events that may be associated

with thrombolytics (Deitcher et al., 2002; Ponec et al., 2001) Exercise caution with patients who have active internal bleeding or have had any of the following:

Surgery (within 48 hours)

Obstetrical delivery (within 48 hours)

Percutaneous biopsy of viscera or deep tissues (within 48 hours)

Puncture of noncompressible vessels (within 48 hours)

Thrombocytopenia

Hemostatic defects (e.g., severe hepatic or renal disease)

Any condition in which bleeding constitutes a significant hazard or would be particularly difficult to manage because of its location

High risk for embolic complications (e.g., venous thrombosis in the region of the catheter)

6. The use of TPA in patients with infected catheters may release a localized infection into the systemic circulation. Therefore TPA should be used with caution in patients with known or suspected catheter-related infections.

EQUIPMENT

2-mg Cathflo Activase vial: contains 2.2 mg of TPA (which includes a 10% overfill)

Three 10-ml syringes

10 ml of sterile water for injection (SWFI)

20 ml of normal saline (for catheter assessment and flushing)

Alcohol wipes

PATIENT PREPARATION

Perform a thorough assessment, to include:

1. Ruling out external mechanical catheter obstruction
2. Ruling out patient position-related mechanical catheter obstruction
3. Ruling out obstruction due to lipid or drug precipitate
4. Review of cautions for TPA treatment

PROCEDURAL STEPS (Genentech, 1996)
TPA Reconstitution

1. Using a 10-ml syringe and aseptic technique, withdraw 2.2 ml of SWFI, and then inject the SWFI into the Cathflo Activase vial, directing the diluent stream into the powder. Slight foaming may occur; allow vial to stand until large bubbles dissipate.
2. Mix by gently swirling the vial contents until they are completely dissolved, which should occur within 3 minutes. *Do not shake.* The resulting solution should be pale yellow to colorless transparent solution, which contains 1 mg/ml of Cathflo Activase.
3. Because Cathflo Activase contains no preservatives, it should be reconstituted immediately before use. The solution may be used for intracatheter instillation within 8 hours of reconstitution if it is stored at 2°-30° C (36°-86° F).

TPA Instillation

1. Using the same 10-ml syringe, administer the appropriate dose of solution from the reconstituted vial per Table 73-1. Instill the dose of Cathflo Activase into the occluded catheter.

TABLE 73-1

CATHFLO ACTIVASE DOSING

Patient weight	Dose
≥30 kg	2 mg in 2 ml
≥10 to <30 kg	110% of the internal lumen volume of the catheter, not to exceed 2 mg in 2 ml

From Genentech (1996). *Cathflo Activase (alteplase) 2 mg prescribing Information.* San Francisco: Author.

2. Wait 30 minutes and then assess catheter function by attempting to withdraw blood. If the catheter is functional, then aspirate 4-5 ml of blood to remove the Cathflo Activase and residual clot and gently irrigate the catheter with a 10-ml syringe containing 0.9% sodium chloride solution.
3. If catheter function is not restored after 30 minutes, then relock the catheter and assess again after 120 minutes. At 120 minutes after the first instillation, again assess catheter function. If the catheter is functional, follow the same irrigation process described in step 2 above. If catheter function has not been restored, the 0 mg dose of Cathflo Activase may be repeated, following the same steps described above.

COMPLICATIONS

1. The most serious adverse events reported in the clinical trials were sepsis, gastrointestinal bleeding, and venous thrombosis. There were no reports of intracranial hemorrhage. No allergic-type reactions were observed in the patients treated with TPA (Deitcher et al., 2002; Ponec et al., 2001).
2. The goal is to prevent serious bleeding through careful screening. Assessment and prompt treatment are also critical to minimize the effects of bleeding when it does occur. Should serious bleeding occur (e.g., intracranial, gastrointestinal, retroperitoneal, pericardial), treatment with Cathflo Activase should be stopped, and the drug should be withdrawn from the catheter.

PATIENT TEACHING

1. Report symptoms that occur with Cathflo Activase instillation.
2. Report any bleeding.

REFERENCES

Deitcher, M.R., Fesen, M.R., Kiproff, P.M. et al. (2002). Safety and efficacy of alteplase for restoring function in occluded central venous catheters: results of the cardiovascular thrombolytic to open occluded lines trial. *Journal of Clinical Oncology, 20*(1), 317-324.

Genentech (1996). Cathflo ACTIVASE (alteplase) 2mg prescribing information. San Francisco: Author.

Ponec, D., Irwin, D., Haire, W.D. et al. (2001). Recombinant tissue plasminogen activator (alteplase) for restoration of flow in occluded central venous access devices: a double-blind placebo-controlled trial: the cardiovascular thrombolytic to open occluded lines (COOL) efficacy trial. *Journal of Vascular and Interventional Radiology, 12*(8), 951-955.

Blood Product Administration

Administration of Blood Products

Mike D. McMahon, RN, BSN

This procedure contains information on administering red blood cells (RBCs), whole blood, platelets, plasma, and cryoprecipitate. See Procedures 75-78 for information regarding blood filters, massive transfusion, fluid warmers, and blood and fluid pressure infusers.

GENERAL PRINCIPLES (American Association of Blood Banks [AABB], 1999)

1. The intended recipient must be positively identified before a transfusion is started. This is the single most important step in preventing transfusion reactions.
2. Risks versus benefits need to be explained to the patient. Informed consent may be required by specific institutions.
3. The plastic blood component container should not be vented.
4. A filter designed to retain blood clots and particles must be used in the transfusion.
5. Components should be mixed thoroughly before administration.
6. No medications or solutions should be added to, or transfused concurrently with blood components except normal saline solution. Plasma compatible with A, B, and O blood types; 5% albumin; plasma protein fraction; or any calcium free isotonic electrolytic solution may be used with the approval of the physician.
7. Lactated Ringer's solution or other electrolyte solutions containing calcium should never be administered concurrently with a blood component mixed with an anticoagulant containing citrate, because calcium binds to citrate.
8. Needles and intravenous (IV) catheters used for infusion may be as small as 23 G, but the recommended size is 18 or 19 G.
9. If the fitness of any component is questioned on visual inspection, it should be returned to the blood bank for further evaluation.
10. If the blood component container is entered for any reason, the component expires after 4 hours at room temperature.
11. All blood or blood components that are not used within 30 minutes must be stored in a monitored refrigerator that has been approved by the blood bank.
12. Blood components should not be heated above the level that hemolysis can occur (42° C,107.6° F).
13. The patient's religious beliefs may prohibit the administration of blood or blood products.

PATIENT PREPARATION

1. Obtain informed consent per the policy of the institution. Most policies waive consent in emergency situations.

2. Establish vascular access (see Procedures 63-72); a normal saline solution on Y blood tubing is indicated for most blood products.
3. Obtain specimens for type and cross-match as required. Adhere to institutional policy regarding labeling of the specimen, and complete necessary blood bank forms.
4. Assess and document vital signs, including temperature.
5. Document preexisting hematuria and pain in the chest, back, or abdomen.

RED BLOOD CELLS

Red blood cells, also known as RBCs or packed red blood cells, are prepared by removing 80%-90% of the plasma from whole blood. Therefore there are no significant amounts of clotting factors or platelets in RBCs. Each unit contains 250-300 ml.

Indication

To increase the oxygen-carrying capacity of the circulatory system in the presence of acute or chronic blood loss, usually resulting from acute hemorrhage, surgical blood loss, or chronic anemia (Eberst, 2000).

Contraindications and Cautions

1. Removal of the plasma reduces the chance of adverse reactions from RBCs that might occur with the use of whole blood; however, transfusion reactions may still occur.
2. Always have a second person check typing; cross matching, expiration date, any special processing, such as irradiation; and client identification. Document these data according to the hospital's policy. Most major or fatal transfusion reactions result from type mismatches caused by a clerical error, administration of blood to the wrong patient, or incorrect identification of the blood component (Puget Sound Blood Center and Program [PSBCP], 2002; Hoffman, 2002). In emergency situations, O-negative blood can be administered until cross-matched blood is available. Male patients and postmenopausal female patients may receive O-positive blood.
3. Monitor fluid balance carefully in patients at risk for fluid overload.
4. Do not allow the RBCs to stand at room temperature longer than 30 minutes before administration.
5. Infusion time should not exceed 4 hours. The longer the RBCs are left at room temperature, the greater the danger of bacterial proliferation and RBC hemolysis (PSBCP, 2002).

Equipment

Blood administration set, Y type (170- to 260-micron filter)

Procedural Steps

1. Check the expiration date on the blood.
2. Identify the patient according to your hospital's procedure. With another nurse, check the blood record with the patient's identification (Wooldridge-King, 2001).
3. Invert the RBCs gently several times to suspend them.

4. Spike the RBCs with one tail of the Y blood set. Make sure the upper drip chamber is half full to prevent damage to the RBCs (Figure 74-1).
5. Close the roller clamp on the normal saline tail and open the roller clamp on the RBCs. A gentle squeeze on the filter helps start the flow of blood.
6. Infuse slowly for the first 15-30 minutes while observing the patient for reactions. Most serious reactions occur during this time. This step assumes that the patient is not in need of multiple, rapid, life-sustaining transfusions.
7. After 15-30 minutes, reassess the vital signs and adjust the flow rate to the desired speed.
8. Continue the assessments of the patient (always include the vital signs) throughout the transfusion as needed, according to the patient's condition and the number of units being administered.
9. After the infusion is complete, reassess the vital signs and flush the tubing with normal saline solution. If the transfusion therapy is complete, either discontinue the IV or hang the prescribed solution with new IV tubing.

Age-Specific Considerations

1. Fluid overload is of concern in both elderly and young patients. Your hospital blood bank may be able to separate full units of RBCs and whole blood into smaller units. This allows the full unit to be used while maintaining the integrity of the blood bag (American Association of Blood Banks, 1999).
2. There is a risk of viral infection during a transfusion. Cytomegalovirus infection can be found in 50%-80% of the population, which results in a large pool of infected blood. This is a concern in the neonatal patient because it can lead to such problems as pneumonia and death (Parker, 2002).

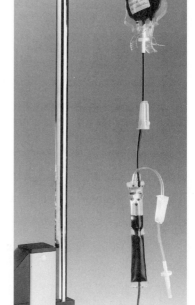

FIGURE 74-1 Red blood cells on Y tubing with upper chamber half full.

3. Neonates may be transfused with a packed RBC unit that has a hematocrit of 70%-90% (Strauss, 2000).

WHOLE BLOOD
Whole blood may be either stored or fresh. Whole blood is rarely used in any hospital setting. There is a rapid loss of platelets and coagulation factor within 72 hours from collection. The only normal use is for exchange transfusions in neonates (Eberst, 2000). Likewise, the use of whole blood is rarely indicated now, because all clotting factors, plasma, RBCs, and platelets are available as individual components.

Indications
1. To increase the oxygen-carrying capacity of the blood
2. To replace volume in a patient in shock
3. To replace a blood component that is unavailable individually

Contraindications and Cautions
1. Whole blood has the same contraindications and cautions as RBCs,
2. Whole blood has a volume of 500 ml per unit and places the patient at a higher risk for fluid overload than RBCs.

Equipment, Procedural Steps, and Age-Specific Considerations
The equipment, procedural steps, and age-specific considerations for whole blood are identical to those for RBCs; see these sections in this procedure under Red Blood Cells.

ALBUMIN
Albumin is a circulating protein found in both the serum and the extravascular area. The primary function of albumin is the maintenance of normal colloid oncotic pressure. Albumin solutions are available in 5% and 25% solution concentrations. Preparation of an albumin solution includes heat inactivation for 10 hours at a temperature of 60° C, which eliminates the risk of viral infection (Eberst, 2000). The use of albumin is controversial and has limited indications (Eberst, 2000; Davidson & Chern, 1999).

Indications
1. To replace volume after an acute loss, a therapeutic phlebotomy, or a plasma exchange
2. To correct hypoalbuminemia
3. May be used to improve intravascular volume in patients who have severe burns or who are developing signs of edema (Eberst, 2000).

Contraindications and Cautions
1. In the presence of a disease process that increases capillary permeability, such as sepsis and acute respiratory distress syndrome, albumin may leak into the pulmonary system and aggravate pulmonary edema.
2. Albumin is very expensive when compared with the cost of crystalloid solutions.

Equipment
Use the vented administration set supplied with the glass vial of albumin.

Procedural Steps
1. Check that the proper solution is being used (5% or 25%). Albumin does not have to be ABO compatible.
2. The 25% solution is usually delivered concurrently with crystalloid solution, whether it is administered directly or inserted in piggyback fashion into another line.
3. Infuse the 5% solution as fast as it can be tolerated. The 25% solution should be administered over 20-60 minutes.

Age-Specific Considerations
Colloids are difficult to titrate, so the risk of fluid overload in both young and elderly patients is a serious consideration.

PLATELET CONCENTRATION
Platelets play an important role in blood coagulation and thrombus formation. They are obtained by centrifugation of whole blood. They are available in single or multiple-dose units in a 30- to 50-ml bag and are usually ordered 4-10 units at a time. Your blood bank may pool the entire order into one bag.

Indication
To increase platelets in the presence of thrombocytopenia (low platelet count) of any etiology

Contraindications and Cautions
1. Platelets must be infused rapidly or they lose their viability. Call the blood bank only when you are ready to administer the platelets (PSBCP, 2002).
2. Transfusion reactions are possible owing to the plasma in which the platelets are stored.
3. Platelet transfusions during massive trauma should be based on laboratory values and patient presentation, not on amount of blood transfused (Raife & Friedman, 2002).
4. Platelets must be transfused through a filter.
5. Pooled and aphaeresis units must be infused within 4 hours of mixing.
6. Check the unit for clumps or aggregates. If these are found, knead the unit gently until the clumps disappear. If clumps do not disappear with gentle kneading, return the unit to the blood bank. The color of the platelets may range from clear to straw to light strawberry.

Equipment
Blood administration set, Y type with filter
60-ml syringe
Three-way stopcock
250-ml bag, or larger, of normal saline solution

Procedural Steps

1. Prime the blood administration set with a normal saline solution and place a three-way stopcock at the distal end of the tubing (just in front of the IV catheter).
2. Check the platelet blood type versus the patient's blood type. It is not necessary to have the same ABO type, but it is preferred, especially in those who weigh less than 40 kg (Eberst, 2000).
3. Rh-negative women who are of childbearing age should be transfused with Rh-negative platelets (Eberst, 2000).
4. Hang the platelet bag on one tail of the Y set.
5. Close the normal saline-solution line roller clamp and open the platelet line.
6. Run the infusion slowly for the first 15 minutes, as with other blood products, and watch closely for any transfusion reactions. After this, the infusion rate can be moved up to 4-8 ml/kg per hour according to the patient's tolerance (PSBCP, 2002).
7. If platelets do not run at a sufficient speed, attach the syringe to the 3-way stopcock (Figure 74-2). Turn off the stopcock to the patient and withdraw the platelets into the syringe. Close the stopcock to the IV line, open it to the patient, and inject the platelets at 5-10 ml/min.
8. When the platelet pack is empty, close its roller clamp, open the normal saline solution, and flush the line to infuse all the platelets.
9. Assess and document the vital signs.

FRESH FROZEN PLASMA

Fresh frozen plasma (also known as FFP, FP, or frozen plasma) is an unconcentrated source of all the clotting factors except platelets. It is needed to restore appropriate levels of factors V and VIII. It comes in a 100- to 300-ml bag. Three types of plasma are available for use (Raife & Friedman, 2002):

- Standard FFP with significant retesting done for viral infections
- Donor-retested plasma, in which the plasma is held until the donor returns after several months to be tested for blood-borne pathogens
- Solvent/detergent (S/D)-treated plasma that is pooled then treated to disrupt viral envelopes and repackaged

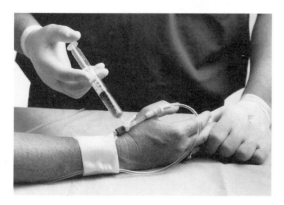

FIGURE 74-2 Administering platelets with a syringe via three-way stopcock.

Indications

1. To correct coagulation deficiencies for which specific factor concentrates are unavailable
2. To correct a bleeding tendency of unknown cause or one associated with liver failure
3. To correct coagulopathy and active bleeding, such as may occur during massive transfusion or in disseminated intravascular coagulation
4. To reverse warfarin effect
5. Not indicated solely for volume expansion (Eberst, 2000)

Contraindications and Cautions

1. The required thawing time for FFP is 30-40 minutes, after which it must be used immediately or stored in a monitored refrigerator that has been approved by the blood bank.
2. A filter must be used for FFP transfusion.
3. Transfusion reactions can occur owing to the presence of antibodies and antigens.
4. Administration of FFP must take place within 4 hours of thawing.

Equipment

Blood administration set, Y type
Normal saline IV fluid

Procedural Steps

1. Identify the patient and the blood type and double check the unit of plasma with another person to make sure it is correct. It should be the same type. Document the double-checked data according to the institutional policy.
2. Inspect the bag for leaks and the color of the infusion. The color of the solution should range from yellow or straw to light green to orange, and it should be clear (PSBCP, 2002).
3. Spike the plasma with the other tail of the Y set.
4. Close the roller clamp on the normal saline solution, open up the plasma, and regulate the drip rate.
5. Run the infusion slowly for the first 15 minutes, as with other blood products, and watch closely for any transfusion reactions. After this, the infusion rate can be moved up to 4-8 ml/kg per hour according to the patient's tolerance (PSBCP, 2002).
6. Assess and document the vital signs.

CRYOPRECIPITATED ANTIHEMOPHILIAC FACTOR (CRYOPRECIPITATE)

Cryoprecipitate is prepared from FFP and may be frozen for up to 1 year. Each single donor unit or bag contains factor VIII, von Willebrand factor, fibrinogen, factor XIII, and fibronectin in 10-15 ml of plasma. Each bag is prepared from 10 donors and is prescribed at a dose of two to four bags per 10 kg in body weight (Eberst, 2000).

Indication

To control bleeding by replacing clotting factors in the presence of the following:

1. Hemophilia A, when factor VIII concentrates are not available
2. Factor VIII deficiency
3. von Willebrand's disease
4. Hypofibrinogenemia, disseminated intravascular coagulation
   Cryoprecipitate is also used as fibrin glue surgical adhesives.

Contraindications and Cautions
1. Infuse only at room temperature.
2. Use only a plastic syringe, because factor VIII may bind to the surface of a glass syringe.
3. Cryoprecipitate must be given through a filter.
4. Transfusion reactions can occur.

Equipment
Blood administration set, Y type with filter
Normal saline IV fluid
Three-way stopcock
30-ml plastic syringe

Procedural Steps
1. Initiate an IV line with a normal saline solution and Y blood set at a keep-vein-open (KVO) rate.
2. Inspect the bag for leaks and examine the solution. It is normal for the solution to be cloudy (PSBCP, 2002).
3. Hang the cryoprecipitate on the other tail of the Y blood set. NOTE. Cryoprecipitate is usually given in doses greater than one unit (often 10 units in adults). The cryoprecipitate is usually diluted in the laboratory when the units are pooled together.
4. Infuse slowly for the first 15 minutes and watch for a transfusion reaction. Then, adjust the drip rate to infuse at a rate of 4-8 ml/kg per hour.
5. If necessary, the three-way stopcock and syringe may be used to infuse. Refer to the administration of platelets, covered earlier in this procedure.
6. Flush the IV line with a normal saline solution after the cryoprecipitate is finished.
7. Assess and document the vital signs.

Age-Specific Consideration
If the patient is younger than 1 year of age, ABO-Rh–compatible cryoprecipitate units are to be given (PSBCP, 2002).

COMPLICATIONS
1. Hemolytic-transfusion reactions can be either immediate or delayed. Acute hemolysis can occur when recipient plasma antibodies react with the donor RBC antigens. Both acute and delayed hemolytic reactions are potentially life-threatening events. Hemolytic reactions occur in 1 of every 21,000 to 1 million units of blood transfused (Parker, 2002; Eberst, 2000). A fatal transfusion reaction occurs in 1 of every 100,000 units (Eberst, 2000).
   a. Signs and symptoms of hemolytic reactions occur almost immediately and include chills, apprehension; headache; fever; pain in the back, the

abdomen, and the chest, or at the infusion site; respiratory distress; hypotension; peripheral circulatory collapse; and shock. Hemoglobin is present in the plasma and urine.

b. In the anesthetized patient, the only signs that may indicate a reaction are abnormal bleeding, hypotension regardless of the volume replacement, respiratory failure, and tubular necrosis (Eberst, 2000).

c. Stop the transfusion immediately. Prime new IV tubing with a normal saline solution and replace the blood-filled tubing.

d. Place the patient on oxygen if supplemental flow is not yet being given.

e. Save the blood bag and the tubing, notify the blood bank, and follow your institution's policy regarding transfusion reactions.

f. Contact the physician for further instructions. Some additional interventions may include placing a Foley catheter to track the urinary output more accurately and giving a diuretic, such as furosemide.

g. Administer IV fluids to achieve a urine output of 100 ml/hr to help prevent renal failure (Parker, 2002; Wooldridge-King, 2001).

2. Allergic reactions and fever occur in about 1 of every 100 units of blood. These usually occur as a result of the interaction of host antibodies with donor plasma proteins. Allergic reactions are rarely serious and do not justify the routine use of washed red cells (Parker, 2002). An emergent anaphylactic reaction is much rarer, occurring in 1 of every 20,000 transfusions (Eberst, 2000). An allergic reaction is most likely to occur with administration of whole blood or plasma because the plasma contains many antibodies and antigens.

a. Signs and symptoms commonly include a skin rash, urticaria, edema, and pruritus. Less frequent reactions are dyspnea, wheezing, and, occasionally, anaphylaxis.

b. Stop the transfusion immediately.

c. Save the blood bag and the tubing, notify the blood bank, and follow your institution's policy for transfusion reaction.

d. Contact the physician for additional interventions. Usually, a parenteral antihistamine is prescribed.

3. Transfusion-related acute lung injury (TRALI). This reaction occurs within 4 hours of the initiation of transfusions. Symptoms are the same as acute respiratory distress syndrome and may require intubation and mechanical ventilation (Hoffman, 2002; Parker, 2002).

4. Febrile nonhemolytic transfusion reactions. This reaction is reflected by 1° C rise in temperature and chills during or after transfusion. Treatment usually consists of stopping the transfusion and administrating antipyretics and diphenhydramine if allergic components are present. Blood samples should be drawn and the cross-matching reperformed. Patients with underlying cardiovascular disease are at risk for more severe outcomes (Hoffman, 2002; Parker, 2002).

5. Circulatory overload and pulmonary edema can occur.

6. Hyperkalemia may develop because of the build-up of extracelluar potassium in banked blood. In most cases, this is a theoretic consideration, not an actual event (Davidson & Chern, 1999). Hyperkalemia from transfusions mostly occurs in neonates and patients with renal disease (Eberst, 2000).

7. Hypocalcaemia is another potential problem caused by large amount of citrate containing blood and blood products. Normally, this problem is self-limiting and mild (Wooldridge-King, 2001).

8. Infectious diseases, such as hepatitis, cytomegalovirus, Epstein-Barr virus, and human immunodeficiency virus, may be transmitted via blood products.

9. Bacterial contamination of donor blood is very rare.

PATIENT TEACHING

Report immediately any chills, itching, feeling of warmth, difficulty breathing, or pain in the back, the abdomen, the chest, or at the IV site.

REFERENCES

American Association of Blood Banks (AABB) (1999). *Technical manual*, 13th ed. Arlington, VA: Author.

Davidson, S.J., & Chern, I.M. (1999). Transfusion therapy in emergency medicine (pp. 1033-1038). In Schwartz, G.R. (Ed.), *Principles and practice of emergency medicine*. Baltimore: Williams & Wilkins.

Doctor, M.D. (2000). Blood transfusions and component therapy (pp. 1391-1399). In Tintinalli, J.E., Kelen, G.D., & Stapszynski, J.S. (Eds.), *Emergency medicine* New York: McGraw-Hill.

Hoffman, G.L. (2002). Blood and blood components (pp. 48-52). In Marx, J.A. Hockberger, R.S., Watls, R.M., et al. (Eds.), *Rosen's emergency medicine: concepts and clinical practice*, 5th ed St. Louis: Mosby.

Parker, C.J. (2002). Adverse reactions to blood transfusions (pp. 450-454). In Rakel, R.E., & Bope, E.T. (Eds.), *2002 Conn's current therapy*. Philadelphia: W.B. Saunders.

Puget Sound Blood Center and Program (PSBCP). (2002). *Blood and Blood Components Reference Manual*. Seattle: Author. Available at http://www.psbc.org/medical/default.htm.

Raife, T.J., & Friedman, K.D. (2002). Therapeutic use of blood components (pp. 450-454). In Rakel, R.E., & Bope, E.T. (Eds.), *2002 Conn's current therapy*. Philadelphia: W.B. Saunders.

Strauss, R.G. (2000). Blood and blood component transfusions (pp. 1499-1500). In Behrman, R.E., Kliegman, R.M., & Jenson, H.B. (Eds.), *Textbook of pediatrics*. Philadelphia: W.B. Saunders.

Wooldridge-King, M. (2001). Blood and blood component administration (pp. 757-764). In Lynn-McHale, D.J., & Carlson, K.K. (Eds.), *AACN procedure manual for critical care*, 4th ed. Philadelphia: W.B. Saunders.

Blood Filters

Mike D. McMahon, RN, BSN

See Procedure 74 for information about specific blood components.

INDICATION

To remove clots and debris from blood components. All blood products should be administered through a standard filter (170-260 microns) (Eberst, 2000; Puget Sound Blood Center and Program [PSBCP], 2002).

CONTRAINDICATIONS AND CAUTIONS

1. Microaggregate filters (20-40 microns) slow down the infusion rate and have not been proven to be of value (PSBCP, 2002).
2. Four hours is a reasonable time for use of blood tubing and filters (American Association of Blood Banks [AABB], 1999), but some institutions may change it after each unit of blood delivered.
3. Each filter may be used for two to four units of blood (AABB, 1999).
4. To prevent air entrapment in the filter, never squeeze the drip chamber when the tubing clamp is open.
5. Do not use a filter for platelet infusion if it has previously filtered red blood cells. The trapped cells can block the passage of the platelets.

EQUIPMENT

Blood products as prescribed
Normal saline intravenous (IV) fluid
Y-type blood or solution set

PROCEDURAL STEPS

1. Most in-line Y blood sets prime like normal IV tubing. Fill the drip chamber, the filter area, and the tubing from the normal saline solution bag. Clamp the patient line and the solution line.
2. Ensure that the filter is completely saturated with fluid so that it can function properly.
3. Insert the filter spike into the blood bag.
4. Close the patient clamp and hold the blood bag and the filter upright, with the blood bag slightly above the level of the normal saline solution. Open the blood clamp slowly to allow the blood to enter the drip chamber. Close the solution clamp.
5. Suspend the blood bag on the IV stand.
6. Open the patient-line clamp to the desired rate.

COMPLICATIONS

1. All blood and blood components must be delivered through a filter. This is to prevent accidental delivery of clots and debris (AABB, 1999; PSBCP, 2002).

2. During rapid resuscitation, the filter may clog, making it necessary to change the filter or tubing sooner than recommended to achieve the desired flow rates.

REFERENCES

American Association of Blood Banks (AABB). (1999). *Technical manual*, 13th ed. Arlington, VA: Author.

Eberst, M.E. (2000). Blood transfusions and component therapy (pp 1391-1399). In Tintinalli, J.E., Kelen, G.D., & Stapszynski, J.S. (Eds.), *Emergency medicine*. New York: McGraw-Hill.

Puget Sound Blood Center and Program (PSBCP). (2002). *Blood and blood components reference manual*. Seattle: Author. Available at http://www.psbc.org/medical/default.htm.

PROCEDURE 76

Massive Transfusion

Mike D. McMahon, RN, BSN

Massive blood transfusion is defined as the infusion of half of the patient's blood volume at one time (Davidson & Chern, 1999) or transfusion of the patient's normal blood volume within a 24-hour period (Eberst, 2000).

INDICATION
To treat severe hemorrhagic shock.

CONTRAINDICATIONS AND CAUTIONS
1. The patient's religious beliefs may prohibit the administration of blood or blood products. Jehovah's Witnesses prohibit treatment with whole blood, autologous and allogenic red blood cells (RBCs), fresh frozen plasma, platelets, and hemoglobin solutions (Dasen et al., 2000).
2. Warm all fluids to be administered during a massive transfusion (see Procedure 77).

EQUIPMENT
Normal saline intravenous (IV) fluid and blood products, as prescribed
IV catheters (large bore: 16 G or larger for peripheral access; 7.5 French or larger for central access)
IV tubing (Y blood or trauma tubing)
Fluid warmer
Pressure infuser or pressure bags

PATIENT PREPARATION

1. Make sure that a blood specimen has been sent for typing and crossmatching (T&C) and that the patient has a blood-bank identification band.
2. Establish peripheral IV access using short large-bore (14-G) catheters before considering a central line (Gin-Shaw & Jorden, 2002). If the peripheral circulation has collapsed, then proceed to a cutdown, a percutaneous femoral approach, or a central approach (see Procedures 65-69).
3. While establishing IV access, have an assistant prime the IV tubing (Y blood or trauma tubing) with a normal saline solution. Other types of IV tubing have smaller internal diameters and are unsuitable for massive transfusions. *If the IV fluid is to be infused under pressure, the air in the fluid bag should be removed with a needle and a syringe to avoid an air embolism.*
4. The use of a macropore (170-260 micron) filter and a fluid warmer are necessary to reduce the adverse effects of the rapid infusion of blood products (Eberst, 2000).
5. Micropore filters slow the rate of blood administration and should be avoided if rapid infusion is necessary. Although micropore filters relieve the lungs of the responsibility of filtering microaggregates from the blood circulation, there does not appear to be any benefit in the reduction of acute respiratory distress syndrome (Davidson & Chern, 1999).

PROCEDURAL STEPS

1. Give the initial crystalloid fluid bolus of 20 ml/kg over 15 minutes to a pediatric patient (Cantor & Leaming, 2002) and 1-2 L to the adult patient (Kline, 2002). Assess the patient's response to the fluid bolus.
2. If there is a no response or the response is transient, repeat the fluid bolus and check with the blood bank on the availability of cross-matched blood.
3. When the crystalloid infusion exceeds 30 ml/kg (2-3 L) for the adult patient, blood should be administered (Gin-Shaw & Jorden, 2002) (see Procedure 74). Warm all blood and IV fluids to prevent hypothermia (see Procedure 77). Pressurized infusion may also be indicated (see Procedure 78). When it is available, typed and cross-matched blood is preferred; next in order of preference is type-specific blood. In emergencies, O-negative RBCs may be used in any patient. Any male patient or a female patient who is past childbearing age may receive O-positive RBCs (Hoffman, 2002; Davidson & Chern, 1999).
4. Consider starting RBC infusion immediately if the patient presents with central nervous system trauma or a Glasgow Coma Score of <9 (Kline, 2002).
5. Blood from the chest may be autotransfused if it is available in patients with a thoracic injury (see Procedures 79-83). Because of the risk of fecal contamination, only blood from the chest cavity should be used (Stern & Bobek, 2001).
6. Vital signs, skin perfusion, end-tidal carbon dioxide concentration (EtCO$_2$), pulse oximetry, and urinary output should be monitored frequently to assess the patient's response to fluid resuscitation.
7. After every 5 units of red blood cells, send laboratory specimens for complete blood count (CBC), prothrombin time (PT), partial thromboplastin time (PTT), and fibrinogen level to help guide the administration of additional blood products.
8. The cause of the fluid or blood loss must be identified and corrected as soon as possible.

AGE-SPECIFIC CONSIDERATIONS

1. In pediatric patients, intraosseous needle placement should be attempted if peripheral venous access cannot be obtained within 60-90 seconds (Tobias, 1999) (see Procedure 70).
2. Neonates are at increased risk of developing citrate toxicity (Eberst, 2000).
3. Neonates and pediatric patients are at risk for circulatory overload because of their small baseline blood volume.

COMPLICATIONS

1. Bleeding is the most frequent complication of massive transfusion. This is due in part to the transfusion of multiple units of blood, but it is also due to the complications of hypovolemia, such as hypothermia, sepsis, and disseminated intravascular coagulation (DIC) (Eberst, 2000). Platelet transfusions should be considered when the patient continues to bleed after surgical repair or in a patient who has a platelet count lower than 20,000/ml. Prophylactic treatment should be based on laboratory values, not on amount of blood transfused (Raife & Friedman, 2002).
2. Hypothermia occurs if fluids and blood are not warmed. This is frequently the overlooked cause of impaired hemostasis (Davidson & Chern, 1999).
3. Hypocalcemia is caused by citrate binding of ionized calcium in whole blood. Most patients can tolerate citrate loads of up to 1 unit every 5 minutes (Hoffman, 2002). Electrocardiograph changes are not reliable indicators in the trauma setting. Patients who receive more than 5 units should have serum calcium levels checked. If serum calcium level is subnormal, calcium gluconate, 5-10 ml, should be given by slow IV push (Eberst, 2000).
4. Citrate toxicity is evidenced by acute hypocalcemia.
5. Hyperkalemia
6. Acid-base imbalance, or acidosis, in the trauma patient is caused by increased lactic acid production as a result of shock and poor perfusion. Additionally, the citric and lactic acid levels increase over time in banked blood (American Association of Blood Banks, 1999). This may alter oxygen-carrying ability.
7. For blood reactions, see Procedure 74.

REFERENCES

American Association of Blood Banks. (1999). *Technical manual*, 13th ed. Arlington, VA: Author.

Cantor, R.M., & Leaming, J.M. (2002). Pediatric trauma (pp. 267-281). In Marx, J.A., Hockberger, R.S., Walls, R.M., et al. (Eds.), *Rosen's emergency medicine: concepts and clinical practice*, 5th ed. St. Louis: Mosby.

Dasen K.R., Niswander, D.G., & Schlenker, R.E. (2000). Autologous and allogenic blood products for unanticipated massive blood loss in a Jehovah's Witness. *Anesthesia and Analgesia, 90*, 553-555.

Davidson, S.J., & Chern, I.M. (1999). Transfusion therapy in emergency medicine (pp. 1033-1038). In Schwartz, G.R. (Ed.), *Principles and practice of emergency medicine*. Baltimore: Williams & Wilkins.

Eberst, M.E. (2000). Blood transfusions and component therapy (pp. 1391-1399). In Tintinalli, J.E., Kelen, G.D., & Stapszynski, J.S. (Eds.), *Emergency medicine*. New York: McGraw-Hill.

Gin-Shaw, S.L., & Jorden, R.C. (2002). Multiple trauma (pp. 242-255). In Marx, J.A., Hockberger, R.S., Walls, R.M., et al. (Eds.), *Rosen's emergency medicine: concepts and clinical practice*, 5th ed. St. Louis: Mosby.

Hoffman, G.L. (2002). Blood and blood components. In Marx, J.A., Hockberger, R.S., Walls, R.M.,
    et al. (Eds.), *Rosen's emergency medicine: concepts and clinical practice*, 5th ed. (pp. 48-52).
    St. Louis: Mosby.
Kline, J.A. (2002). Shock (pp. 33-47). In Marx, J.A., Hockberger, R.S., Walls, R.M., et al. (Eds.),
    Rosen's emergency medicine: concepts and clinical practice, 5th ed. St. Louis: Mosby.
Raife, T.J., & Friedman, K.D. (2002). Therapeutic use of blood components. In Rakel, R.E.,
    & Bope, E.T. (Eds.) *2002 Conn's current therapy* (pp. 450-454). Philadelphia: W.B. Saunders.
Stern, S.A., & Bobek, E.M. (2001). Resuscitation: management of shock (pp. 75-102). In Ferrera, P.C.,
    Colucciello, S.A., Marx, J.A., et al. (Eds.), *Trauma management: an emergency medicine
    approach*. St Louis: Mosby.
Tobias, J.D. (1999). Traumatic injury and burns (pp. 273-286). In Tobias, J.D. (Ed.), *Pediatric crit-
    ical care: the essentials*. Armonk, NY: Futura.

PROCEDURE 77

Blood and Fluid Warmers

Mike D. McMahon, RN, BSN

See Procedures 74-76 and 78 for information on blood products, blood filters,
massive transfusion, and pressure infusers.

INDICATIONS
Warming intravenous (IV) fluids and blood products is indicated in the following
situations:
1. To prevent iatrogenic hypothermia when large quantities of IV fluid and blood
   products are administered
2. To provide core rewarming in the presence of hypothermia. Ten liters of fluid
   warmed to 40° C can raise a patient's temperature by 1.4° C (Lapointe &
   Rueden, 2002).
3. To prevent coagulopathy in the trauma patient related to administration of
   unwarmed fluids and blood (Gin-Shaw & Jorden, 2002)

CONTRAINDICATIONS AND CAUTIONS
Hemolysis can occur with excessive warming (42° C, 107.6° F) (American
Association of Blood Banks, 1999).

EQUIPMENT
    IV fluid or blood as prescribed
    Blood/fluid warmer
    IV administration set compatible with warmer

PATIENT PREPARATION

1. Establish venous access (see Procedures 63-72).
2. Attach a short (20 cm or less) extension set to the IV cannula. This prevents the IV site from being disturbed when the blood tubing is being changed.

PROCEDURAL STEPS

Level 1 fluid warmer (Sims Level 1, Inc., 1998a) (Figure 77-1)

The Level 1 fluid warmer is a countercurrent heat exchanger; warmed fluid flows through a tube that surrounds the IV tubing.

1. Push the bottom end of the heat exchanger into the socket labeled "1."
2. Insert the heat exchanger into the guide. Slide the top socket, labeled "2," down over the top of the tube until it clicks.
3. Insert the filter/gas vent into its holder, labeled "3."
4. Plug in and turn on the machine. The display panel should have a green "system operational" indicator light.
5. Ensure that all the tubing connections are tight.
6. When infusing fluid under pressure, remove all the air from the fluid bag by withdrawing the air with a needle and a syringe to avoid an embolism.
7. Close all the IV clamps, spike the IV bag, and hang it on the IV pole.
8. Open the clamp above the drip chamber and squeeze the drip chamber until it is half full.

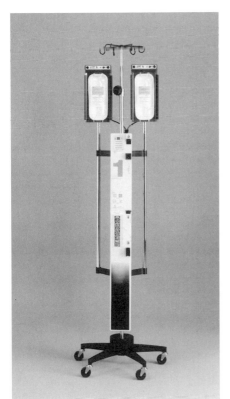

FIGURE 77-1 Level 1 fluid warmer, model 1025. (The model 1000 is identical except that it does not include the pressure infusers.) (Courtesy Sims Level 1, Inc., Rockland, MA.)

9. Open the last two clamps, remove the end cap, and prime the remaining tubing.
10. Close the distal clamp to cause the filter/gas vent to self-prime. Gently tap the filter or gas vent against the cabinet to remove all the trapped air.
11. Connect the system directly to the IV catheter to achieve the optimal flow rate. The Level 1 System 1000/1025 can warm fluid to 37°-42° C at a rate of up to 1 L/min (60,000 ml/hr).
12. When infusing blood products, replace the filter/gas vent or tubing set every 3 hours or sooner if the filter becomes clogged or the air is vented slowly.
13. *To activate the pressure infuser (present on model 1025) (Sims Level 1, 1997), do the following:*
    a. To prevent an air embolism, remove all the air from the IV bag with a 20-ml syringe and a needle, or use a needle to vent the air out of the injection port while squeezing the inverted bag. Spike the bag and prime the IV tubing.
    b. Ensure that the venous access is made with a 14-G or larger cannula.
    c. Flip the toggle switch on the pressure infuser to the "off" position.
    d. Open the hinged latch on the right side of the infuser and hang the solution on the post at the top of the door. For blood or 500-ml bags of IV solution, use the post mounted on the inside of the door.
    e. Close the door and latch it. Open all the clamps in the IV tubing and close the clamp to the opposite spike tail.
    f. Flip the toggle switch to the "on" (+) position. Observe the pressure gauge to see whether a pressure of approximately 300 mm Hg is achieved. The pressure is not adjustable.
    g. When the fluid infusion is complete, flip the switch to the "off" (−) position and open the door. Remove the bag and repeat steps a through f. Manual decompression of the infuser bladder facilitates the insertion of a new IV bag.
14. PF-1 blood filter: The PF-1 is a 340-micron blood filter that prolongs the life of the 170-micron filter incorporated into the Level 1 tubing (Figure 77-2). Spike the blood bag with the PF-1 filter and then spike the PF-1 filter with the spike on the tubing set. Replace the PF-1 filter with each unit of blood.
15. Y-30 connector: Simultaneous infusion into two different IV sites can be achieved with the Y-30 connector. The Y-30 connector is added to the distal end of the tubing set and primed. The connector may be added even if two sites are not in use. Prime both tails and clamp off one. This ensures fast access to the warmed fluid if another site is obtained.
16. D-60HL tubing: Slow infusion rates increase the likelihood that much of the heat may be lost between the fluid warmer and the patient. The D-60HL tubing system, however, has a warm water jacket surrounding the full length of the tubing to allow the infusion of the warmed solution at rates as low as 75 ml/hr.
17. Troubleshooting alarms:
    a. The "check disposables" alarm indicates that a part of the tubing is not fully inserted into the warmer. Check the tubing at the points labeled "1," "2," and "3."
    b. The "add water" alarm signals a low water level in the circulating bath. Turn off the machine and remove the plug from the front of the machine.

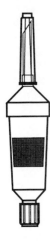

FIGURE 77-2 PF-1, 340-micron prefilter for blood. (Courtesy Sims Level 1, Inc., Rockland, MA.)

Add distilled water to the reservoir until it is full, as evidenced by the window in the front. (Sterile water is frequently distilled and may be used; however, the water does not need to be sterile.)
  c. The "over temperature" alarm signals excessive heating. Turn off the fluid warmer and remove it from service until it can be inspected and serviced.

HotLine Fluid Warmer (Sims Level 1, Inc., 1998b)

The HotLine uses a tubing half-set, which connects to the distal portion of any conventional IV tubing. Heating results from the warm water's flowing around an inner lumen, which carries the IV fluids or blood.

1. Check the water level in the tank and plug the warmer into the power outlet.
2. Push the two extended tubes into the socket on the side of the warmer (Figure 77-3). A snap should be felt.
3. Turn on the power switch. If the warmer is functioning properly, a green "operating" light comes on and the water temperature gauge starts to increase.
4. The water flow should be visible in the outer lumen. Check to make sure that this lumen becomes fully primed before connecting it to the IV line.
5. Connect the IV tubing to the warmer set and prime the inner lumen with fluid.
6. Open and set the fluid rate with the roller clamp on the IV tubing set.

FloTem IIe (CVC/DataChem, Inc., 2000)

This warmer uses dry-heat technology that places IV tubing between metal heating plates (Figure 77-4).

1. Prime the IV tubing.
2. Place the tubing into the indented channel on the heating plate.
3. Close the warmer and turn on the power switch. The unit achieves the required temperature within 2 minutes.
4. A green power light is visible on the front of the unit along with the heated temperature of the fluid.
5. An audible alarm sounds if the temperature exceeds 41.5° C, and power to the coils is stopped. If the temperature reaches 42.5° C, the entire unit shuts off.

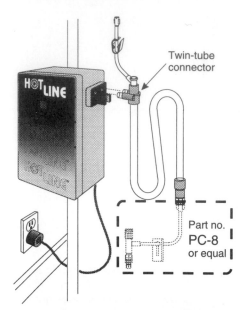

FIGURE 77-3 HotLine fluid warmer. (Courtesy Sims Level 1, Inc., Rockland, MA.)

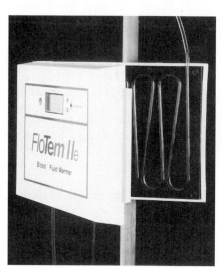

FIGURE 77-4 FloTem IIe blood and fluid warmer. (Courtesy CVC/DataChem, Indianapolis, IN.)

Warmflo FW-538 Fluid Warmer (formerly Alton Dean) (Nellcor, 2002) (Figure 77-5)

This warmer employs a stainless steel foil heat-exchanger cassette. The cassette sits between two microprocessor-controlled heating plates.

1. The warmer displays specific operating instructions on the liquid crystal diode (LCD) screen. To start the warmer, press the "on" button and follow the instructions on the screen.

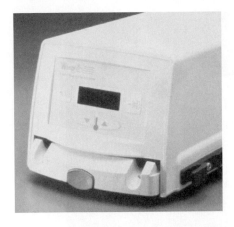

FIGURE 77-5 Warmflo blood and fluid warmer (formerly Alton Dean). (Courtesy Mallinckrodt Medical [Nellcor, division of Tyco], St. Louis.)

2. To remove the cassette, press the "eject" button and follow the instructions on the screen.
3. To turn the warmer off, press the "off" button and follow the instructions on the screen.
4. To change the temperature set point, press the ▼ or ▲ button.
5. Fluid may be pressurized up to 500 mm Hg. For pressurized infusion, do the following:
   a. *To prevent an air embolism, remove all the air from the IV bag with a 20-ml syringe and a needle,* or use a needle to vent the air out of the injection port while squeezing the inverted bag. Spike the bag and prime the IV tubing.
   b. Place the IV bag in the infuser compartment and close and latch the door.
   c. Turn the toggle switch on the bottom of the infusor to the "on" (+) position. The pressure infuser can then be activated by the warmer at the appropriate time.
   d. To increase the pressure, turn the regulator knob clockwise (right). To decrease infusion pressure, turn the regulator knob counterclockwise (left) one turn. Turn the toggle switch "off" and then "on" again to allow the pressure to stabilize. Repeat if necessary.

Thermal Angel TA-200 (Estill Medical Technologies, 2002) (Figure 77-6)
This device is a battery-operated in-line warmer. It is a disposable unit capable of warming fluids for 72 hours.
1. Visually inspect the sterile packing to make sure there is no damage to the packing, device, or extension tubing.
2. Using aseptic technique, open the packages.
3. Connect the IV tubing from the fluid bag to the female end of the warming unit.
4. Connect the extension tubing to the male end of the device, located at the opposite end.
5. Connect the power cable between the unit and the battery. The battery must be charged before use—do not charge the battery while it is connected to the warming device.

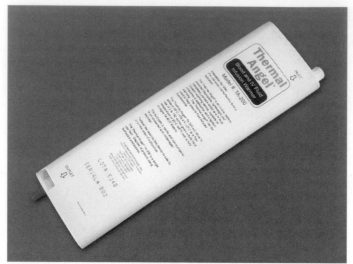

FIGURE 77-6 Thermal Angel TA-200. (Courtesy Estill Medical Technologies.)

6. The green LED will light when the battery is properly connected.
7. Prime the IV tubing and connect it to the patient's IV site.
8. Each battery will supply enough energy for warming 2-4 L of fluid or 1-3 units of blood. When the battery is depleted, another battery can be connected to the device to continue the warming. The warming device will operate for up to 72 continuous hours, at which point it will not respond to new batteries.

Fenwal Blood Warmer (Figure 77-7)

NOTE: This device is no longer manufactured, but the tubing sets are still available from Baxter.

1. Plug in the warmer with the door closed. If the unit does not activate, press the reset switch at the rear of the unit. Approximately 2 minutes are required for the unit to warm to 32°-37° C.
2. Obtain the Fenwal blood warmer tubing. Close the clamp on the tubing.
3. Open the warmer. Hold the warmer bag so the outlet chamber (which goes up) is in the left hand and the right edge is in the right hand.
4. Mount the bag on the top and the bottom support pins of the blood warmer.
5. Ensure that the bag is flat and smooth against the back panel of the warmer.
6. Close the door and fasten the latch. NOTE: Do not open the door once you have infused the fluid or blood through the warming bag, because the bag distends and you cannot close the warming door again.
7. Prime the blood administration set with a normal saline solution and attach it to the Fenwal tubing.
8. Open the clamp on the upper tubing that has the drip chamber of the Fenwal tubing. Squeeze this drip chamber and hold until the normal saline solution appears in the chamber at the point of the white line (on the blood warmer); release the chamber and flush the remainder of the tubing.
9. Attach the tubing to the IV site.
10. Hang the blood and infuse as prescribed.

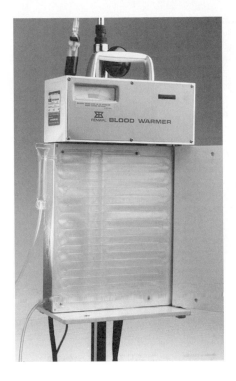

FIGURE 77-7 Fenwal blood warmer. (Courtesy Baxter, Deerfield, IL.)

11. After the blood is infused, flush the warming tubing with the normal saline solution to remove all blood from the warming chamber.

AGE-SPECIFIC CONSIDERATIONS

1. Infants and children, because of the proportion of their surface area to their body weight (Cantor & Leaming, 2002), and the elderly are especially susceptible to hypothermia. Blood and IV fluids should be warmed if rapid infusion is indicated.
2. Slower infusion rates (indicated for small children and the elderly) result in a loss of heat between the warmer and the patient. Use of the Level 1 HotLine or the D-60HL tubing with the system 1000/1025 can overcome this limitation.

COMPLICATIONS

1. Hemolysis
2. Sepsis
3. Air injection if a pressure infuser is used; this may occur if all the air is not removed from the bag before pressurization
4. Drop in fluid temperature with either slow infusion rates or as the distance between the warmer and the patient increases

REFERENCES

American Association of Blood Banks (AABB). (1999). *Technical manual*, 13th ed. Arlington, VA: Author.

Cantor, R.M., & Leaming, J.M. (2002). Pediatric trauma. In Marx, J.A., Hockberger, R.S., Walls, R.M., et al. (Eds.), *Rosen's emergency medicine: concepts and clinical practice*, 5th ed. (pp. 267-281). St. Louis: Mosby.

CVC/DataChem Inc. (1995). *FloTem IIe fluid warmer: instructions for use*. Indianapolis, IN: Author.

Estill Medical Technologies. (2002). Product literature. Available from www.thermalangel.com/html/products-thermalangelinstructions.html.

Gin-Shaw, S.L., & Jorden R.C. (2002). Multiple trauma (pp. 242-255). In Marx, J.A., Hockberger, R.S., Walls, R.M., et al. (Eds.), *Rosen's emergency medicine: concepts and clinical practice*, 5th ed. St. Louis: Mosby.

Lapointe, L.A., & Rueden, K.T. (2002). Coagulopathies in trauma patients. *AACN Clinical Issues*, *13*(2), 192-203.

Nellcor. (2002). *Warmflo® fluid warming system brochure*. Pleasanton, CA: Author.

Sims Level 1, Inc. (1998a). *Level 1 fluid warmer: instructions for use*. Rockland, MA: Author.

Sims Level 1, Inc. (1998b). *HotLine fluid warmer: instructions for use*. Rockland, MA: Author.

Sims Level 1, Inc. (1997). *Operator's & service manual: pressure infusion system, model H-25*. Rockland, MA: Author.

PROCEDURE 78

Blood and Fluid Pressure Infusers

Mike D. McMahon, RN, BSN

NOTE: The Level 1 (Sims) blood and fluid warmer has an integrated pressure infuser on some models. See Procedure 77 for information and operating instructions.

INDICATION
To infuse blood products and/or intravenous (IV) fluids rapidly to treat intravascular volume deficit or pulseless electrical activity (PEA).

CONTRAINDICATIONS AND CAUTIONS
1. Frequent assessment of blood pressure, pulse, skin temperature, capillary refill, urinary output, central venous pressure, or pulmonary artery wedge pressure (if available) is required to evaluate the response to fluid resuscitation.
2. Because they are not compressible, glass IV containers and some autotransfusion devices cannot be used with pressure infusers.

3. Make sure that there are no in-line restrictions, such as small bore T and Y adapters and stopcocks, in the IV tubing. If these connectors have small lumens, they restrict the flow.
4. Remove all the air from the IV bag to prevent an air embolism.
5. Iatrogenic hypothermia may result from the rapid infusion of room temperature IV fluids or refrigerated blood products; warm the blood and IV fluids if rapid infusion is necessary (see Procedure 77).
6. Do not use a blood pressure cuff as a pressure device for delivering blood products. The cuff can cause uneven pressure on the bag, leading to rupture of the bag or damage to the contents (Puget Sound Blood Center and Program, 2002).
7. Many long-term implanted ports or tunneled catheters should not be used with pressure infusers; check manufacturer's specifications before administering pressurized fluid through one of these devices.

EQUIPMENT
18-G needle
20-ml syringe (optional)
Pressure infuser:
   Manual pressure bag
   Warmflo automatic pressure infuser (formerly Alton Dean) (Nellcor, a division of Tyco)

PATIENT PREPARATION
1. Establish an IV access, preferably with a 14-G or larger catheter (see Procedures 63-70). Use of a large-bore catheter prevents red blood cell hemolysis as the blood passes through the catheter (Hoffman, 2002). If the patient has a preexisting IV site, assess the site for signs of problems, such as redness, pain, and swelling.
2. Ensure that the IV tubing is blood or trauma tubing. Blood tubing allows a 200% fluid flow rate, and trauma tubing allows a 500% or greater fluid flow rate than regular IV tubing (Neff, 1993).

PROCEDURAL STEPS
Manual Bag (Figure 78-1)
1. To prevent an air embolism, remove all the air from the IV bag with a 20-ml syringe and a needle, or use a needle to vent the air out of the injection port while squeezing the inverted bag. Spike the bag and prime the IV tubing.
2. Invert and insert the IV bag through the lower opening of the pressure cuff.
3. Insert the loop at the top end of the pressure cuff through the eye of the IV bag.
4. Suspend the cuff and the solution bag by the strap on the IV pole.
5. Check the security of the IV tubing connections at the bag and at the IV site.
6. Inflate to the desired pressure, but do not exceed 300 mm Hg. This is to prevent damage to the red blood cells, disruption of the delivery system, and complications at the IV site.
7. Maintain the desired pressure by squeezing the bulb pump as the fluid or blood is infused.
8. When the blood bag is empty, clamp the line and then flush any blood from the line with normal saline solution.

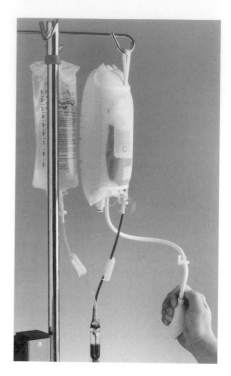

FIGURE 78-1 Manual pressure bag.

9. Remove the empty solution bag by releasing the pressure in the bag.
10. After removing the bag, finish deflating the pressure bag manually. This facilitates insertion of the next bag of solution.

Warmflo Automatic Pressure Infuser (Formally Alton Dean) (Nellcor [a Division of Tyco], 2003) (Figure 78-2)

These devices require that a source of compressed gas be connected to the device.

1. To prevent an air embolism, remove all the air from the IV bag with a 20-ml syringe and a needle, or use a needle to vent the air out of the injection port while squeezing the inverted bag. Spike the bag and prime the IV tubing.
2. Turn the on/off switch to the "off" position.
3. Plug the air hose into the air or the oxygen outlet.
4. Open the door and hang the IV solution bag on the hang tab. If a 500-ml bag is being used, line up the bottom of the bag with the bottom of the door.
5. Close the door and lock it with the latch.
6. Hang the pressure infuser on an IV pole.
7. Turn the regulator knob to the left (counterclockwise) until it stops.
8. Turn the on/off switch to the "on" position. A hissing sound is heard as the air bladder behind the solution bag fills.
9. While monitoring the pressure gauge, turn the regulator knob to the right (clockwise) until the desired pressure is reached.

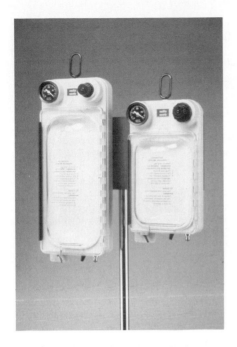

FIGURE 78-2 Warmflo Automatic Pressure Infuser. (Courtesy Mallinckrodt Medical [Nellcor, division of Tyco], St. Louis, MO.)

10. If the pressure exceeds 300 mm Hg, or if you wish to decrease the pressure, keep the switch "on." Then turn the regulator knob to the left and observe the pressure reading in the gauge. Once the selected pressure is reached, turn the infuser toggle switch to "off" and then back to "on" and check the pressure reading. The gauge may need to be tapped lightly after an adjustment.

11. To increase the pressure (do not turn off the infuser), turn the regulator knob to the right until the desired pressure is reached. Do not exceed 300 mm Hg to prevent damage to the container or cells.

12. To remove the IV bag, turn the toggle switch to the "off" position. Open the door and remove the bag.

AGE-SPECIFIC CONSIDERATIONS

1. Elderly patients or those who have a chronic disease (renal or liver disease, heart failure) must be resuscitated cautiously with fluids because of their impaired ability to deal with a fluid overload. At the same time, elderly patients poorly tolerate hypotension and hypovolemia (Birnbaumer, 2002).

2. Neonates and pediatric patients are at risk for circulatory overload because of their small baseline blood volume.

3. Elderly and pediatric patients are at increased risk of iatrogenic hypothermia; warm the fluids if a rapid infusion is necessary (see Procedure 77).

COMPLICATIONS

1. Air embolization
2. Volume overload
3. Infiltration of IV fluid

4. Manual cuff devices must be inflated carefully. Some older devices are capable of generating pressures up to 1000 mm Hg without alerting the user (Health Devices, 1995).
5. Iatrogenic hypothermia can occur if unheated solutions are administered rapidly.

REFERENCES

Birnbaumer, D.M. (2002). Geriatric trauma (pp. 281-286). In Marx, J.A., Hockberger, R.S., Walls, R.M., et al. (Eds.), *Rosen's emergency medicine: concepts and clinical practice*, 5th ed. St. Louis: Mosby.

Health Devices. (1995). Use of pressure infusion with Level 1 Technologies L-10 gas eliminators and HotLine fluid warmers. *Health Devices, 24*, 478-479.

Hoffman, G.L. (2002). Blood and blood components (pp 48-52). In Marx, J.A., Hockberger, R.S., Walls, R.M., et al. (Eds.), *Rosen's emergency medicine: concepts and clinical practice*, 5th ed. St. Louis: Mosby.

Neff, J.A. (1993). Perfusion: cardiac and vascular injuries (pp. 195-262). In Neff, J.A., & Kidd, P.S. (Eds.), *Trauma nursing: the art and science*. St. Louis: Mosby.

Nellcor. (2003). Warmflo® Pressure Infusor. www.nellcor.com/prod/.

Puget Sound Blood Center and Program (PSBCP). (2002). *Blood and blood components reference manual*. Seattle: Author. Available at http://www.psbc.org/medical/default.htm.

PROCEDURE 79

General Principles of Autotransfusion

Deborah A. Upton, RN, BSN, CEN
and Jean A. Proehl, RN, MN, CEN, CCRN

Autotransfusion includes preplanned donation of blood before elective surgery, autotransfusion after cell washing in the operating room, and emergency autotransfusion of pleural or mediastinal blood without cell washing. This procedure describes the emergency autotransfusion of pleural blood without cell washing.

INDICATION

To return shed autologous blood to the patient with a massive hemothorax. The advantages of using autotransfused blood include warmth and immediately availability, perfect compatibility with the patient and no risk of transfusion reaction, no risk of blood-borne disease transmission to the patient, and decreased demand on the stored blood supply. Indications include:

1. Massive hemothorax

2. Myocardial rupture
3. Great vessel rupture
4. Chest trauma where there is a known history of transfusion reactions
5. Chest trauma for which patient, for religious or other reasons, refuses banked blood

Some autotransfusion systems require assembly or insertion into the chest-drainage system; therefore, consider routinely setting the autotransfusion component for patients who are at high risk for hemothorax. Otherwise, blood that drains immediately on chest-tube insertion may be lost to recovery. Some systems (Atrium and Argyle) offer the option of closed loop collection and reinfusion.

CONTRAINDICATIONS AND CAUTIONS

1. If contamination of the pleural blood from gastrointestinal contents is suspected, the risk of sepsis is significant. When the possibility exists of a communication between the abdomen and the chest (e.g., diaphragmatic disruption from a gunshot or stab wound), the risks and benefits of autotransfusion must be considered. Prophylactic broad-spectrum antibiotics are usually given if gastrointestinal contamination of autotransfused blood is suspected.
2. Wounds more than 4 hours old.
3. Reinfusion of collected blood should occur within 6 hours of initiating the collection (American Association of Blood Banks [AABB], 2001).
4. Autotransfusion is contraindicated in the presence of coagulopathy, malignant neoplasm, enteric contamination of thoracic cavity, or infection (systemic, pulmonary, pericardial, or mediastinal) (Atrium Medical Corporation, 2001).
5. Only blood collected in the autotransfusion unit should be reinfused. Any collected in the chest-drainage device should not be reinfused. Blood collected by use of the Atrium system is an exception because it is collected in a sterile chamber and is later transferred to a bag for reinfusion.

PROCEDURAL STEPS

1. Insert a large-bore chest tube(s) (see Procedure 41).
2. Prepare the autotransfuser for blood collection (see Procedures 80-83).
3. Inject an anticoagulant into the collection unit (optional). The use of an anticoagulant is not mandatory, because the blood is frequently defibrinated by friction in the pleural cavity. However, if blood loss and recovery are rapid, the blood may still clot. Anticoagulants do not dissolve clots; they prevent them. Hence, if clots form in the collection chamber, the blood is not available for autotransfusion. Some sources report no difficulty in autotransfusing blood without an anticoagulant (Kharasch et al., 1994). If an anticoagulant is used, instill it as soon as possible during or before the blood collection. Common anticoagulant options include the following:
   a. Citrate phosphate dextrose (CPD) is a commonly used anticoagulant. Fourteen milliliters of CPD for every 100 ml of blood is recommended (AABB, 2002). Because it is difficult to estimate the amount of blood in a patient's chest, one approach is to instill enough CPD to anticoagulate one unit of blood initially (60-70 ml). When one unit of blood has been collected (about 500 ml total volume of blood plus CPD), it may be reinfused,

or additional CPD may be added to continue the collection. The CPD injection may be facilitated by the use of a volume-control intravenous chamber; run the desired amount of CPD into the chamber and then infuse the CPD via the intravenous tubing to the injection port.

    b. Citrate phosphate dextrose adenine (CPDA-1) administered as 14 ml per 100 ml of blood is recommended (AABB, 2002). Instill as described in step 3a above.

4. Collect blood.

5. When 500-1000 ml of blood has been collected, prepare for reinfusion (see Procedures 80-83).

6. Ongoing evaluation of the patient who is being autotransfused includes evaluation of laboratory data to include hematocrit, prothrombin time (PT), partial thromboplastin time (PTT), platelet count, and arterial blood gases.

AGE-SPECIFIC CONSIDERATIONS

1. For pediatric patients, if an anticoagulant is used, administer a proportionately smaller amount (based on the amount you plan to collect before the recovery for reinfusion).

2. Lower wall suction levels (5-15 mm Hg) may decrease hemolysis in young children (Kharasch et al., 1994).

COMPLICATIONS

1. Hematologic complications include decreased platelet count and fibrinogen level, prolonged prothrombin time and partial thromboplastin time, and red blood cell hemolysis. These complications usually occur with massive autotransfusion (greater than 1-1.5 times the patient's blood volume in pediatric patients) (Atrium Medical Corporation, 2001; Kharasch et al., 1994).

2. Nonhematologic complications include bacteremia and microembolism (Atrium Medical Corporation, 2001; Kharasch et al., 1994).

3. Rapid reinfusion of citrate-containing blood can result in citrate toxicity, hypocalcemia, and myocardial depression. Signs and symptoms of citrate toxicity include tingling around the mouth, stomach cramps, dysrhythmias, hypokalemia, alkalosis, circumoral cyanosis, and hypotension.

REFERENCES

American Association of Blood Banks (AABB). (2002). *Technical manual*, 14th ed. Bethesda, MD: Author.

American Association of Blood Banks (AABB). (2001). *Standards for perioperative autologous blood collection and administration*. Bethesda, MD: Author.

Atrium Medical Corporation. (2001). *Chest drain autotransfusion* (package insert). Hudson, NH: Author.

Kharasch, S.J., Millham, F., & Vinci, R.J. (1994). The use of autotransfusion in pediatric chest trauma. *Pediatric Emergency Care, 10*, 109-112.

Autotransfusion Devices: Pleur-Evac

Deborah A. Upton, RN, BSN, CEN
and Jean A. Proehl, RN, MN, CEN, CCRN

Pleur-Evac is a registered trademark of the Deknatel Product Group, Genzyme Surgical Products.

The information in this procedure should be used in conjunction with the information in Procedure 79.

INDICATIONS
See Procedure 79.

CONTRAINDICATIONS AND CAUTIONS
Refer to Procedure 79.

EQUIPMENT
Pleur-Evac chest-tube drainage system and autotransfusion unit
Blood tubing with filter
Suction setup
Anticoagulant (optional)
18-G needle (optional)
60-ml syringe or intravenous (IV) tubing with volumetric chamber
(optional)

PATIENT PREPARATION
Insert a large-bore chest tube (see Procedure 41).

PROCEDURAL STEPS (Deknatel, 1988)
1. Prepare the chest-drainage unit (see Procedure 46).
2. Attach the autotransfusion bag if the unit is not ready for autotransfusion. The autotransfusion bag (A-1500) is attached to the side of the Pleur-Evac chest tube drainage system. Use the foot hook and the ATS hanger on the side of the unit (Figure 80-1).
   a. Close the two white clamps on the top of the A-1500 replacement bag.
   b. Close the white clamp on the Pleur-Evac patient tubing and milk the blood distally from the tubing into the Pleur-Evac.
   c. Detach the red and the blue connectors.
   d. Remove the red protective cap from the collection tubing on the A-1500 replacement bag and connect it to the patient chest-drainage tubing using the red connectors.

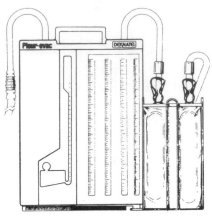

FIGURE 80-1 Pleur-Evac autotransfusion unit, set up to collect blood. (Courtesy Deknatel, Fall River, MA.)

    e. Remove the blue protective cap from the tubing on the A-1500 replacement bag and connect it to the Pleur-Evac tubing using the blue connectors.
    f. Open all the clamps and make sure all the connections are airtight.
    g. Inject an anticoagulant into the collection bag (optional). A 60-ml syringe or a volumetric IV chamber can be used to instill the anticoagulant.
3. Collect blood.
4. To discontinue collection:
    a. Use the high-negativity relief valve to reduce excessive negativity.
    b. Close the white clamps on the patient tubing and on top of the autotransfusion bag.
    c. Detach all the red and the blue connectors.
    d. Attach the red and the blue connectors on top of the autotransfusion bag.
    e. Securely attach the red and the blue connectors by joining the patient tube (red) to the Pleur-Evac tube (blue).
    f. Open the white clamps on the patient tube so that the drainage can be collected in the Pleur-Evac.
    g. Remove the autotransfusion bag from the Pleur-Evac by removing the collection-bag frame from the hanger on the side of the unit. Disconnect the foot hook from the Pleur-Evac unit and slide the bag off the wire frame.
5. To change the autotransfusion bag, refer to preceding steps 2a-g.
6. Prepare for reinfusion (Figure 80-2) by doing the following:
    a. Invert the bag so that the spike port points upward, remove the protective cap, and insert a blood filter into the spike port by using a constant twisting motion (see Procedure 75).
    b. Remove the air from the bag. Keeping the unit inverted, squeeze all the air from the bag carefully through the filter and the drip-chamber assembly. Close the infusion set clamp, invert the autotransfusion bag, suspend it from an IV pole by using the plastic strap, open the infusion set, and flush the administration line carefully to remove all of the air.
7. *Reinfusion:* Attach the distal end of the infusion set assembly to the IV line and infuse the blood by using gravity or pressure. A pressure infuser that wraps around the bag is best suited for the A-1500 replacement bag when a pressure reinfusion is indicated. Be sure to remove all air from the bag before infusing under pressure.

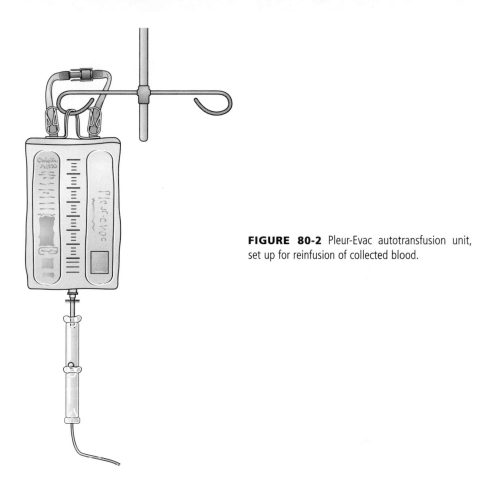

FIGURE 80-2 Pleur-Evac autotransfusion unit, set up for reinfusion of collected blood.

AGE-SPECIFIC CONSIDERATION

Although the Pleur-Evac autotransfusion system is designed for adult use, it can be used for pediatric patients. The amount of anticoagulant used should be proportionate to the amount of blood collected or anticipated.

COMPLICATIONS

1. Refer to Procedure 79.
2. An air embolism is a potential complication during autotransfusion with this system. To reduce the risk of an air embolism, the collected blood must be properly prepared for reinfusion by removing all the air from the blood bag before hanging it for reinfusion.

REFERENCE

Deknatel, Inc. (1988). *Pleur-Evac adult-pediatric single use chest drainage unit* (product insert). Fall River, MA. Author.

Autotransfusion Devices: Thora-Klex

Deborah A. Upton, RN, BSN, CEN
and Jean A. Proehl, RN, MN, CEN, CCRN

Thora-Klex is a registered trademark of Deknatel DSP Worldwide, Inc. (Fall River, MA).

The information in this procedure should be used in conjunction with the information in Procedure 79.

INDICATION
See Procedure 79.

CONTRAINDICATIONS AND CAUTIONS
Refer to Procedure 79.

EQUIPMENT
Thora-Klex autotransfusion unit
Thora-Klex chest drainage unit
Blood tubing with filter
Suction setup
Anticoagulant (optional)
18-G needle (optional)
60-ml syringe or intravenous tubing with volumetric chamber (optional)

PATIENT PREPARATION
Insert a large-bore chest tube (see Procedure 41).

PROCEDURAL STEPS (Deknatel DSP, 1996)
1. Prepare the chest-drainage unit (see Procedure 47).
2. Disconnect the Thora-Klex chest-drainage unit from the suction device.
3. Attach the autotransfusion unit.
   a. Close both clamps on the top of the autotransfusion unit (Figure 81-1).
   b. Attach the autotransfusion unit to the chest-drainage unit by lining up the bottom leg and the Easy-Link lock of the Easy-Link adapter with their respective receptacles on the chest-drainage unit. Push down until the Easy-Link lock clicks into position.
   c. Remove the protective seal from the quick-disconnect locking connector located midway on the Thora-Klex unit patient tube.
   d. Clamp or crimp the chest tube to stop the flow of blood.
   e. Separate the connector by twisting the quick-disconnect locking connector counterclockwise and pulling it apart.

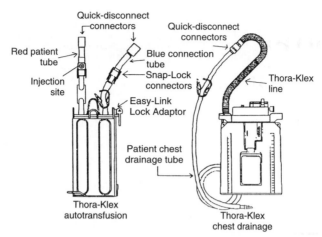

FIGURE 81-1 Thora-Klex chest drainage system and autotransfusion bag. (Courtesy Deknatel DSP, Fall River, MA.)

 f. Using an aseptic technique, remove the red cover from the collection tubing and insert the corresponding red color-coded connector of the patient tube, making sure that the connector is locked into place by twisting it clockwise. Repeat the insertion and locking of the blue connectors (Figure 81-2).

 g. Open all the clamps.

 h. Reconnect the unit to the suction device.

 i. Inject an anticoagulant through the anticoagulant port (optional). Add the anticoagulant by inserting a needle through the latex injection port of the filter housing. Alternatively, twist and remove the injection port fitting and insert a Luer-Lok to add the anticoagulant. A 60-ml syringe or a volumetric intravenous chamber can be used to instill the anticoagulant.

4. Collect blood.

5. Prepare for reinfusion.

 a. Disconnect the Thora-Klex chest-drainage unit from the suction device.

 b. Clamp the patient tube and both clamps on the autotransfusion unit.

 c. Separate the red and the blue connectors and attach the tubes at the top of the autotransfusion unit.

 d. Link the patient tubes together at the quick-disconnect locking connector or attach another collection bottle as discussed in steps 3b-i.

 e. Release the clamp on the patient tube.

 f. Reconnect the unit to the suction device.

 g. Remove the Easy-Link adapter bracket by twisting it slightly. Unhook the top from the wire frame.

 h. Slide the bag off the wire frame.

 i. Invert the bag and remove the blue cap from the spike port (Figure 81-3).

 j. Spike the bag with the blood tubing (see Procedure 75).

 k. Remove all the air from the blood bag by squeezing the inverted bag until the air is ejected and the drip chamber is half full.

 l. Invert the bag and hang it by using the plastic strap.

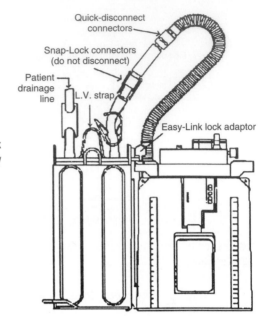

FIGURE 81-2 Assembled Thora-Klex autotransfusion kit system. (Courtesy Deknatel DSP, Fall River, MA.)

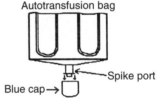

FIGURE 81-3 Autotransfusion bag spike port. (Courtesy Deknatel DSP, Fall River, MA.)

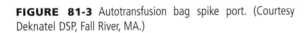

m. Infuse the collected blood. For faster infusion, use a pressure infuser (see Procedure 78). Be sure to remove all air from the bag before administration under pressure.

AGE-SPECIFIC CONSIDERATION

The Thora-Klex autotransfusion system is designed for adult use, but it can be used for pediatric patients. The amount of anticoagulant used should be proportionate to the amount of blood collected or anticipated.

COMPLICATIONS

1. Refer to Procedure 79.
2. An air embolism is a potential complication during autotransfusion with this system. To reduce the risk of air embolism, the collected blood must be properly prepared for reinfusion by removal of all air from the blood bag before hanging it for reinfusion.

REFERENCE

Deknatel DSP. (1996). *Thora-Klex autotransfusion system with Easy-Link.* Fall River, MA: Author.

Autotransfusion Devices: Argyle

Deborah A. Upton, RN, BSN, CEN
and
Jean A. Proehl, RN, MN, CEN, CCRN

Argyle is a registered trademark of Sherwood Medical (St. Louis, MO).

The information in this procedure should be used in conjunction with the information in Procedure 79.

INDICATION

See Procedure 79.

The Argyle autotransfusion system allows for the reinfusion of blood by using a continuous reinfusion method. This technique is generally not suitable for emergency department use, but it may be acceptable for a patient who belongs to a religious group, such as the Jehovah's Witnesses, that opposes blood transfusion.

CONTRAINDICATIONS AND CAUTIONS

See Procedure 79.

EQUIPMENT

    Argyle autotransfusion chest-drainage unit (Thora-Seal III, Aqua-Seal, or
        Sentinel Seal)
    Autotransfusion accessory unit (Figure 82-1)
    Suction device setup
    Anticoagulant of choice (optional)
    18-G needle (optional)
    60-ml syringe or intravenous (IV) tubing with volumetric chamber
        (optional)
    Microembolus blood filter, IV pump, and blood-compatible pump tubing
        (continuous-infusion method only)

PATIENT PREPARATION

Insert a chest tube (see Procedure 41).

PROCEDURAL STEPS (Sherwood Medical, 1992a, b)

1. Prepare the chest-drainage unit as described in Procedure 48. The aspiration vacuum should not exceed -25 cm H_2O.
2. If not preattached, attach the autotransfusion unit to the chest-drainage unit by using the hooks and the Velcro closure. Connect the tubing so that the autotransfusion bag is in line between the patient and the chest-drainage unit (match the connectors: blue to blue and white to white) (Figures 82-2 and 82-3).

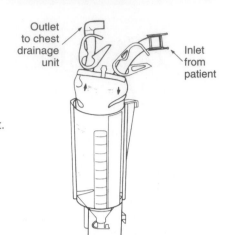

FIGURE 82-1 Autotransfusion accessory unit. (Courtesy Sherwood Davis & Geck, St. Louis, MO.)

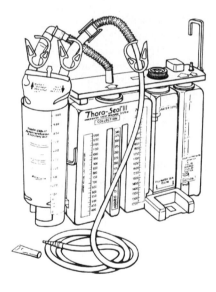

FIGURE 82-2 Thora-Seal III autotransfusion chest-drainage system. (Courtesy Sherwood Davis & Geck, St. Louis, MO.)

3. (Optional) Use a 60-ml syringe or IV tubing with a volumetric chamber to add an anticoagulant to the drainage-collection chamber through the injection port located on the top of the blood-collection bag.
4. Collect the blood.
5. Reinfusion via gravity includes the following steps:
    a. Close all the tubing clamps and detach the blue and the white connectors. Place a new autotransfusion unit in line, or reconnect the patient directly to the chest-drainage unit by connecting the blue and the white connectors. Open all the clamps.
    b. Attach the blue and the white connectors on the top of the autotransfusion bag. Remove the autotransfusion bag from the plastic tower.
    c. Prime the blood tubing with saline solution (see Procedure 75).

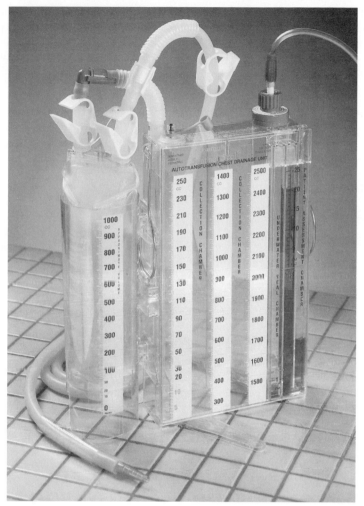

FIGURE 82-3 Sentinel Seal autotransfusion chest-drainage unit. (Courtesy Sherwood Davis & Geck, St. Louis, MO.)

    d. Spike the port at the bottom of the autotransfusion bag with the primed blood tubing. Hang the bag on an IV stand.

    e. Open the roller clamp and initiate the transfusion. If pressurized infusion is anticipated, remove all the air from the autotransfusion bag. Reinfusion pressure should not exceed 150 mm Hg (see Procedure 78).

6. The continuous-reinfusion method includes the following steps:

    a. When adequate blood has collected in the autotransfusion bag, prime the blood-compatible pump tubing with normal saline solution.

    b. Spike the port at the bottom of the autotransfusion bag with the primed pump tubing.

c. Lower the IV pump as close to the level of the chest-drainage unit as possible. The chest-drainage unit must remain below the level of the patient's chest.
d. Set the pump to reinfuse the blood at a rate approximating the drainage rate. Monitor the amount of blood in the autotransfusion bag carefully, and discontinue autotransfusion when there is 50 ml or less in the collection bag.

AGE-SPECIFIC CONSIDERATION
The Argyle autotransfusion system is designed for adult use, but it can also be used for pediatric patients. The anticoagulant ratio should be proportionate to the volume of blood recovered and reinfused.

COMPLICATIONS
1. See Procedure 79.
2. An air embolism is a potential complication during autotransfusion with this system. To reduce the risk of an air embolism, the collected blood must be properly prepared for reinfusion by removing all of the air from the blood bag before hanging it for reinfusion.

REFERENCES
Sherwood Medical. (1992a). *Aqua-Seal autotransfusion accessory unit* (instruction card). St. Louis: Author.
Sherwood Medical. (1992b). *Thora-Seal III autotransfusion accessory unit* (instruction card). St. Louis: Author.

PROCEDURE 83

Autotransfusion Devices: Atrium

Deborah A. Upton, RN, BSN, CEN
and Jean A. Proehl, RN, MN, CEN, CCRN

The information in this procedure should be used in conjunction with the information in Procedure 79.

INDICATION
See Procedure 79.

The Atrium autotransfusion system also allows for reinfusion of blood using a "closed-loop" technique. This technique is generally not suitable for emergency department use but may be acceptable to a patient who belongs to a religious group, such as the Jehovah's Witnesses, that opposes blood transfusion.

CONTRAINDICATIONS AND CAUTIONS

See Procedure 79.

EQUIPMENT

Atrium chest-drainage unit 2050 (blood-recovery system)
Atrium ATS blood-recovery bag (self-filling bag 2450 or in-line bag 2550)
Suction setup
Sterile saline solution or sterile water (saline solution is recommended for all continuous ATS applications)
Anticoagulant of choice (optional)
18-G needle (optional)
60-ml syringe or intravenous (IV) tubing with volumetric chamber (optional)
Blood tubing and filter
IV pump, microembolus blood filter, blood-compatible pump tubing (closed-loop technique only)

PATIENT PREPARATION

Insert a chest tube (see Procedure 41).

PROCEDURAL STEPS (Atrium, 1996)

1. Prepare the Atrium blood-recovery chest-drainage unit as described in Procedure 49. Sterile saline solution is recommended for blood-recovery procedures. These units have an additional access line for autotransfusion (ATS access line), which allows access to the drainage unit without disconnecting the chest drain or interrupting the patient drainage (Figure 83-1).

2. (Optional) As soon as significant bloody drainage is noted, add the selected anticoagulant to the drainage-collection chamber through the grommet located on the top of the drain or the ATS bag. The anticoagulant should be added directly to the ATS collection system during setup or simultaneously with the blood collection. Swab the injection site on top of the drain or on the ATS bag and use an 18-G or smaller needle and syringe (or IV tubing that has a volumetric chamber) to add the anticoagulant. The controlled doses for anticoagulant citrate dextrose (ACD), as recommended by the manufacturer, are noted in the Table 83-1.

3. For self-filling ATS bags (Figure 83-2), do the following:
   a. Turn off the suction.
   b. Close the chest drain ATS access-line clamp and remove the spike port cap before attaching the bag.
   c. Insert the ATS bag spike into the chest-drain ATS access line spike port by using a twisting motion. Position the ATS bag below the base of the chest drain to facilitate filling.
   d. Open both clamps and hold the ATS bag 2-4 inches below the base of the chest drain. Gently bend the ATS bag upward to activate blood transfer.

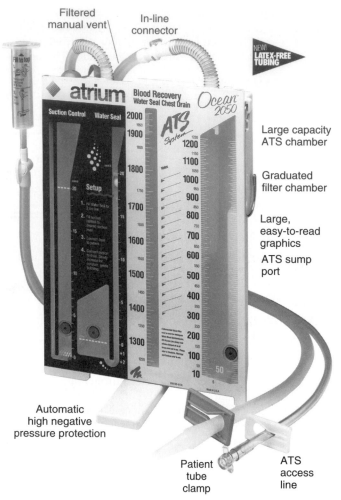

FIGURE 83-1 Atrium 2050 blood recovery system. (Courtesy Atrium, Hudson, NH.)

TABLE 83-1

THE MANUFACTURER'S RECOMMENDED DOSES OF ANTICOAGULANT CITRATE DEXTROSE-A

Blood Volume Expected	Amount of ACD-A	
	1:7 ratio	1:20 ratio
Low volume, 140-250 ml	20-35 ml	7-12.5 ml
Incremental volume, over 250 ml	14 ml/100 ml blood	5 ml/100 ml blood
Moderate volume, 250-500 ml	40-70 ml	12.4-25 ml
Large volume, 500-1000 ml	70-140 ml	70-140 ml

Atrium (1996). *Atrium autotransfusion guide*. Hudson, NH: Author.

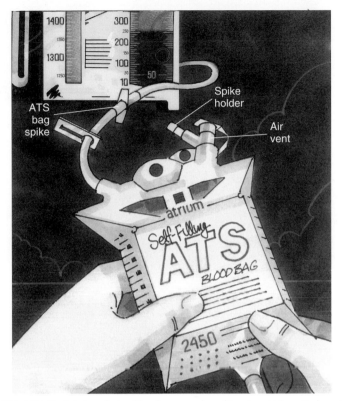

FIGURE 83-2 Autotransfusion blood recovery bag. (Courtesy Atrium, Hudson, NH.)

   e. To disconnect the ATS bag, close both clamps, remove the ATS spike, and
      insert it into the ATS bag spike holder. Recap the ATS access line spike
      port and place the access line in the holder located on top of the chest
      drain. The ATS bag is ready for infusion.
4. For in-line ATS bags (Figure 83-3):
   a. Open the patient tube clamp and move it next to the in-line connector for
      easy setup and visual checks.
   b. Close the patient-tube clamp and separate the connector by depressing the
      connector lock.
   c. Remove the cap from the female ATS-bag connector and insert it into the
      male patient-tube connector.
   d. Remove the second ATS-bag cap and insert the male ATS bag connector
      into the female chest-drain connector.
   e. Open both in-line ATS-bag clamps before opening the patient-tube clamp.
      Open the patient-tube clamp after both ATS-bag clamps have been opened.
   f. To remove the in-line ATS bag from the chest drain, close the patient-tube
      clamp and both ATS bag clamps. Disconnect the chest-drain side first, and
      then disconnect the patient-side connector. Place the male patient-tube

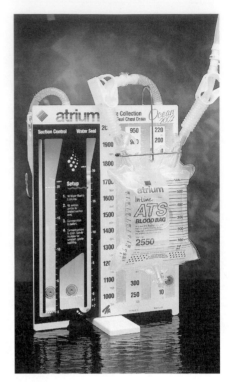

FIGURE 83-3 In-line autotransfusion bag. (Courtesy Atrium, Hudson, NH.)

connector into the female chest-drain connector and open the patient tube clamp. Reconnect the ATS bag connectors to each other. The ATS bag is ready for reinfusion.

5. Reinfusion requires the following steps:
   a. Prime the blood tubing with saline solution (see Procedure 75).
   b. Invert the ATS bag with the spike port pointing up and remove the tethered cap. Insert the blood filter spike into the ATS bag spike port by using a firm twisting motion. Hang the ATS bag on an IV stand.
   c. Open the air vent and initiate the transfusion.

6. The closed-loop technique (not usually used in the emergency department) (Figure 83-4) requires the following steps:
   a. For direct reinfusion of shed autologous blood via a blood-compatible infusion pump, a microembolus blood filter and a nonvented, blood-compatible IV pump tubing are required. Position the IV pump as close to the chest-drainage unit as possible. Prime the tubing with saline solution according to the directions of the pump manufacturer, spike the ATS access line with the blood tubing setup, and connect it to an injection port on a preexisting IV site. Program the pump to deliver the blood at approximately the same rate that it is draining from the chest.

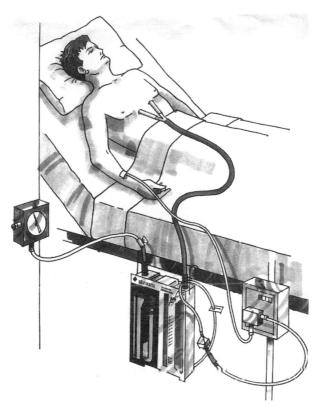

FIGURE 83-4 Closed-loop setup using an intravenous infusion pump. (Courtesy Atrium, Hudson, NH.)

AGE-SPECIFIC CONSIDERATION

The Atrium autotransfusion system is designed for adult use, but it can also be used for pediatric patients. The anticoagulant ratio should be proportionate to the volume of blood recovered and reinfused.

COMPLICATIONS

See Procedure 79.

REFERENCE

Atrium. (1996). *Atrium autotransfusion guide.* Hudson, NH: Author.

Electrical Therapy

Defibrillation

Mike D. McMahon, RN, BSN

Defibrillation is also known as direct-current countershock, electrical counter-shock therapy, unsynchronized cardioversion, or "defib." The word *defibrillate* refers to an effect on the heart and is not synonymous with delivery of a shock from a defibrillator. This section deals with manual use of defibrillators only; see Procedure 86 for information on the automatic external defibrillator.

Since 1996, external defibrillators have been available with two different types of energy waveforms, the monophasic and the biphasic. In a monophasic defibrillator, the electrical current travels in one direction between the paddles or electrodes. In a defibrillator that has a biphasic waveform, the electrical current starts in one direction and then reverses direction part way through (Figure 84-1). This allows the peak current delivered by a biphasic shock to be lower than the same peak current delivered by a monophasic shock. This development of the biphasic defibrillation waveform follows from implanted cardiac defibrillators, in which biphasic waveforms have become the standard for use (Dell'Orfano & Naccarelli, 2001). The American Heart Association (AHA, 2000) has not made a recommendation for optimal biphasic defibrillation energy levels, but biphasic shock energies of ≤200 joules are safe and effective. Since the publication of the 2000 AHA guidelines, further data have emerged demonstrating good results for cardioversion of atrial fibrillation and defibrillation of ventricular fibrillation with biphasic shocks up to 360 joules (Jain & Wheelan, 2002).

INDICATIONS
1. To terminate ventricular fibrillation
2. To terminate pulseless ventricular tachycardia

CONTRAINDICATIONS AND CAUTIONS
1. Rapid defibrillation is crucial to increase the patient's chance of survival. For each minute that passes, there is a 7%-10% reduction of successful defibrillation (AHA, 2000).
2. Successful defibrillation depends on the metabolic state of the myocardium. Factors that affect the metabolic state include severe hypothermia, hypoxia, acidosis, and electrolyte imbalances.
3. Transthoracic impedance, or resistance, to current flow can affect the ability to defibrillate the myocardium. Factors that determine transthoracic impedance are the following:
   a. Energy level: More current flows with higher energy levels. The American Heart Association (2000) recommends that the first defibrillation attempt be performed at 200 joules if a monophasic device is used. For the biphasic device, levels that are clinically equivalent to the 200 joules in the monophasic device should be used. Because the transthoracic impedance declines

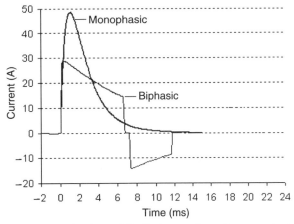

FIGURE 84-1 Monophasic and biphasic defibrillation waveforms. The monophasic waveform is generated from a 200-J shock and reaches a peak current of 48 amps. The biphasic waveform is generated from a 150-J shock and its peak current is 28 amps. (Modified from Walker, R.G., Melnick, S.B., Chapman, F.W., et al. [2003]. Comparison of six clinically used external defibrillators in swine. *Resuscitation, 57,* 73-83.)

with repeated shocks, even with the same energy level, if there is no rhythm change on the monitor, the second defibrillation should be administered immediately, using an energy level from 200-300 joules *or the clinically equivalent biphasic shock.* If after a quick assessment of the patient's rhythm you determine that the patient is still in ventricular fibrillation or that the patient has pulseless ventricular tachycardia, a third shock of 360 joules *or the clinically equivalent biphasic shock* is delivered.
   b. Electrode or paddle size: For adults, the defibrillation electrodes or paddles range from 8.5-12 cm in diameter. Total area of the two electrodes should not exceed 150 cm^2.
   c. Correct electrode or paddle placement is an important factor in determining the success of defibrillation.
   d. The more shocks delivered and the shorter the interval between shocks, the lower the transthoracic impedance.
   e. Delivering shocks during exhalation lowers impedance.
   f. Use of a conductive gel lessens the transthoracic impedance. Too little conductive gel may result in skin burns, whereas too much conductive gel may lead to arcing of the current between the paddles. Disposable defibrillation electrodes are manufactured with a gel coating, which is the conductive medium.
4. Remove the nitroglycerin ointment or patches from the patient's chest because they may also allow an inappropriate path for the current.
5. The defibrillation electrodes should be placed at least 5 inches away from a pacemaker generator. Damage can occur if the generator is directly defibrillated. The generator may also absorb the discharged current and thus reduce the chance of successful defibrillation.

6. Defibrillation may become necessary during noninvasive pacing. This may require turning off the pacemaker before the external defibrillation may be performed. Most devices that provide both noninvasive pacemakers and defibrillation disable the pacemaker function when defibrillation is selected. Defibrillating a noninvasively paced patient may require disconnecting the pacemaker from the patient before externally defibrillating. If hard-paddle defibrillation or pacing electrodes have already been applied, hard paddles should neither touch the disposable electrodes nor lie on top of them.

7. Implantable cardioverter defibrillator (ICD) is an implanted electronic device used in patients who are at high risk for ventricular fibrillation or ventricular tachycardia. An ICD is designed to monitor cardiac rhythms and deliver countershocks if ventricular fibrillation or ventricular tachycardia is identified. If ventricular tachycardia or ventricular fibrillation is present despite an ICD, an external shock should be given immediately. Place the paddles or electrodes at least 5 inches from the ICD. The internal ICD electrodes may cover a section of the epicardium and interfere with the current flow to the heart. If shocks delivered up to 360 joules *or a clinically equivalent biphasic shock* fail to defibrillate the patient, change the paddle or defibrillation electrode placement to an alternative site (anteroposterior or axillary-axillary).

8. Hypothermia. On initial presentation, ventricular fibrillation should be treated with defibrillation. If there is no success with the initial shock, rewarming should be started. Most attempts at defibrillation are unsuccessful when the patient's core temperature is below 28°-30° C (Danzl, 2002).

EQUIPMENT
Cardiac monitor defibrillator
Electrocardiograph (ECG) electrodes
ECG cable
Strip-chart recorder
Strip-chart recording paper
Disposable defibrillation electrodes or hard paddles
Defibrillation gel or pads (if paddles are used)

PATIENT PREPARATION
1. Remove the patient from wet or metallic surfaces.
2. If possible, quickly obtain a hard copy of the preshock rhythm.

PROCEDURAL STEPS
1. Identify the ventricular fibrillation or the pulseless ventricular tachycardia through a three-lead ECG monitoring system (lead I, II, or III), through the hard paddles ("quick look"), or through the disposable defibrillation electrodes.
2. Turn on the defibrillator, making sure the synchronized selection is off.
3. Select an energy level. The first defibrillation is performed with 200 joules *or a clinically equivalent biphasic shock*, many defibrillators are preset at 200 joules.
4. Charge the defibrillator.
5. Ensure the proper placement of the paddles or the defibrillation electrodes on the chest (Figure 84-2).

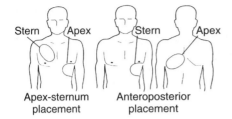

FIGURE 84-2 Placement options for defibrillation paddles or electrodes; apex-sternum or antero-posterior placement may be used. (Courtesy Medtronic Physio-Control Corporation, Redmond, WA.)

Paddles: Apply the conductive gel on the hard paddles, rubbing the paddles together to spread the gel over the surfaces of both paddles. Ensure the proper paddle placement and exert 25-30 pounds of pressure on each paddle. The goal is to ensure the maximal contact between the chest wall and the paddle. Be sure that there is no path of gel between the paddles; otherwise, an energy arc may occur.

Defibrillation electrodes: Disposable defibrillation electrodes are manufactured with a gel coating. The AHA (2000) recommends placing the anterior electrode to the right of the upper sternal border below the clavicle, and the apex electrode to the left of the nipple line with the center of the electrode in the midaxillary line. The anteroposterior placement is also acceptable for defibrillation, but this may take more time, because the patient must be turned for placement of the posterior electrode. The anterior electrode is placed over the precordium, and the posterior electrode is placed behind the heart at the left scapular line at the inferior angle of the scapula. Ensure proper placement for an adequate adherence to the chest wall.

6. State "Clear" loudly, and visually assess that all personnel have no direct or indirect contact with the patient.
7. Deliver a countershock by depressing both discharge buttons simultaneously, or, in the case of disposable electrodes, press the "SHOCK" button on the device.
8. Observe the postshock rhythm. If the ventricular fibrillation or the pulseless ventricular tachycardia persists, immediately deliver another shock at 200-300 joules *or a clinically equivalent biphasic shock.* Deliver a third shock at 360 joules *or a clinically equivalent biphasic shock* if the second shock is unsuccessful and proceed with advanced cardiac life-support recommendations. If an organized rhythm results from the defibrillation, check the pulse and obtain a hard copy of the postshock rhythm.

AGE-SPECIFIC CONSIDERATIONS

1. Ventricular fibrillation is rare in infants and children, but it can occur as a result of respiratory arrest. Two joules per kilogram is the initial energy delivered to defibrillate, and the strength should be doubled for repeated shocks (AHA, 2000). The AHA (2000) states that biphasic energy settings should be the same as for monophasic defibrillators. There are inadequate data to recommend effective lower doses.
2. For infants and children who weigh more than 10 kg, the AHA recommends using adult electrodes or paddles because the smaller pediatric electrodes increase transthoracic impedance (AHA, 2000).

3. In children and infants, regardless of the paddle size, the paddles must not touch each other (AHA, 2000).
4. If hard paddles are used, enough pressure should be applied to the paddles so that complete contact with the chest wall is ensured.
5. Neonatal and pediatric patients may be propped on their side and an antero-posterior paddle placement may be used (AHA, 2000). This may be most helpful if only adult paddles or disposable electrodes are available.

COMPLICATIONS

1. Skin irritation, redness, or burns may result if an inadequate conductive medium is used or if there are multiple countershocks.
2. Arcing of the current may occur if the defibrillation gel is spread across the chest wall.
3. A current literature search does not yield any references to bystander death due to contact with a patient being defibrillated. There have been documented cases of harm requiring hospitalization.

REFERENCES

American Heart Association (AHA). (2000). Guidelines 2000 for cardiopulmonary resuscitation and emergency cardiovascular care. *Circulation, 102* (suppl. I).
Danzl, D.F. (2002). Accidental hypothermia (pp. 1979-1996). In Marx, J.A., Hockberger, R.S., Walls, R.M., et al. (Eds.). *Rosen's emergency medicine: concepts and clinical practice*, 5th ed. St. Louis: Mosby.
Dell'Orfano, J.T., & Naccarelli, G.V. (2001). Update on external cardioversion and defibrillation. *Current Opinion in Cardiology, 16,* 54-57.
Jain, V.C., & Wheelan, K. (2002). Successful cardioversion of atrial fibrillation using 360-joules biphasic shock. *American Journal of Cardiology, 90,* 331-332.

PROCEDURE 85

Synchronized Cardioversion

Mike D. McMahon, RN, BSN

Synchronized cardioversion is also known as cardioversion, direct-current synchronized countershock, and electrical synchronized countershock therapy. The goal of synchronized cardioversion is to deliver a defibrillation shock outside the relative refractory period of the electrocardiogram (ECG) cycle (Barnason, 2003), protecting the patient from going into ventricular fibrillation.

Cardioversion may be performed with either a monophasic or a biphasic waveform (see Procedure 84). The cardioversion energies given below are all monophasic. If the defibrillator is a biphasic unit, use the clinically equivalent energy dose as provided by the manufacturer. Jain and Wheelan (2002) presented three case studies in which 360 joules of biphasic energy were used without adverse effects.

INDICATIONS

1. To terminate ventricular tachyarrhythmias in a patient who has a pulse. Patients who are *stable* are given oxygen and antiarrhythmic medications as the first line of treatment. Synchronized cardioversion is used if these methods fail (American Heart Association [AHA], 2000). Patients who are unstable with signs and symptoms related to tachycardia, including chest pain, dyspnea, decreased level of consciousness, low blood pressure (less than 90 mm Hg systolic), pulmonary congestion, congestive heart failure, ischemia, or infarction, are prepared for immediate synchronized cardioversion if the ventricular rate is greater than 150 beats/min. A brief trial of antiarrhythmic medications is sometimes used during setup for the cardioversion. When the ventricular rate is less than 150 beats/min, synchronized cardioversion is used after failed trials of medications according to advanced cardiac life support guidelines. Wide-complex tachycardias of uncertain type may be treated in similar fashion.

2. In the stable patient with narrow-complex supraventricular tachycardia, cardioversion is used only if medication administration and vagal maneuvers fail to convert the rhythm to a normal sinus rhythm. Cardioversion is avoided in patients with known histories of impaired cardiac function (ejection fraction <40%) (AHA, 2000).

3. To terminate atrial fibrillation and atrial flutter. Synchronized cardioversion is used as a first-line therapy for atrial rhythms with a rapid ventricular response (>100 beats/min) accompanied by clinical distress (AHA, 2000). See cautions for patients who have had atrial fibrillation and atrial flutter for longer than 48 hours.

CONTRAINDICATIONS AND CAUTIONS

1. Airway protection may be necessary, especially when the patient is sedated. Intubation equipment and materials must be readily available.

2. The hemodynamic status must be monitored continuously. A sudden deterioration may warrant rapid synchronized cardioversion or an unsynchronized countershock.

3. Premedication with sedative and analgesic medications is warranted if the patient's condition permits.

4. Remove any nitroglycerin ointment or patches from the chest because they may allow an inappropriate path for the current.

5. If possible, digoxin should be withheld on the day of treatment with synchronized cardioversion because digoxin levels in the toxic range increase the risk of ventricular tachycardia and ventricular fibrillation after cardioversion. Patients receiving a maintenance dose of digoxin therapy can be safely treated with cardioversion (Bolton, 2000).

6. If the patient is stable, electrolyte imbalances should be corrected before synchronized cardioversion is administered. Hypokalemia can predispose patients to postshock dysrhythmias after cardioversion (Hambach, 2001).

7. Cardioversion is not used in the treatment of atrial fibrillation and atrial flutter in a patient with underlying valvular disease or chamber enlargement, or those patients with onset of the dysrhythmia longer than 72 hours because there is a risk of embolization of a mural thrombus (Yealy & Delbridge, 2002). Rate control through medication is the best initial treatment.
8. If the patient's condition permits, intravenous access should be established before this procedure (see Procedure 63).
9. Paddle or electrode placement must be modified if the patient has a permanent pacemaker or an implanted cardioverter defibrillator (ICD). Place the paddles or electrodes at least 5 cm from the implanted device. The internal ICD electrodes may cover a section of the epicardium and interfere with the current flow to the heart. If shocks delivered up to 360 J or clinically equivalent biphasic shocks fail to convert the rhythm, change the paddle or electrode placement to alternative sites (anteroposterior or axillary-axillary).

EQUIPMENT

Cardiac monitor/defibrillator with synchronization capability
ECG electrodes and cable
Strip chart recorder and paper
Disposable defibrillation electrodes or hard paddles
Defibrillation gel or pads
Supplies and equipment for resuscitation (i.e., a crash cart)

PATIENT PREPARATION

1. When the patient's condition permits, a standard 12-lead ECG should be obtained (see Procedure 59). If this is not possible, obtain a hard-copy rhythm strip. Allow the patient access to the bathroom to empty his/her bladder. Remove dentures to prevent them from obstructing the patient's airway (Barnason, 2003).
2. Administer sedation, analgesia, or both as prescribed (Barnason, 2003).
3. Verify that informed consent has been obtained (not applicable in emergency situations).
4. Remove the patient from any wet or a metallic surfaces.

PROCEDURAL STEPS

1. Turn on the monitor/defibrillator.
2. Attach the monitor leads and ensure the proper display of the patient's rhythm.
3. Depress the SYNC button to activate the synchronized mode. Note that the default setting in some defibrillators can be set to the synchronized mode after each attempt. Other machines need to be reset to deliver a subsequent synchronized countershock.
4. Look for markers on the QRS complex that indicate that the defibrillator is in the SYNC mode (Figure 85-1).
5. Adjust the R-wave gain on the monitor to ensure that SYNC markers occur on each QRS complex.
6. Select an energy level of 100 J or a clinically equivalent biphasic level as prescribed.
7. Position the electrodes or paddles on the patient (Figure 85-2).

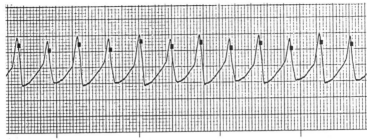

FIGURE 85-1 Appropriate SYNC marker placement on the QRS complex. (Courtesy Medtronic Physio-Control Corporation, Redmond, WA.)

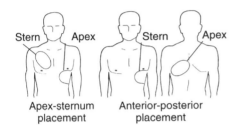

Apex-sternum   Anterior-posterior
placement   placement

FIGURE 85-2 Placement options for paddles or electrodes; apex-sternum or anteroposterior placement may be used. (Courtesy of Medtronic Physio-Control Corporation, Redmond, WA.)

Paddles: Apply a conductive gel on the hard paddles and rub the paddles together to spread the gel over the surfaces of both paddles. Make sure that the paddles are placed correctly and that each paddle is receiving 25-30 lb of pressure. The goal is to ensure the maximal contact between the chest wall and the paddle. Be sure that there is no path of gel between the paddles; otherwise, an energy arc may occur.

Defibrillation electrodes: Disposable defibrillation electrodes are pregelled. The AHA (2000) recommends placing the anterior electrode to the right of the upper third of the sternum below the clavicle and the apex electrode to the left of the nipple line below the axilla. An anteroposterior placement is also acceptable. The anterior electrode is placed over the precordium, and the posterior electrode is placed behind the heart at the left scapular line at the inferior angle of the scapula. Ensure the proper placement for adequate adherence to the chest wall.

8. Charge the defibrillator and state "Clear" loudly. Visually confirm that no personnel have direct or indirect contact with the patient.
9. Deliver a countershock by depressing the discharge button until the energy is delivered. When using paddles, depress both of the discharge buttons simultaneously and hold them down until discharge occurs; this may take several milliseconds.
10. Check the monitor. If a dysrhythmia persists, increase the energy level to 200 J or a *clinically equivalent biphasic level* and deliver another shock. A third shock at 300 J or a *clinically equivalent biphasic level* and a fourth shock at 360 J or a *clinically equivalent biphasic level* are recommended if the rhythm does not convert (AHA, 2000). Remember to check that the

SYNC mode is active after each attempt. Some defibrillators can be set to remain in SYNC mode after each discharge. If cardioversion is successful, record the vital signs, obtain a hard copy of the postshock rhythm, and repeat the 12-lead ECG.

11. If the patient has an implanted pacemaker or ICD, the device should be interrogated after the cardioversion to verify functionality (Fuster & Ryden, 2001).

AGE-SPECIFIC CONSIDERATIONS

1. The pediatric patient with a tachydysrhythmia may present with a history of poor feeding, tachypnea, pallor, and lethargy (Corrall, 2000).

2. For pediatric patients, the initial energy level is 0.5-1.0 J/kg; the dose is doubled for subsequent shocks. The AHA (2000) states that biphasic energy settings should be the same as for monophasic defibrillators. There are inadequate data to recommend effective lower doses.

3. Paroxysmal supraventricular tachycardia is the most common rapid rate dysrhythmia seen in children. Ventricular tachycardia and atrial fibrillation and flutter occur infrequently in children and are usually related to congenital or rheumatic heart disease or to dilated cardiomyopathy (Corrall, 2000).

4. If vascular access is available, consider treating the pediatric patient with unstable supraventricular tachycardia first with adenosine before cardioversion (Primm & Reamy, 2002).

5. For infants and children who weigh more than 10 kg, the AHA recommends using adult electrodes or paddles because the smaller pediatric electrodes increase transthoracic impedance (AHA, 2000).

6. In children and infants, regardless of the paddle size, the paddles must not touch each other (AHA, 2000).

7. If you are using hard paddles for a pediatric patient, apply enough pressure to the paddles so there is complete contact with the chest wall.

8. Neonatal and pediatric patients may be propped on their side and an anteroposterior paddle placement may be used (AHA, 2000). This may be helpful if only adult paddles or disposable electrodes are available.

COMPLICATIONS

1. Inappropriate sensing of the QRS complex may result in improper timing of the discharge of the current. This may result in ventricular tachycardia or fibrillation, especially if the current is delivered while superimposed on a T wave. An unsynchronized countershock at 200 J or a clinically equivalent biphasic shock should be given immediately if ventricular fibrillation occurs. If this is needed, make sure that the SYNC function is turned off or there will be a delay in delivering the defibrillation shock.

2. Burns may occur if the conductive medium is insufficient or excessive. Proper pressure applied to the paddles and proper positioning decrease this risk. The risk of burns increases with multiple shocks.

3. A pulmonary embolus is a rare complication that usually occurs in a patient who has been in chronic atrial fibrillation. This risk can be minimized with anticoagulant therapy administered before cardioversion.

4. Embolic cerebrovascular events occur rarely as a result of cardioversion, but they are also a risk in conditions for which synchronized cardioversion is undertaken, especially if the atrial wall motion is compromised.

5. A current literature search does not yield any references to bystander death due to contact with a patient being defibrillated. Gibbs et al. (1990) have documented cases of harm requiring hospitalization.
6. Muscle soreness may be experienced by some patients.
7. Transient elevations in creatine phosphokinase (CPK) and lactate dehydrogenase may be noted, but more specific cardiac markers, such as CPK-MB and troponin, are rarely abnormal (Bolton, 2000).
8. Transient ST-segment elevation may be noted after cardioversion. These changes typically resolve within less than 5 minutes (Bolton, 2000).

PATIENT TEACHING

1. The procedure should be explained as the delivery of a small electrical impulse to the heart. Patients need to be aware of the possibility that multiple attempts may have to be made.
2. Patients should be informed that this procedure is performed while they are awake (unless general anesthesia is used) but that sedation with medication produces a relaxed and usually drowsy state.
3. Patients do want to know how the shock feels. Some patients report a brief, very sharp pain. The sedative usually erases the memory of this pain.
4. Aftereffects may include redness of the skin and minimal soreness of the chest wall.
5. Patients who are discharged from the emergency department should be instructed to seek emergency care promptly if they experience chest pain, shortness of breath, lower-extremity swelling, dizziness, weakness, or changes in vision or speech.

REFERENCES

American Heart Association (AHA). (2000). Guidelines 2000 for cardiopulmonary resuscitation and emergency cardiovascular care. *Circulation, 102* (suppl I).

Barnason, S. (2003). Cardiovascular emergencies (pp. 450-604). In Newberry, L. (Ed.). *Sheehy's emergency nursing,* 5th ed. St. Louis: Mosby

Bolton, E. (2000). Disturbances of cardiac rhythm and conduction (pp. 169-193). In Tintinalli, J.E., Kelen G.D., & Stapszynski, J.S. (Eds.). *Emergency medicine.* New York: McGraw-Hill.

Corrall, C.J. (2000). Pediatric heart disease (pp. 774-786). In Tintinalli, J.E., Kelen, G.D., & Stapszynski, J.S. (Eds.). *Emergency medicine.* New York: McGraw-Hill.

Fuster, V., & Ryden, L.E., Asinger, R.W., et al. (2001). ACC/AHA/ESC Guidelines for the management of patients with atrial fibrillation: executive summary. *Journal of the American College of Cardiology, 38,* 1231-1265.

Gibbs, W., Eisenberg, M., & Damon, S.K. (1990). Dangers of defibrillation: injuries to emergency personnel during patient resuscitation. *American Journal of Emergency Medicine, 8,* 101-104.

Hambach, C. (2001). Cardioversion (pp. 211-218). In Lynn-McHale, D.J., & Carlson, K.K. (Eds.), *AACN procedure manual for critical care,* 4th ed. Philadelphia: W.B. Saunders.

Jain, V.C., & Wheelan, K. (2002). Successful cardioversion of atrial fibrillation using 360-joules biphasic shock. *The American Journal of Cardiology, 90,* 331-332.

Primm, P.A. & Reamy, R.R. (2002). Cardiopulmonary resuscitation (pp. 18-27). In Strange, G.R., Ahrens, W., Lelyvled, S., et al. (Eds.). *Pediatric emergency medicine: A comprehensive guide.* New York: McGraw-Hill.

Yealy, D.M., & Delbridge, T.R. (2002). Dysrhythmias (pp. 1053-1098). In Marx, J.A. Hockberger, R.S., Walls, R.M., et al. (Eds.). *Rosen's emergency medicine: concepts and clinical practice,* 5th ed. St. Louis. Mosby.

Automated External Defibrillator Operation

Mike D. McMahon, RN, BSN

INDICATION

Automated external defibrillators (AEDs) are for use on patients who are in cardiac arrest. They differ from manual defibrillators in that the decision to deliver shock is made by the device, not the user, thus allowing a minimally trained individual to treat a sudden cardiac arrest. The AHA (2000) has set a high-priority goal to increase the survivability of sudden cardiac arrest by recommending that the first shock be delivered within 5 minutes of activation of emergency medical service. Further, it is a class I recommendation that hospitals be able to provide defibrillation within 3 minutes from time of collapse. AEDs are now present in many public locations and on most airplanes.

CONTRAINDICATIONS AND CAUTIONS

1. Most AEDs are for use in patients who are older than 8 years of age or greater than 25 kg. See Age-Specific Considerations for exceptions.
2. AEDs are designed for use in patients who are in cardiac arrest. The device is not to be placed on a patient who is conscious or has a pulse or respirations. AEDs cannot differentiate from a cardiac rhythm that is generating a pulse from one that is not. One exception is the use of an AED by a health care professional to monitor a patient's cardiac rhythm when no other monitor is available (e.g., on an airplane).
3. The defibrillation pads should be placed in the same positions as for manual defibrillation (see Procedure 84). The anterior electrode should be placed to the right of the upper sternal border below the clavicle, and the apex electrode to the left of the nipple line with the center of the electrode in the midaxillary region. The device's algorithms for determining shockability are based on these positions.
4. Some AEDs are fully automatic and do not have a "SHOCK" button. These devices deliver defibrillation energy to the patient without the user's pressing any buttons. Make sure that no one is touching the patient while the device is preparing to delivery energy.

EQUIPMENT

AED (Figure 86-1)
Disposable defibrillation electrodes

PATIENT PREPARATION

1. Remove the patient from any standing water, and expose and dry the chest.

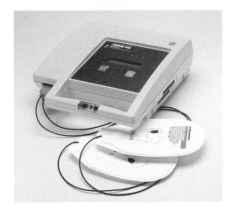

FIGURE 86-1 LIFEPAK 500. (Courtesy Medtronic Physio-Control, Redmond, WA.)

2. Remove any transdermal patches from areas where the defibrillation electrodes are to be attached.

PROCEDURAL STEPS

The AHA (2000) recommends the following steps for the operation of an AED:
1. Power on the AED.
2. Attach electrode pads to the patient in the standard apex-sternum locations. If the patient has an implanted pacemaker or an automatic implantable cardioverter-defibrillator, place the electrodes at least 1 inch away from the device (AHA, 2000).
3. Analyze the rhythm.
4. Clear the victim and press the SHOCK button (if advised).
5. After three shocks or after any "no shock advised" message, check for signs of circulation.
6. If no signs of circulation are present, perform cardiopulmonary resuscitation for 1 minute.
7. Press Analyze and repeat three shocks if needed.

Currently, multiple AEDs are available. Devices range from those with three-button function (Power, Analyze, Shock) to those that are always on and deliver energy without user intervention. Most devices also allow the user to customize functions of the defibrillator to meet local requirements. Users may be able set a range of energy to be delivered, change the time between series of shocks, and choose what, if any, verbal commands will be delivered by the device. Some devices can be used in AED mode only, and others allow the user to override the automated function and manually deliver a shock for defibrillation. For specific details, see the manufacturer's operating instructions for each device.

AGE-SPECIFIC CONSIDERATION

Currently, Medtronic Physio-Control and Philips Medical Systems (Figure 86-2) have AEDs that are cleared by the US Food and Drug Administration for use in the pediatric (<8 years of age) population. These devices use specially designed electrodes that reduce the defibrillation energy delivered by the AED to the

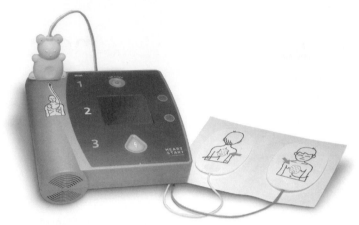

FIGURE 86-2 Heartstream FR2 with pediatric use electrodes. (Courtesy Philips Electronics)

patient by approximately one third the set charge. Because the AED delivers a full charge, pediatric electrodes used for manual defibrillation should not be used on the pediatric patient.

COMPLICATIONS

1. Skin irritation, redness, or burns may result if the defibrillation pads are not completely adhered to the patient's chest or if there are multiple counter-shocks.
2. A current literature search does not yield any references to bystander death due to contact with a patient being defibrillated. There have been documented cases of harm requiring hospitalization (Gibbs et al., 1990).
3. Using pediatric AED electrodes on an adult patient may prevent successful defibrillation because of the reduced energy that is delivered. Conversely, using anything but the specially designed AED pediatric electrodes on the pediatric patient will deliver full energy to the patient.
4. AEDs cannot differentiate between pulsed and pulseless cardiac rhythms. This can lead to defibrillation of a patient who is awake.

REFERENCES

American Heart Association (AHA). (2000). Guidelines 2000 for cardiopulmonary resuscitation and emergency cardiovascular care. *Circulation, 102* (suppl. I).

Gibbs, W., Eisenberg, M., & Damon, S.K. (1990). Danger of defibrillation: Injuries to emergency personnel during patient resuscitation. *American Journal of Emergency Medicine, 8,* 101-104.

Emergency Management of the Patient With an Automatic Implantable Cardiac Defibrillator

Mike D. McMahon, RN, BSN

Automatic implantable cardiac defibrillators (AICDs) have become more prevalent in the patient population. First brought into service into 1980, now more than 50,000 units are implanted each year. These devices have become a standard of care for patients who are at high risk for sudden cardiac arrest and sustained ventricular tachycardia (Hayes & Zipes, 2001). The currently available devices (dual chamber) combine the functions of an internal defibrillator and that of an implanted pacemaker. Additional models are being developed for the treatment of tachycardiac rhythms originating in the atrium (Gold, 2000). The patient or family usually carries information about the specific device that is in place.

The devices are connected to cardiac lead wires and continually monitor the electrocardiogram (ECG) cycle. Because the defibrillation leads are in direct contact with the myocardium, lower energy levels are necessary. AICDs can be set to deliver up to 40 J of biphasic energy should the patient go into ventricular fibrillation, but most patients need only 15-20 J to restore the heart rhythm to normal sinus. These devices are also capable of delivering lower energy for cardioversion and antitachycardic pacing (Bessman, 2000).

INDICATIONS

Patients who have AICDs may present to the emergency department under the following circumstances:

1. After cardiac arrest with successful defibrillation by the device. Treat patients who have had a cardiac arrest and undergone successful resuscitation the same as any other arrest patient. The cardiology department should be notified so that the AICD event can be downloaded. If the patient is conscious, information about the number of shocks delivered, any symptoms preceding the defibrillation, and the patient's activity around the event should be elicited (Bessman, 2000).

2. In cardiac arrest with the device having properly functioned, but with the heart rhythm unable to be converted to a perfusing rhythm. If the patient arrives in cardiac arrest, external defibrillation may be required if the AICD has stopped its defibrillation function. AICDs shut down the defibrillation function after a set number of defibrillations on the basis of a preprogrammed algorithm. Place the defibrillation pads or electrodes at least 2

inches away from the implanted device. The epicardial patches used in the older AICD may protect the heart from external defibrillation, and alternate (anteroposterior) positions may be needed (Wood et al., 2000). Most current models use transvenous electrodes, eliminating the need for epicardial patches (Niemann, 2002).

3. Successful and unsuccessful correction of tachycardic rhythms. The underlying tachycardic rate may fall out of the range that the AICD is programmed to respond to.

4. Inadvertent firing of the defibrillator. This can be related to external stimuli, such as poorly grounded electrical equipment (Sabaté et al., 2001). Gold (2000) has found that chest wall muscle movement, such as hand gripping, Valsalva maneuver, and deep breaths, can cause the AICD to discharge.

5. In the emergency department for another problem not related to the AICD, but undergoing procedures that may damage or disrupt the device.

CONTRAINDICATIONS AND CAUTIONS

1. Strong magnetic fields, such as from magnetic resonance imaging, cause the AICD to not respond in the event that the patient has a rhythm of ventricular fibrillation or ventricular tachycardia.

2. Electrocautery devices can damage the AICD. Make sure that everyone is aware of the patient's implanted device.

3. The epicardial pads used by the AICD can shield the heart, making external defibrillation more difficult. Higher external defibrillation energy or alternate pad/paddle placement may be needed to convert the patient's heart rhythm.

4. The AICD may need to be deactivated in the postresuscitation period. This is to prevent discharge due to recurrent ventricular dysrhythmias caused by metabolic changes during the arrest (Niemann, 2002).

EQUIPMENT

ECG monitor
12-lead ECG
Doughnut (round)–shaped magnet
External cardiac defibrillator

PROCEDURAL STEPS
Deactivating the AICD

Placing a doughnut-shaped magnet on top of the pulse generator can inhibit the defibrillation component of most AICDs. Second-generation devices require that the magnet be placed on the generator for 30 seconds, and then the magnet can be removed. Third-generation devices require that the magnet remain on the device for the entire time that the defibrillation function is stopped (Bessman, 2000). The underlying pacemaker functions in the AICD are not affected by the magnet (Martin et al., 2001).

1. To deactivate the AICD, place a doughnut-shaped magnet over the AICD pulse generator.

2. The magnet will stop the device from delivering defibrillation energy, but it will not stop the pacemaker function of the device.

3. After the magnet is removed, 12-lead electrocardiography should be performed to record the current state of the device.
4. All patients require follow-up with their cardiologist to check out the functions of the device.

COMPLICATIONS

With the defibrillation function turned off, no defibrillation shocks will be delivered if the patient goes into ventricular fibrillation or tachycardia. An external monitor/defibrillation should always be present when this procedure is performed.

PATIENT TEACHING

Patients may have questions about devices that they should avoid or use caution around. The following list is condensed from websites created by Medtronic, St. Jude Medical, and Guidant (2002). The patient should be directed to contact the cardiologist for any concerns they may have regarding their AICD.

Medical Equipment

Most medical equipment is safe for use around patients who have an AICD. This includes most diagnostic x-ray equipment, including fluoroscope, dental and chest x-ray machines, computed tomographic scans, mammographs, and ultrasonic dental cleaners.

The following procedures should be avoided until the patient's cardiologist has been consulted:
- Magnetic resonance imaging
- Electrical nerve and muscle stimulators (transcutaneous electrical nerve stimulation units)
- Diathermy
- Electrocautery
- Lithotripsy, if the AICD is in the treatment field

General Household and Office Items
- Any household item in good repair is safe to use. The items should have three prongs or polarized prongs (i.e., one prong is larger than the other).
- Do not put magnets or products containing magnets close to the AICD.
- Avoid bringing power tools like drills or saws close to the chest area.
- When working with tools or appliances, be careful in situations in which you could be injured if you become dizzy or receive a therapeutic shock from your ICD.

Security Systems
- Walk through the screening areas at a normal pace and do not linger in these areas.
- If you are being searched with a hand wand, ask the screener to avoid the AICD.
- If dizziness or weakness occurs, move away from the screening devices.

Industrial Areas

- Large industrial equipment, such as generators, electric motors, and arc welders, often generate strong electromagnetic fields that can interfere with an AICD.
- Make sure that the equipment is properly grounded before working near it.

REFERENCES

Bessman, E.S. (2000). Invasive monitoring, pacing techniques, and automatic and implantable defibrillators (pp. 111-118). In Tintinalli, J.E., Kelen, G.D., & Stapszynski, J.S. (Eds.), *Emergency medicine*. New York: McGraw-Hill.

Gold, M.R. (2000). ICD therapy in the new millennium. *Cardiology Clinics, 18*(2), 375-387.

Guidant. Available at *http://www.guidant.com/products/AICD.shtml*.

Hayes, D.L., & Zipes, D.P. (2001). Cardiac pacemakers and cardioverter-defibrillators (pp. 775-814). In Braunwald, E., Zipes, D.P., & Libby, P. (Eds.), *Heart disease*, 6th ed. Philadelphia: W.B. Saunders Company.

Martin, C.M., Morton, P.G., & Nace, M.A. (2001). Implantable cardioverter-defibrillator (pp. 257-263). In Lynn-McHale, D.J. & Carlson, K.K. (Eds.), *AACN procedure manual for critical care*, 4th ed. Philadelphia: W.B. Saunders Company.

Medtronic. http://www.medtronic.com/patients/heart.html.

Niemann, J.T. (2002). Implantable cardiac devices (pp. 1099-1110). In Marx, J.A., Hockberger, R.S., Walls, R.M., et al. (Eds.), *Rosen's emergency medicine: concepts and clinical practice*, 5th ed. St. Louis: Mosby.

Sabaté, X., Moure, C., Nicolás, J., Sed, M., & Navarro, X. (2001). Washing machine associated 50 Hz detected as ventricular fibrillation by an implanted cardioverter defibrillator. *Journal of Pacing and Clinical Electrophysiology, 24*(8), 1281-1283.

St. Jude Medical. Available at *http://www.stjudemedical.com/4.0/4.3/4.3.shtm*.

Wood, M.A., Belz, M.K., & Ellenbogen, K.A. (2000). Cardiac pacemakers and implantable defibrillators in the intensive care unit setting (pp. 1061-1070). In Shoemaker, W.C., Ayres, S.M., Grenvik, A., & Holbrook, P.R. (Eds.), *Textbook of critical care*, 4th ed. Philadelphia: W.B. Saunders.

Cardiac Pacing

Transcutaneous Cardiac Pacing

Mike D. McMahon, RN, BSN

Transcutaneous cardiac pacing is also known as TCP, noninvasive cardiac pacing, external cardiac pacing, precordial cardiac pacing, temporary pacing, or external transthoracic pacing.

INDICATIONS
1. To provide emergency pacing in patients with hemodynamically unstable bradycardias.
   a. Signs and symptoms of hemodynamic instability include systolic blood pressure lower than 80 mm Hg, altered mental status, angina, acute myocardial infarction, chest pain, shortness of breath, congestive heart failure, and pulmonary edema (American Heart Association [AHA], 2000).
   b. Simultaneous initiation of TCP and pharmacologic therapy may stabilize the patient more rapidly.
   c. TCP may be used as a prophylactic treatment in patients who have a high risk of atrioventricular block (Bessman, 2000).
2. To provide emergency cardiac stimulation in patients who have bradyasystolic cardiac arrest.
   a. TCP is a class IIb intervention (acceptable, possibly helpful) for asystole, but it must be performed early to have any chance at success (AHA, 2000).
   b. TCP is most effective in patients who have a normal myocardium and whose cardiac arrest is due to a drug overdose, electrolyte abnormalities, or acidosis.
3. To increase the heart rate in patients with a myocardial infarction who may present with bradycardia-dependent life-threatening ventricular rhythms (Hollander, 2000).
4. To provide overdrive pacing in patients who have supraventricular and ventricular tachycardias that are resistant to pharmacologic therapy or electrical cardioversion.
   a. TCP is a class IIa intervention for overdrive pacing of tachycardias refractory to drug therapy or electrical cardioversion (AHA, 2000).
5. To provide temporary pacing to patients when transvenous pacing is contraindicated, for instance, in patients who have sepsis, immunosuppression, or severe vascular disease, as well as those who have undergone or will undergo transplantation (Paschall & McErlean, 2001).

CONTRAINDICATIONS AND CAUTIONS
1. Misinterpreting a fine ventricular fibrillation as asystole may lead to inappropriate pacing when defibrillation is indicated.

2. TCP is contraindicated in severe hypothermia because the bradycardia may be physiologic as a result of a decreased metabolic rate (AHA, 2000).
3. TCP is relatively contraindicated in bradyasystolic arrest that lasts longer than 20 minutes because the chance of success is low.
4. Check the manufacturer's guidelines regarding the length of time the pacing electrodes may be used for continuous pacing.

EQUIPMENT

Transcutaneous pacemaker with monitor
Multifunction cable or pacing cable
Pacing electrodes
Electrocardiogram (ECG) cable
ECG electrodes
Monitor recorder paper
Advanced life support equipment
Sedatives or analgesics as indicated

PATIENT PREPARATION

1. A simple explanation of the purpose and procedure for TCP should be given to the conscious patient. A description of the sensations, including discomfort, that are associated with TCP, and the sedation and analgesia options may be discussed. The sensation at low-current levels has been described as a superficial tingling and at high current levels as a deep thumping. The patient may require continuous reassurance during the procedure.
2. Administer sedatives or analgesics as indicated and prescribed.
3. Place the ECG electrodes on clean, dry skin. Lead II gives a clearer picture of the pacing artifact (see Procedure 58). The ECG cable must be connected for the pacemaker to operate in the demand mode.
4. Obtain a hard-copy strip of the baseline rhythm along with vital signs.

PROCEDURAL STEPS

1. Following the manufacturer's recommendations, attach the multifunction or pacing electrodes in either the anterior-anterior (sternum-apex) position (Figure 88-1) or the anteroposterior position (Figure 88-2). The skin should be clean and dry. Remove lotions and ointments with soap and water and dry the skin completely afterward. No other cleaning agents should be used. Excessive hair should be clipped rather than shaved. Shaving causes microabrasions and increases the likelihood of skin burns. The electrodes should not be placed over wires, drains, dressings, ECG electrodes, implanted cardioverters/defibrillators, pacemakers, or medication patches. Rolling the electrodes onto the skin decreases the amount of air trapped beneath and improves electrical conduction. Press firmly on the adhesive area around the periphery to increase adherence. Press gently on the gelled area to remove any trapped air and to ensure good skin coupling.
2. Select the pacing mode (demand or asynchronous). In some pacemakers, the mode is automatically "demand" if the ECG cable is attached. It switches to "asynchronous" when the ECG electrodes or cable is removed.
   a. Demand mode. The demand mode is used when the patient has an underlying rhythm. The pacemaker delivers a pacing stimulus only when the

patient's intrinsic heart rate falls below the preset rate. Correct sensing of the intrinsic R wave must be ensured. Some pacemakers mark each sensed R wave, whereas others flash a symbol each time an R wave is sensed. The sensitivity is increased by increasing the ECG gain until all intrinsic R waves are seen.

   b. Asynchronous mode. The asynchronous (fixed rate) mode should be used only in emergency situations when the patient has no underlying rhythm or when an ECG cannot be obtained (Zoll Medical Corporation, 2002). In this mode, the pacemaker disregards the patient's intrinsic rhythm and delivers a pacing stimulus at the preset rate. There is a risk that a lethal arrhythmia may be generated if the pacing energy occurs during the vulnerable period of ventricular repolarization (Bessman, 2000).

3. Select the pacing rate. The rate range is typically 60-100 beats/min.

4. Set the output (mA) on zero and turn the pacemaker on.

   a. For a patient in a comprised hemodynamic state, but not in arrest, determine the capture threshold and set the maintenance pacing output. Beginning at zero milliamperes (mA), increase the output until the electrical capture is seen. Electrical capture is evidenced by a wide QRS complex (>0.12 msec) and broad T wave following the pacing artifact (Figure 88-3). Capture thresh-

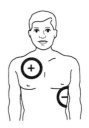

FIGURE 88-1 Anterior-anterior electrode placement. In female patients, position the negative electrode under the breast. (Modified from illustrations supplied by Medtronic Physio-Control Corporation, Redmond, WA.)

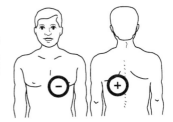

FIGURE 88-2 Anteroposterior electrode placement. In female patients, position the negative electrode under the breast. (Modified from illustrations supplied by Medtronic Physio-Control Corporation, Redmond, WA.)

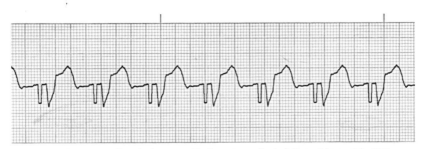

FIGURE 88-3 Electrical capture. Each pacing spike is followed by a wide QRS.

olds typically range from 40-80 mA. Maintenance pacing outputs should be set about 10% above the threshold (Zoll Medical Corporation, 2002).
  b. For patients without a pulse, the device should be set to maximum output when it is turned on (AHA, 2000). If capture of the heart rate is achieved at the maximum energy, the device should be turned down until loss of capture occurs, and then increased to 110% of capture energy.
5. Hypoxia, acidosis, pericardial effusion, and tamponade may lead to higher capture thresholds (Del Monte & Gamrath, 1996). The identification of electrical capture may be difficult in the presence of ECG signal distortion (Figure 88-4). An artifact increases in size as the current is increased. Positioning the ECG electrodes as far as possible from the pacing electrodes may reduce the signal distortion. Sometimes changing the lead being monitored minimizes the distortion (Del Monte & Gamrath, 1996).
6. Assess the patient for mechanical capture by palpating a pulse. A Doppler, a pulse oximeter, or both may also assist in identifying and confirming the mechanical capture (Del Monte & Gamrath, 1996).
7. Document the electrical capture with a rhythm strip indicating the pacemaker settings. Document the mechanical capture with vital signs.
8. Assess the patient's comfort level. Most patients have difficulty tolerating pacing currents above 50 mA. Sedation and analgesia should be used for conscious patients.
9. TCP is a bridge to a more definitive treatment. The patient should be prepared for the insertion of a transvenous pacemaker.

AGE-SPECIFIC CONSIDERATIONS

1. Severe bradycardias in children are usually the result of hypoxia and hypoventilation (Primm & Reamy, 2002). These issues should be addressed before pharmacologic agents or pacing is attempted.
2. Minimal heart rates indicating possible need for pacing are the following (Conway, 1997):
  a. Infant: less than 55 beats/min
  b. Child: less than 45-50 beats/min
  c. Adolescent: less than 40 beats/min

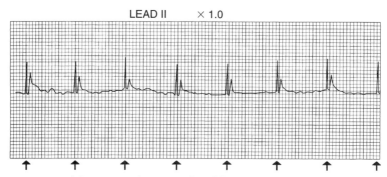

LEAD II   × 1.0

FIGURE 88-4 Signal distortion. Each pacing spike is followed by a signal-distortion artifact that must be distinguished from electrical capture. (From Del Monte, L., & Gamrath, B. [1996]. *Noninvasive pacing: what you should know,* 2nd ed. [p. 25]. Redmond, WA: Medtronic Physio-Control Corporation.)

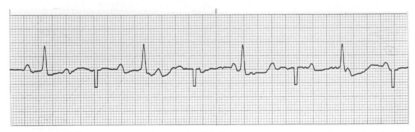

FIGURE 88-5   Failure to capture. Pacing stimuli fail to capture in a patient in complete heart block.

3. Consider using TCP in children who have primary bradycardia secondary to congenital defects or after heart surgery (AHA, 2000).
4. As with adults, discomfort during TCP is a major drawback to its use. Sedation and artificial ventilation should be considered.
5. Smaller sized pacing electrodes are available for patients who weigh <15 kg. (Zoll Medical Corporation, 2002). The smaller the pacing electrode, the higher the resistance. Therefore using a larger electrode is beneficial as long as the adherence is good and the electrodes do not touch.
6. Placement of pacing electrodes in the pediatric population does not differ from that in the adult population (Primm & Reamy, 2002). Be sure that the pacing electrodes do not touch; use of the smaller pacing electrodes or an anteroposterior position may be necessary to ensure this in infants and small children.
7. Pediatric patients are at a higher risk for skin breakdown when TCP is used for longer than 30 minutes. In newborns and infants, the area under the pads should be inspected regularly for signs of thermal damage to the skin (Zoll, Medical Corporation 2002).

COMPLICATIONS

1. Failure to capture is evidenced by pacer spikes that do not induce the wide QRS of an electrical capture (Figure 88-5). A capture threshold may change over time and should be determined frequently when the patient is dependent on a pacemaker (Del Monte & Gamrath, 1996).
2. Undersensing occurs when the pacemaker does not sense an intrinsic QRS and delivers a pacing spike. Failure to sense is recognized by competition between the pacing rhythm and the intrinsic rhythm and by a short interval between the native QRS and the pacing spike (Figure 88-6). If the pacer fails to recognize all the intrinsic QRS complexes, it operates as if it were in the asynchronous mode.
3. Oversensing is due to an inappropriate inhibition of the pacing by electrical signals from outside the heart (Figure 88-7). Extracardiac electrical signals include muscle artifact and electromagnetic signals in the environment. These may be corrected by decreasing the ECG size, which decreases the sensitivity to the native QRS. If the problem persists, it may be necessary to operate the pacemaker in the asynchronous mode to obtain reliable pacing (Del Monte & Gamrath, 1996).

▶ 20 : 49 01APR96   LEAD II   X0 . 2   DIAG   PACE RATE 70

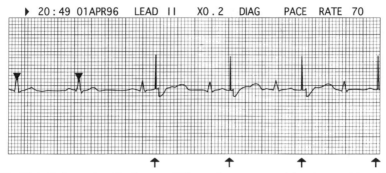

FIGURE 88-6 Undersensing. The first two QRS complexes are sensed, but the remaining QRS complexes are not of sufficient amplitude to be detected. The pacemaker fires even though the patient's intrinsic rate is greater than the set pace rate. (From Del Monte, L., & Gamrath, B. [1996]. *Noninvasive pacing: what you should know,* 2nd ed. [p. 29]. Redmond, WA: Medtronic Physio-Control Corporation.)

▶ 18 : 20   01 MAY 95 PACE @ 80,   45 MA LEAD II   X 1 . 0

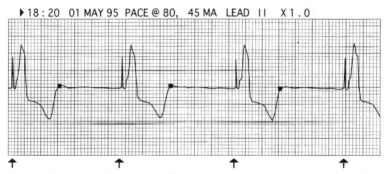

FIGURE 88-7 Oversensing. The set rate is 80, but the actual paced rate is 45. Note the sense marker on the T wave, which inappropriately inhibits the pacemaker. The next paced pulse is late, which disrupts the timing cycle of the pacemaker. (From Del Monte, L., & Gamrath, B. [1996]. *Noninvasive pacing: what you should know,* 2nd ed. [p. 29]. Redmond, WA: Medtronic Physio-Control Corporation.)

4. Loss of the ECG monitoring lead causes the pacing device to default to asynchronous mode. This can lead to pacing energy being delivered during the heart's vulnerable period.

PATIENT TEACHING

1. Report increasing discomfort related to the pacing impulses.
2. Touching the patient during TCP does not cause any harm. A small shock hazard does exist, and the pacing energy can be felt.
3. Some pacing devices continue to deliver pacing energy when the electrodes are removed from the patient. As in item 2, there is a shock hazard, but there is no risk of harm to the user.

REFERENCES

American Heart Association (AHA). (2000). *Textbook of advanced cardiac life support.* Dallas: Author.

Bessman, E.S. (2000). Invasive monitoring, pacing techniques, and automatic and implantable defibrillators (pp. 111-118). In Tintinalli, J.E., Kelen, G.D., & Stapszynski, J.S. (Eds.), *Emergency medicine*. New York: McGraw-Hill.

Conway, S.P. (1997). Pediatric pacemakers for patients with complete heart block. *Dimensions of Critical Care Nursing, 16* (1), 29-39.

Del Monte, L., & Gamrath, B. (1996). *Noninvasive pacing: what you should know*, 2nd ed. Redmond, WA: Physio-Control Corporation.

Hollander, J.E. (2000). Intervention strategies for acute coronary syndromes (pp. 366-374). In Tintinalli, J.E., Kelen, G.D., & Stapszynski, J.S. (Eds.), *Emergency medicine*. New York: McGraw-Hill.

Paschall, F.E., & McErlean, E.S. (2001). Temporary transcutaneous (external) pacing (pp. 271-277). In Lynn-McHale, D. J., & Carlson, K.K. (Eds.) *AACN procedure manual for critical care*, 4th ed. Philadelphia: W.B. Saunders.

Primm, P.R., & Reamy, R.R. (2002). Cardiopulmonary resuscitation (pp. 18-27). In Strange, G.R., Ahrens, W.R., Lelyveld, S., & Schafermeyer, R.W. (Eds.), *Pediatric emergency medicine*. New York: McGraw-Hill.

Zoll Medical Corporation. (2002). *Zoll M series operator's guide*. Burlington, MA: Author.

PROCEDURE 89

Temporary Transvenous Pacemaker Insertion

Patricia A. DeWitt, RN, MSN

INDICATIONS

1. To maintain an adequate heart rate in the presence of hemodynamically compromising bradycardias, including complete heart block, symptomatic second-degree block, symptomatic sick-sinus syndrome, drug-induced bradycardias, permanent pacemaker failure, temporary epicardial pacemaker failure, postoperative cardiac surgery, idioventricular bradycardias, symptomatic atrial fibrillation with slow ventricular response, refractory bradycardia during resuscitation of patients who are in hypovolemic shock, and bradyarrhythmias with malignant ventricular escape mechanisms (Becker, 2001)

2. To provide pacing readiness in an acute myocardial infarction. Dysrhythmias accompanying acute myocardial infarction include symptomatic bradycardia, complete heart block, new bundle branch block, and alternating bundle branch block (Becker, 2001).

3. To suppress or terminate supraventricular tachycardia or ventricular tachycardia that is refractory to pharmacologic therapy or electrical cardioversion
4. To diagnose dysrhythmias by simultaneous recording of surface electrocardiogram (ECG) and either atrial or ventricular electrograms or both (Hayes & Holmes, 1993)
5. To maintain temporary pacing in the setting of Lyme disease and myocarditis with high-degree atrioventricular (AV) block (Mitrani et al., 2001)
6. After radiofrequency ablation of the AV junction (Mitrani et al., 2001)
7. To provide a bridge to permanent pacing
8. To suppress bradycardia-induced ventricular dysrhythmias in patients with prolonged QT syndrome (Becker, 2001)
9. To treat chronotropic incompetence accompanying cardiogenic shock (Becker, 2001)
10. To manage of tachyarrhythmias with overdrive pacing (Mitrani et al., 2001)

CONTRAINDICATIONS AND CAUTIONS

1. Transcutaneous pacing is preferred in patients who have received or may receive thrombolytic therapy (AHA, 2003).
2. Asynchronous pacing is contraindicated in patients who have an intrinsic rhythm (Medtronic, 1996).
3. Overdriving ventricular tachycardias using high-rate burst pacing is contraindicated in the ventricle because it may result in life-threatening arrhythmias (Medtronic, 1996). In some temporary pacer models, a high rate of burst pacing can be achieved only in the asynchronous mode and may result in R-on T, leading to ventricular fibrillation.
4. Transvenous pacing is relatively contraindicated in a bradyasystolic arrest that lasts longer than 20 minutes because the chance of success is low (AHA, 2003).
5. Right-sided heart catheterization may induce transient right bundle branch block (Ellenbogen & Wood, 2001).
6. Electrical safety precautions include the following:
   a. Properly grounded hospital equipment
   b. Insulated metal parts on the generator or pacing catheter
   c. Rubber gloves for handling the exposed terminal wires
   d. Not touching the electronic equipment and the patient or the pacing system simultaneously
   e. Adaptors for shrouded electrode pins to articulate with older model pacemakers.
7. Pacing the severely hypothermic patient who is bradycardic may precipitate fibrillation secondary to irritation. Bradycardia may be physiologic in these patients because of decreased metabolic demand. The hypothermic ventricle, once fibrillating, is resistant to defibrillation (AHA, 2003).

EQUIPMENT

Percutaneous sheath introducer kit (jugular, subclavian, or femoral insertion site; a 6-French introducer can accommodate a 5-French bipolar balloon-tipped catheter)
Cutdown tray (brachial insertion site only)
Sterile towels and drapes

Sterile gowns, gloves, masks, and caps for everyone at the bedside (recommended)

Temporary pacemaker generator (single or dual chamber)

Extension cables

9-volt battery

Pacing lead (a balloon-tipped, flow-directed, bipolar catheter is usually used; unipolar and pacing pulmonary artery catheters are also available)

12-lead ECG with a male-to-male connector or an alligator clip

Cardiac monitor/defibrillator/pacemaker

Advanced life support equipment

Fluoroscopy equipment (optional)

PATIENT PREPARATION
1. Place the patient on continuous ECG monitoring (see Procedure 58).
2. Obtain a baseline 12-lead ECG (see Procedure 59).
3. Position the patient on the fluoroscopy table, if applicable.

PROCEDURAL STEPS
1. Clip the hair at the insertion site. Shaving is avoided because it predisposes to infection.
2. Don a mask, a gown, a cap, and sterile gloves.
3. *Prepare the skin with a povidone-iodine solution and drape the area with sterile towels.
4. *Insert the introducer via the percutaneous or the cutdown technique (see Procedures 66, 67, 68, and 69). In an emergency situation, the preferred approach is the percutaneous technique via the subclavian site or the internal jugular insertion site, both of which offer ease and speed of insertion. The right internal jugular approach provides a straight line into the right ventricle. There are risks associated with the subclavian insertion site, including bleeding due to an inadvertent puncture of the subclavian artery and pneumothorax (Mitrani et al., 2001). The brachial-vein approach site is problematic because the catheter tends to be unstable and the patient experiences discomfort. The femoral site carries the greatest risk of thrombosis, phlebitis, and infection.
5. *Insert the pacemaker catheter using one of the following techniques.
   a. *Emergency placement:* The pacemaker and the extension cable are attached to the pacing catheter. The tip, or the distal electrode, of the pacing catheter is connected to the negative pole of the pacemaker. The ring, or the proximal electrode, is connected to the positive pole of the pacemaker. The pacemaker is turned on and advanced blindly. Contact with the right ventricular endocardium is indicated by capture. The right internal jugular approach is used because it provides the straightest route to the right ventricle (Figure 89-1).
   b. *Urgent insertion via ECG monitoring:* Place the limb electrodes of the 12-lead ECG in the standard positions. The V_1 electrode is connected with alligator clips or a male-to-male connector to the distal terminal of the

---

*Indicates portions of the procedure usually performed by a physician or an advanced practice nurse.

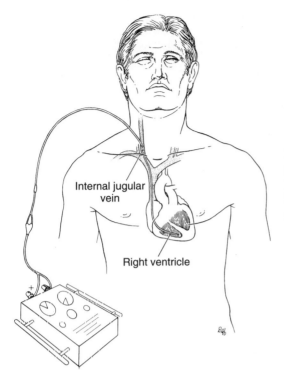

FIGURE 89-1 Internal jugular placement and setup for temporary transvenous pacing. (From Rosen, P., & Sternbach, G.L. [1983]. *Atlas of emergency medicine,* 2nd ed. [p. 101]. Baltimore: Williams & Wilkins.)

Internal jugular vein

Right ventricle

pacing catheter. The standardization of the ECG machine may have to be decreased to half or quarter standard because the electrical activity sensed at the tip of the pacing catheter is of greater magnitude when it is recorded internally. As the pacemaker tip approaches and enters the right atrium, the P wave becomes larger. When the catheter tip enters the right ventricle, the P wave diminishes in size and the QRS complex becomes larger. When the tip of the pacing catheter is against the wall of the right ventricle, the P wave disappears and the QRS complex becomes very large and shows ST-segment elevation. The ST elevation is the marker of an appropriate catheter position (Figure 89-2).

   c. *Fluoroscopic insertion:* Proper positioning of the patient and the fluoroscopic machine is necessary for tracking the advancement of the catheter tip; therefore, continuous communication between the physician and the assistant is essential. The final catheter position is at the right ventricular apex. Most rigid catheter or brachial insertions require the use of a fluoroscope for safe and proper placement in the right ventricle. The confirmation of the catheter position by ECG may be made as described previously in step 5b.

6. Every 5 minutes, monitor the patient's tolerance of the procedure, vital signs, and rhythm. If the pacing catheter induces ventricular ectopy during the insertion, inform the physician. Amiodarone or lidocaine and a defibrillator should be available to treat ectopy that does not abate by withdrawing the catheter from the right ventricle.

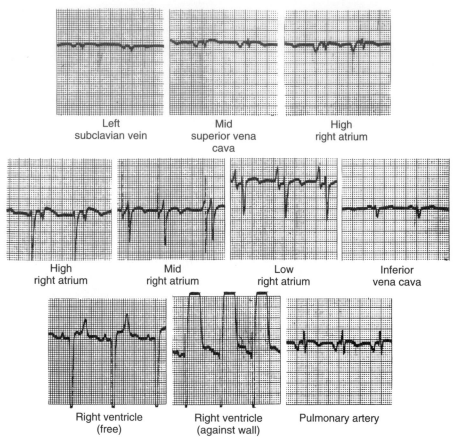

FIGURE 89-2 Pacemaker placement by electrocardiographic monitoring. (From Bing, O.H.L., Mc Dowell, J.W., Hantman, J., et al. [1972]. Pacemaker placement by electrocardiographic monitoring. *New England Journal of Medicine, 287,* 651.)

7. When the endocardial placement is achieved with ECG or fluoroscopic guidance, connect the pacing catheter to the generator directly or via a connecting cable. The distal lead, or the tip, is connected to the negative terminal of the pacemaker. The proximal lead, or the ring, is attached to the positive terminal of the pacemaker. The electrode lead pins on the catheter may be protected by a shroud in compliance with U.S. Food and Drug Administration rulings. The shrouded connector pin requires a universal adapter to connect with older pin that accepts pacemakers and pacemaker cables (Figure 89-3).

8. The pacing mode and the pacemaker settings are directed by the physician, and the pacemaker is turned on. The pacemaker rate is set higher than the patient's intrinsic rate. An initial rate of 80-100 beats/min is selected for most patients. The mode of pacing is determined by the type of catheter used and the clinical situation.

Step 1. Insert and secure
adaptor to cable

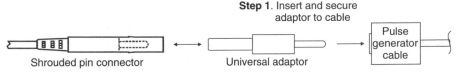

Shrouded pin connector   Universal adaptor

Pulse generator cable

FIGURE 89-3 Pacing catheter shrouded pin connector inserts into the universal adaptor. The universal adaptor converts the connection to an unshrouded pin which articulates with most pulse generators. (Courtesy Edwards Lifesciences LLC, Irvine, CA.)

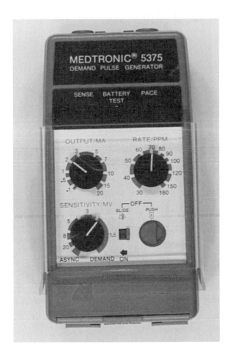

FIGURE 89-4 An example of an older-model single-chamber temporary pacemaker.

a. *Asynchronous pacing:* In a pulseless, asystolic patient, the ventricular asynchronous mode is used initially. The milliampere (mA) setting in this mode should be at the maximum, which is 20-25 mA, depending on the model of generator used. The milliamperes may be reduced after capture is achieved. Newer models of pacemakers have an "Emergency On" key, which automatically turns on the pacemaker in the asynchronous mode at a rate of 80 mA with maximal output settings. Older models require a manual setting. See Figures 89-4, 89-5, and 89-6 for examples of pacemakers.

b. *Demand pacing:* In patients who are stable or who have been stabilized with transcutaneous pacing, the demand mode is used. Sensitivity settings are the default settings of the pacer model, or they may be set manually. Ventricular sensitivity is the strength of the native QRS that the pacemaker can sense. Ventricular sensitivity is between the maximum, which

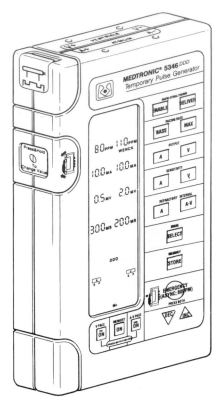

FIGURE 89-5 An example of key pad–controlled, dual-chamber, temporary pacemaker with rapid atrial pacing capacity. (Courtesy Medtronic, Inc. [1993]. *Pulse generator model 5346 technical manual* [p. 2]. Minneapolis, MN.)

is the lowest number, and 2 millivolts (Medtronic, 1996). This sensitivity ensures that even a small native QRS can be sensed by the pacemaker. The milliampere output is increased until continuous capture is achieved, which is the threshold. The maintenance pacing output is set at 1.5-2 times the threshold output required to achieve capture (Figure 89-7).

9. Assess the patient's response to the pacing by continuously monitoring the ECG and by checking the patient's vital signs, neurologic status, and urine output.
10. *Secure the pacing catheter to the skin with a suture.
11. Place a sterile dressing over the insertion site.
12. Secure the pacing leads by looping and taping them to the outside of the dressing. Secure the generator to the patient, and ensure electrical safety as mentioned in the Contraindications and Cautions.
13. Obtain a chest x-ray film so that the physician can verify the lead placement and evaluate the patient for a pneumothorax or hemothorax.

AGE-SPECIFIC CONSIDERATIONS

1. Severe bradycardias in children are usually the result of hypoxia or hypoventilation (Del Monte, 2001; AHA, 2003). Oxygenation, airway intervention, and

---

*Indicates portions of the procedure usually performed by a physician or an advanced practice nurse.

1. Pace/sense LEDs
2. Lock/unlock key
3. Lock indicators
4. Rate dial
5. Atrial output dial
6. Ventricular output dial
7. Menu parameter dial
8. Parameter selection key
9. Menu selection key
10. Pause key
11. Power on key
12. Power off key
13. Emergency/asynchronous pacing key
14. Lower screen
15. Ventricular output graphics
16. Atrial output graphics
17. Upper screen
18. Rate graphics
19. Setup indicators
20. DDI indicator
21. Low battery indicator
22. Setup labels

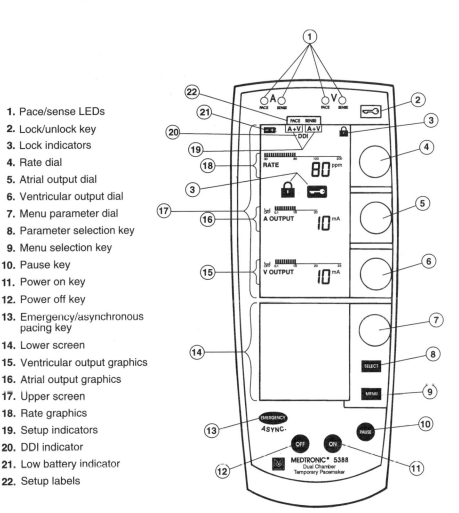

FIGURE 89-6 An example of a dial- and key pad–controlled, dual-chamber temporary pacemaker. (Courtesy Medtronic, Inc. [1996]. *Dual chamber temporary pacemaker model 5388 technical manual* [p. 3-3]. Minneapolis, MN.)

ventilation should be addressed before pharmacologic agents or pacing are attempted.
2. Minimal heart rates indicating the possible need for pacing are the following (Conway, 1997):
   a. Infant: less than 55 beats/min
   b. Child: less than 45-50 beats/min
   c. Adolescent: less than 40 beats/min
3. Consider pacing in children with primary bradycardia due to congenital defects, complete heart block, abnormal sinus node function, drug overdose, or failing implanted pacemaker, as well as those who have undergone heart surgery (AHA, 2003).

COMPLICATIONS
Related to the Patient-Pacer Interface

1. Failure to achieve capture is evidenced by pacer spikes that fail to induce a wide QRS complex (Figure 89-8). The capture threshold may change over time and should be determined frequently when the patient is pacemaker dependent (Del Monte & Gamrath, 1996).

2. Undersensing occurs when the pacemaker does not sense an intrinsic QRS and delivers a pacing spike. Failure to sense is recognized by a competition between the pacing rhythm and the intrinsic rhythm and by a short native QRS to the pacing spike interval (Figure 89-9). If the pacer fails to recognize all the intrinsic QRS complexes, it operates as if it is in the asynchronous mode.

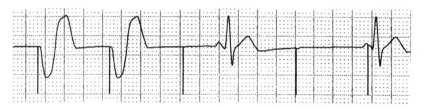

FIGURE 89-7 Ventricular capture in a single-chamber pacemaker. Each pacing spike is followed by a wide QRS complex.

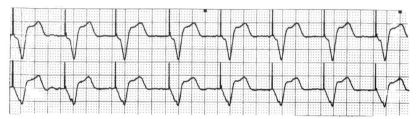

FIGURE 89-8 Intermittent failure to capture. Some pacing spikes are not followed by wide QRS complexes. (Courtesy Medtronic, Inc. [1996]. *Temporary pacing workshop instructor guide* [overhead S-5]. Minneapolis, MN.)

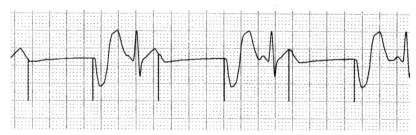

FIGURE 89-9 Undersensing. The pacer fails to sense the intrinsic beats (beats 2 and 4) and fires prematurely. The pacer also does not capture, because the spike has fallen during the refractory period. (Courtesy Medtronic, Inc. [1996]. *Temporary pacing workshop instructor guide* [Overhead S-6]. Minneapolis, MN.)

3. Oversensing is due to an inappropriate inhibition of pacing by the electrical signals from outside the heart (Figure 89-10). Extracardiac electrical signals include a muscle artifact and electromagnetic signals in the environment. These may be corrected by decreasing the ECG size, thereby decreasing the sensitivity to the native QRS. If the problem persists, it may be necessary to operate the pacemaker in the asynchronous mode to obtain reliable pacing (Del Monte & Gamrath, 1996).

Related to Insertion

1. Hemothorax and pneumothorax associated with subclavian and jugular insertion (Ellenbogen & Wood, 2001)
2. Bleeding that is difficult to control associated with femoral and subclavian insertion
3. Myocardial perforation, which may lead to cardiac tamponade or diaphragmatic pacing. This is more common with brachial or femoral catheters and is more likely with rigid catheters (Ellenbogen & Wood, 2001).
4. Myocardial irritability, which may cause ventricular dysrhythmias
5. Transient bundle branch block
6. Failure to achieve capture because of malpositioning of the catheter in the inferior vena cava or the pulmonary artery
7. Arterial trauma and air embolism (Ellenbogen & Wood, 2001)

Related to Catheter Maintenance

1. Local myocardial edema and inflammation, causing an increase over time in the threshold to achieve capture
2. For long-term temporary pacing, the femoral vein should be avoided in order to prevent infection (Mitrani et al., 2001).

Related to Equipment

1. Generator or battery failure, or both, possibly resulting in failure to fire, capture, or sense
2. Lead displacement, possibly resulting in failure to sense or capture, usually associated with brachial and femoral insertion
3. Poor connections, possibly resulting in failure to fire, sense, or capture

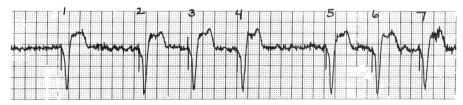

FIGURE 89-10 Oversensing. Pacing spikes 2 and 5 occur late because of oversensing of myopotentials. (Courtesy Medtronic, Inc. [1996]. *Temporary pacing workshop instructor guide* [Overhead S-7]. Minneapolis, MN.)

PATIENT TEACHING

1. Bed rest and restriction of movement at the hip are required with femoral insertion. Immobilization of the arm is required with brachial insertion. Other insertion sites do not require movement or position restrictions.
2. Do not move or manipulate the pacemaker or the wire.
3. Report dizziness, lightheadedness, or weakness immediately.

REFERENCES

American Heart Association. (2003). *ACLS principles and practice: the reference textbook.* Dallas: Author.

Becker, D.E. (2001). Temporary transvenous pacemaker insertion (perform). (pp. 278-284). In Lynn-McHale, D.J. & Carlson, K.K. (Eds.), *AACN procedure manual for critical care,* 4th ed., Philadelphia, W.B. Saunders.

Bing, O.H.L., McDowell, J.W., Hantman, J., et al. (1972). Pacemaker placement by electrocardiographic monitoring. *New England Journal of Medicine, 287,* 651.

Conway, S.P. (1997). Pediatric pacemakers for patients with complete heart block. *Dimensions of Critical Care Nursing, 16* (1), 29-39.

Del Monte, L. (2001) Pediatric pacing. Trainers of Emergency Services. May/June 2001. Available at www.kpemsc.org/toes. Accessed 6/30/02.

Del Monte, L., & Gamrath, B. (1996). *Noninvasive pacing: what you should know,* 2nd ed. Redmond, WA: Physio-Control Corporation.

Ellenbogen, K.A., & Wood, M. (2001). *Cardiac pacing,* 3rd ed. Boston: Blackwell Scientific Publications.

Hayes, D.L., & Holmes, D.D., Jr. (1993). Temporary cardiac pacing. In Furman, S., Hayes, D.L., & Holmes, D.R., Jr. (Eds.), *A practice of cardiac pacing* (pp. 231-260). Mt. Kisco, NY: Futura.

Medtronic. (1996). *Dual chamber temporary pacemaker model 5388 technical manual.* Minneapolis: Author.

Mitrani, R.D., Myerburg, R.J., & Castillanos, A. et al. (2001). Cardiac pacemakers (pp. 963-992). In Fuster, V., Alexander, R.W., O'Rourke, R.A., et al (Eds.), *Hurst's the heart,* 10th ed. New York: McGraw-Hill.

Invasive Hemodynamic Monitoring

Central Venous Pressure Measurement via Manometer

Lucinda W. Rossoll, BSN, MS, CEN, CCRN, ARNP

Central venous pressure is also known as CVP or right atrial pressure (RAP).

INDICATIONS

1. To monitor volume status and right ventricular function
2. To guide the administration of fluids, diuretics, and vasoactive drugs when other invasive monitoring options are not available

CONTRAINDICATIONS AND CAUTIONS

1. Increases in CVP may occur as a result of increased cardiac output, right ventricular infarct or failure, increased vascular volume, cardiac tamponade, tension pneumothorax, constrictive pericarditis, or pulmonary hypertension. Falsely elevated CVP measurements may occur in the setting of a pneumothorax, positive-pressure ventilation, or chronic obstructive pulmonary disease (COPD).
2. Dislocation of the tip of the central line from the superior vena cava or improper manometer positioning causes inaccurate readings.
3. Decreases in CVP may be due to hypovolemia, drug-induced vasodilation, or shock of any etiology.

EQUIPMENT

CVP water manometer
Intravenous (IV) fluid and tubing
Felt-tip marker

PATIENT PREPARATION

1. See Procedures 66 and 67 for information about central line insertion.
2. Place the patient in the supine position with the head of the bed flat or elevated no more than 30 degrees.
3. Locate and mark the phlebostatic axis with the felt-tip marker to ensure that the same zero reference point is used for consistent measurements. The phlebostatic axis is found by locating the junction of the fourth intercostal space and the midaxillary line (Figure 90-1).

PROCEDURAL STEPS

1. Turn the stopcock off to the manometer and flush the tubing with IV fluid (Figure 90-2, *A*).
2. Attach the manometer tubing to the central venous line and flush to ensure patency.

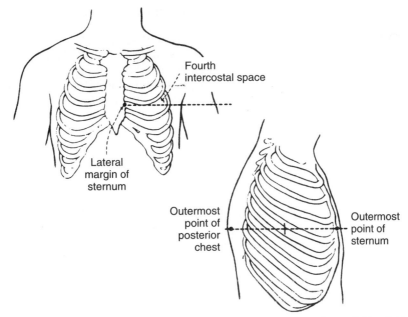

FIGURE 90-1 Level of the right atrium or phlebostatic axis. (From Wood, S.L., & Mansfield, L.W. [1976]. Body position upon pulmonary artery and pulmonary capillary wedge pressures in noncritically ill patients. *Heart and Lung, 5,* 84.)

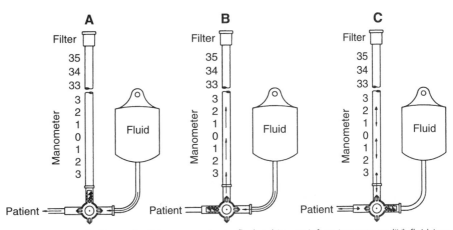

FIGURE 90-2 A, Stopcock off to manometer to flush tubing or infuse intravenous (IV) fluid into patient. **B,** Stopcock off to patient to fill manometer. **C,** Stopcock off to IV fluid to read central venous pressure. (Courtesy Medex, Afaron Healthcare Company, Incorporated, Hilliard, OH.)

3. Position the zero mark on the water manometer at the phlebostatic angle. The manometer can be either secured to an IV pole or hand held at the point of reference.
4. Turn the stopcock off to the patient and open it between the IV solution and the manometer. Allow the manometer to fill with IV fluid up to the 25-cm level. Note that the faster the IV fluid is running, the faster the manometer fills. Avoid letting the fluid run out the top of the manometer, because contamination of the manometer may result (see Figure 90-2, *B*).
5. Turn the stopcock off to the IV fluid and open between the patient and manometer. This causes the fluid level to fall and fluctuate with respirations (Figure 90-2, *C*).
6. Take the CVP reading when the fluid level stabilizes. The reading should be taken from the base of the meniscus at the end of expiration. If the patient is spontaneously breathing, the fluid in the manometer slightly drops with inspiration; end-expiration is seen when the fluid in the manometer rises. In a ventilated patient, the fluid height in the manometer increases during inspiration and drops at end-expiration.
7. Turn the stopcock off to the manometer and run the IV fluids through the central venous line as prescribed (see Figure 90-2, *A*).
8. Document the reading and the patient's position.
9. Normal CVP ranges from 3-11 cm H_2O. When monitoring CVP, it is the trend of the reading that is most significant. The CVP trend, combined with the clinical assessment, determines the appropriate interventions.

COMPLICATIONS

1. As with other procedures using central venous catheters, complications may include infection, phlebitis, venous thrombosis, and air embolism.
2. Occlusion of the catheter caused by improper positioning of the stopcock results in slowing or cessation of IV fluid administration through the central venous line.
3. Hemorrhage may result from disconnection of the tubing from the central venous catheter.

PATIENT TEACHING

Report any tubing disconnections or blood in the tubing immediately.

Arterial Line Insertion and Monitoring

Lucinda W. Rossoll, BSN, MS, CEN, CCRN, ARNP

An arterial line is also known as an "A-line" or an "art line."

INDICATIONS

1. To monitor arterial pressure accurately and continuously in patients who are, or who have the potential to become, hemodynamically unstable.
2. To monitor the response to vasoactive drugs.
3. To facilitate frequent sampling of arterial blood gases (ABGs) and other laboratory specimens.
4. To determine derived hemodynamic parameters, such as the mean arterial pressure (MAP). This is helpful for calculating and maintaining cerebral perfusion pressure.

CONTRAINDICATIONS AND CAUTIONS

1. Knowledge and understanding of the arterial line monitoring system, the waveforms, and how to obtain accurate values is necessary for the registered nurse assisting with insertion and monitoring of the A-line.
2. Significant blood loss may occur if the tubing is disconnected.
3. Close patient monitoring is necessary for any patient with an A-line in place, and monitoring alarms should always be on to alert the nurse of hemodynamic changes or system malfunction.
4. Avoid A-line insertion in extremities with injuries that may compromise distal circulation.

EQUIPMENT

Arterial catheter or 18- to 20-G, 1- to 2-inch intravenous (IV) catheter
Sterile gloves
Antiseptic solution
Lidocaine 1% (without epinephrine) for local anesthesia
3-ml syringe for lidocaine
18-G 1½ inch needle (to draw up lidocaine)
25-G ½ inch needle (to administer lidocaine)
Flush solution with 1-4 units of heparin/ml (amount of heparin per institutional policy) in 250- to 500-ml bag of normal saline
Cardiac monitor with hemodynamic monitoring capability
Recorder (preferably analog recorder)
Pressure transducer cable

413

*Microdrip IV tubing
*Pressure tubing with continuous flush device
*Pressure transducer (if not already part of the pressure tubing setup)
*Pressure extension tubing
*Long pressure extension tubing (for pole-mounted transducer)
*Two or three (three-way) stopcocks (number used depends on how blood draws are performed, i.e., one or two stopcock method)
*Dead-end caps (nonvented) for stopcock ports
Pressure-infuser bag or cuff
Armboard
Pole-mounted transducer holder (optional)
Level (optional)
4-0 nylon sutures
Dressing supplies per institutional protocol, e.g., tincture of benzoin, adhesive tape, and occlusive dressing

PATIENT PREPARATION

1. Establish cardiac monitoring (see Procedure 58).
2. Check with the physician regarding the site to be cannulated. The radial, ulnar, brachial, or femoral artery may be selected. The radial artery is usually used

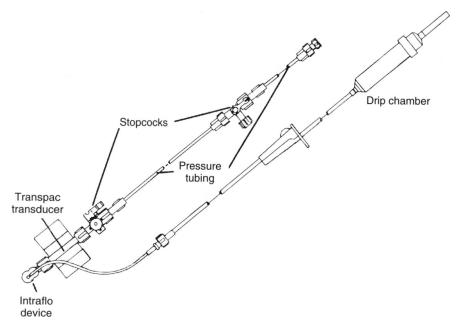

FIGURE 91-1 Preassembled disposable transducer and tubing for pressure monitoring. (Courtesy Abbott Critical Care Systems, North Chicago, IL.)

---

*Preassembled tubing or transducer sets are available with these components integrated (Figure 91-1).

for arterial pressure monitoring because it generally has good collateral circulation, is easily accessible, and does not require extremity immobilization, which restricts patient movement, as the other sites frequently do. The patient's collateral circulation to the hand may be assessed before insertion of the radial or ulna line by use of the Allen test (Procedure 21) or a Doppler ultrasound device (Procedure 52).

3. Position the extremity in extension.

4. Cleanse the area to be cannulated with an antiseptic solution.

PROCEDURAL STEPS

1. Turn on the hemodynamic monitor and attach the transducer cable. Set the scale on the 200 mm Hg range.

2. Prepare the pressure monitoring system as follows:

   a. Spike the flush solution with the IV pressure tubing and remove all air from the bag. Attach the flush solution to the microdrip IV tubing portion of the pressure tubing set and fill the drip chamber half full to prevent air from entering the system.

   b. If you do not use preassembled transducer and tubing sets:

      i. After spiking the flush solution and flushing the IV tubing, attach the IV tubing to the transducer.

      ii. Place two stopcocks onto the transducer and attach to the short extension tubing.

      iii. If the transducer is to be pole mounted, add a stopcock onto the transducer and add a long piece of pressure extension tubing, then add the two stopcocks and the short pressure tubing.

      iv. Attach two stopcocks and add an extension set to the end.

   c. Prime the tubing and the transducer to remove all the air from the system. This is accomplished by opening the roller clamp and activating the flush device (pigtail) according to the manufacturer's directions. Work your way down the system from the flush solution, and flush each stopcock until all air is flushed through the fenestrated (vented) cap. Replace the vented caps with nonvented caps on each side port of the stopcock as the stopcock is flushed. Continue until all the air is removed from the system and all the stopcocks are flushed. The flush device, also known as the continuous-flow device, allows a flow rate of 3-5 ml/hr (usual rate is 3 ml/hr) to maintain patency of the system. Turn each stopcock so they are on to both the patient and the transducer.

   d. Place the flush solution in the pressure bag and pressurize it to 300 mm Hg. This step is not performed before step c, because the increased pressure causes rapid flushing and increased turbulence, which may trap air bubbles in the system and cause a damped waveform.

   e. Position the transducer. If the patient-mounted option is being used, keep the transducer on the same plane as the right atrium (Campbell, 1997). For a pole-mounted transducer, secure the transducer on the IV pole at the level of the right atrium so that the stopcock at the air-fluid interface (the same stopcock that is used to open the system to atmospheric pressure) is at the level of the phlebostatic axis (use a level to guide placement). The phlebostatic axis is found by locating the junction of the fourth intercostal space and the midaxillary line (see Procedure 90, Figure 90-1).

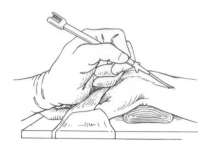

FIGURE 91-2 Insertion of a radial artery cannula. (From Rosen, P., & Sternbach, G.L. [1983]. *Atlas of emergency medicine,* 2nd ed. [p. 97]. Baltimore: Williams & Wilkins.)

f. Zero balance the transducer. Zero balancing the system to the atmospheric pressure negates the effects of the atmospheric pressure. To prevent erroneous pressure readings, zero the system before and after the pressure system is attached to the patient, with any significant change in the waveform and the values, whenever the system is disconnected, and at the beginning of each shift. To zero, turn the stopcock next to the transducer off to the patient and open the port to air (this is known as the air-fluid interface). Zero the monitor according to the manufacturer's directions. Once the monitor is zeroed, flush the open stopcock port and replace the dead-ender cap. Turn the stopcock on to the patient and on to the transducer. Some monitors may also need to be calibrated; if this is the case, do so according to the manufacturer's directions.

3. *Cleanse the insertion site with antiseptic solution and infiltrate the insertion site with a local anesthetic (optional).

4. *Cannulate the artery with the catheter and remove the inner wire. Allow the catheter to back fill with blood (Figure 91-2).

5. Connect the pressure tubing to the catheter and secure it tightly via the Luer-Lok connection.

6. Activate the flush device to clear the line of any blood resulting from the backflow.

7. *Suture the catheter in place.

8. Cleanse the site with an antiseptic solution, apply tincture of benzoin around the insertion site, use adhesive tape to secure the catheter in place, and cover with a sterile or occlusive dressing (as per institutional policy).

9. Observe and record the arterial pressure waveform (Figure 91-3) on the monitor and note the digital blood pressure reading. Many protocols require checking the cuff pressure to ensure the accuracy of the arterial measurement. In low-flow states, such as hypotension, lower pressure readings are obtained with a cuff pressure rather than A-line pressures, and higher cuff pressure readings are obtained in high-flow states, such as sepsis. Darovic & Franklin (1999) caution against the inconsistent practice of accepting a cuff pressure reading one time and an A-line pressure another. There is no need to correlate cuff pressures with monitor pressures if the square wave shows an optimally damped system. See square wave information under Complications, number 3.

---

*Indicates portions of the procedure usually performed by a physician or an advanced practice nurse.

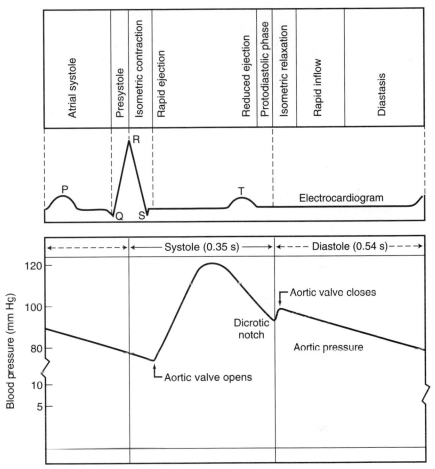

Atrial systole | Presystole | Isometric contraction | Rapid ejection | Reduced ejection | Protodiastolic phase | Isometric relaxation | Rapid inflow | Diastasis

R

P

T   Electrocardiogram

Q   S

Systole (0.35 s) ⟶   ⟵ – – – Diastole (0.54 s)– – – ⟶

120

Blood pressure (mm Hg)

100

Aortic valve closes

Dicrotic
notch

80   Aortic pressure

Aortic valve opens

10

5

FIGURE 91-3 Arterial pressure waveform. (From Smith, R.N., & de Asla, R.A. [1988]. Instrumentation. In Kinney, M.R., Packa, D.R., & Dunbar, S.B. [Eds.], AACN's *clinical reference manual for critical care nursing,* 2nd ed. [p. 48]. St. Louis: Mosby.)

10. Maintain a continuous display of the pressure tracings. This allows for early detection of hemodynamic changes in the patient or catheter disconnection.
11. Turn on the monitor alarms to limits based on the patient's clinical condition.
12. To withdraw blood for ABG analysis, use either the one-stopcock or the two-stopcock method.
    a. Two-stopcock method
        i. Attach a 10-ml syringe to the stopcock most distal to the insertion site (distal stopcock). Attach the heparinized ABG syringe to the stopcock closest to the patient (proximal stopcock).
        ii. Turn the distal stopcock off to the transducer and turn it on to the patient. Withdraw 10 ml of blood to clear any heparinized blood from the line. Turn the stopcock off to the 10-ml syringe.

    iii. Turn the proximal stopcock off to the transducer and on to the patient. Withdraw 1 ml of blood into the ABG syringe. Turn the stopcock off to the ABG syringe. Remove the ABG syringe and purge any air before capping it and placing it on ice.

    iv. Reinfuse the blood in the 10-ml syringe (optional). Turn the distal stopcock off to the transducer, turn it on to the patient, reinfuse the blood, and turn the stopcock off to the syringe port. If reinfusion is not desired, leave the stopcock closed, remove the 10-ml syringe, and discard it.

    v. Flush both stopcocks as described in Procedural Step 2c. and cap them with sterile deadender caps.

b. One-stopcock method

    i. Attach a 10-ml syringe to the stopcock closest to the catheter site.

    ii. Turn the stopcock off to the transducer and turn it on to the patient. Withdraw 10 ml of blood to clear any heparinized blood from the line. Turn the stopcock off to the 10-ml syringe. Remove and discard the 10-ml waste syringe.

    iii. Attach the heparinized ABG syringe to the port. Turn the stopcock off to the transducer and turn it on to the patient. Withdraw 1 ml of blood into the ABG syringe. Turn the stopcock off to the ABG syringe. Remove the ABG syringe and purge any air before capping it and placing it on ice.

    iv. Flush the stopcock as described in Procedural Step 2c and cap it with a sterile dead-ender cap.

AGE-SPECIFIC CONSIDERATIONS

1. In the pediatric population, the dorsalis pedis, posterior tibial, axillary, or temporal artery may also be cannulated (Steinhart, 1997).

2. In infants, catheter patency may be maintained with a 1- to 3-ml/hr continuous infusion of heparinized saline (1 unit heparin/ml) using an intraflow system and an IV pump (Figure 91-4) (Steinhart, 1997).

COMPLICATIONS

1. An air embolism can be introduced into the circulation if the tubing and transducer are not flushed properly before connection to the cannula. If air bubbles persist despite tight connections, check the flush device and stopcocks for cracks.

2. Severe blood loss, or exsanguination, may occur if the connections are not tightly secured or the catheter is dislodged.

3. Damping of the waveform may occur if the cannula lodges against the vessel wall or if there is clot formation, kinking of the catheter, or air trapped between the transducer diaphragm and the dome diaphragm (Figure 91-5). Slight readjustment of the cannula may free it from its position against the vessel wall. If a clot is suspected, aspirate with a syringe to attempt to remove the clot. Never inject into the line because a clot may become dislodged into the circulation. If air is entrapped in the transducer and cannot be cleared, replace the transducer assembly. To ensure accurate and consistent pressure readings:

a. Level and zero the transducers as outlined in procedural steps 2e and 2f. Inaccurate pressure readings may occur if the transducer is placed incor-

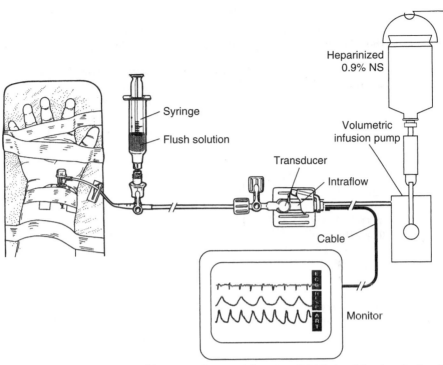

FIGURE 91 4 Pediatric arterial line setup. (From Steinhart, C.M. [1997]. Arterial catheterization. In Dieckmann, R.A., Fiser, D.H., & Selbst, S.M. [Eds.], *Pediatric emergency and critical care procedures* [p. 218]. St. Louis: Mosby.)

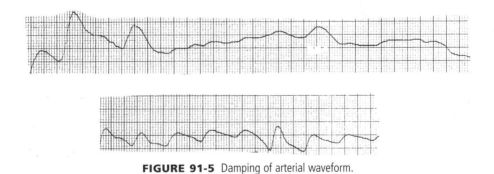

FIGURE 91-5 Damping of arterial waveform.

rectly. If the transducer is above the level of the right atrium, the pressure reading will be falsely low. If the transducer is below the level of the right atrium, the pressure reading will be falsely elevated. To prevent inaccurate pressure readings, level before and after the pressure system is attached to the patient, any change in bed height, any significant change in the waveforms and their values, whenever the system is disconnected, and at the beginning of each shift.

b. Check the dynamic response. The dynamic response is used to ensure that the monitoring system is accurately reproducing the patient's pressure signal at the monitor. This is achieved by evaluating the square wave. With the pressure bag inflated to 300 mm Hg, activate the fast flush quickly.

   i. The system is optimally damped when the resulting waveform exceeds the upper limits of the scope followed by a negative deflection and a small overshoot. It then returns to the patient's pressure waveform (Figure 91-6, *A*).

   ii. The system is overdamped if the fast flush results in a waveform that does not exceed the upper limits of the scope, followed by a slow return to the baseline (Figure 91-6, *B*). This gives a false-low systolic pressure. The most common cause is a stopcock or inadequate pressure on the system, allowing the blood to back up.

   iii. The system is underdamped if the fast flush results in a waveform that goes above and below the limits of the scope, with several more positive and negative deflections occurring before returning to baseline. If the system is underdamped, it gives falsely elevated systolic values. This can be due to excessive catheter length, fast heart rate, or high pressures that cause a "ringing" in the system (Figure 91-6, *C*). Commercial devices that attach to the pressure system are available to assist in controlling underdamping.

   iv. If the system is under damped or overdamped and cannot be corrected, monitor the mean arterial pressure because this measurement is not affected by catheter movement within the vessel or by poor dynamic response and will provide a reliable trend (Darovic & Franklin, 1999).

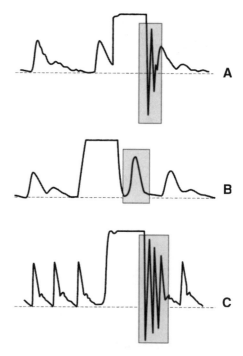

FIGURE 91-6 A, Optimal square wave test. The fast flush trace ends with a small undershoot, followed by a small overshoot, and the oscillations cease before the next patient waveform. **B,** Overdamped square wave. The fast flush trace slowly returns to the next patient waveform without any oscillations. **C,** Underdamped square wave. The fast flush trace has oscillations that continue into the next waveform. (Courtesy Baxter Healthcare Corporation, Edwards Critical Care Division, Santa Ana, CA.)

4. Infection may occur if poor aseptic technique is used, if there are openings in the system that allow entrance and promote growth of bacteria (e.g., blood not cleared from the port after the blood is drawn or after failure to apply sterile dead-end caps to the unused ports) or if the catheter is left in for a prolonged period of time.
5. Median nerve damage may occur if the wrist remains dorsiflexed.
6. A hematoma, with possible nerve compression at the insertion site, may occur.

PATIENT TEACHING
1. Use care when moving about in bed so as not to disconnect the system.
2. Report any disconnections or dampness around the site immediately.

REFERENCES
Campbell, B. (1997). Arterial waveforms: monitoring changes in configuration. *Heart and Lung*, *26*, 204-214.
Darovic, G.O., & Franklin, C. (1999). *Handbook of hemodynamic monitoring*, Philadelphia: W.B. Saunders.
Steinhart, C.M. (1997). Arterial catheterization (pp. 213–219). In Dieckmann, R.A., Fiser, D.H., & Selbst, S.M. (Eds.), *Pediatric emergency and critical care procedures*. St. Louis: Mosby.

PROCEDURE 92

Pulmonary Artery Catheter Insertion

Lucinda W. Rossoll, BSN, MS, CEN, CCRN, ARNP

The pulmonary artery (PA) catheter is also known as a Swan-Ganz catheter or a flow-directed, balloon-tipped, thermodilution catheter. Pulmonary artery occlusive pressure (PAOP) is also known as pulmonary capillary wedge pressure (PCWP) or "wedge" pressure.

INDICATIONS
1. To provide a continuous and reliable method of monitoring right atrial, pulmonary artery, and pulmonary wedge pressures in hemodynamically unstable patients and patients with pulmonary or cardiac conditions. This information

may help determine underlying pathology, for example, with septic shock there is hypotension with low systemic and peripheral vascular resistance and high cardiac output.
2. To determine cardiac output using the thermodilution method
3. To obtain mixed venous samples for analysis of an intrapulmonary shunt, an intracardiac shunt, and oxygen consumption
4. To monitor interventions such as the titration of vasoactive and inotropic medications and the administration of fluids and diuretics.

CONTRAINDICATIONS AND CAUTIONS
1. There are no absolute contraindications for insertion of a PA catheter. Caution should be used in patients with prolonged bleeding times, hypercoagulable states, mechanical tricuspid valve, left bundle branch block, or recurrent sepsis.
2. Knowledge and understanding of the hemodynamic monitoring system, the PA catheter, and the waveforms, as well has how to accurately obtain readings from the waveforms, are essential for the registered nurse assisting with the insertion and monitoring of the PA catheter.

EQUIPMENT
Level
Pressure-infuser bag or cuff
*8.5-French or larger introducer (most introducers now come with a side port for continuous fluid administration)
Intravenous (IV) fluid and tubing of choice for the side port
*Percutaneous sheath
Antiseptic solution
Flush solution with 1-4 units of heparin/ml (amount of heparin per institutional policy) in 500-ml bag of normal saline
Pressure transducer cable(s) (the number needed depends on the number of waveforms to be monitored continuously)
Pole-mounted transducer holder
†Pressure tubing with continuous flush device
†Pressure transducer(s) (the number needed depends on the number of waveforms to be monitored continuously)
†Pressure extension tubing
†Two stopcocks (three-way)
†Dead-end caps for stopcock ports
Cardiac monitor with hemodynamic monitoring capability
Recorder (preferably analog recorder)
Cardiac output monitor with thermodilution setup
Indelible felt-tip marker
Sterile caps, gloves, gowns, and masks
Sterile drapes
*Suture
*Lidocaine 1% (without epinephrine) for local anesthesia

---

*Indicates equipment that may come in a prepackaged introducer kit.
†Indicates equipment that may come prepackaged in a pressure tubing and transducer set.

*3-ml syringe (for lidocaine)
*18-G 1½-inch needle (to draw up lidocaine)
*25-G ½-inch needle (for administration of lidocaine)
*Scalpel
Dressing supplies per institutional protocol, such as tincture of benzoin, adhesive tape, and occlusive dressing
Cardiopulmonary resuscitation equipment, including a temporary pacemaker (may be a transcutaneous pacemaker)
100 mg of lidocaine for IV use in the event of a dysrhythmia
7.5-French PA catheter (Figure 92-1)
Sterile basin (optional, see Procedural Step 8)
Sterile water or normal saline (optional, see Procedural Step 8)

PATIENT PREPARATION

1. Establish cardiac monitoring (see Procedure 58).
2. Establish a peripheral IV line because there is the potential for cardiac dysrhythmias during catheter insertion (see Procedure 63).
3. Position the patient. For an internal jugular (IJ) or subclavian (SC) insertion, the patient should be placed in a slight Trendelenburg position with a rolled

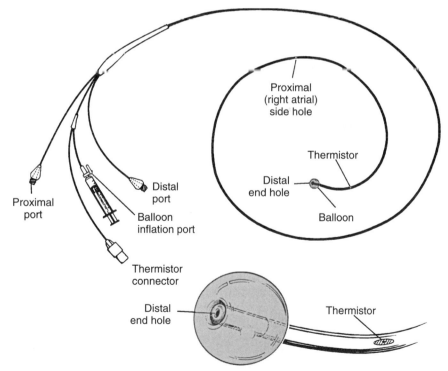

FIGURE 92-1 A flow-directed thermodilution pulmonary artery catheter. (Courtesy Spacelabs Medical, Inc, Issaquah, WA.)

---

*Indicates equipment that may come in a prepackaged introducer kit.

towel under the shoulder on the side in which the catheter will be inserted. For a femoral vein insertion, the patient should be in the supine position. Infrequently, a median basilic vein or a lateral cephalic vein in the antecubital fossa may be used.

4. Mark the phlebostatic axis with the felt-tip marker to ensure that the same zero reference point is used for consistent measurements. The phlebostatic axis is found by locating the junction of the fourth intercostal space and the midaxillary line (see Procedure 90, Figure 90-1).

PROCEDURAL STEPS

1. Turn on the hemodynamic monitor and attach the transducer cable. Set the scale on the 40 to 60 mm Hg range.

2. Assemble and flush the pressure monitoring system as outlined in steps a-c. (Figure 92-2). Two or three transducers may be used, depending on the number of pressures that need to be monitored.

   a. Spike the flush solution with the IV pressure tubing and remove all air from the bag. Attach the flush solution to the pressure tubing set, and fill the drip chamber half full to prevent air from entering the system.

   b. Prime the tubing and the transducer to remove all the air from the system. This is accomplished by opening the roller clamp and activating the flush device (pigtail) according to the manufacturer's directions. Work down the system from the flush solution and flush each stopcock until all air is flushed through the fenestrated cap. Replace the vented caps with nonvented caps on each side port of the stopcock as the stopcock is flushed. Continue until all the air is removed from the system and all the stopcocks are flushed. The flush device, also known as the continuous-flush device, allows a flow rate of 1-5 ml/hr (usual rate is 3 ml/hr) to maintain patency of the system Turn each stopcock on to the patient and on to the transducer.

   c. Place the flush solution in the pressure bag and pressurize it to 300 mm Hg. This step is not performed before step 3, because the increased pressure causes rapid flushing and increased turbulence, which may entrap air bubbles in the system and cause a damped waveform.

3. Attach the transducer cable(s) to the transducer(s) and monitor.

4. Level the transducer(s). Inaccurate pressure readings may occur if the transducer is placed incorrectly. If the transducer is above the level of the right atrium (RA), the pressure reading will be falsely low. If the transducer is below the level of the RA, the pressure reading will be falsely elevated. To prevent inaccurate pressure readings, level before and after the pressure system is attached to the patient, any change in bed height, any significant change in the waveforms and their values, whenever the system is disconnected, and at the beginning of each shift. Using a level to guide placement, secure the transducer to the pole, so that the stopcock at the air-fluid interface (the same stopcock that is used to open the system to atmospheric pressure) is at the level of the phlebostatic axis.

5. Zero balance the transducer. Zero balancing the system to the atmospheric pressure negates the effects of the atmospheric pressure. To prevent erroneous pressure readings, zero the system before and after the pressure system is attached to the patient, with any significant change in the waveforms and the

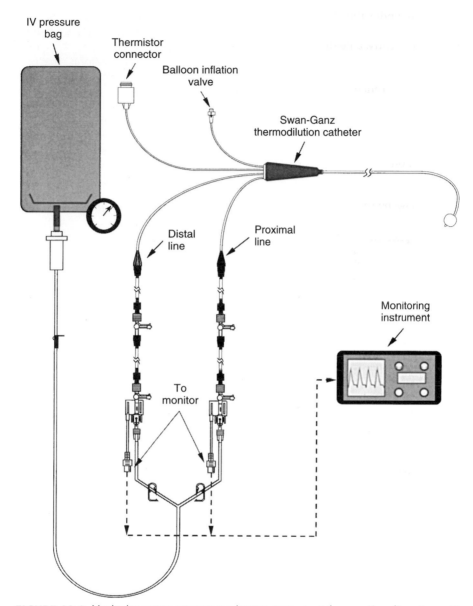

FIGURE 92-2 Monitoring system set up to monitor two pressures at the same time. (From Arone, M. [2001]. Single and multiple pressure transducer systems [p. 477]. In Lynn-McHale, D.J., & Carlson, K.K. (Eds.), *AACN procedure manual for critical care*, 4th ed. Philadelphia: W.B. Saunders.)

values, whenever the system is disconnected, and at the beginning of each shift. To zero, turn the stopcock next to the transducer off to the patient and to air (this is known as the air-fluid interface). Zero the monitor according to the manufacturer's directions. Once the monitor is zeroed, flush the open open the port stopcock port and replace the dead-ender cap. Turn the stopcock on to the patient and on to the transducer. Some monitors may also need to be calibrated; if this is the case, do so according to the manufacturer's directions.

6. Close the stopcock to air and cover it with a nonvented cap.
7. Place the sterile sheath over the catheter before testing the balloon. This protects the balloon from damage during placement of the sheath. The sheath allows the catheter to be repositioned and may prevent contamination of the PA catheter.
8. Check the catheter balloon for leaks by inflating it to the recommended inflation volume, usually 0.8-1.5 ml of air. The balloon should inflate symmetrically and have no air leaks (i.e., stay inflated). If a right-to-left shunt is suspected, extra caution is warranted to prevent an air embolism. In this instance, the inflated balloon may be tested for an air leak by placing it into a basin of sterile water and looking for air bubbles.
9. Connect the proximal and distal lumens of the catheter to the pressure tubing and flush the air out of the catheter.
10. Don sterile gowns, masks, and gloves.
11. *Cleanse the insertion site with an antiseptic solution.
12. *Infiltrate the insertion site with local anesthetic.
13. *Cannulate the vein by using the technique required for that particular insertion site, and insert the introducer (see Procedures 66, 67, and 68).
14. *Advance the catheter through the introducer about 15-20 cm until it is in the RA, where the RA waveform can be seen (Figure 92-3). The physician asks for the balloon to be inflated at this point.
15. Monitor and record the distal lumen waveform during insertion. Keep the physician informed of the catheter's location in the heart, and document the opening pressures. After the PAOP is measured, take the syringe off the balloon port to allow the balloon to deflate passively, and position the stopcock so that the balloon cannot be inflated accidentally. The balloon must be deflated so that it does not obstruct the distal blood flow and cause a pulmonary infarct (Table 92-1 shows normal adult pressures).
16. Observe the ECG tracing for dysrhythmias during the insertion. Premature ventricular contractions (PVCs) and ventricular tachycardia are frequently observed as the catheter passes through the RA to the right ventricle (RV). These usually resolve if the catheter is withdrawn or when it has passed through the RV.
17. *Suture the introducer in place and document the number of centimeters that the catheter is inserted at the level of the introducer. The catheter is marked with a thin black line for each 10 cm, and there is a thick black line for every 50 cm.
18. Obtain a chest x-ray film to check the catheter placement and to rule out a pneumothorax. If the catheter needs to be repositioned, manipulate it within the sterile sleeve and recheck the placement with an x-ray film.
19. To ensure accurate and consistent pressure readings:
    a. Level and zero the transducers as outlined above (steps 6 and 7).
    b. The pressure readings may be taken in the supine position with the head of the bed positioned from 0 to 45 degrees (Lynn-McHale & Preuss, 2001).

*Indicates portions of the procedure usually performed by a physician or advanced practice nurse.

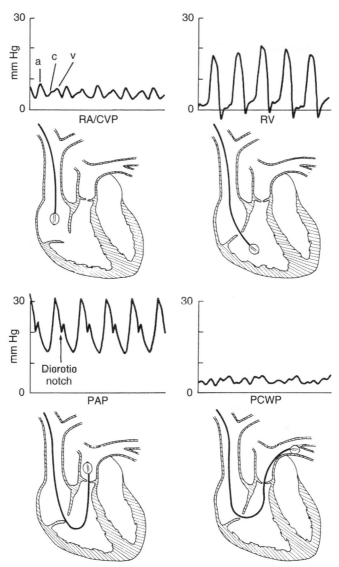

FIGURE 92-3 Right-sided heart pressures and waveforms. Pulmonary artery pressures and waveforms. (Courtesy Abbott Critical Care Systems, Morgan Hills, CA.)

The air-fluid interface in the transducer must remain level with the phlebostatic axis if the position is changed.

c. Take the readings at end expiration when the intrapleural and atmospheric pressures are about the same. This provides a more consistent and accurate reading.

d. The dynamic response is used to ensure that the monitoring system is accurately reproducing the patient's pressure signal at the monitor. This is

TABLE 92-1

NORMAL ADULT VALUES

Parameter	Normal Adult Range
Right atrium pressure (RAP)	Mean 2-6 mm Hg
Right ventricle pressure (RVP)	15-30 // 0-5 mm Hg
Pulmonary artery pressure (PAP)	15-30 // 10-15 mm Hg
Pulmonary artery occlusive pressure (PAOP)	Mean 4-12 mm Hg
Mixed venous oxygen (SvO$_2$)	60%-75%
Cardiac output (CO)	4-8 L/min
Cardiac index (CI)	2.5-4 L/min/m^2
Systemic vascular resistance (SVR)	900-1400 dynes/sec/cm^{-5}

Data from Daily, E.K., & Schroeder, J.S. (1994). *Techniques in bedside hemodynamic monitoring*, 5th ed. St. Louis: Mosby.

achieved by evaluating the square wave. With the pressure bag inflated to 300 mm Hg, activate the fast flush quickly. If the system is optimally damped, the resulting waveform exceeds the upper limits of the scope, followed by a negative deflection and a small overshoot. It then returns to the patient's pressure waveform (see Procedure 91, Figure 91-6, *A*).

e. The system is overdamped if the fast flush results in a waveform that does not exceed the upper limits of the scope, followed by a slow return to the baseline (see Procedure 91, Figure 91-6, *B*). This gives a false-low systolic pressure. The most common cause is a stopcock or inadequate pressure on the system, allowing the blood to back up.

f. The system is underdamped if the fast flush results in a waveform that goes above and below the limits of the scope, with several more positive and negative deflections occurring before returning to baseline. If the system is underdamped, it gives falsely elevated systolic values. This can be due to excessive catheter length, fast heart rate, or high pressures that cause a "ringing" in the system (see Procedure 91, Figure 91-6, *C*). Commercial devices that attach to the pressure system are available to assist in controlling underdamping.

20. Maintain a continuous display of all pressure tracings. This allows for early detection of hemodynamic changes in the patients or catheter malposition.

21. To obtain cardiac output by the thermodilution method, inject a bolus of cold or room-temperature fluid into the RA through the proximal port of the catheter. The temperature change in the blood, when sensed by the thermistor over a period of time, gives the cardiac output in liters per minute. The amount, the temperature, and the number of injections used should be achieved according to the institutional protocol.

22. Measurements of mixed venous blood may be performed by continuous monitoring with an oximetric, fiberoptic catheter or by sampling the blood from the catheter. To obtain a mixed venous sample, aspirate 2½ times the dead space (approximately 3 ml) from the distal lumen of the catheter to clear the lumen of the heparin solution. Attach an arterial blood-gas syringe to the catheter and obtain the sample. Slow aspiration is imperative while the

lumen is cleared, and while the sample is obtained. This avoids mixing the mixed venous blood sample with the oxygenated blood from the pulmonary circulation. Flush the lumen with the heparinized solution after sampling to clear the catheter of blood and to prevent clotting of the lumen.

AGE-SPECIFIC CONSIDERATIONS

1. For children who weigh less than 15-18 kg, use a 6.0-French introducer; a 5- to 5.5-French PA catheter for children weighing 14-18 kg; and 7-French for children weighing 18-20 kg (Hazinski, 2002). In very small children, the injectate port of the catheter may not be in the RA, and a shorter catheter may be needed.
2. A PA catheter may be indicated in a pediatric patient who has sepsis or who is in shock that does not respond to fluid therapy and inotropic support, as well as to monitor the effects of a new drug that may cause cardiovascular instability. A PA catheter may be indicated in a child with pulmonary hypertension, but the risk of PA rupture must be weighed against the benefit of the information gathered.
3. A PA catheter insertion is contraindicated in pediatric patients who have large intracardiac shunts. Caution should be used in children with serious dysrhythmias, severe coagulopathies, and low cardiac output, in whom the balloon may not be able to float through the RV (Daily & Schroeder, 1994).
4. Normal resting values in children are not the same as those in adults, and they depend on the age of the child (Table 92-2).
5. The small lumens in the 5-French catheter are easily occluded by fibrin, making it imperative to maintain a continuous flush system at all times.

COMPLICATIONS

1. A pneumothorax may result from internal jugular or subclavian insertion.
2. A hemothorax or hematoma may result from vascular damage. If a hematoma appears on one side of the neck, observe the patient for airway obstruction and do not attempt cannulation on the opposite side of the neck.
3. An air embolism may occur during the time of insertion or if there is a loose connection anywhere in the system.

TABLE 92-2
NORMAL PEDIATRIC VALUES

	Newborn	Child
Right atrium	Mean, 0-4 mm Hg	Mean, 0-4 mm Hg
Right ventricle	50/3 mm Hg	30/3 mm Hg
Pulmonary artery	50/30 mm Hg	30/12 mm Hg
Pulmonary artery occlusive pressure	Mean, 4-8 mm Hg	Mean, 4-8 mm Hg
Cardiac output*	4-8 L/min	4-8 L/min
Cardiac index*	3.3-6 L/min/m^2	3.3-6 L/min

Data from Hazinski, M.F. (1992). *Nursing care of the critically ill child,* 2nd ed. St. Louis: Mosby; Toro-Figueroa Figueroa, L.O., & Levine, D.L. (1997). Pulmonary artery catheterization pp. 203-212. In Dieckmann, R.A., Fiser, D.H., & Selbst, S.M. (Eds.), *Pediatric emergency and critical care procedures.* St. Louis: Mosby.
*Cardiac index is preferred over cardiac output in children because It factors in the child's size.

4. Cardiac dysrhythmias may occur (as previously discussed). In a patient with a preexisting left bundle-branch block, irritation of the right bundle branch may result in right bundle-branch block and lead to complete heart block. If the waveforms and pressure values indicate that the catheter has migrated back into the RV, inflate the balloon to cushion the tip of the catheter. This protects the RV from irritation by the catheter resulting in dysrhythmias. Notify the physician.

5. Pulmonary artery perforation may occur during insertion of the catheter if it is advanced too far with an underinflated balloon or if the balloon is overinflated during PAOP measurement. Inflate the balloon slowly and stop when the PAOP appears. Use caution in patients with high PA pressures when obtaining PAOP, because the high pressures may drive the PA catheter into the smaller vessels, resulting in infarction and/or hemorrhage.

6. Pulmonary infarction may result from frequent or prolonged PAOP measurements or migration of the catheter. The balloon should not be inflated for longer than three cycles, the time it takes to obtain the measurement. If the waveforms and pressure values indicate that the catheter had migrated into "wedge" position, reposition the patient and/or have the patient cough. If the catheter is still wedged, make sure the balloon is deflated and pull the catheter back to the PA position. Notify the physician. Do not flush the wedged PA catheter as this could lead to rupture of the PA.

7. Damage to the intracardiac structures may occur if the balloon is withdrawn while inflated.

8. Cardiac tamponade may occur if the RA or RV is perforated.

9. The balloon may rupture if there have been multiple inflations or if the catheter has been in place for a prolonged period of time. If the balloon ruptures, withdraw the air until blood is seen in the syringe and then close off the port. The catheter should be removed because the pieces of the ruptured balloon may come free and produce an embolus. In a patient with a right-to-left shunt, there is a greater chance for an air embolism to occur if the balloon ruptures. Use carbon dioxide to inflate the balloon in this situation because carbon dioxide is easily dispersed in the blood if the balloon should rupture (Hazinski, 2002). If an air embolism is suspected, place the patient in the left lateral Trendelenburg position, have the patient perform the Valsalva maneuver, and administer high-flow oxygen.

10. Infection or sepsis may occur in a catheter left in for a prolonged period of time. The catheter and sheath may be left in place for 5-7 days, as long as there are no signs or symptoms of catheter-related infection (Darovic & Kumar, 1999).

11. Thrombus formation may occur on the catheter tip or around the catheter and may lead to venous occlusion.

12. Endocarditis may occur during a prolonged PA catheter insertion.

13. Knotting or coiling of the catheter may occur. This is more frequent with the small-sized catheters or during a prolonged insertion time.

14. Neurovascular compromise may occur from a catheter inserted femorally or peripherally. Monitor the peripheral pulses.

15. Heparin-induced thrombocytopenia (nonheparinized PA catheters are available).

PATIENT TEACHING

1. Request assistance for position changes so that the catheter is not displaced.
2. Report any tubing disconnections or dampness around the site immediately.

REFERENCES

Daily, E.K., & Schroeder, J.S. (1994). *Techniques in bedside hemodynamic monitoring*, 5th ed. St. Louis: Mosby.

Darovic, G.O., & Kumar, A. (1999). Catheter and infusion-related sepsis (pp. 188). In Darovic, G.O., & Franklin, C.M. (Eds.), *Handbook of hemodynamic monitoring*. Philadelphia: W.B. Saunders.

Hazinski, M.F. (1992). *Nursing Care of the critically ill child*, 2nd ed. st. Louis, Mosby.

Hazinski, M.F. (2002). Pediatric evaluation and monitoring considerations. In Darovic, G.O. (Ed.), *Hemodynamic monitoring: invasive and noninvasive clinical applications*, 3rd ed. Philadelphia: W.B. Saunders.

Lynn-McHale, D.J., & Preuss, T. (2001). Pulmonary artery catheter insertion (assist) and pressure monitoring. In Lynn-McHale, D.J., & Carlson, K.K. (Eds.), (2001). *AACN procedure manual for critical care*, 4th ed. (pp. 439-456). Philadelphia: W.B. Saunders.

Toro-Figueroa, L.O., & Levine, D.L. (1997). Pulmonary artery catheterization (pp. 203-212). In Dieckmann, R.A., Fiser, D.H., & Selbst, S M (Eds), *Pediatric emergency & critical care procedures*. St. Louis: Mosby.

Neurologic Procedures

Positioning the Patient With Increased Intracranial Pressure

Ruth L. Schaffler, PhD(c), CEN, ARNP

INDICATIONS
1. To minimize increased intracranial pressure (ICP) in the presence of a head injury, a brain lesion, or other neurologic disorders
2. To facilitate venous drainage from the head

CONTRAINDICATIONS AND CAUTIONS
1. Avoid the prone and Trendelenburg positions. Some controversy exists as to whether the patient should be placed in a flat position, and ICP monitoring may be indicated. Types of monitoring devices available may include bolts or screws, cannulas, and fiberoptic probes (Brain Trauma Foundation, 2000; Bullock et al., 2000) (see Procedure 95).
2. Head elevation is commonly used to reduce ICP; however, this practice has been challenged. Some investigators argue that although head elevation lowers ICP, it also contributes to decreased cerebral perfusion pressure (CPP); others rationalize that a horizontal position increases CPP. Data suggest a moderate approach of head elevation between 15 and 30 degrees, which reduces ICP significantly without impairing CPP (Winkelman, 2000). Adequate blood flow to the brain is dependent on the CPP, which is the difference between the mean arterial pressure (MAP) and the ICP.

$$CPP = MAP - ICP$$

3. The patient's head should remain in a neutral position without rotation to the left or right, flexion, or extension of the neck.
4. Elevating the head of the bed more than 40 degrees may contribute to postural hypotension and decreased cerebral perfusion (Brain Trauma Foundation, 2000).
5. Minimize noxious stimuli. Warn the patient before you touch him or her, explain the procedures, and use gentle movements. Do not jar the bed, make loud noises, or use bright lights.
6. Plan turning or positioning activities separately from other nursing interventions. Allow at least 15 minutes between each activity to avoid a cumulative effect of ICP increases.
7. Head elevation is contraindicated in hypotensive patients because it further compromises CPP (Brain Trauma Foundation, 2000).

8. Spinal immobilization should be maintained until the patient's spine has been cleared of fracture per institutional protocol (see Procedure 115).

EQUIPMENT
Stretcher or hospital bed
Towel rolls or foam blocks (optional)
Cervical collar (optional)

PROCEDURAL STEPS
1. Place the patient in a supine position.
2. Maintain the head in a neutral position without flexion, extension, or rotation. If a cervical collar is used, be sure it does not obstruct the venous return via the jugular veins. Towel rolls or foam blocks can be used to support the head if necessary.
3. Place the bed or stretcher in the prescribed position.
4. Align the torso and the lower extremities. Avoid extreme hip flexion, which may increase intraabdominal pressure.
5. A padded footboard at the end of the stretcher or bed can prevent the patient from sliding or shifting positions when the head of the bed is elevated (Figure 93-1).
6. Padded side rails may be needed for seizure precautions.
7. If the patient must remain on a backboard, use a reverse Trendelenburg position to elevate the patient's head (Figure 93-2). Make sure the board cannot slide off of the foot of the stretcher or bed.

AGE SPECIFIC CONSIDERATIONS
The use of restraints and immobilization devices for maintaining body position may compound the patient's agitation and lead to increased ICP; this is especially true in young children.

COMPLICATIONS
1. Neck flexion or extension, or rotation of the head to the left or right, increases ICP by obstructing venous outflow.
2. Abnormal posturing may be stimulated by the position of the head in relation to gravity or by excessive noxious stimuli.
3. Pooling of secretions or skin breakdown may occur if the patient is not turned every 2 hours.
4. Turn and move the patient gently. Pain or agitation can increase ICP.

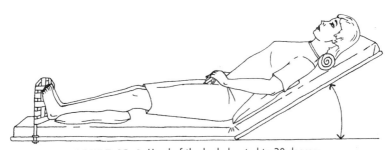

FIGURE 93-1 Head of the bed elevated to 30 degrees.

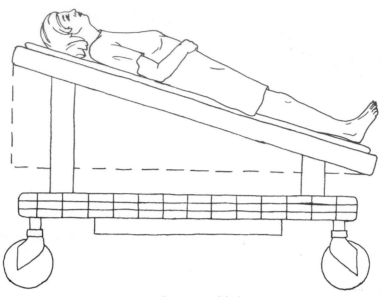

FIGURE 93-2 Reverse Trendelenburg position.

PATIENT TEACHING

1. Conscious patients should report increasing headache, nausea, or visual disturbances.
2. Explain that positioning is used along with other interventions to control the intracranial pressure. The position is to be changed every 2 hours.
3. Family members should be advised not to give the patient additional fluids or to change the position of the bed without asking the nurse.

REFERENCES

Brain Trauma Foundation. (2000). Part I: *Guidelines for the management of severe traumatic brain injury*. Retrieved June 10, 2002, from http://www.braintrauma.org.

Bullock, R.M., Chestnut, R.M., Clifton, G.L., Ghajar, B.C., Marion, D.W., Narayan, R.J., Newell, D.W., Pitts, L.H., Rosner, M.J., Walters, B.C., & Wilberger, J.E. (2000). Part 1: guidelines for the management of severe traumatic brain injury. *Journal of Neurotrauma, 17*, 450-553.

Winkelman, C. (2000). Effect of backrest position on intracranial and cerebral perfusion pressures in traumatically brain-injured adults. *American Journal of Critical Care, 9*, 373-382.

Lumbar Puncture

Lucinda W. Rossoll, BSN, MS, CEN, CCRN, ARNP

Lumbar puncture is also known as LP, spinal tap, or spinal puncture.

INDICATIONS
1. To assist in the diagnosis of meningitis or encephalitis in febrile patients exhibiting an acute alteration in mental status.
2. As part of fever work-up in a febrile infant less than 3 months old without any obvious source of infection.
3. To assist in the diagnosis of subarachnoid hemorrhage (SAH). If SAH is highly suspected and computed tomography (CT) of the head results are negative, LP may be required for diagnosis.
4. To instill medication, blood, or radiopaque contrast material into the subarachnoid space for the diagnosis or treatment of central nervous system (CNS) disorders.
5. To measure cerebrospinal fluid (CSF) pressure.
6. To diagnose acute or chronic demyelinating disease (e.g., Guillain-Barré, multiple sclerosis) or malignancies (e.g., carcinomatous meningitis, lymphomatous meningitis) (Simon & Brenner, 2002).

CONTRAINDICATIONS AND CAUTIONS
1. If an LP is performed in the presence of elevated intracranial pressure, herniation of the supratentorial area or through the foramen magnum may occur and may result in serious injury or death, because fluid drainage increases the pressure gradient between the supratentorial and lumbar spaces. In a patient with a history of a progressive deterioration of mental status, a worsening headache, localizing neurologic signs, or papilledema, a computed tomographic scan should precede the LP.
2. Positioning patients with excessive neck flexion may cause respiratory compromise, especially in children. Monitoring oxygen saturation via pulse oximetry can alert the nurse to problems during the procedure.
3. Performing an LP in an anticoagulated or thrombocytopenic patient may result in a spinal epidural hematoma.
4. A superficial infection at the puncture site could cause meningitis or an epidural or subdural empyema. Lumbar puncture through infected tissue is contraindicated.

EQUIPMENT
Sterile drape and towels
Gauze dressings
21- to 25-G, 2½- to 3-inch spinal needle with stylet
1% lidocaine with epinephrine

25-G, ⅝-inch needle and 21- or 22-G, ½- and 1-inch needles for anesthetic infiltration

3-5 ml syringe

Manometer with three-way stopcock (extension tubing optional)

Four collection tubes

Adhesive gauze patch

Antiseptic solution

NOTE: Preassembled kits containing all or some of these supplies are available.

PATIENT PREPARATION

1. Obtain a blood glucose level.
2. Assist the patient into a lateral decubitus position, with the shoulders and pelvis perpendicular to the stretcher. The patient should then flex or curl the back and maintain this position to separate the lumbar spinous processes. It may help to provide a small pillow for the head. The nurse should remain to assist with proper positioning, especially in children and infants and in uncooperative adults.
3. If the patient has bony deformities or is obese, a sitting position with head and arms resting over a padded bedside table may help to identify landmarks. This position can be maintained during the LP. Patients with bony deformities may need fluoroscopic guidance for the puncture.
4. If time allows, a topical anesthetic, such as EMLA, may be used over the insertion site.

PROCEDURAL STEPS

1. *Palpate the back to identify the spinous process levels. The level of L3-L4, L4-L5, or L5-S1 can be used safely, because they avoid the spinal cord, which ends at the level of L2-L3. The posterior iliac crest is even with L3-L4 (Figure 94-1). The site may be marked with an indentation from a fingernail or a skin marker.
2. *Cleanse the back in a circular fashion with an antiseptic solution.

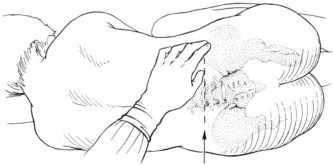

L3–L4 interspace

FIGURE 94-1 Patient position for lumbar puncture and the relationship of the posterior iliac crest to the spinous processes. (From Rosen, P., & Sternbach, G.L. [1983]. *Atlas of emergency medicine,* 2nd ed. [p. 149]. Baltimore: Williams & Wilkins.)

---

*Indicates portions of the procedure usually performed by a physician or an advanced practice nurse.

3. *Attach the sterile drape to the patient's back with the adhesive strips.
4. *Infiltrate the skin and the subcutaneous tissue with the anesthetic solution via the 25-G needle. Infiltrate the interspinous spaces with the anesthetic solution at the intended puncture site via the 22-G needle.
5. *Identify the intended puncture site and insert the spinal needle at the midline with the bevel parallel to the axis of the spine. The needle is often angled slightly cephalad. The patient feels pressure but should not feel pain.
6. *A pop may be felt once the needle passes the ligamentum flavum, and it is advisable at this point to remove the stylet and to check for the CSF every 2 mm or so to avoid passing through the subarachnoid space into the ventral epidural space. If the epidural space is entered, the patient may feel pain from the puncture of a nerve root, and a traumatic tap is likely, because of the venous plexus within the epidural space (Simon & Brenner, 2002).
7. *Once CSF is noted at the hub of the needle, attach the manometer and the three-way stopcock to measure CSF opening pressure. Extension tubing may be used between the needle and the manometer to allow greater flexibility, but the pressure should be measured at zero on the manometer at the level of the needle. The patient should relax the legs and the neck to help avoid falsely elevated pressures. Have the patient breathe quietly, and read the pressure when it comes to a rest and fluctuates only slightly with each breath. Normal CSF pressure is 50-200 mm H_2O (Lavoie & Saucier, 2002).
8. *Collect CSF specimens in the four collection tubes (Figure 94-2). Fluid from the manometer may be drained into the first tube. Usually, 1-2 ml is placed in each tube. The first tube is sent for a culture and sensitivity test, Gram's stain, and red blood cell count (if a traumatic tap is suspected, comparison with tube No. 4 is needed); the second tube is tested for glucose and protein determination; the third tube may be used for antibodies, antigens, or other specialized examinations (e.g., tuberculosis or fungal cultures); and the last tube is exam-

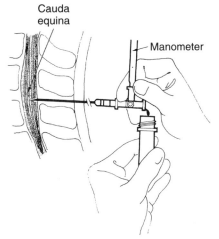

Cauda
equina

Manometer

FIGURE 94-2 Technique for collection of cerebral spinal fluid samples from a spinal needle with the manometer attached. The manometer may also be removed and the fluid collected directly from the spinal needle hub. (From Simon, R., & Brenner, B. [2002]. *Emergency procedures and techniques*, 4th ed. [p. 199]. Baltimore: Williams & Wilkins.)

---

*Indicates portions of the procedure usually performed by a physician or an advanced practice nurse.

TABLE 94-1

BASIC DIFFERENTIATION OF CEREBROSPINAL FLUID FINDINGS IN VIRAL AND BACTERIAL MENINGITIS

	Viral	Bacterial
WBC	Elevated, lymphocytes predominant	Very high, neutrophils predominant
Protein	Normal-to-mild increase	High
Glucose	Usually normal	Low (<60% of blood value)

WBC, White blood cell.

ined for the cell count (white and red blood cells). A fifth tube may be collected for cytology if necessary. Normal CSF findings include the following (Lavoie & Saucier, 2002):

   a. Clear, colorless fluid
   b. White blood cell count: <5/mm^3
   c. Total protein count = 15-45 mg/dl (adults). Numerous processes elevate protein level, including blood in the CSF, but levels above 500 mg/dl may indicate meningitis or other disease.
   d. Glucose is normally 60%-70% of the blood-glucose level; a decreased level may implicate disease of the central nervous system and is a useful indicator in differentiating viral from bacterial meningitis (Table 94-1).
 9. *Reinsert the stylet and slowly remove the spinal needle. Apply pressure to the site with a gauze pad, and then apply the adhesive gauze pad.
10. The patient should remain flat for at least 2 hours. Prone positioning may help reduce CSF leakage and thereby decrease the likelihood of post-LP headache.
11. Observe the patient for any changes in the level of consciousness (in case of worsening meningitis or possible herniation), altered motor or sensory status in the lower extremities, bladder dysfunction (spinal subdural hematoma), or complaints of headache.

AGE-SPECIFIC CONSIDERATIONS

1. Use 1.5-inch spinal needle for infants and toddlers (Zorc, 2001). A 21-gauge butterfly needle may be used for neonates (Simon & Brenner, 2002).
2. When positioning children, avoid excessive neck flexion, because this may occlude the airway and lead to respiratory compromise or arrest. A nurse should be in the room with the infant or toddler during the procedure, and oxygen saturation should be monitored. Excessive neck flexion may also impede CSF return.
3. The infant may be placed in the upright position with the thighs against the abdomen and the neck flexed forward. The infant may be stabilized against your torso and the arms immobilized with your hands (Emergency Nurses Association, 1998).

---

*Indicates portions of the procedure usually performed by a physician or an advanced practice nurse.

4. If the child is struggling or crying, CSF pressures may be falsely elevated. The upper limits of normal pressure in children are 110 mm H_2O for neonates and 200 mm H_2O for infants and young children (Zorc, 2001).
5. If a child cannot cooperate, consider the use of conscious sedation. Avoid ketamine because it can increase intracranial pressure (Zorc, 2001).

COMPLICATIONS

1. To differentiate between a traumatic tap and an SAH, compare the cell count of the first tube with that of the last tube. If a decrease in the number of red blood cells is noted, it is likely a traumatic tap rather than an SAH. Hemolyzed blood causes positive xanthochromia in the CSF if the SAH occurs at least 4 hours before the LP.
2. A spinal subdural hematoma may occur in thrombocytopenic patients or in elderly patients whose CSF was removed too rapidly or in too large a volume.
3. The use of a large spinal needle (18-20 G) creates a greater chance of CSF leakage and is often associated with headache (Simon & Brenner, 2002). If a significant postprocedural headache develops, a blood patch (injection of autologous blood into the epidural space) may be necessary.
4. Herniation of the transtentorial area or through the foramen magnum (rare).
5. A spinal epidural hematoma is rare, but it may occur in anticoagulated patients.
6. In a dry tap, no CSF is obtained.
7. An infection is usually related to an inadequate aseptic technique or a puncture through irritated or infected tissue. A local infection, meningitis, or epidural or subdural empyema may result.

PATIENT TEACHING

1. Monitor temperature and report it if it is greater than 101° F (38.3° C).
2. Take an analgesic or a prescribed medication for headache. Report a severe or prolonged headache.
3. Remain flat for at least 2 hours after the procedure. A prone position may help prevent a spinal headache.
4. Drink fluids to help replace CSF and prevent spinal headache.

REFERENCES

Emergency Nurses Association. (1998). *Emergency nursing pediatric course*, 2nd ed. Des Plaines, IL: Author.

Lavoie, F.W., & Saucier, J.R. (2002). Central nervous system infections (pp. 1527-1541). In Marx, J.A., Hockberger, R.S., Walls, R.M., et al. (Eds.), *Rosen's emergency medicine: concepts and clinical practice*, 5th ed. St. Louis: Mosby.

Simon, R.R., & Brenner, B.E. (2002). *Emergency procedures and techniques*, 4th ed. Baltimore: Williams & Wilkins.

Zorc, J.J. (2001) Lumbar puncture (pp. 43-47). Goepp, J.G., & Hostetler, M.A. (Eds.), *Procedures for primary care pediatricians*, St. Louis: Mosby.

Intracranial Pressure Monitoring

Reneé Semonin Holleran, RN, PhD, CEN, CCRN, CFRN, SANE

Intracranial pressure monitoring devices are also known as bolts, screws, and ventriculostomy catheters.

INDICATIONS

To measure intracranial pressure (ICP), which allows for calculation of cerebral perfusion pressure (CPP). CPP is an important indicator of cerebral blood flow. ICP monitoring may be useful in patients with the following conditions (Sullivan, 2001a; Sullivan, 2001b; American Association of Neurological Surgeons, 2000; Salim & Khoo, 2002):

1. Severe head injury (Glasgow Coma Scale ≤7) in patients who are hemodynamically unstable, so that computed tomography (CT) cannot be obtained because of prolonged resuscitative or operative interventions
2. Severe head injury with normal computed tomographic scan in the presence of two or more of the following: age >40 years, unilateral or bilateral motor posturing, systolic blood pressure <90 mm Hg
3. Severe head injury in patients in whom computed tomography/magnetic resonance imaging (MRI) demonstrates diffuse injury
4. Anoxic event that may contribute to secondary cerebral injury (e.g., near-drowning)
5. To monitor the effects of specific interventions (hyperventilation, diuresis) on the patient's ICP/CPP

CONTRAINDICATIONS AND CAUTIONS

1. Severe coagulopathy and chronic coagulopathy (hemophilia, von Willebrand disease) are absolute contraindications to ICP monitor insertion because of the high risk of intracranial hemorrhage (Salim & Khoo, 2002).
2. Relative contraindications include infection, open wounds of the scalp and skull near the planned insertion site, and immunosuppression. Small or effaced ventricles are a relative contraindication for ventriculostomy (Salim & Khoo, 2002).
3. The resuscitation process may make it difficult to set up and obtain accurate ICP readings, and other resuscitation priorities may preclude placement of an ICP monitoring device in the emergency department.
4. Kinked tubing, air bubbles, catheter movement, failure to properly zero the transducer, and loose connections can contribute to inaccurate readings.
5. An intraventricular catheter (IVC) can become occluded with blood or brain tissue and cease to function.
6. A fiberoptic or pressure-sensing ICP monitor is easily damaged and cannot be calibrated once inserted.

EQUIPMENT

Razor or hair clippers
Antiseptic solution
Sterile drapes and towels
No. 11 scalpel
Local anesthetic
10-ml syringe; 18-, 25-, and 27-G needles for local anesthesia (optional)
Twist drill
Nonbacteriostatic saline
3-ml syringe
Analgesics and sedatives as prescribed
ICP monitoring system options:
    Becker drainage system (fluid-filled system)
    Fiberoptic (Camino fiberoptic system)
    Transducer and cable for specific monitoring system being used
Monitor, calibrated, with ICP monitoring setup
Suture, needle carrier, scissors
Topical antibiotic
Sterile occlusive dressing

PATIENT PREPARATION

1. A conscious patient requires sedation and/or analgesia for this procedure. At a minimum, the area of insertion should be anesthetized with a local anesthetic.
2. Perform and document a baseline neurologic assessment, including the Glasgow Coma Scale and motor and sensory responses. Calculate and record the patient's mean arterial pressure (MAP).
3. Consider using restraints to prevent the patient from dislodging the monitor (see Procedure 192).
4. Calibrate the monitoring equipment according to the manufacturer's recommendations.
5. Place the patient in a supine position.
6. Administer analgesia and sedation as prescribed.
7. *Cleanse the site with an antiseptic solution, shave or clip hair, and infiltrate the site with a local anesthetic. There are five common places that an ICP monitor may be placed inside of the head, as well as many access devices available (Figure 95-1). The location and type of device are determined by the neurosurgeon (Table 95-1), depending on the advantages and disadvantages of each.

PROCEDURAL STEPS

1. *Incise down to the skull. Use a small twist drill to make a hole in the skull, aiming toward the ipsilateral medial canthus (see Procedure 96). Place the monitor as follows (Salim & Khoo, 2002):
    a. *Ventricular catheter: Penetrate the dura and insert the ventricular catheter with the stylet in place through the brain tissue until it is in the ventricle. Remove the stylet. Free flow of cerebrospinal fluid (CSF) confirms placement.

---

*Indicates portions of the procedure usually performed by a physician or an advanced practice nurse.

   b. *Subarachnoid bolt:* Insert the bolt into the subarachnoid space.
   c. *Subdural monitor:* Place the catheter or the fiberoptic monitor in the subdural space.
   d. *Epidural monitoring:* Place the epidural sensor between the skull and the dura.
   e. *Intraparenchymal monitoring:* Penetrate the dura and insert the sensor catheter into the brain tissue to a predetermined distance.

2. Irrigate the wound gently to remove blood and bony debris.
3. Attach the device to the calibrated monitoring system. Observe for an appropriate waveform (Figure 95-2). A ventricular drainage system requires that the sliding graduated-flow chamber be set at zero. The transducer is then aligned with a reference point at the anatomic level of the foramen of Monro. This is a point lateral to the canthus of the eye or the top of the ear

TABLE 95-1

ADVANTAGES AND DISADVANTAGES OF DIFFERENT INTRACRANIAL MONITOR LOCATIONS

Site	Advantages	Disadvantages
Epidural	Low infection risk	Cannot drain CSF
	Decreased risk of brain injury	Readings may be inaccurate
Subdural	Accurate readings	Increased risk of infection
	Easy to insert	Bolt may become obstructed by blood or brain tissue
Subarachnoid	Easy and quick to insert	May leak CSF
	Useful for patient with cerebral edema when the ventricles cannot be accessed	May become occluded
Intraparenchymal	Can be inserted quickly	Requires a fiberoptic system that is expensive and easily damaged
	Accurate and reliable readings	
Intraventricular	Most likely to display whole-brain pressures	Highest risk of infection
	Allows for drainage and sampling of CSF	CSF drainage requires constant nursing monitoring
	Accurate and reliable readings	Takes longer to insert and has more potential for injury to brain tissues

CSF, Cerebrospinal fluid.
Data from Luckmann, J. (Ed.). (1997). *Saunders manual of nursing care.* Philadelphia: W.B. Saunders; Mitchell, P. (1994). Central nervous system I: closed head injuries (pp. 383-434). In Cardona, V, et al. (Eds.), *Trauma nursing: from resuscitation through rehabilitation,* 2nd ed. Philadelphia: W.B. Saunders.

FIGURE 95-1 Sites for intracranial pressure monitoring. (From Youmans, J.R. [1996]. *Youmans neurological surgery,* 4th ed. [p. 505]. Philadelphia: W.B. Saunders.)

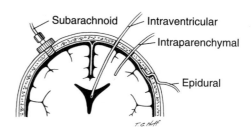

---

*Indicates portions of the procedure usually performed by a physician or an advanced practice nurse.

(University Hospital Patient Care Services, 2001) (Figure 95-3). Consult with the neurosurgeon for specific positioning information. For fluid-coupled monitors, the transducer may be zeroed before or after insertion. Fiberoptic and sensor systems must be zeroed before insertion (Sullivan, 2001a).

4. Once a good waveform is established, assist with wound closure and apply an antibiotic ointment and a sterile occlusive dressing.
5. Monitor and document the ICP.
   a. Document the initial ICP, quality of the waveform, and appearance of the cerebrospinal fluid. Normal ICP is 1-15 mm Hg (50-200 cm H_2O). However, like blood pressure, ICP is a dynamic, not static, number.

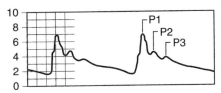

FIGURE 95-2 Normal intracranial pressure waveform at a rapid chart speed. The waveform should resemble an arterial blood pressure waveform. P1 is the percussion wave, P2 is the tidal wave, and P3 is the dicrotic wave. (From Youmans, J.R. [1996]. *Youmans neurological surgery,* 4th ed. [p. 497]. Philadelphia: W.B. Saunders.)

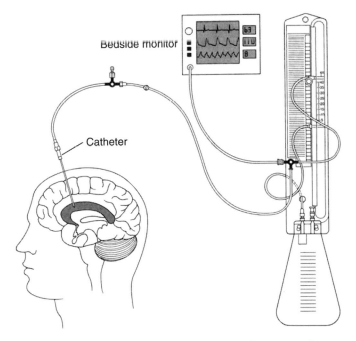

FIGURE 95-3 Intraventricular catheter attached to closed system for intracranial pressure monitoring and cerebral spinal fluid drainage. (From McNair, N. [1996]. Intracranial pressure monitoring [p. 298]. In Clochesy, J., Breu, C., Cardin, S., et al. [Eds.], *Critical care nursing,* 2nd ed. Philadelphia: W.B. Saunders.)

b. Calculate the CPP. CPP = MAP − ICP. Normal CPP is greater than 60-70 mm Hg.
c. The ICP waveform should fluctuate with respirations and heartbeats.

AGE-SPECIFIC CONSIDERATIONS

1. Neonates and infants with open sutures may not benefit from ICP monitoring because of their thin and pliable skulls (Bergsneider & Becker, 1995).
2. In infants and small children, the occipital or coronal approach is recommended because of their open sutures, fontanelles, and thin skull bones (Montague, 1990).
3. In children with an internal shunt, a shunt reservoir can be used to measure ICP as well as drain cerebrospinal fluid (Montague, 1990).
4. Normal ICP varies with age as follows: newborns, 0.7-1.5 mm Hg; infants, 1.5-6.0 mm Hg; children, 3.0-7.5 mm Hg (Vernon-Levett, 2001).

COMPLICATIONS

1. Iatrogenic epidural hematoma (Salim & Khoo, 2002).
2. Occlusion of a ventricular catheter by blood or brain tissue can occur. If the blockage is distal to a port that can be used for flushing, flush the system *away* from the patient and toward the drainage bag. If the blockage is proximal to the drainage port, notify the physician.
3. If a break in the sterile system occurs, notify the physician.
4. If a dampened waveform appears, check for the presence of air bubbles or loose connections. Flush the system with solution in the direction *away* from the patient and toward the drainage bag. Check that all connections are intact.
5. If the ICP waveform is lost or the catheter is not draining, check that all equipment is functioning. Recalibrate the monitor. If the waveform is still inadequate, notify the physician.
6. Monitor for signs and symptoms of infection, including fever, redness, or drainage at the insertion site; headache; nuchal rigidity; or seizures.

PATIENT TEACHING

1. Remain in a supine position so the monitor functions accurately. Do not touch or manipulate the ICP device.
2. Allow visitors to talk to and touch the patient, but try to keep external stimulation to a minimum.

REFERENCES

American Association of Neurological Surgeons (AANS): The brain trauma foundation: joint section on neurotrauma and critical care. (2000). Guidelines for the management of severe traumatic brain injury. *Journal of Neurotrauma*, *17*, 6-7.

Bergsneider, M., & Becker, D. (1995). Intracranial pressure monitoring (pp. 311-315). In Ayers, S., Grenvick, A., Holbrook, P.R. (Eds.), *Textbook of critical care*, 3rd ed. Philadelphia: W.B. Saunders.

Montague, D. (1990). Intracranial pressure measurements (pp. 879-887). In Blumer, J. (Ed.), *A practical guide to pediatric intensive care*. St. Louis: Mosby.

Salim, A., & Khoo, L. (2002). Intracranial pressure monitoring. In Shoemaker, W.C., Velamahos, G.C., & Demetriades, D. (Eds.), *Procedures and monitoring for the critically ill*. Philadelphia: W.B. Saunders.

Sullivan, J. (2001a). Intracranial bolt insertion (pp. 551-560). In Lynn-McHale, D., & Carlson, K.K. (Eds), *AACN procedure manual for critical care*, 4th ed. Philadelphia: W.B. Saunders.

Sullivan, J. (2001b). Intraventricular catheter insertion, monitoring, care, troubleshooting, and removal (pp. 561-569). In Lynn-McHale, D., & Carlson, K.K. (Eds), *AACN procedure manual for critical care*, 4th ed. Philadelphia: W. B. Saunders.

University Hospital Patient Care Services (2001). *Intraventricular pressure monitoring and drainage system.* Cincinnati, OH: Author.

Vernon-Levett, P. (2001). Intracranial dynamics (pp. 323-368). In Curley, M.A.Q., & Maloney-Harmon, P.A. (Eds.), *Critical care nursing of infants and children*, 2nd ed. Philadelphia: W.B. Saunders.

PROCEDURE 96

Burr Holes

Dawn A. Smith, RN, MS, CEN

Burr holes are also known as skull trephination or twist drill holes.

INDICATIONS
1. To place an intracranial pressure (ICP) monitoring device (see Procedure 95).
2. To relieve increased ICP in a patient with a suspected epidural or subdural hematoma when the following conditions exist (Simon & Brenner, 2002):
   a. The patient is nonresponsive to conventional first-line interventions to decompress the brain tissue and prevent brain herniation (such as occurs in hyperventilation or hyperosmolar or diuretic therapy), and
   b. The patient also exhibits a rapidly deteriorating neurologic status manifested by a unilateral dilated and fixed pupil and contralateral hemiparesis or hemiplegia, and
   c. An operating room and/or a neurosurgeon is not available, and transport time is lengthy.

CONTRAINDICATIONS AND CAUTIONS
1. Therapeutic burr holes are rarely placed in the emergency department. The optimal environment for hematoma evacuation is in the controlled atmosphere of an operating room.
2. Make sure there is a secure and patent airway before inserting the burr holes; intubation is preferred.

3. Patients with hemophilia who are taking anticoagulants or who have other known or suspected coagulopathies require special treatment. Obtain baseline coagulation studies and prepare to administer vitamin K and fresh frozen plasma to decrease intracranial bleeding.
4. Therapeutic burr holes should not be attempted in patients who have intracranial hematomas without signs of tentorial herniation, such as flaccid extremities and bilateral fixed, dilated pupils, or when a neurosurgeon is immediately available (Winfield, 1992).
5. If a therapeutic burr hole is successful in releasing a hematoma, the patient's mental status may lighten and he or she may become combative. Be prepared to administer sedatives and analgesics.

EQUIPMENT
Burr hole or craniotomy tray, which includes the following:
    Hand drill with bits (or twist drill) and drill stop
    Knife handle with No. 10, 11, or 15 blade
    Two curved hemostats
    Dural suction tip
    Scalp or dural hook
    Self-retaining retractors
    Sterile towels and drapes
    NOTE: Disposable trays are commercially available.
Local anesthetic with epinephrine (optional)
Syringes and needles for local anesthesia
Electric hair clippers or razor
Antiseptic solution
Gauze dressings
Hemostatic agents (Gelfoam)
Bone wax
Monopolar disposable coagulator
Suture material
    3-0 chromic gut
    4-0 nylon

PATIENT PREPARATION
1. Insert a gastric tube to decompress the stomach and help prevent aspiration (see Procedure 101).
2. Maintain cervical spine precautions if injury has not been ruled out. If no cervical spine precautions are needed, place the patient in the supine position with the head of the bed elevated 15-20 degrees (Simon & Brenner, 2002). For a therapeutic burr hole, turn the head so that the side of the head with the dilated pupil is parallel to the floor and is on the upper side (Winfield, 1992). Pupillary changes occur on the same side as the hematoma in most patients. If possible, place a sandbag or rolled towel under the patient's shoulder to help prevent kinking of the neck and venous outflow obstruction, which may increase ICP (Figure 96-1).
3. Shave the insertion site. If an epidural hematoma is suspected after trauma, a temporal burr hole is usually attempted first on the side of the dilated

pupil. Burr holes for intracranial monitoring devices are usually placed through the top of the head.

4. Cleanse the insertion site with an antiseptic solution.
5. Administer sedatives or paralytics as prescribed.

PROCEDURAL STEPS

1. *Anesthetize the site with a local anesthetic (optional depending on the level of consciousness of the patient).
2. *Drape the area to provide a sterile field.
3. *Palpate the superficial temporalis artery to determine its course through the skin. The temporal burr hole site is located just above the root of the zygomatic arch and one finger breadth anterior to the external ear (Simon & Brenner, 2002) (Figure 96-2).
4. *Using the scalpel, make a 3- to 4-mm vertical skin incision at the temporal site (Figure 96-3). Minimal bleeding is usually encountered and may be controlled by the application of direct pressure with a gauze dressing.
5. *Expose the burr hole site and place a self-retaining retractor (Figure 96-4). Spreading the self-retaining retractor usually results in a complete hemosta-

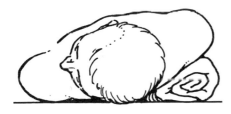

FIGURE 96-1 Patient position for emergency temporal burr hole. (From Winfield; J. [1992]. Emergency temporal burr hole in patients with clinical signs of progressive tentorial herniation [p. 219] In Jastremski, M S, Dumas, M., & Penalver, I., (Eds.), *Emergency procedures.* Philadelphia: W.B. Saunders.)

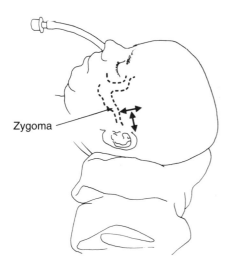

Zygoma

FIGURE 96-2 The temporal burr hole is placed just above the root of the zygomatic arch and one finger breadth anterior to the external ear. (From Simon, R., & Brenner, B. [2002]. *Emergency procedures and techniques,* 4th ed. [p. 190]. Baltimore: Williams & Wilkins.)

---

*Indicates portions of the procedure usually performed by a physician or an advanced practice nurse.

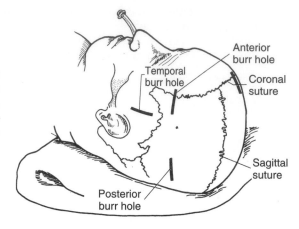

FIGURE 96-3 Placement of burr holes and incision sites. (From Simon, R., & Brenner, B. [2002]. *Emergency procedures and techniques,* 4th ed. [p. 190]. Baltimore: Williams & Wilkins.)

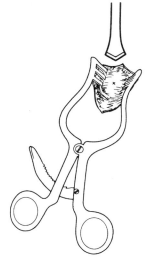

FIGURE 96-4 Use of a self-retaining retractor to expose burr hole site. (From Simon, R., & Brenner, B. [2002]. *Emergency procedures and techniques,* 4th ed. [p. 191]. Baltimore: Williams & Wilkins.)

sis. If bleeding continues, hemostats or a cautery can be used to stop the sources of the bleeding (Winfield, 1992).

6. *Using either the standard hand-held drill or a twist drill with a drill stop (Figure 96-5), introduce the drill bit perpendicular to the site and rotate the drilling in a clockwise motion to penetrate to the inner table of the skull. At this site, the skull is 3 to 8 mm thick and has three layers, so the drilling passes through three stages (difficult, easy, then difficult again) as it approaches the inner table (Winfield, 1992).

7. *Using a saline-filled syringe, gently irrigate the bone dust from the site.

8. *Inspect the extradural site for a hematoma. Dark red, clotted blood usually indicates an epidural hematoma. Use the dural suction tip to assist in evacuating the clotted material (Figure 96-6). If the exposed dura begins to pulsate,

---

*Indicates portions of the procedure usually performed by a physician or an advanced practice nurse.

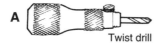

A

Twist drill

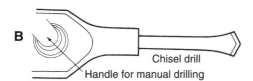

B

Chisel drill

Handle for manual drilling

FIGURE 96-5 A, Hand-held twist drill. **B,** Chisel drill bit. (From Simon, R., & Brenner, B. [2002]. *Emergency procedures and techniques,* 4th ed. [p. 189]. Baltimore: Williams & Wilkins.)

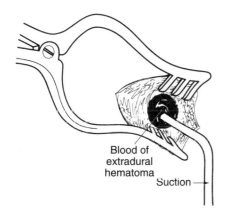

Blood of extradural hematoma

Suction

FIGURE 96-6 Once the extradural space is entered, a hematoma may be visualized. Use suction to remove any clots or hemorrhaging present. (From Simon, R., & Brenner, B. [2002]. *Emergency procedures and techniques,* 4th ed. [p. 192]. Baltimore: Williams & Wilkins.)

the procedure is finished and the incision may be closed (Winfield, 1992). If bright red blood is present, an active bleed is indicated and needs to be located and clamped until further intervention can be provided. Gelfoam strips may also be placed as a temporary measure to promote hemostasis.

9. *A bluish tinge usually indicates a subdural hematoma. Insert the dural hook through the outer layer of the dura, pull it upward, and incise with a No. 11 blade to release the accumulated blood. Suction may be needed to evacuate the clot. Use a low-vacuum setting to prevent damage to the brain tissue. If bleeding continues, small pieces of Gelfoam may be applied to the area.

10. *If no clot is seen, repeat the procedure at one of the other sites.

11. Apply a loose gauze dressing over the site and prepare the patient for transport to the operating room or a tertiary care facility for definitive treatment.

12. Assess and document the neurologic status.

COMPLICATIONS

1. Potential damage to the underlying brain tissue if the drill is advanced too far while the burr hole is being placed. This can usually be prevented by use of a drill stop.

2. Infection or subdural empyema

---

*Indicates portions of the procedure usually performed by a physician or an advanced practice nurse

3. Laceration of an artery or sinus perforation
4. Broken drill bit
5. False-positive or false-negative tap
6. Release of a tamponaded epidural may result in further bleeding and patient deterioration.

REFERENCES

Simon, R., & Brenner, B. (2002). *Emergency procedures and techniques*, 4th ed. Baltimore: Williams & Wilkins.

Winfield, J. (1992). Emergency temporal burr hole in patients with clinical signs of progressing tentorial herniation (pp. 217-221). In Jastremski, M.S., Dumas, M., & Penalver, L. (Eds.), *Emergency procedures*. Philadelphia: W.B. Saunders.

PROCEDURE 97

Tongs or Open-Back Halo for Cervical Traction

Daun A. Smith, RN, MS, CEN

Tongs for cervical spine traction are also known as Gardner-Wells tongs, skull tongs, caliper traction, or tongs.

INDICATIONS
1. To reduce and stabilize an unstable cervical spine secondary to fracture, subluxation, dislocation, arthritis, or neoplasm
2. To provide continuous traction and stabilization for an unstable cervical spine

CONTRAINDICATIONS AND CAUTIONS
1. Pins should not be inserted over skull fractures or through infected tissue.
2. The cervical collar should be kept in place during tong or halo application. When the traction is established and cervical spine films have been cleared, the hard cervical collar may be removed (Botte et al., 1995).
3. Addition or deletion of traction weights should be supervised by a physician.
4. Avoid sudden movements of the traction apparatus, patient, or bed.
5. Cervical tongs and open-back halos usually take 24 hours to become seated. The stability of the device should be assessed and documented frequently for the first 24 hours.

EQUIPMENT

Razor or clippers
Antiseptic solution
Sterile gauze dressings
Syringes and needles for local anesthetic
Local anesthetic for infiltration
Sterile open-back halo ring in appropriate size with sterile halo pins and
    halo torque wrenches
or
Sterile cervical tong set
(Both the cervical tongs and the halo apparatus can be obtained in a form
    compatible with the use of magnetic resonance imaging.)
Bed with pulley or traction system attached (e.g., Roto-Rest bed, Stryker
    frame)
Weights: assorted sizes—1, 2, 3, 5 lb
Weight holder, usually a C- or an S-hook

NOTE: Various tongs are available for insertion. This procedure discusses the Gardner-Wells tongs. Gardner-Wells tongs feature spring-loaded points for assisting in cervical traction (Gardner, 1973) and are easily placed on the patient in the emergency department (Figure 97-1). Tong selection is usually by physician preference or availability.

Open-back halo traction devices are also easily applied in the emergency department and may be attached to traction via a pulley or immediately fitted to a halo vest in the stable patient.

PATIENT PREPARATION

1. Assess and document neurologic status.
2. Shave or clip a small area of hair from the scalp at selected sites for tong or halo pin insertion.
3. Cleanse the area with an antiseptic solution.
4. *Infiltrate the pin insertion sites with a local anesthetic.
5. Instruct the patient to report immediately any increased pain, paresthesia, or difficulty in breathing during or after the insertion.
6. Consider sedation so that the patient may be comfortable yet remain awake enough that peripheral neurologic status may be monitored during the application of the immobilization device (see Procedure 181).

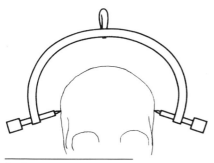

FIGURE 97-1 Gardner-Wells tongs. (From Simon, R., & Brenner, B. [2002]. *Emergency procedures and techniques,* 4th ed. [p. 203]. Baltimore: Williams & Wilkins.)

---

*Indicates portions of the procedure usually performed by a physician or an advanced practice nurse.

PROCEDURAL STEPS
Gardner-Wells Tongs

1. *Apply points of tongs below the temporal ridges and in line with the external auditory meatus. Tighten each side alternately until the spring-loaded mechanism extends approximately 1 mm on each side (Figure 97-2). This indicates a squeezing pressure of 30 pounds (Simon & Brenner, 2002).
2. *Gently rock the tong back and forth to ensure that it is securely seated in the scalp.
3. *Connect the S-hook on the tongs to the pulley rope. Cervical flexion and extension may be obtained by adjusting the height of the pulley (Gardner, 1973).
4. *Place the desired amount of weight onto the weight holder. Ten pounds is usually needed for the head, and an additional 5 lb per disk space is required

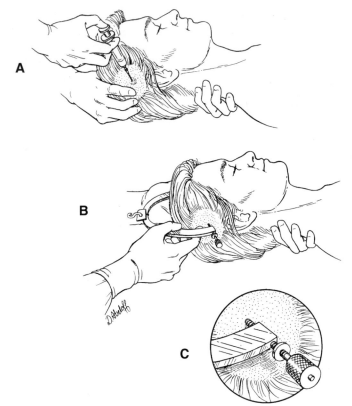

FIGURE 97-2 A, Anesthetizing the insertion site. **B,** Placement of Gardner-Wells tongs. **C,** Indicator of spring-loaded pins extends 1 mm on each side when a squeeze pressure of 30 lb has been obtained. (From Rosen, P., & Sternbach, G.L. [1983]. *Atlas of emergency medicine,* 2nd ed. [p. 153]. Baltimore: Williams & Wilkins.)

---

*Indicates portions of the procedure usually performed by a physician or an advanced practice nurse.

for reduction. Additional weight may be needed to overcome severe muscle spasm in the neck or upper back.

5. Obtain a radiograph to check alignment 5-10 minutes after each weight or position change.

6. To prevent rotation of the head, place sandbags under the projecting points of the tongs. This is especially important in odontoid fractures (Simon & Brenner, 2002).

7. Perform pin site care according to institutional guidelines.

Open-Back Halo

1. *Measure the patient's head circumference, and select the appropriate-sized halo according to the manufacturer's guidelines.

2. *Select pin sites. Anterior pins should be placed 1 cm above the lateral third of each eyebrow. Posterior pins should be placed in the lateral occipital areas at approximate positions of 4 o'clock and 8 o'clock (midforehead = 12 o'clock) (Botte et al., 1995).

3. *Keep the halo sterile so that contamination does not occur as each pin is passed through the ring and into the skin and the skull.

4. *Place the halo using positioning pins or padding, so that there is approximately 1 cm of clearance from the head below the equator of the skull but above the top of the ear.

5. *Insert the four skull pins and turn until finger-tight, as perpendicular to the skull as possible (Figure 97-3).

6. *Advance each pin through the skin into the skull using torque wrenches. During the anterior pin placement, the patient's eyes should be closed (to prevent difficulty in closing the eyes after the pin placement). Tighten diagonally opposite pairs of pins at alternating 2 inches per pound intervals until the desired torque of 8 inches per pound is reached (The torque wrenches stop functioning when the desired pressure is reached.) (Figure 97-4).

7. *Gently place pin locks or locknuts according to the manufacturer's guidelines.

8. Apply traction as described for the Gardner-Wells tongs.

9. Obtain postprocedure cervical spine films.

10. Perform pin site care according to institutional guidelines.

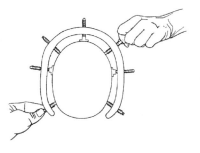

FIGURE 97-3 Insertion of halo pins until "finger-tight." (Courtesy Ace Medical Company, El Segundo, CA.)

---

*Indicates portions of the procedure usually performed by a physician or an advanced practice nurse.

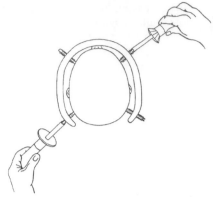

FIGURE 97-4 Tightening alternate halo pins with torque wrenches. (Courtesy Ace Medical Company, El Segundo, CA.)

AGE-SPECIFIC CONSIDERATIONS

1. Less weight is needed for traction in small children; 1-2 lb may be adequate for upper cervical injuries. Be careful not to use excessive weight, which may result in overdistraction.
2. Patient cooperation in remaining immobile is paramount. In children, cooperation must be obtained in a manner appropriate to the child's developmental level (see Procedure 193).

COMPLICATIONS

1. Pin loosening
2. Infection
3. Pin site pain
4. Penetration of the skull and dura
5. Loss of immobilization
6. Dysphagia
7. Bleeding at pin sites
8. Nerve injury secondary to excessive traction or inadequate traction
9. Sensory deprivation secondary to restrictions from the halo device

PATIENT TEACHING

1. Report nausea immediately.
2. Report increased pain at the insertion site, neck, or across the shoulders.
3. Avoid sudden movements because mobility of the neck and head is severely restricted.

REFERENCES

Botte, M.J., Byrne, T.P., Abrams, R.A., & Garfin, S.R. (1995). The halo skeletal fixator: current concepts of application and maintenance. *Orthopedics, 18,* 463-467.

Gardner, W. (1973). The principle of spring-loaded points for cervical traction. *Journal of Neurosurgery, 39,* 543.

Simon, R.R., & Brenner, B.E. (2002). *Emergency procedures and techniques,* 4th ed. Baltimore, MD: Williams & Wilkins.

Abdominal and Genitourinary Procedures

Diagnostic Peritoneal Lavage

Jean A. Proehl, RN, MN, CEN, CCRN

Diagnostic peritoneal lavage (DPL) is also known as "belly tap," "peri dial," "peri" lavage, and peritoneal lavage.

INDICATIONS

1. To help diagnose intraabdominal bleeding or viscous perforation after abdominal trauma, especially in patients who are unable to contribute to the physical examination because of paralysis, unconsciousness, or intoxication or in patients in whom the examination is equivocal because of lower rib, pelvis, or lumbar spine fractures
2. To evaluate patients at risk for intraabdominal trauma who are about to undergo lengthy anesthesia for nonabdominal surgical or radiographic procedures
3. To assess patients with undiagnosed hypotension after trauma
4. To provide core rewarming for moderately to severely hypothermic patients (temperature <32° C [90° F])

CONTRAINDICATIONS AND CAUTIONS

1. Computed tomography or ultrasonography of the abdomen is performed instead of peritoneal lavage in many situations.
2. If abdominal surgery is already indicated because of physical examination or clinical presentation, there is no need to perform peritoneal lavage.
3. Multiple prior abdominal surgeries increase the risk of adhesions, which may cause the intestines to adhere to the abdominal wall and result in viscous perforation when the catheter is introduced.
4. Pregnancy of more than 12 weeks' gestation is a relative contraindication; if performed, peritoneal lavage should be superior to the uterus by the open technique (American College of Surgeons [ACS], 1997).
5. Pelvic fractures may cause false-positive results; therefore, a supraumbilical insertion site should be chosen.
6. Because insertion of the catheter through a hematoma may cause false-positive results, an alternative site should be chosen.
7. Peritoneal lavage does not rule out retroperitoneal injuries (pancreas or duodenum), perforation of a hollow viscous, or diaphragmatic disruption.
8. Morbid obesity, advanced cirrhosis, and preexisting coagulopathy are relative contraindications to DPL (ACS, 1997).

EQUIPMENT

Razor or clippers
Antiseptic solution
Scalpel (nos. 10, 11, or 15)

Mosquito forceps
Gauze sponges
1% lidocaine (with epinephrine)
10-ml syringe, 18-G or 25- to 27-G needles for local anesthesia
1000 ml of warmed (36.6°-37.7° C) normal saline or lactated Ringer's solution
Peritoneal dialysis catheter (with or without trocar) or catheter, dilator, and spring-wire guide assembly
Nonvented intravenous (IV) tubing without a backcheck valve or cystoscopy tubing
Sterile drapes or towels
20-ml syringe
Blood collection tubes (optional, for transport of lavage specimens to the laboratory)
Needle holder
4-0 nylon suture
Antibiotic ointment
Adhesive tape
NOTE: Preassembled kits containing much of this equipment are available.

PATIENT PREPARATION

1. Insert an indwelling urinary catheter (Procedure 107) to decompress the bladder and to prevent bladder perforation when the catheter is introduced. The peritoneal dialysis catheter should not be inserted until this step is completed unless the cutdown technique with direct visualization of the peritoneum is used (Simon & Brenner, 2002.)
2. Insert a gastric tube (Procedure 101) to decompress the stomach and to prevent stomach perforation during catheter insertion.
3. If possible, complete any abdominal radiographs before the procedure, because air may enter the abdomen and confuse any future abdominal films.
4. Place the patient in the supine position.
5. *Shave the abdomen or clip the hair and cleanse it with antiseptic solution. The usual site for catheter insertion is midline, one third of the distance between the umbilicus and the symphysis pubis. The umbilical or supraumbilical areas may also be used.

PROCEDURAL STEPS

1. *Drape the abdomen with sterile towels.
2. *Infiltrate the insertion site with lidocaine. In general, lidocaine with epinephrine is used to help control bleeding at the site. Absolute hemostasis at the site is essential to help prevent false-positive results.
3. *Insert the catheter into the peritoneal space via guide wire or trocar. For the trocar technique, incise through the abdominal skin and the subcutaneous tissue and insert the trocar/catheter through the abdominal wall. If conscious, the patient may assist by tensing the abdominal muscles as the catheter is inserted. This facilitates catheter passage through the muscles and helps prevent viscous perforation. If desired, towel clips may be used to pro-

---

*Indicates portions of the procedure usually performed by a physician or an advanced practice nurse.

vide traction on the abdomen of unconscious or uncooperative patients. Alternatively, the catheter may be inserted over a guide wire (Seldinger technique). The guide wire is passed through an 18-G needle inserted into the abdomen. The use of a guide wire is associated with a lower risk of complications than the standard percutaneous technique (Simon & Brenner, 2002).

4. *For core rewarming or cooling, insert two catheters; one is used to infuse constantly and the other is used to drain the solution. This is more time efficient than infusing and draining via the same catheter.

5. If the lavage is for diagnostic purposes, attach a 20-ml syringe and aspirate. If 20 ml of blood is aspirated, the lavage is considered positive and is stopped at this point (ACS, 1997; Simon & Brenner, 2002).

6. Attach the primed IV tubing to the catheter (Figure 98-1). The IV tubing should not contain a backcheck valve because this prevents the fluid from being siphoned out of the abdomen. If the tubing is vented, the fluid may leak from the vent, or a water seal may form and prevent fluid return. Cystoscopy tubing allows much faster infusion and drainage. To connect the catheter to the cytoscopy tubing, push the end of the connecting tubing into the sleeve of the cystoscopy tubing. Tying a suture around the distal end of the sleeve of the cystoscopy tubing tightens the connection (optional).

7. Infuse 1 L of sterile warmed normal saline solution or lactated Ringer's solution. Room temperature solutions may cause or worsen hypothermia. Stopping

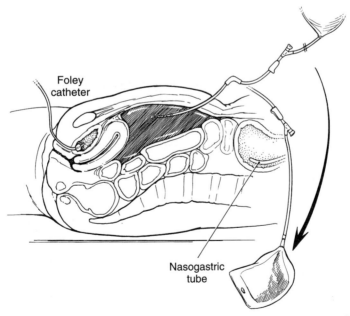

FIGURE 98-1 Lavage catheter in peritoneal space. (From Rosen, P., Chan, T.C., Vilke, G.M., & Sternbach, G. [2001]. *Atlas of emergency procedures.* [p. 111]. St. Louis: Mosby.)

---

*Indicates portions of the procedure usually performed by a physician or an advanced practice nurse.

the infusion before the drip chamber is dry facilitates siphoning of the fluid. Monitor urinary catheter and chest tube drainage for evidence of lavage fluid because this may assist with a diagnosis of diaphragm or bladder rupture.

8. If the patient's condition allows, leave the fluid in the peritoneal space for 5-10 minutes. Palpate the abdomen or gently rock the patient from side to side to help distribute the fluid throughout the peritoneal cavity.

9. Lower the IV bag to the floor and allow the fluid to siphon out of the abdomen. If the fluid does not return, make sure the appropriate tubing has been used. If necessary, cut off a backcheck valve or vent and drain the fluid into a basin. Then try repositioning the patient. The physician may reposition the catheter or insert another catheter to facilitate drainage. Additional fluid may also be instilled to encourage fluid return. Typically, 70%-90% of the fluid should be returned. Any fluid left in the abdomen is absorbed through the peritoneum and should be added to the patient's parenteral fluid intake.

10. Obtain laboratory specimens from the IV bag when the fluid return is finished. Commonly ordered tests include red blood cell count (RBC), white blood cell count (WBC), Gram's stain, and amylase. The fluid is placed in the same specimen tubes that would be used if the tests were being performed on blood. Some laboratories also accept the fluid in the IV bag or syringes. Positive findings include the following (ACS, 1997; Simon & Brenner, 2002):
RBC >100,000/mm^3
WBC >500/mm^3
Amylase >100 U/dl
Bacteria present on Gram's stain
Another, less accurate, method is to attempt to read newsprint through the returned fluid in the IV tubing. If the fluid is so bloody that newsprint cannot be read, the lavage is considered positive.

11. *Remove the catheter and suture the wound. If a laparotomy is indicated, the wound should not be sutured, and a sterile dressing should be applied. If the findings are equivocal, the catheter may be left in place, the wound sutured, and the lavage repeated 2-3 hours later.

12. Place a thin layer of an antibiotic ointment and a dry sterile dressing over the wound.

AGE-SPECIFIC CONSIDERATIONS

1. Children require sedation and analgesia. If a child is too young to cooperate with the procedure without deep sedation, DPL should not be performed. The patient should undergo computed tomographic scanning or, if the patient is unstable, DPL in the operating room under general anesthesia (Henneman, 1997).

2. Because distressed children tend to swallow air, which leads to stomach distention, it is essential that a gastric tube be inserted before the dialysis catheter is inserted.

3. Withdrawal of 10 ml of blood is considered positive for a child (Simon & Brenner, 2002).

4. Infuse 15-20 ml/kg of normal saline solution or lactated Ringer's solution in children (ACS, 1997; Simon & Brenner, 2002).

---

*Indicates portions of the procedure usually performed by a physician or an advanced practice nurse.

5. Trocars are not used in children; use a percutaneous approach instead.

COMPLICATIONS

1. Perforation of abdominal organs or blood vessels, resulting in peritonitis or hemorrhage
2. False-positive results, which may result from bleeding at the insertion site, bleeding within the muscle sheath, or pelvic fractures
3. Inadequate fluid return or false-negative results as a result of incorrect catheter placement
4. Wound infection or dehiscence, hematoma
5. Evisceration or incisional hernia

PATIENT TEACHING

1. Keep the wound clean and dry, and observe for signs of infection.
2. Have the sutures removed in 8-10 days.
3. Notify the nursing or medical staff if abdominal pain, tenderness, rigidity, or fever increases.

REFERENCES

American College of Surgeons, Committee on Trauma. (1997). *Advanced trauma life support course*. Chicago: Author.

Henneman, P.L. (1997). Diagnostic peritoneal lavage (pp. 604-606). In Dieckmann, R.A., Fiser, D.H., & Selbst S.M. (Eds.), *Pediatric emergency and critical care procedures*. St. Louis: Mosby.

Simon, R.R., & Brenner, B.E. (2002). *Emergency procedures and techniques*, 4th ed. Baltimore: Lippincott Williams & Wilkins.

PROCEDURE   99

Paracentesis

Lucinda W. Rossoll, BSN, MS, CEN, CCRN, ARNP

INDICATIONS

1. Abdominal paracentesis is a sterile procedure used to obtain peritoneal fluid for analysis, to diagnose new-onset ascites, or to diagnose infection in a patient with ascites.

2. To promote comfort and improve cardiorespiratory and gastrointestinal status by relieving intraabdominal pressure.

CONTRAINDICATIONS AND CAUTIONS

1. Bleeding. Coagulopathies, thrombocyctopenia, and portal hypertension with abdominal collateral circulation increase the chance of hemorrhage.
2. Caution in patients with multiple prior abdominal surgeries and adhesions as the intestines may be adhered to abdominal wall and result in viscous perforation during introduction of the needle.
3. An open supraumbilical or ultrasound-assisted approach is preferred during a second- and third-trimester pregnancy (Marx, 2004).
4. Caution in patients with infection at the insertion site.

EQUIPMENT

Antiseptic solution
Sterile drapes/towels
2-in sterile needle with inner trocar or intravenous (IV) catheter with stylet, size 10, 12, or 14
3-ml syringe and 18-G, 27-G × 1½-inch needle for local anesthesia
1% lidocaine with epinephrine
10-ml syringe
60-ml syringe
Scalpel, no. 11 blade
Sterile gauze sponges
Four empty 1000-ml vacuum bottles or other drainage collection container (e.g., bag, bottle)
Three-way stopcock
Nonvented IV tubing without a backcheck valve, or 36-inch pressure tubing
Four sterile tubes or cytology bottles for specimens
Male-to-male IV tubing connecter
Sterile dressing/tape/antibiotic ointment
NOTE: Preassembled trays with some or all of these supplies are available.

PATIENT PREPARATION

1. Have the patient void immediately before the procedure or if the patient is unable to void, place an indwelling catheter (see Procedure 107) to decompress the bladder and prevent perforation of the bladder during introduction of the needle.
2. Position the patient upright on the side of the bed or chair or in high or semi-Fowler's position. This helps fluid to accumulate in the lower abdomen. Alternatively, a lateral decubitus position may be used.

PROCEDURAL STEPS

1. Cleanse the abdomen with antiseptic solution.
2. *Drape the abdomen with the sterile drapes or towels.

---

*Indicates portions of the procedure usually performed by a physician or an advanced practice nurse.

3. *Infiltrate the insertion site with lidocaine.
4. *An incision is made midline 2 cm below the umbilicus, or alternatively, in a patient with midline scarring, either lower quadrant medial to the anterior superior iliac crest and 4-5 cm cephalad (Marx, 2004).
5. *Attach a 10-ml syringe to the catheter. The catheter is inserted slowly in 5-cm increments through the abdominal wall until peritoneal fluid is aspirated. Continuous aspiration during insertion is to be avoided because this may pull the bowel toward the needle. Remove the inner trocar or stylet.
6. Fluid may be drained by gravity drainage, by aspiration with 60-ml syringe, or by vacuum drainage.
   a. The paracentesis kit may come with a bag and tubing for fluid drainage by gravity, or IV tubing may be attached to the needle and the fluid is allowed to drain into a collection device. NOTE: Nonvented IV tubing should be used because fluid may leak from the vent in vented tubing. The IV tubing should not contain a backcheck valve because this would prevent the drainage of the fluid.
   b. A three-way stopcock may be attached to the needle and fluid aspirated by a 60-ml syringe.
   c. Pressure tubing may be attached to the needle. Attach a male-to-male adapter to the other end of the tubing and attach a needle. The needle is inserted into a vacuum bottle, and the fluid is removed by vacuum. If regular IV tubing is used, the vacuum may collapse the tubing.
   Limit drainage to 1-2 L to minimize the risk of shock secondary to fluid shifts. Marx (2004) questioned this limit, citing reports in which up to 6 L have been removed in 15 minutes without complication. Some practitioners may administer colloids to maintain intravascular volume.
7. Collect laboratory specimens in sterile containers. Commonly ordered laboratory tests include cell count, albumin, culture, and Gram's stain (Marx, 2004).
8. When needle is withdrawn, apply a thin layer of antibiotic ointment and dressing or as per institutional protocol.
9. Watch for and report bleeding, fluid leakage, or scrotal edema after procedure.
10. Check vital signs frequently to detect the onset of any hypotensive complications early. Recommendations are every half hour for 2 hours after the procedure, then hourly for 2 hours, then every 4 hours for 24 hours.

AGE-SPECIFIC CONSIDERATION

An older patient may not be able to tolerate sitting at the side of the bed for the period of time needed for procedure and may be placed in high or semi-Fowler's or lateral decubitus position.

COMPLICATIONS

1. Perforation of abdominal organs (bladder, bowel or stomach) or blood vessels, resulting in hemorrhage or peritonitis
2. Infection at insertion site

---

*Indicates portions of the procedure usually performed by a physician or an advanced practice nurse.

3. Shock secondary to fluid and electrolyte shifts
4. Leaking of peritoneal fluid at the puncture site. If leakage continues, a suture may be placed at the site.

REFERENCE

Marx, J.A. (2004). Peritoneal procedures (pp. 841-859). In Roberts, J.R., & Hedges, J.R. (Eds.) *Clinical procedures in emergency medicine*, 4th ed. Philadelphia: W.B. Saunders.

PROCEDURE 100

Intraabdominal Pressure Monitoring

Lucinda W. Rossoll, BSN, MS, CEN, CCRN, ARNP

Compartment syndrome is defined as a condition in which there is increased pressure within a closed space that compromises the function of organs and tissues within that space. Abdominal compartment syndrome occurs from elevated intraabdominal pressure, when the contents of the abdomen expand, leading to decreased venous return, decreased cardiac output, and dysfunction of the organs contained in the abdominal cavity. Normal intraabdominal pressure (IAP) is 2-10 mm Hg. Mildly elevated pressure is defined as 10-20 mm Hg and the physiologic effects of the pressure are compensated for. Moderately elevated pressure is 20-40 mm Hg, and severe is 40 mm Hg and higher (Harrahill, 1998). When IAP pressure is >25 mm Hg, renal dysfunction can occur. Abdominal pressure can be measured directly with an intraperitoneal catheter or indirectly via a gastric balloon or urinary bladder pressure measurement (gold standard).

IAP pressure is measured indirectly by measuring bladder pressure. The bladder acts as a pressure reservoir, a compliant structure that reflects pressure changes. There is a significant correlation between bladder pressure and abdominal pressure.

INDICATIONS

IAP monitoring is indicated for any condition that may produce elevated pressures in the abdomen, such as blunt abdominal trauma, abdominal aortic aneurysm rupture, bleeding, large hematoma, abdominal packing, bowel obstruction, abscess, peritonitis, visceral edema, ascites, tumors, burn eschar, or use of a pneumatic antishock garment.

CONTRAINDICATIONS AND CAUTIONS

Bladder pressure may not be accurate in a patient with a small or noncompliant bladder, or a patient in Trendelenburg or reverse Trendelenburg position.

EQUIPMENT

    500- to 1000-ml bag of normal saline
    Cardiac monitor with hemodynamic monitoring capability
    Pressure transducer cable
    IV tubing
    Pressure tubing, 12 inch
    Pressure transducer (if not already part of the pressure tubing setup)
    Pressure extension tubing
    Long pressure extension tubing (for pole-mounted transducer)
    Four-way stopcock or two three-way stopcocks
    Dead-end caps (nonvented) for stopcock ports
    Pressure-infuser bag or cuff
    Pole-mounted transducer holder (optional)
    Level (optional)
    60-ml Luer-Lok syringe
    18-G needle or IV catheter
    Clamp
    Povidone-iodine pads, swab sticks, or alcohol pad
    Urinary catheter with closed drainage bag

PATIENT PREPARATION

Place patient in a supine position, as flat as possible to negate downward pressure of abdominal organs that may falsely elevate pressure readings.

PROCEDURAL STEPS

1. Prepare the pressure monitoring system as follows (Figure100-1):
   a. Spike the normal saline solution with the IV tubing.
   b. Attach the four-way stopcock or the two three-way stopcocks (connected together) to the pressure transducer and attach the IV tubing to the stopcock. If two three-way stopcocks are used, one side port is the air-fluid interface and the other holds the 60-ml syringe.
   c. Attach the pressure tubing to the other end of the transducer.
   d. Attach the 18-G needle to the pressure tubing.
   e. Attach the 60-ml syringe to the side port of the stopcock.
   f. Flush the stopcock, pressure tubing, and transducer with normal saline. Cap each port with a nonvented cap after flushing.
2. Level the air side of the stopcock (air-fluid interface) to the top of the symphysis pubis.
3. Turn on the monitor and select either the 30– or the 60–mm Hg scale.
4. Connect transducer to the monitor and zero balance the transducer. Zero balancing the system to the atmospheric pressure negates the effects of the atmospheric pressure. To prevent erroneous pressure readings, zero the

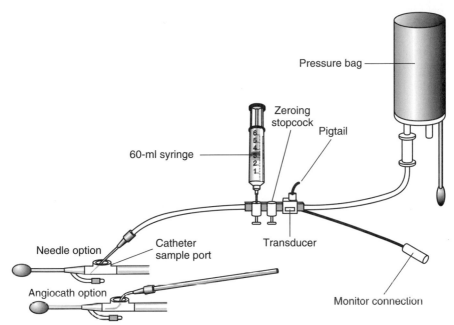

FIGURE 100-1 Intraabdominal pressure monitoring set-up using two three-way stopcocks in place of a four-way stopcock. (From Gallagher, J.J. [2001]. Intra-abdominal pressure monitoring [p. 676]. In McHale, D.J., & Carlson, K.K. (Eds.), *AACN procedure manual for critical care*, 4th ed. Philadelphia: W.B. Saunders.)

system before and after the pressure system is attached to the patient, with any significant change in the waveform and the values, whenever the system is disconnected, and at the beginning of each shift. To zero, turn the four-way stopcock off to the patient and open to the transducer and to air (air-fluid interface). Zero the monitor according to the manufacturer's directions. Once the monitor is zeroed, flush the open stopcock port and replace the dead-ender cap. Turn the stopcock on to the patient and on to the transducer.

5. Clamp the drainage bag tubing distal to the sampling port.
6. Cleanse port with alcohol.
7. Insert the 18-G needle into the sampling port of the drainage tubing or insert the 18-G IV catheter and thread the catheter into the port.
8. Instill 50 ml of sterile normal saline into the urinary catheter through the sampling port.
9. Briefly release the clamp to allow fluid from the bladder to fill the tubing and remove air from the system.
10. Run a strip of the waveform and read the mean IAP at end-expiration.
11. Document the reading and patient position (flat or supine).
12. Remove the needle and unclamp the drainage system. If an IV catheter is used, it may be left in place.

COMPLICATIONS
Urinary tract infection

REFERENCE

Harrahill, M. (1998). Intra-abdominal pressure monitoring. *Journal of Emergency Nursing, 24,* 465-466.

PROCEDURE 101

Insertion of Orogastric and Nasogastric Tubes

Lucinda W. Rossoll, BSN, MS, CEN, CCRN, ARNP

Orogastric and nasogastric tubes are also known as Levin, Lavacuator, Salem sump, Ewald, enteric, or feeding tubes.

INDICATIONS

1. To decompress the stomach through the removal of air or gastric contents
2. To instill fluid (lavage fluid, activated charcoal, tube feedings) into the stomach
3. To facilitate clinical diagnosis through analysis of gastric contents

CONTRAINDICATIONS AND CAUTIONS

1. In the presence of head trauma, maxillofacial injury, or anterior fossa skull fracture, there is the potential for inadvertent penetration of the brain via the cribriform plate or ethmoid bone if the tube is inserted nasally. In these instances, the orogastric route is used.
2. Caution should be used when inserting the tube in a patient with a potential cervical spine injury; the patient's head should be manually immobilized for this procedure.
3. If the patient has esophageal varices, there is a risk of inadvertent esophageal rupture and hemorrhage as a result of tube placement.
4. The smallest possible tube appropriate to the intervention or task should be used, because smaller tubes place less stress on the esophageal sphincter.
5. Do not irrigate a Salem sump tube through the blue air vent.
6. If tetracaine is used for intranasal anesthesia, the dose should not exceed 20 mg (Noorily et al., 1995).

EQUIPMENT

60-ml catheter-tip syringe
Water-soluble lubricant gel or 2% lidocaine jelly
Bite block or oral airway
Tongue blade
pH paper (optional)
Stethoscope
Emesis basin
Cup of water with straw (optional)
1-inch tape, benzoin, or commercial tube holder
Specimen container (optional)
Orogastric or nasogastric tube (Figure 101-1)

NOTE: The type and the size of the tube chosen relate to the size of the patient and the reason for the tube placement. Large-bore tubes are desirable for rapid removal of gastric contents. Smaller-bore tubes are chosen for diagnostics and for removal of air and gastric secretions. The single-lumen tube (Levin) is nonvented; it is used for gastric decompression, lavage, or feeding and should not be attached to suction. The double-lumen tube (Salem sump tube) is chosen if constant air flow and controlled suction force are desired.

Optional for nasopharyngeal anesthesia: Atomizer or mucosal atomization device (MAD, Wolfe Tory Medical, Inc., Salt Lake City, UT) with a 10-ml syringe.

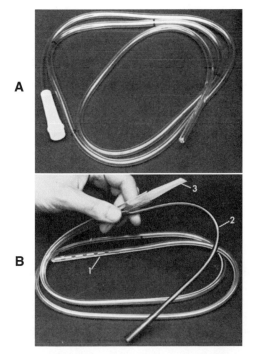

FIGURE 101-1 Two varieties of gastric tubes. **A,** Large-bore tube (Lavacuator, Levin, or Ewald tube). **B,** Salem sump tube: *1,* Gastric end with suction eyes; *2,* air vent tube; *3,* adaptor to connect gastric lumen to suction. (From Samuels, L.E. [2004]. Nasogastric and feeding tube placement [p. 794]. In Roberts, J.R., & Hedges, J.R. [Eds.], *Clinical procedures in emergency medicine,* 4th ed. Philadelphia: W.B. Saunders.)

Analgesic (tetracaine, lidocaine) and vasoconstrictor are administered as prescribed (oxymetazoline, phenylephrine).

PATIENT PREPARATION

1. Position alert patients in an upright or high Fowler's position. Position obtunded or unconscious patients head down, preferably lying on the left side.
2. If the nasogastric route is to be used, choose the largest naris. Have the patient occlude one nostril at a time and take a breath through the open nostril; select the nostril with the best air flow.
3. Estimate the length of the tube needed to reach the stomach by measuring the tube either from the tip of the nose to the earlobe and down to the xiphoid process or from the tip of the nose to the umbilicus. Mark the length (Figure 101-2).
4. The obtunded or unconscious patient requiring gastric lavage for drug overdose should be intubated to prevent aspiration.
5. If prescribed, apply a topical anesthetic to reduce pain during tube placement. Lidocaine jelly may be applied the inside of the nose with a cotton swab. Alternatively, anesthetics, such as tetracaine or lidocaine, with or without a vasoconstrictor, such as oxymetazoline, may be sprayed into the nose and posterior pharynx with an atomizer (Noorily et al., 1995; Wolfe et al., 2000).

PROCEDURAL STEPS

1. *Nasogastric placement:*
   a. Curve the tube by wrapping the end of the tube (4-6 inches) around finger.
   b. Lubricate the tip of the tube, choose the largest naris, and thread the tube through the naris, with the curved end pointing downward. Aim down and back toward the pharynx with the patient's head flexed forward (Figure 101-3).

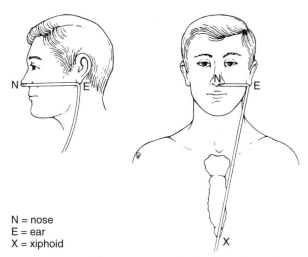

N = nose
E = ear
X = xiphoid

FIGURE 101-2 Measurement of the nasogastric tube. (From Smeltzer, S.C., & Bare, B.G. [2002]. *Brunner & Suddarth's Textbook of Medical-Surgical Nursing,* 9th ed. [p. 835]. Philadelphia: Lippincott Williams & Wilkins.)

c. When the tube reaches the nasopharynx, resistance may be felt. Apply gentle pressure downward to advance the tube. Try to rotate the tube to see whether it will advance. Do not force the tube. If tube still meets resistance, withdraw the tube and try the other side.

d. When the tube reaches the pharynx, the patient should flex the head forward. Flexing forward is desirable for tube passage in the alert, unconscious, or obtunded patient because it closes off the upper airway to facilitate insertion.

e. Advance the tube while the patient swallows (either mimicking swallowing or swallowing a small amount of fluid from a cup or straw) until the previously noted level or mark is reached. If the patient coughs, gags, or begins to choke, pull the tube back to let the patient rest. If patient continues to gag, use a tongue blade to check the back of the pharynx to see if the tube is coiled in the back of the pharynx. If tracheal or bronchial intubation is suspected, withdraw the tube before reattempting insertion.

2. *Orogastric placement:*
   a. In the uncooperative patient, place an oral airway or bite block in the mouth before attempting to place the tube. This prevents the patient from biting the tube and obstructing the flow or severing the tube.
   b. Lubricate the tip of the tube and pass it through the lips and over the tongue, aiming down and back toward the pharynx with the patient's head flexed forward (Figure 101-4).
   c. Advance the tube with the patient's swallowing motion until the previously noted mark is reached.

3. Center and secure the tube in place with adhesive tape or with a gastric tube holder. Do not tape the tube to the forehead because this places undue pressure on the nares, resulting in tissue ulceration.

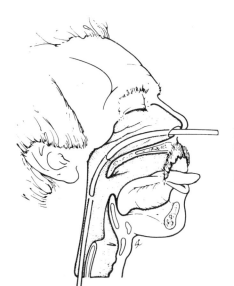

FIGURE 101-3 Placement of a nasogastric tube. (From Smith, S., Duell, D., & Martin, B. [2004]. *Clinical nursing skills,* 6th ed. [p. 601]. Upper Saddle River, NJ: Pearson Education.)

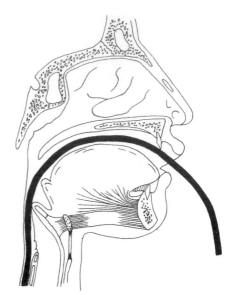

FIGURE 101-4 Placement of an orogastric tube.

4. Verify the tube position. Metheny & Titler (2001) recommend verifying tube placement by using methods a and b below. Hawks (1997) recommends verification of tube placement by using two of the following methods. End tidal CO_2 detection may also be used to check tube placement (see Procedure 26).
   a. Chest x-ray study is the best way to confirm tube placement (Metheny & Titler, 2001).
   b. Aspiration of gastric contents and assessment of the aspirate appearance. Gastric contents may be cloudy, green, tan, brown, bloody, or off-white.
   c. Auscultate over the epigastrium for air while instilling 30 ml of air. NOTE: This traditional method may be inaccurate. Metheny & Titler (2001) report that there is little scientific evidence to support the use of this method and that the literature contains numerous reports of its ineffectiveness.
   d. Aspirating a small amount of the gastric contents for measurement of the pH of the aspirant; gastric pH usually has an acidic range of 1-5 (Metheny & Titler, 2001).
   e. Small-bore feeding tubes present challenges in verifying placement. A chest x-ray study or pH test of the aspirate is recommended (Chen et al., 1996).

AGE-SPECIFIC CONSIDERATIONS
1. Nasogastric tubes should not be placed in infants because they are obligate nose breathers; use the orogastric route instead.
2. The diameter of the air passages of the nasopharynx is smaller in children, and their tongues are disproportionally large for the oral cavity.
3. Children in distress swallow large amounts of air. This can result in gastric distention, which can compromise an efficient abdominal examination as well as effective ventilation; therefore gastric decompression is a high-priority intervention.

4. Gastric dilation is common in children after traumatic injury and in children being ventilated via bag-valve-mask and may compromise ventilation or lead to vomiting and aspiration.

COMPLICATIONS

1. Hypoxia, cyanosis, or respiratory arrest as a result of inadvertent intubation of the trachea
2. Cardiac compromise as a result of vagal response secondary to gagging
3. Injury to the spinal cord if movement occurs during tube insertion in a patient with a spinal injury
4. Intracranial placement if a tube is placed through the nose in a patient with head or facial fractures
5. Nasal irritation or skin erosion, rhinorrhea, sinusitis, esophagitis, esophago-tracheal fistula, gastric ulceration, or pulmonary and oral infections from prolonged tube placement
6. Epistaxis from trauma during tube insertion
7. Vomiting and aspiration resulting in aspiration pneumonia secondary to a gagging response as the tube is passed
8. Aspiration secondary to incorrect tube position. Reassess tube position before instilling any medication, feeding, or irrigating.
9. Pharyngeal paralysis, vocal cord paralysis, and rupture of esophageal varices

PATIENT TEACHING

1. Report any respiratory difficulty or displacement of the tube immediately.
2. Do not manipulate or reposition the tube.

REFERENCES

Chen, C.A., Paxton, P., & Williams-Burgess, C. (1996). Feeding tube placement verification using gastric pH measurement. *Online Journal of Knowledge Synthesis for Nursing, 3*, No. 34, Document 10.

Hawks, J.H. (1997). Nursing care of the client with gastric disorders (pp. 1748-1785). In Black, J.M., & Matassarin-Jacobs, E. (Eds.). *Medical-surgical nursing: clinical management for continuity of care*, 5th ed. Philadelphia: W.B. Saunders.

Metheny, N.A., & Titler, M.G. (2001). Assessing placement of feeding tubes. *American Journal of Nursing, 101*(5), 36-45.

Noorily, A.D., Noorily, A.H., & Otto, R.A. (1995). Cocaine, lidocaine, tetracaine: which is best for topical nasal anesthesia? *Anesthesia and Analgesia, 81*, 724-727.

Smith, S., & Duell, D. (1989). *Clinical nursing skills*, 2nd ed. Norwalk, CT: Appleton & Lange.

Wolfe, T.R., Fosnocht, D.E., & Linscott, M.S. (2000). Atomized lidocaine as topical anesthesia for nasogastric tube placement: a randomized, double-blind, placebo-controlled trial. *Annals of Emergency Medicine, 35*, 421-425.

Gastric Lavage for Gastrointestinal Bleeding

Joni Hentzen Daniels, MSN, RN, CEN, CCRN, CNS and Margo E. Layman, MSN, RN, RNC, CN-A

In a gastrointestinal (GI) emergency, the primary clinical concern should be hemodynamic stability. Older persons are far more likely than younger adults to experience significant morbidity and death from untreated GI conditions or emergencies. In the Unites States, for example, 85% of deaths from peptic ulcer disease occur in persons aged 65 and older (Swaim, 1999).

INDICATIONS

1. To control an acute upper GI hemorrhage when other interventions are not immediately available. Other interventions may include electrocoagulation, injection sclerotherapy, photocoagulation (laser technology), vasoactive infusion (usually vasopressin), octreotide infusion, and transcatheter embolization.
   NOTE: Gastric lavage is still being performed to control acute GI hemorrhage, but its therapeutic value has not been proved. In many facilities, emergency departments have access to endoscopy units capable of performing esophagogastroduodenoscopy, the primary method of identifying the site of upper GI hemorrhage. Another small study suggests that irrigation is useful for patients with an upper GI bleed who have ulcers with clots (Laine et al., 1996).
2. To remove irritating gastric secretions and prevent nausea and vomiting through gastric decompression
3. To obtain information on the site and rate of bleeding
4. To help evacuate clots (Laine et al., 1996)

CONTRAINDICATIONS AND CAUTIONS

1. In the presence of GI hemorrhage, irrigation can knock the clot off a bleeding vessel and cause further bleeding, resulting in shock.
2. If the patient has a gag reflex but is obtunded or if the patient does not have a gag reflex, there is risk of aspiration if vomiting occurs during lavage. Endotracheal intubation should be considered in order to protect the airway.
3. Controversy exists regarding the use of iced or room-temperature solution. Some authors believe that iced solution causes a local vasoconstriction, resulting in decreased bleeding and in clot formation. Others maintain that cold temperatures stimulate hydrochloric acid production, thereby adding to gastric irritation. Iced solutions may cause hypothermia and prolong bleeding times; room-temperature solutions have been shown effective in clearing the stomach and promoting hemostasis (Thomas, 2001).

EQUIPMENT

Gastric tube (usually a large 32-to 26-French gastric lavage tube)
Irrigation tray
Stethoscope
Adhesive tape
Gloves, protective apron or gown, goggles, mask
Lubricating jelly (lidocaine gel may be used if ordered for patient comfort)
Cetacaine spray (may be ordered to locally numb the throat for comfort)
60-ml catheter-tip syringe
Tincture of benzoin
Normal saline or tap water
Bite block
Suction equipment

PATIENT PREPARATION

1. Protect the patient's airway from aspiration by endotracheal intubation if indicated (Procedures 9-11). Place the patient in left side-lying or semi-Fowler's position.
2. Have suction equipment readily available.
3. Place the patient on the cardiac monitor, pulse oximeter (Procedure 23) and assess the vital signs every 5-10 minutes.
4. Insert at least one large-bore intravenous line; two lines are preferred. Send blood samples for type and crossmatch as indicated (see Procedures 61 and 63).
5. Insert a gastric tube in the mouth or nose using lubricating jelly. If the gastric tube is inserted via the mouth, a bite block with a hole for the tube to pass through is preferable (Procedure 101).

PROCEDURAL STEPS

1. Pour normal saline or tap water into an irrigation container (Pinaka & Affronti, 2001).
2. Draw up the solution using a 60-ml syringe and inject it into the gastric tube. Alternatively, use a preassembled lavage setup. Infuse approximately 200-300 ml.
3. Aspirate or drain the solution from the stomach and discard it into a measured basin.
4. Repeat until active bleeding stops or until the patient is transferred to endoscopy.
5. Measure the volumes of irrigant and aspirant, and document as intake and output.

AGE-SPECIFIC CONSIDERATIONS

1. Comorbid conditions and decreased physiologic reserves make persons aged 65 and older particularly vulnerable to the adverse consequences of acute blood loss. Because of age-related changes, including decreased cardiovascular reserve and a higher risk for hemorrhage, any evidence of GI bleeding in an older patient demands diligent intervention (Swaim, 1999).
2. Be especially watchful of the older patient presenting with complaints consistent with GI bleeding who does not exhibit tachycardia in the presence of beta-blocker use.

COMPLICATIONS

1. Perforation of esophageal varices
2. Mallory-Weiss tear resulting from repeated vomiting, a sharp increase in intraabdominal pressure from overdistention of the stomach, or aggressive insertion of the lavage tube
3. Aspiration of gastric contents into an unprotected airway
4. Systemic hypothermia if the lavage is prolonged or large quantities of cold irrigant are used

REFERENCES

Laine, L., Stein, C., & Sharma, V. et al. (1996). A prospective outcome study of patients with clot in an ulcer and the effect of irrigation. *Gastrointestinal Endoscopy, 43,* 107-110.

Pinaka, J.D., & Affronti, J. (2001). Management principle of gastrointestinal bleeding. *Primary Care Clinics in Office Practice, 28,* 557-571.

Swaim, M.W. (1999). GI emergencies: rapid therapeutic responses for older patients. *Geriatrics, 54*(6), 20-22, 25-26, 29-30.

Thomas, R.H. (2001). Gastric lavage in hemorrhage and overdose (pp. 664-673). In Lynn-McHale, D.J., & Carlson, K.K. (Eds.). *AACN procedure manual for critical care,* 4th ed. Philadelphia: Saunders.

PROCEDURE 103

Gastric Lavage for Removal of Toxic Substances

Lin Courtemanche, RN, CSPI and
Jean A. Proehl, RN, MN, CEN, CCRN

Gastric lavage for removal of toxic substances is also known as gastric decontamination, orogastric lavage, gastric emptying, or stomach pumping.

INDICATION

To remove potentially toxic, orally ingested substances from patients who have ingested a life-threatening amount of a toxic substance less than 60 minutes before the procedure (American Academy of Clinical Toxicology [AACT] et al., 1997a). Contact your Poison Control Center for current recommendations regarding the treatment of specific ingestions.

CONTRAINDICATIONS AND CAUTIONS

1. "Gastric lavage should not be employed routinely in the management of poisoned patients" (AACT et al., 1997a). No conclusive clinical evidence has demonstrated improved outcomes with lavage, and significant morbidity may result from the lavage procedure itself. Gastric lavage should be considered when the ingestion is potentially life-threatening and when the procedure can be performed within 60 minutes of the ingestion (AACT et al., 1997a). Gastric lavage may be beneficial when it is performed more than 60 minutes after the ingestion of substances that are sustained-release formulations, substances known to form concretions, or substances with anticholinergic properties, all which slow gastric emptying. Research has indicated that some patients have a satisfactory clinical outcome without gastric emptying because administration of activated charcoal and aggressive supportive care are sufficient treatment (Bosse et al., 1995; Kulig et al., 1985; Merigan et al., 1990; Pond et al., 1995). Small-to-moderate ingestions of most substances do not require gastric lavage if activated charcoal can be given promptly, and these substances are bound to activated charcoal (Olson, 1999).

2. "Single dose activated charcoal should not be administered routinely in the management of poisoned patients" (AACT et al., 1997b). Administration of activated charcoal should be considered for potentially toxic ingestions of substances known to adsorb to charcoal; the greatest benefit of charcoal occurs with administration within 1 hour of the ingestion (AACT et al., 1997b).

3. "Routine use of a cathartic in combination with activated charcoal is not endorsed" (AACT et al., 1997c).

4. Gastric lavage may actually push tablets into the duodenum instead of removing them (Bayer & McKay, 1996).

5. Gastric lavage is contraindicated in caustic ingestions (risk of esophageal perforation). Lavage in hydrocarbon ingestions is contraindicated (risk of aspiration) unless a significant toxin is involved (e.g., camphor, halogenated hydrocarbons, aromatic hydrocarbons, metals, pesticides) (AACT et al., 1997a; Phillips et al., 1993).

6. Lavage is contraindicated for patients who have ingested large or sharp foreign objects or drug packets.

7. Patients without a gag reflex or who are obtunded, comatose, or convulsing require intubation before lavage to help prevent aspiration (AACT et al., 1997a). Activated charcoal should not be administered unless the patient has an intact or protected airway (AACT et al., 1997b).

EQUIPMENT

Pharyngeal suction equipment
Pulse oximeter
Endotracheal intubation supplies (if indicated)
Restraints (if indicated and prescribed)
Gastric tube, 36-40 French
Bite block
60-ml irrigating syringe with catheter tip
Lavage tubing setup (commercially available or may be constructed with
    Y-cystoscopy tubing, suction extension tubing, and enema bags)

Tubing clamps
Warm tap water or normal saline solution
Activated charcoal

PATIENT PREPARATION

1. Set up pharyngeal suction equipment (see Procedure 31).
2. Initiate pulse oximetry monitoring (see Procedure 23) and cardiac monitoring (see Procedure 58).
3. Restrain the patient as indicated and prescribed (see Procedure 192).
4. Intubate the patient if indicated (Procedures 9-12).
5. Place the patient on the left side in the Trendelenburg position (left lateral decubitus position with the head down) to promote the return of the lavage fluid, help prevent aspiration, and decrease movement of the gastric contents into the duodenum (Ellenhorn et al., 1997; Gorelick, 1997) (Figure 103-1).

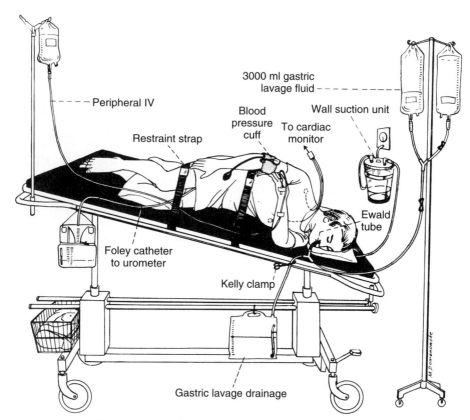

FIGURE 103-1 Correct positioning for patient undergoing gastric lavage. The patient is shown uncovered with side rails down for illustration purposes only. The patient should be covered to maintain body temperature and preserve privacy; side rails should be up for safety. (From Luckman, J., & Sorenson, K. [1987]. *Medical-surgical nursing: a psychophysiologic approach,* 3rd ed. [p. 1934]. Philadelphia: W.B. Saunders.)

6. Assemble the lavage tubing and prime it with fluid. Insert a large-bore oro-gastric tube (see Procedure 101). Place a bite block to keep the patient from biting the tube.

PROCEDURAL STEPS

1. Aspirate the stomach contents and save the initial sample for a toxin screen.
2. Unclamp the tubing between the fluid bag and the patient, and instill 150-200 ml of warmed (38° C) fluid. Using larger aliquots of fluid may move the gastric contents into the duodenum (Ford et al., 2001). Warming the fluid helps prevent hypothermia and may increase the efficacy of emptying (Gorelick, 1997). Reclamp the tubing.
3. Unclamp the tubing between the patient and the drainage source, and allow the fluid to drain into the bucket by use of gravity. If no fluid returns, use the syringe to pull the fluid and the particles gently through the tube. Position change may assist with fluid return. Do not use continuous suction to remove the fluid, because this may result in gastric mucosal damage. Allow the lavage fluid to drain by gravity until the recovered lavage solution is clear of particulate matter. Keep a running tally of the fluid input and output.
4. Repeat steps 1 and 2 until the fluid return is clear of stomach contents. If no gastric contents return, it is likely that the substance is in the small intestine or that large pill fragments are present and cannot traverse the tube.
5. If prescribed, instill activated charcoal (50-100 g for adults) before removing the lavage tube (see Contraindications and Cautions). Routine use of a cathartic is not recommended. The administration of a cathartic alone has no role in the management of poisoned patients. Based on available data, the routine use of cathartics with activated charcoal is not recommended. There are no published clinical data supporting the efficacy of cathartics in reducing ingestant bioavailability or improvement in patient outcome (AACT, 1997c).
6. With suction available, remove the tube with the patient in a lateral recumbent position; observe for vomiting.

AGE-SPECIFIC CONSIDERATIONS

1. Children are more prone to the vagal stimulation associated with endotracheal and gastric intubation and gastric lavage; monitor the heart rate carefully and consider premedication with atropine.
2. Use the largest gastric tube that can safely be inserted. Usual recommendations are for 16-22 French in infants, 24-32 French in children, and 36-42 French in adolescents and adults (Dart, et al., 2000).
3. Instill 10 ml/kg of lavage fluid per aliquot for pediatric patients. Warm normal saline solution is recommended instead of water in young children because of the risk of water intoxication and hyponatremia (Ellenhorn et al., 1997; Gorelick, 1997).
4. The activated charcoal dose for children is 1 g/kg for infants who are younger than 1 year and 1-2 g/kg for children 1-12 years. Charcoal with sorbitol is not recommended.

COMPLICATIONS

1. Inadvertent tracheal intubation.

2. Laryngospasm, decreased arterial oxygen saturation, aspiration pneumonia (Pond et al., 1995; Ford, 2001)
3. Sinus bradycardia, ST elevation on electrocardiogram (Pond et al., 1995; Ford, 2001)
4. Diarrhea, ileus (Pond et al., 1995)
5. Esophageal or gastric perforation or laceration
6. Hypothermia, especially in children (Gorelick, 1997)
7. Electrolyte imbalance if large amounts of nonisotonic solutions are used (Gorelick, 1997; Phillips et al., 1993)
8. Vomiting resulting in pulmonary aspiration of stomach contents if the airway is unprotected

REFERENCES

American Academy of Clinical Toxicology (AACT); European Association of Poison Centres and Clinical Toxicologists. (1997a). Position statement: gastric lavage. *Clinical Toxicology, 35,* 711-719.

American Academy of Clinical Toxicology (AACT); European Association of Poison Centres and Clinical Toxicologists. (1997b). Position statement: single-dose activated charcoal. *Clinical Toxicology, 35,* 721-741.

American Academy of Clinical Toxicology (AACT); European Association of Poison Centres and Clinical Toxicologists. (1997c). Position statement: cathartics. *Clinical Toxicology, 35,* 743-752.

Bayer, M.J., & McKay, C. (1996). Advances in poison management. *Clinical Chemistry, 42,* 1361-1366.

Bosse, G.M., Barefoot, J.A., Pfeifer, M.P., & Rodgers, G.C. (1995). Comparison of three methods of gut decontamination in tricyclic antidepressant overdose. *Journal of Emergency Medicine, 13,* 203-209.

Dart, R.C., Hurlbut, K.M., Kuffner, E.K., & Yip, L. (Eds.). (2000). *The 5 minute toxicology consult.* Philadelphia: Lippincott Williams & Wilkins.

Ellenhorn, M.J., Schonwald, S., Ordog, G., & Wasserberger, J. (1997). *Ellenhorn's medical toxicology: Diagnosis and treatment of human poisoning,* 2nd ed. Baltimore, MD: Williams & Wilkins.

Ford, M.D., Delaney, K.A., Ling, L.J., & Irickson, T. (2001). *Clinical toxicology.* Philadelphia: W.B. Saunders Company.

Gorelick, M. (1997). Gastric emptying (pp. 557-562). In Dieckmann, R.A., Fiser, D.H., & Selbst, S.M. (Eds.). *Pediatric emergency and critical care procedures.* St. Louis: Mosby.

Kulig, K., Bar-Or, D., Cantrill, S., Rosen, P., & Rumack, B. (1985). Management of acutely poisoned patients without gastric emptying. *Annals of Emergency Medicine, 14,* 562-567.

Merigan, K.S., Woodard, M., Hedges, J.R., et al. (1990). Prospective evaluation of gastric emptying in the self-poisoned patient. *American Journal of Emergency Medicine, 8,* 479-483.

Olson, K. (Ed.) (1999). *Poisoning and drug overdose,* 3rd ed. (pp. 47-50). Stamford, CT: Appleton & Lange.

Phillips, S., Gomez, H., & Brent, J. (1993). Pediatric gastrointestinal decontamination in acute toxin ingestion. *Journal of Clinical Pharmacology, 33,* 497-507.

Pond, S.M., Lewis-Driver, D.J., Williams, G.M., et al. (1995). Gastric emptying in acute overdose: a prospective randomized controlled trial. *Medical Journal of Australia, 163,* 345-349.

Toll, L.L. & Hurlbut, K.M. (Eds.). POISINDEX® System. MICROMEDEX, Greenwood Village, Colorado, Edition 117; expires 9/2003.

Whole Bowel Irrigation

Lin Courtemanche, RN, CSPI and
Jean A. Proehl, RN, MN, CEN, CCRN

Whole bowel irrigation (WBI) has become an accepted method to remove some poisons and drugs from the gut; however, it is rarely used. It involves cleansing the entire gastrointestinal (GI) tract by instillation of large volumes of bowel-cleansing preparation containing electrolyte-balanced, nonabsorbable solution (usually polyethylene glycol, i.e., GoLYTELY, Colyte, Nulytely). This solution is given at high flow rates and produces rapid catharsis, clearing most matter from the GI tract within hours. There is no conclusive evidence that WBI improves outcomes for poisoned patients.

INDICATIONS

To decontaminate the GI tract when other methods are ineffective or inadequate. "There is no conclusive evidence that WBI improves the outcomes of poisoned patients" (American Academy of Clinical Toxicology [AACT] et al., 1997). Contact your Poison Control Center for current recommendations regarding the treatment of specific ingestions. Indications for WBI may include the following (AACT et al., 1997; Bayer & McKay, 1996; Gorelick, 1997; Phillips et al., 1993; Olson, 1999):

1. Substances that are not well bound by activated charcoal (e.g., iron, lithium, lead, zinc)
2. Medications that are slowly released over 12-24 hours (sustained-release preparations), especially when serum drug levels continue to rise or the patient continues to deteriorate
3. Massive ingestions, with a significant delay in presentation
4. Toxic solid object (e.g., drug-filled packets or vials, or condoms filled with heroin or cocaine such as those found in body packers)

CONTRAINDICATIONS AND CAUTIONS

1. WBI is contraindicated in the presence of significant GI hemorrhage, bowel obstruction, perforation, ileus, absent gag reflex, uncontrollable intractable vomiting, hemodynamic instability, or compromised unprotected airway (AACT et al., 1997; Gorelick, 1997; Phillips et al., 1993).
2. Nausea and bloating are common; vomiting with aspiration is a risk. Anal irritation and discomfort secondary to diarrhea are common (Dart et al., 2000).
3. The patient must remain sitting on a commode for a prolonged time (4-6 hours), so this procedure is not appropriate for patients who are potentially clinically unstable or at risk for a depressed level of consciousness (Olson, 1999).
4. Aggressive use of antiemetics may be required to control vomiting. Metoclopramide or ondansetron may be used (Dart et al., 2000).

5. Polyethylene glycol electrolyte solution decreases the adsorptive capacity of activated charcoal and therapeutic drugs (Gorelick, 1997; Olson, 1999; Dart et al., 2000).

EQUIPMENT

Gastric tube (if indicated)
Enteral feeding bag (if indicated)
Bedside commode or bedpan
2-8 L of a polyethylene glycol–balanced electrolyte solution (PEG-EBS) (e.g., GoLYTELY, Colyte)

PATIENT PREPARATION

1. Insert a gastric tube if the patient is unwilling or unable to drink the prescribed amount of solution (see Procedure 101). Most patients have difficulty drinking an adequate amount of solution at the required rate, and gastric intubation facilitates the procedure (AACT et al., 1997; Hoffman, 1992).
2. Place the patient on a commode; an upright posture aids in evacuation of the bowel (Hoffman, 1992; Howland, 1994). If the patient cannot sit on a commode, a bedpan may be used with the patient's head elevated.

PROCEDURAL STEPS

1. Administer the polyethylene glycol–balanced electrolyte solution either orally or by gastric tube at a rate of 1-2 L/hr (Bayer & McKay, 1996; Olson, 1999; Dart et al., 2000). Start at the lower amount and increase to 2 L/hr as the patient tolerates it.
2. If vomiting occurs, slow the administration rate, and gradually increase the rate as tolerated. Antiemetics may be prescribed to control vomiting.
3. Continue administration of the solution until the rectal effluent is clear. This process varies in time according to the substance and amount being removed. If a radiopaque substance (iron, lithium) was ingested, continue until there is no radiographic evidence of toxin remaining in the GI tract.
4. If no rectal effluence is removed, stop after 4 L (Olson, 1999).

AGE-SPECIFIC CONSIDERATIONS

1. The pediatric dose for WBI is 500 ml/hr (20-35 ml/kg/hr) for children 1-6 years of age and 1 L/hr for children 6-12 years of age (Olson, 1999; Haddad, 1998).
2. If no rectal effluence is removed, stop after 100 ml/kg (Olson, 1999).

COMPLICATIONS

1. Aspiration, nausea, vomiting, abdominal cramping, bloating, or distention (AACT et al., 1997). These effects can be decreased by keeping the head of the bed elevated or slowing the rate of administration. Consider administering an antiemetic (Gorelick, 1997; Phillips et al., 1993; Rumack et al., 1998). Metoclopramide is recommended if an antiemetic is indicated because it relaxes the lower esophageal sphincter as well as improves GI mobility (Hoffman, 1992).
2. Hypoglycemia may occur if WBI use exceeds 6 hours (Phillips et al., 1993).
3. Rectal irritation can be decreased by discouraging the patient from wiping until the procedure has been completed (Hoffman, 1992).

PATIENT TEACHING

1. Sitting up on the commode is important to help move material through the bowel. Notify the nurse immediately if dizziness or light-headedness occurs. If this procedure is used for someone who must lie in the bed, the copious amounts of liquid stool it produces require frequent linen change (Haddad et al., 1998).
2. Frequent wiping may cause rectal irritation; try not to wipe until the entire procedure is finished.
3. The procedure may take 2-6 hours to complete.

REFERENCES

American Academy of Clinical Toxicology (AACT); European Association of Poison Centres and Clinical Toxicologists. (1997). Position statement: whole bowel irrigation. *Clinical Toxicology, 35,* 753-762.

Bayer, M.J., & McKay, C. (1996). Advances in poison management. *Clinical Chemistry, 42,* 1361-1366.

Dart, R.C., Hurlbut, K.M., Kuffner, E.K., & Yip, L. (Eds.) (2000). *The 5 minute toxicology consult.* Philadelphia: Lippincott Williams & Wilkins.

Gorelick, M. (1007). Gut decontamination (pp. 563-566) In Dieckmann, R.A., Fiser, D.H., & Selbst, S.M. (Eds.). *Pediatric emergency and critical care procedures.* St. Louis: Mosby.

Haddad, L.M., Shannon M.W., & Winchester J.F. (1998). *Clinical management of poisoning and drug overdose.* Philadelphia: W.B. Saunders.

Olson, K. (Ed.) (1999) *Poisoning and drug overdose,* 3rd ed. Stamford, CT: Appleton & Lange.

Phillips, S., Gomez, H., & Brent, J. (1993). Pediatric gastrointestinal decontamination in acute toxin ingestion. *Journal of Clinical Pharmacology, 33,* 497-507.

PROCEDURE 105

Balloon Tamponade of Gastroesophageal Varices

Jean A. Proehl, RN, MN, CEN, CCRN

Balloon tubes for the tamponade of gastroesophageal varices are also known as Sengstaken-Blakemore (SB) tube, Minnesota (MN) tube, and Linton-Nachlas (LN) tube.

INDICATIONS

1. To temporarily control severe bleeding from gastroesophageal varices or Mallory-Weiss tears that is unresponsive to other interventions or when other interventions are unavailable or contraindicated.
2. To control bleeding from the rectum, uterus, or aortoesophageal fistula (Amin et al., 1998; Chan et al., 1997; Maxwell-Armstrong et al., 1995). These uses are uncommon and are not addressed in this procedure.

CONTRAINDICATIONS AND CAUTIONS

1. Because of the potential for serious complications, including death, more conservative measures, such as pharmacologic therapy (using octreotide, vasopressin, somatostatin, nitroglycerin) and sclerotherapy, are usually attempted first (Simone, 2001; Simon & Brenner, 2002).
2. Caution should be exercised in the presence of esophageal pathology (e.g., strictures, cancer, caustic ingestion).
3. Air only should be used to inflate the balloons; using water makes the balloon heavy and increases the risk of pressure necrosis of the mucosa (Simon & Brenner, 2002). Also, water is more difficult to remove if emergency deflation of the balloon(s) becomes necessary (Tsarouhas, 1997).
4. Nasal insertion is associated with more complications; therefore the oral route is preferred (Simon & Brenner, 2002).

EQUIPMENT

Gastroesophageal balloon tube. Options include the following:

SB, a triple-lumen, double-balloon tube. One lumen functions as a gastric tube, another is used to inflate or deflate the gastric balloon, and the third is used to inflate or deflate the esophageal balloon.

MN, a quadruple-lumen tube. It is the same as an SB tube, but it also has a lumen that terminates just proximal to the esophageal balloon. This lumen is attached to suction to remove oropharyngeal secretions that accumulate in the esophagus.

LN, a modified Linton tube with a larger gastric balloon and a port to drain the esophagus.

Gastric tube (not necessary if an MN or an LN is used)
Lubricating jelly (anesthetic jelly may be used if prescribed)
Local vasoconstrictor (e.g., oxymetazoline) for nasal passages (optional for nasal route only)
50- to 60-ml catheter-tip syringe
Bite block
Four rubber-shod clamps
Manometer
Y-connector or three-way stopcock
Intermittent suction source
Adhesive tape
Foam rubber to pad nares
Basin of ice to chill tube (optional)
Topical anesthetic (viscous lidocaine, benzocaine, cocaine) (optional)

Catcher's mask or helmet with face mask (football or hockey), or commercial mask or traction setup with 3-5 lb of weight

Normal saline solution

Scissors

PATIENT PREPARATION

1. Intubate the patient to help prevent aspiration (see Procedures 9-12).
2. Empty the stomach via lavage (see Procedure 102). Failure to do so may result in vomiting and aspiration during the tube insertion.
3. Spray a topical vasoconstrictor into the nose (if prescribed).
4. *Anesthetize the conscious patient's nasopharynx (optional). Some sources discourage this practice because anesthetizing the nasopharynx may decrease the gag reflex and increase the risk of aspiration (Tsarouhas, 1997).
5. If possible, place the patient in a left lateral decubitus position (Simon & Brenner, 2002).
6. Emergency endoscopy to diagnose the presence of esophageal varices usually precedes tube placement (Simon & Brenner, 2002).

PROCEDURAL STEPS

1. Inflate both balloons underwater to check for leaks.
2. Stiffen the tube by chilling it in a basin of ice or refrigerating it (optional).
3. *Pass the lubricated tube through the patient's mouth to about the 5-cm mark (Simon & Brenner, 2002). The balloons are folded around the tube to facilitate its passage. A bite block must be placed to prevent the patient from biting through the tube. Endoscopic placement allows the direct visualization of position before balloon inflation (Lin et al., 2000). Coiling of the tube during insertion is not uncommon. To prevent this, a guide wire may be inserted through the gastric aspirate port before insertion (Kaza & Rigas, 2002).
4. Check tube placement by instilling air through the gastric lumen while auscultating over the epigastric area. At this point, the tube position should be further verified by instilling 50-100 ml of air into the gastric balloon and obtaining a chest radiograph (Tsarouhas, 1997). Other options to help ensure proper tube placement include insertion with endoscopy or fluoroscopy.
5. *Instill additional air into the gastric balloon per manufacturer's recommendations (a total of 250-300 ml in SB, 600 ml in LN, 400 ml in MN) and double-clamp the port (Simon & Brenner, 2002). Monitor the patient carefully for chest pain during inflation of the gastric balloon because it may signal that the balloon is inappropriately positioned in the esophagus. In this instance, the balloon should be deflated and the tube advanced further.
6. *Exert gentle traction on the tube to pull the gastric balloon up and compress the varices in the upper stomach. The traction is maintained by fastening the tube to a helmet or catcher's mask placed on the patient or by using a standard traction setup with 3-5 lb of weight.
7. Attach the gastric and esophageal lumens to intermittent suction to evacuate or lavage the stomach and assess for continued bleeding.

---

*Indicates portions of the procedure usually performed by a physician or an advanced practice nurse.

8. *If bleeding continues, inflate the esophageal balloon to 25-45 mm Hg of pressure and double-clamp the port (Simon & Brenner, 2002). Use a manometer and Y-connector to check the pressure in the balloon (Figure 105-1).
   NOTE: The LN tube does not have an esophageal balloon.

9. Insert a small gastric tube through the mouth or the opposite naris to the top of the esophageal balloon and attach to low suction to remove oropharyngeal secretions and assess for proximal bleeding sites.
   NOTE: This is not necessary with the MN or LN tube; simply attach the appropriate port to low intermittent suction.

10. Pad the nares with foam rubber to help prevent pressure necrosis as a result of the tube.

11. Clearly label the ports of the tube so that the gastric balloon is not inadvertently deflated (see Complications).

12. Lavage for gastrointestinal bleeding may continue through the gastric port as prescribed.

13. Sedate and restrain the patient as necessary to prevent the tube from becoming dislodged (see procedure 192).

14. If possible, keep the head of the bed elevated at a 30- to 45-degree angle to help keep the stomach empty, decrease nausea and hiccups, and decrease aspiration risk (Simon & Brenner, 2002).

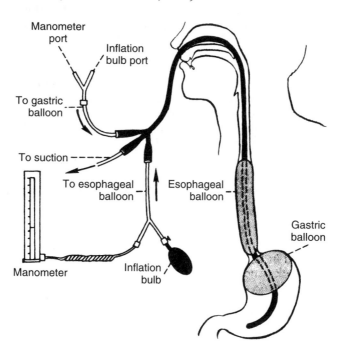

FIGURE 105-1 Measuring balloon pressure in a Sengstaken-Blakemore tube using a manometer. (From Smolen, D. [2001]. Management of clients with hepatic disorders [p. 1242]. In Black, J.M., Hokanson Hawks, J., & Keene, A.M. [Eds.]. *Medical-surgical nursing: clinical management for Positive outcomes,* 6th ed. Philadelphia: W.B. Saunders.)

---

*Indicates portions of the procedure usually performed by a physician or an advanced practice nurse.

15. Check esophageal balloon pressure every 2 hours (Simon & Brenner, 2002). The esophageal balloon may be deflated for 1 hour every 4 hours; it is usually not inflated longer than 8 hours (Dartmouth-Hitchcock Medical Center, 2000).
16. If removal of the tube is necessary, the esophageal balloon is always deflated first.

AGE-SPECIFIC CONSIDERATIONS

1. A pediatric SB tube is used for children younger than 13 years old; the gastric balloon in the pediatric tube holds up to 150 ml of air (Tsarouhas, 1997).
2. Children usually require significant sedation or neuromuscular blockade to tolerate the tube and remain immobile (Simone, 2001).

COMPLICATIONS

1. Airway obstruction as a result of dislodgement of the tube or compression of the trachea (Kelly et al., 1997). Monitor the patient for respiratory distress, aspiration, or chest pain. Never deflate the gastric balloon with the esophageal balloon inflated or while there is traction on the tube. If the tube becomes dislodged and obstructs the airway, cut the ports for both balloons, and quickly remove the tube. Always keep a pair of scissors at the bedside for this purpose.
2. Vomiting and aspiration of gastric contents or oropharyngeal secretions. This can usually be prevented by performing endotracheal intubation, emptying the stomach before tube insertion, maintaining suction on the gastric port, and placing a proximal gastric tube to remove the secretions when an SB tube is used.
3. Atelectasis may result from increased thoracic pressure from the balloon (Simone, 2001).
4. Esophageal erosions or rupture as a result of excess pressure in the esophageal balloon or inflation of the gastric balloon in the esophagus.
5. Persistent hiccups. Elevate the head of the bed to help control hiccups and prevent aspiration (Simon & Brenner, 2002).
6. Cardiac dysrhythmias (Simon & Brenner, 2002).
7. Pulmonary edema from the pressure of the balloons on mediastinal structures (Simon & Brenner, 2002).
8. Irritation or ulceration of the nares. This can be decreased by carefully padding the nares with foam rubber.
9. Impaction of the tube is uncommon but should be suspected if there is any difficulty removing it after balloon deflation (Sarwal & Goenka, 1996).
10. Ruptured balloon(s) with dislodgement, airway obstruction, and or recurrence of bleeding, depending on which balloon(s) rupture.

PATIENT TEACHING

1. Immediately report any chest pain, difficulty breathing, or nausea.
2. Do not pull on the tube or attempt to readjust the tube position.
3. To prevent increased bleeding or movement of the tube, it is important that you lie quietly and not move without assistance.

REFERENCES

Amin, S., Luketich, J., & Wald, A. (1998). Aortoesophageal fistula: case report and review of the literature. *Digestive Diseases and Sciences, 43,* 1665-1671.

Chan, C., Razvi, K., Tham, K.F., & Arulkumaran, S. (1997). The use of a Sengstaken-Blakemore tube to control post-partum hemorrhage. *International Journal of Gynecology & Obstetrics, 58*, 251-252.

Dartmouth-Hitchcock Medical Center (DHMC). (2000). *Minnesota four-lumen tubes (esophagogastric).* Adult Critical Care Policy/Procedure. Lebanon, NH: Author.

Kaza, C.S., & Rigas, B. (2002). Rapid placement of the Sengstaken-Blakemore tube using a guidewire (letter to the editor). *Journal of Clinical Gastroenterology, 34*, 282.

Kelly, D.J., Walsh, F., Ahmed, S., & Synnott, A. (1997). Airway obstruction due to a Sengstaken-Blakemore tube. *Anesthesia and Analgesia, 85*, 219-221.

Lin, T.C., Bilir, B.M., & Powis, M.E. (2000). Endoscopic placement of Sengstaken-Blakemore tube. *Journal of Clinical Gastroenterology, 31*, 29-32.

Maxwell-Armstrong, C.A. Whittaker, S., Pye, G., Steele, R.J.C., & Hardcastle, J.D. (1995). Use of Sengstaken tube to control rectal variceal haemorrhage: illustrated case reports. *Gastroenterology, 2*, 1.

Sarwal, R., & Goenka, M. (1996). Case report: impaction of Sengstaken-Blakemore tube: a rare complication. *Tropical Gastroenterology, 17*, 221-222.

Simon, R.R., & Brenner, R.E. (2002). *Emergency procedures and techniques*, 4th ed. Baltimore: Williams & Wilkins.

Simone, S. (2001). Gastrointestinal critical care problems (pp. 765-804). In Curley, M.A.Q., & Moloney-Harmon, P.A. (Eds.). *Critical care nursing of infants and children*, 2nd ed. Philadelphia: W.B. Saunders.

Tsarouhas, N. (1997). Tube placement (pp. 362-371). In Dieckmann, R.A., Fiser, D.H., & Selbst, S.M. (Eds.). *Pediatric emergency and critical care procedures*. St. Louis: Mosby.

PROCEDURE 106

Diagnostic Bladder Ultrasound

Lucinda W. Rossoll, BSN, MS, CEN, CCRN, ARNP

Diagnostic bladder ultrasound is also known as bladder scanning. The bladder scanner is a portable ultrasound that computes bladder volume with a high degree of accuracy.

INDICATIONS

1. To check bladder volume before and after voiding
2. To diagnose and manage urinary outflow dysfunction
3. To decrease bladder catheterizations to check urine volumes, thus reducing catheter-associated urinary tract infections

4. To assess for the minimum amount of urine volume (10 ml) needed for aspiration and thereby increasing the chances for successful suprapubic aspiration with a minimum number of attempts (Munir et al., 2002)

CONTRAINDICATIONS AND CAUTIONS

1. This procedure is not intended for fetal use or for use on pregnant women.
2. Do not use on patients with open wounds in the suprapubic area.
3. Do not use on a patient with an indwelling catheter in the bladder.
4. Scar tissue, staples, sutures, and incision in the suprapubic area affect the ultrasound transmission.
5. Do not use on patients with ascites.
6. Ovarian cysts, bladder diverticula, or bladder cyst may affect accuracy.

EQUIPMENT

BladderScan (Figure 106-1)
Ultrasound transmission gel or Sontac ultrasound gel pads
Isopropyl alcohol pads or soft cloth moistened with isopropyl alcohol (to clean scan head)
Washcloth (to clean gel off patient)

PATIENT PREPARATION

Position patient in a reclining or supine position.

PROCEDURAL STEPS

1. Clean scanhead with isopropyl alcohol.
2. Turn bladder scanner on.
3. Select the patient gender by pressing the Male/Female button (Figure 106-2). The female gender selection accounts for the uterus; therefore, if the patient has had a hysterectomy, select the male gender.
4. Apply a generous amount of ultrasound gel to the scan head, taking care not to incorporate air bubbles that may interfere with transmission. If the patient

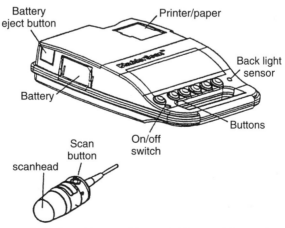

Battery eject button

Printer/paper

Back light sensor

Battery

Buttons

Scan button

On/off switch

scanhead

FIGURE 106-1 BladderScan. (Courtesy Diagnostic Ultrasound Corporation, Bothell, WA.)

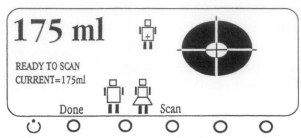

FIGURE 106-2 Bladder scanning screen showing gender selection. Select the male gender for female patients who have had a hysterectomy. (Courtesy Diagnostic Ultrasound Corporation, Bothell, WA.)

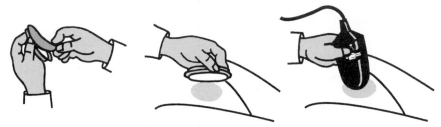

FIGURE 106-3 Application of the Sontac Gel Pad. (Courtesy Diagnostic Ultrasound Corporation, Bothell, WA.)

FIGURE 106-4 Positioning the scanhead. (Courtesy Diagnostic Ultrasound Corporation, Bothell, WA.)

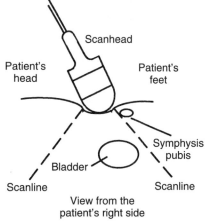

has excessive hair, add some gel directly onto the patient. Alternatively, the Sontac Ultrasound Gel Pad may be applied to the patient immediately superior to the symphysis pubis (Figure 106-3).

5. Place the scanhead about 1 inch or 2.5 cm above the symphysis pubis (the bladder cannot be scanned through the pubic bone) and point it toward the bladder. Point the head icon on the scanhead toward the patient's head

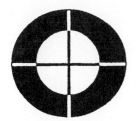

FIGURE 106-5 Aiming icon with crosshairs centered on bladder. (Courtesy Diagnostic Ultrasound Corporation, Bothell, WA.)

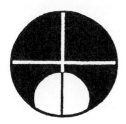

FIGURE 106-6 Aiming icon not centered on bladder indicating that the bladder was not completely scanned. (Courtesy Diagnostic Ultrasound Corporation, Bothell, WA.)

(Figure 106-4). In an obese patient, more pressure may be applied to the scanhead (1-2 inches depression into abdomen).

6. Press the scan button on the scanhead and hold it steady until a beep is heard.
7. The volume measured will be displayed. An aiming screen with crosshairs will be displayed, with the light area on the screen representing the bladder. The crosshairs should be centered on the bladder (Figure 106-5). If the bladder overlaps the side of the crosshairs, the measured volume will be inaccurate (low) (Figure 106-6). Readjust the probe position and rescan until the bladder is properly centered on the aiming screen. Repeat the scan to ensure an accurate measurement.
8. Press "Done" and then "Print" (if hard copy desired).
9. Turn scanner off.
10. Remove gel from patient.
11. Cleanse scanhead.

AGE-SPECIFIC CONSIDERATIONS
The bladder scanner may be used on patients of all ages.

COMPLICATIONS
To date, exposure to pulsed diagnostic ultrasound had not been shown to produce adverse effects (Diagnostic Ultrasound Corporation, 1999-2000).

REFERENCE
Munir, V., Barnett, P., & South, M. (2002). Does the use of volumetric bladder ultrasound improve the success rate of suprapubic aspiration of urine? *Pediatric Emergency Care, 18,* 5.

Urinary Bladder Catheterization

Lucinda W. Rossoll, BSN, MS, CEN, CCRN, ARNP

Urinary bladder catheterization is also known as Foley catheter insertion.

INDICATIONS

1. To obtain a sterile urine specimen for diagnostic purposes when the patient is unable to cooperate or assist in obtaining an adequate specimen
2. To provide bladder drainage for a patient who is unable to void spontaneously
3. To ascertain the residual volume in the bladder after voiding or to facilitate bladder emptying when the patient chronically has large residual volumes after voiding
4. To monitor urine output precisely
5. To obtain a urine specimen for a toxicology screen from the patient who is unable or unwilling to urinate and when it is necessary that the substance ingested or injected be identified as soon as possible
6. To fill the bladder for diagnostic radiologic procedures, such as a pelvic ultrasound or a cystogram
7. To provide a means to deal with incontinence, only after other methods have been proved unsuccessful and when the benefits outweigh the risks
8. To decompress the bladder before surgical procedures or peritoneal lavage

CONTRAINDICATIONS AND CAUTIONS

1. Urinary catheterization should not be performed in a trauma patient with blood at the urinary meatus until a retrograde urethrogram is obtained. The presence of anterior pelvic fractures also requires extra caution.
2. Urinary catheterization should not be performed in a male trauma patient until a rectal examination has been performed to assess for urethral damage by palpating the prostate.
3. Strict aseptic technique should be adhered to when inserting the catheter.
4. A closed sterile drainage bag should be connected to all indwelling catheters.
5. The balloon should never be inflated until urine flow is established, thus ensuring that the catheter is in the bladder and preventing urethral rupture. Gentle pressure on the suprapubic area may help establish urine flow.
6. Institutional policy may require the presence of a chaperone when the nurse is the opposite gender of the patient.

EQUIPMENT

Antiseptic solution
Sterile gloves
Sterile fenestrated drape

Sterile towel
Sterile cotton balls
Sterile forceps
Sterile water-soluble lubricant
Sterile catheter, either straight or indwelling (6-22 French)
Sterile drainage bag
Sterile 10-ml syringe filled with sterile water
Sterile specimen container
Adhesive tape
1% lidocaine jelly (optional)

NOTE: Prepackaged disposable kits that contain equipment for either intermittent or indwelling catheterization are available.

PATIENT PREPARATION
Female
1. Place the patient in the supine position with her knees flexed and separated or with one knee flexed and the other leg flat on the bed.
2. If the patient is unresponsive, unstable, or combative, assistance may be necessary to keep the knees flexed and to prevent contamination of the equipment.
3. If the patient is cooperative but has decreased strength in her legs, have her flex her knees and place the bottoms of her feet together as close to her perineum as possible. This allows her knees to relax against the side rails.

Male
Place the patient in a supine position with head elevated or flat, depending on the patient's comfort, condition, and ability to cooperate.

PROCEDURAL STEPS
Female
1. Put on sterile gloves and place the sterile drape underneath the patient's buttocks, taking care that the gloves are not contaminated. Place the fenestrated drape over the perineum.
2. Open the antiseptic solution packet and pour it over the cotton balls.
3. Attach a prefilled syringe to the balloon port of the catheter (if an indwelling catheter is used). Inflate the balloon and check for leaks. Aspirate to deflate the balloon and leave the syringe attached.
4. Open the package of lubricant and dispense it onto the sterile tray surface. Lubricate 2-3 inches of the catheter.
5. If an indwelling catheter is being inserted, attach it to the drainage bag.
6. Spread the labia majora with one hand (usually the nondominant hand) to expose the urinary meatus. This hand is now considered to be contaminated and should not release the labia until the procedure is complete (Figure 107-1).
7. Grasp an antiseptic-soaked cotton ball with the forceps, and wash the labia majora downward on each side with one cotton ball for each side. Spread the labia minora and repeat. Then wipe directly over the meatus with another antiseptic-soaked cotton ball.
8. Hold the lubricated catheter with the dominant hand a few inches from the tip to ease insertion and to control the direction of the catheter. Allow the distal

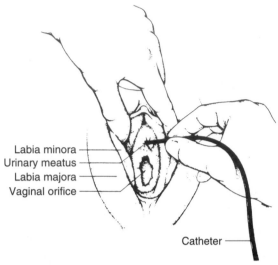

Labia minora
Urinary meatus
Labia majora
Vaginal orifice

Catheter

FIGURE 107-1 Exposing the urinary meatus. (From Nettina, S. [2001]. *The Lippincott manual of nursing practice,* 7th ed. [p. 692]. Philadelphia: Lippincott Williams & Wilkins.)

end of the catheter to rest in the urine container if the end is not attached to a drainage bag. Gently insert the lubricated tip into the urinary meatus until urine begins to flow (about 2-3 inches in an adult; 1 inch in a small child). Then insert the catheter another 1-2 inches. This should ensure that the catheter is in the bladder, thus preventing rupture of the urethra. Never force a catheter during insertion. If you meet resistance, stop and ask the patient to take several deep breaths or to bear down gently. This helps relax the sphincter. If you still meet resistance, seek assistance.

9. Once the catheter is inserted, hold it in place with the hand that has been separating the labia.
10. For an indwelling catheter, inject the water or saline solution into the balloon port. Use the amount of fluid recommended by the manufacturer. A 5-ml balloon requires 9.5-10 ml of fluid to completely fill the balloon and the catheter lumen (Bard, 1997). When inflating the balloon, if resistance or pain is felt, aspirate the fluid back into the syringe, advance the catheter further, and attempt to reinflate the balloon.
11. For a straight catheterization, collect the urine needed in a specimen container; then drain the rest of the urine into the collection receptacle.
12. Hang the drainage bag below the level of the bladder.
13. Attach the catheter to the upper thigh, allowing for some movement. This prevents movement of the catheter and traction on the bladder.

Female Quick Catheter Kit

A quick catheter kit is used to obtain a urine sample. It does not provide complete or continuous drainage.

1. Open the kit and place it on a flat surface. The opened package may be used as a sterile field.

2. Put on the sterile gloves (optional). Open the package of antiseptic solution–soaked swab sticks.
3. Pull the tip of the catheter out of the container until 4-6 inches of the catheter is free. If nonsterile gloves are used, grasp the tip of the catheter through the package to pull the catheter out without contamination. Make sure the cap is screwed on tightly. No lubricant is needed.
4. Spread the labia majora with one hand (usually the nondominant hand) to visualize the urethra. This hand is now considered to be contaminated and should not release the labia until the procedure is complete.
5. Use your other hand to cleanse the labia minora and the meatus with the antiseptic swabs, using one swab for each wipe.
6. Gently insert the catheter into the urethra until urine is seen, and fill the container. If nonsterile gloves are used, be careful to touch only the specimen tube and not the catheter.
7. Remove the catheter from the urethra, then from the container. Close the top of the container.

Male

1. Put on sterile gloves, and place the drape over the patient's thighs. Place the fenestrated drape over the penis
2. Open the antiseptic solution packet and pour it over the cotton balls.
3. Attach a prefilled syringe to the balloon port of the catheter (if using an indwelling catheter). Inflate the balloon, and check for leaks. Aspirate to deflate the balloon, and leave the syringe attached.
4. Open the package of lubricant and dispense it onto the sterile tray surface. Lubricate 2-3 inches of the catheter.
5. If an indwelling catheter is being used, attach it to the drainage bag.
6. Grasp the penis behind the glans (usually with your nondominant hand). This hand is now considered to be contaminated. If the patient is uncircumcised, retract the foreskin.
7. Grasp an antiseptic-soaked cotton ball with the forceps, and wash the meatus and then the glans using a circular motion. Repeat this step, using a new cotton ball until they all are used.
8. Filling the urethra with 1% lidocaine jelly using a syringe is optional; however, this provides more lubrication and some local anesthesia.
9. Hold the penis at a 90-degree angle (perpendicular) to the body with slight tension (Figure 107-2). This straightens the urethra and maintains a sterile field. Hold the catheter in your dominant hand about 4-6 inches from the tip of the catheter, and gently insert the catheter into the meatus until urine begins to flow (6-8 inches in an adult, 1 inch in a small child). The catheter may have to be inserted to the junction of the balloon port to obtain urine flow. When urine flow is established, insert the catheter 1 inch further to ensure that the catheter is in the bladder and not the urethra, thus preventing urethral rupture. Never force the catheter during insertion. If you meet resistance, slightly increase your traction on the penis, ask the patient to bear down as if to pass urine to help relax the sphincter, and apply steady gentle pressure on the catheter. In a male with an enlarged prostate, a coudé catheter may be used to facilitate insertion. If this is unsuccessful, seek assistance.

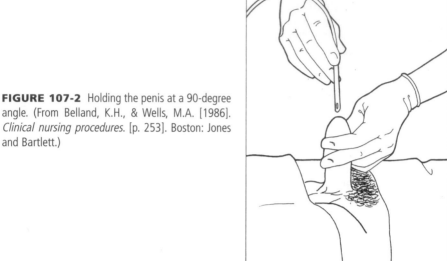

FIGURE 107-2 Holding the penis at a 90-degree angle. (From Belland, K.H., & Wells, M.A. [1986]. *Clinical nursing procedures.* [p. 253]. Boston: Jones and Bartlett.)

10. Once the catheter is inserted, use the hand that has been holding the penis to hold the catheter in place.
11. Replace the foreskin to prevent compromised circulation and painful swelling.
12. For an indwelling catheter, inject water or saline solution into the balloon port. Use the amount of fluid recommended by the manufacturer. A 5 ml-balloon requires 9.5-10 ml of fluid to fill the balloon and the catheter lumen completely (Bard, 1997). When inflating the balloon, if resistance or pain is felt, aspirate the fluid back into the syringe, advance the catheter further, and attempt to reinflate the balloon.
13. For a straight catheterization, collect the urine needed in a specimen container; then drain the rest of the urine into the collection receptacle.
14. Hang the drainage bag below the level of the bladder.
15. Attach the catheter to the upper thigh or the lower abdomen, allowing for some movement. This prevents movement of the catheter and traction on the bladder.

AGE-SPECIFIC CONSIDERATIONS
1. To insert a catheter in a young female, have her flex her knees and place the bottoms of her heels as near the perineum as possible, allowing the knees to relax and separate (Figure 107-3).
2. Catheter sizes for children are as listed below in Table 107-1 (Emergency Nurses Association [ENA], 1998).
3. In an elderly woman who cannot abduct her legs, or in a woman who cannot lie supine, have her lie on her side with upper leg flexed at knee and hip (Figure 107-4).

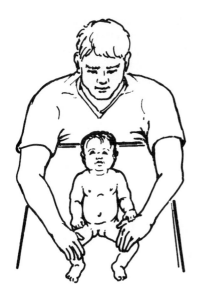

FIGURE 107-3 Position for bladder catheterization in a child. (From Gavula, D.P. [1992]. Bladder catheterization [p. 95]. In Jastremski, M., Dumas, M., & Peñalver, L. [Eds.], *Emergency procedures.* Philadelphia: W.B. Saunders.)

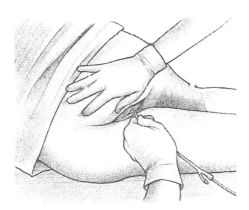

FIGURE 107-4 Side-lying position for urinary bladder catheterization in a female patient. (From Modic, M.B. [1992]. Renal and urological care [p. 566]. In *Springhouse Corporation's nursing procedures.* Springhouse, PA: Springhouse Corporation.)

TABLE 107-1
PEDIATRIC CATHETER SIZES

Age	Size (French)
Neonate	5-8 feeding tube or 6 catheter
6 mo	8
1-3 yr	10
4-7 yr	10-12
8-10 yr	12
11-18 yr	12-18

From Emergency Nurses Association. (1998). *Emergency nursing pediatric course.* Des Plaines, IL: Author.

4. If you are unable to pass the catheter in a male with prostatic hypertrophy, use a larger catheter or one with a coudé tip on the next attempt.
5. If your first attempt to insert a catheter in a female patient is unsuccessful, leave the catheter in place. This helps prevent similar misplacement on the next attempt.

COMPLICATIONS
1. Urethral damage such as strictures or rupture
2. Urinary tract infection
3. Sepsis
4. Catheter obstruction with sediment, mucus, or blood clots leading to acute postobstructive renal failure

PATIENT TEACHING
If the patient is going home with an indwelling catheter, give the following instructions:
1. Wash your hands before and after you handle the catheter.
2. Wash the urinary meatus and the perineal area twice a day with soap and water.
3. Drink at least 8-12 glasses of water a day. If your urine becomes dark, increase the amount of fluid you are drinking.
4. Do not pull on the catheter.
5. Keep the drainage bag lower than your bladder.
6. Wipe all connections with alcohol when changing from leg bag to drainage bag and vice versa.
7. Report any of the following: cloudy or bloody urine, foul-smelling urine, fever.

REFERENCES

Bard Urological Division. (1997). *Foley catheter inflation/deflation guidelines.* Covington, GA: Author.

Emergency Nurses Association. (1998). *Emergency nursing pediatric course*, 2nd ed. Des Plaines, IL: Author.

Suprapubic Urine Aspiration

Lucinda W. Rossoll, BSN, MS, CEN, CCRN, ARNP

Suprapubic aspiration is also known as suprapubic "tap" or suprapubic bladder aspiration.

INDICATION

To obtain a sterile urine specimen for diagnostic purposes when uncontaminated urine cannot be obtained for culture in a child who is younger than 2 years of age, who is not toilet trained, and who has suspected sepsis or fever of unknown origin. Urethral catheterization is the preferred method for obtaining a sterile urine specimen from a child who is older than 2 years of age.

CONTRAINDICATIONS AND CAUTIONS

1. Suprapubic aspiration should not be performed in a child who is older than 2 years of age or who is able to void on command.
2. This procedure should not be performed in a patient who has just voided. The procedure should be delayed for at least 1 hour after voiding.
3. Coagulopathies and leukopenia are relative contraindications (Ogborn, 2001).

EQUIPMENT

Antiseptic solution or antiseptic-soaked swabs
2 × 2 gauze pads
Bandage
Diaper
Lidocaine 1% (with or without epinephrine)
3- or 5-ml syringe
Tuberculin syringe
22-G 1-in needle
22-G 1½-inch needle or 22-G 1½-inch spinal needle
Sterile gloves
Sterile specimen container
Pediatric urine collection bag
Bladder scanner (optional)

PATIENT PREPARATION

1. Wait at least 1 hour after the last void before performing the procedure. This allows enough urine to collect to distend the bladder, making it easier to palpate. A bladder scanner may be used to assess the minimum amount of urine volume (10 ml) needed for aspiration, thereby increasing the chances for successful suprapubic aspiration with a minimum number of attempts (Munir et al., 2002).
2. Remove the diaper. Place a sterile urine collection bag on the patient because the patient may spontaneously void during the procedure.

499

3. Place the patient in a supine position with the knees flexed and the bottoms of the heels as close to the perineum as possible and secure the arms. This position keeps the patient from moving during the procedure, while making it easy to observe and soothe the patient.
4. Allow the patient to use a pacifier or hold onto a security object.

PROCEDURAL STEPS

1. Use the bladder scanner (Procedure 106) to assess whether there is enough urine (10 ml) for aspiration (optional).
2. Wipe the area between the symphysis pubis and the umbilicus twice in a circular motion outward with antiseptic-soaked gauze or swabs. Allow to air dry.
3. *Infiltrate the insertion site with 1% lidocaine using the tuberculin syringe with the 27-G needle.
4. *Attach the 3- or 5-ml syringe to the 22-G 1½-inch needle or the spinal needle, using sterile technique.
5. To prevent urination during the procedure, compress the infant's urethra. If the patient is a boy, place pressure on the penis. In a girl, place digital pressure upward on the urethra from the rectum (Nettina, 2001).
6. *Insert the needle about 1-2 cm above the symphysis pubis at a 15- to 20-degree angle cephalad from the perpendicular (Figure 108-1).
7. *Advance the needle while aspirating until urine is obtained. If urine is not obtained, pull the needle back and advance at a different angle (20 degrees cephalad or caudad). Repeat no more than three times. An ultrasound-guided aspiration may be useful, or wait another hour until more urine is present in the bladder.
8. *Withdraw the needle and the syringe.
9. Hold pressure over the site with gauze for 3 minutes and then apply a small bandage.
10. Apply a clean diaper, and give the child to the parents to comfort.

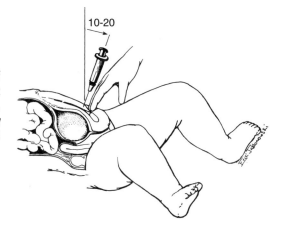

10-20

FIGURE 108-1 Proper placement of the syringe and needle for suprapubic aspiration. (From Bernardo, L.M., & Bove, M. [1993]. *Pediatric emergency nursing procedures.* [p. 138]. Boston: Jones and Bartlett Publishers.)

---

*Indicates portions of the procedure usually performed by a physician or an advanced practice nurse.

11. Place the urine in the sterile container, securing the cap tightly, and transport it to the laboratory.
12. Check periodically for bleeding for 1 hour after the procedure.
13. Discharge the patient after the first void, noting the time of urination and the color of the urine (pink may be expected; report frankly bloody urine to the physician).

COMPLICATIONS
1. Bowel perforation
2. Bladder or abdominal wall hemorrhage. NOTE: Microscopic hematuria is common.
3. Bleeding from the puncture site
4. Infection of the bladder or abdominal wall

PATIENT TEACHING
Report any of the following to the physician or nurse: abdominal pain, bloating, redness or drainage at the insertion site, fever, decreased urine output, bloody urine, or urine with a foul odor.

REFERENCES
Munir, V., Barnett, P., & South, M. (2002). Does the use of volumetric bladder ultrasound improve the success rate of suprapubic aspiration of urine? *Pediatric Emergency Care, 18*, 5.
Nettina, S. (2001). *The Lippincott manual of nursing practice*, 7th ed. Philadelphia: J.B. Lippincott.
Ogborn, C.J. (2001). Urine sampling and access (pp. 43-47). In Goepp, J.G., & Hostetler, M.A. (Eds.). *Procedures for primary care pediatricians*. St. Louis: Mosby.

PROCEDURE 109

Suprapubic Catheter Insertion

Lucinda W. Rossoll, BSN, MS, CEN, ARNP

Suprapubic catheterization is also known as suprapubic bladder drainage or a cystostomy. It may be performed at the bedside, in the operating room, or during a cystoscopy.

INDICATIONS

To provide temporary or continuous urinary drainage in the following circumstances:

1. Instead of long-term urethral catheterization in the presence of urethral injury
2. In patients with strictures or prostatic obstruction that makes urethral catheterization impossible
3. In patients with pelvic fractures

CONTRAINDICATIONS AND CAUTIONS

1. Caution should be exercised in the presence of coagulopathy or previous lower abdominal surgery (may use ultrasound to guide placement).
2. Contraindications include nondistended bladder, pregnancy, bladder cancer, or pelvic irradiation (Quek & Stein, 2002).
3. Gross hematuria with clots may occlude the catheter.

EQUIPMENT

*Prepackaged suprapubic catheter set (Figure 109-1)
Drainage bag (bedside bag or a leg bag)
Sterile gloves
Antiseptic solution
Sterile drapes
No. 11 scalpel
1% lidocaine for local anesthesia
Syringe and needles for local anesthesia

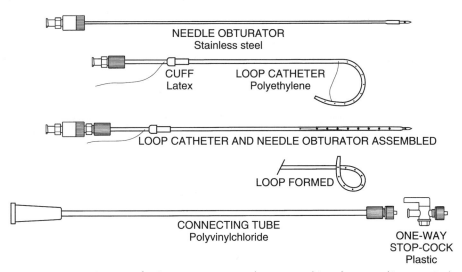

FIGURE 109-1 Contents of a Stamey percutaneous loop suprapubic catheter set. (Courtesy Cook Urological Incorporated, Spencer, IN.)

---

*Several types of suprapubic catheters and kits are available. The method of insertion differs slightly, depending on the type of catheter being used, but the basic principles remain the same (Quek & Stein, 2002).

Needle holder
4-0 nylon suture
Drain sponge
Adhesive tape
Antibiotic ointment

PATIENT PREPARATION

1. Fill the bladder (if not already distended) with sterile saline solution via a urethral catheter or have the patient drink fluids until the bladder is filled. This makes it easier to locate the bladder by palpation.
2. Place the patient into a supine position and expose the abdomen. A rolled towel or a blanket under the hips may be helpful.

PROCEDURAL STEPS

1. Cleanse the insertion area with an antiseptic solution.
2. *Infiltrate the insertion area with local anesthesia.
3. *Make a small midline incision about 2-3 cm above the symphysis pubis but below the upper edge of the bladder. No incision is necessary if the catheter is inserted via a needle and guide wire set.
4. *For patients without a history of prior lower abdominal surgery, insert the catheter vertically. For patients with past lower abdominal surgery, insert the catheter at a 30-degree angle toward the symphysis pubis. Gradually advance the catheter in a caudal direction via a guide wire, needle, or cannula until urine is seen. Then continue 4-5 cm beyond that point or until the flange is against the skin. If a percutaneous loop catheter is used, pull the string to secure the retentive loop into its fully closed position (Figure 109-2). Wrap the drawstring around the catheter shaft several times and tie. Cut off the excess drawstring, and unroll the latex cuff to cover the knotted drawstring. If the catheter needs to be removed, cut the catheter and the drawstring below the latex cuff to free the catheter loop (Cook Urological Inc., 1987). If a urinary catheter is to be inserted, use a 16 Fr and inflate balloon with 7-10 ml of sterile water to hold the catheter in place.
5. Secure the catheter with adhesive tape or sutures. Some suprapubic catheters have a balloon to hold them in place; others are self-retaining winged catheters that have two to four wings to hold them in place.
6. Connect the catheter to a drainage bag and allow the bladder to empty.
7. Apply tincture of benzoin to the catheter shaft and the abdomen. Secure the catheter to the lateral abdomen with adhesive tape.

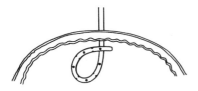

FIGURE 109-2 Retention loop of the suprapubic catheter in its fully closed position within the dome of the bladder. (Courtesy Cook Urological Incorporated, Spencer, IN.)

*Indicates portions of the procedure usually performed by a physician or an advanced practice nurse.

COMPLICATIONS

1. Bowel or peritoneal perforation
2. Infection at the insertion site or in the bladder
3. Skin breakdown around the insertion site
4. Kinking of the catheter
5. Leakage of urine around the insertion site

PATIENT TEACHING

1. Clean and dress the incision site every day. Soap and water or a swab with sterile antiseptic may be used to clean the site. Clean incision site using a circular motion, starting at the insertion site and moving outward (Perry & Potter, 2002).
2. If the catheter becomes obstructed, return to the urologist. Do not try to remove the tube yourself.
3. Call your urologist or return to the emergency department if you experience any of the following:
   a. Uncontrolled urine leakage
   b. Skin breakdown
   c. Redness or foul, purulent drainage at the insertion site
   d. Foul smelling, cloudy, or bloody urine
   e. Abdominal pain
   f. Fever
4. Drink at least 1500 ml of fluids a day (if no fluid restriction) because the small-bore catheter can easily become obstructed by clots, mucus, or sediment (Perry & Potter, 2002).

REFERENCES

Cook Urological Incorporated. (1987). *Stamey percutaneous loop supracatheter set product information.* Spencer, IN: Author.
Perry, A.G., & Potter, P.A. (2002). *Clinical nursing skills & techniques,* 5th ed. St. Louis: Mosby.
Quek, M.L., & Stein, J.P. (2002). Suprapubic urinary tube placement (pp. 139-145). In Shoemaker, W.C., Velamahos, G.C., & Demetriades, D. (Eds.). *Procedures and monitoring for the critically ill.* Philadelphia: W.B. Saunders.

Pelvic Examination

Lucinda W. Rossoll, BSN, MS, CEN, CCRN, ARNP

Pelvic examination is also known as vaginal examination, per vaginal examination, and PV.

INDICATIONS

1. To assist in the diagnosis of intraabdominal pathology in the female patient with abdominal pain
2. To obtain specimens to diagnose vaginal and uterine infections

CONTRAINDICATIONS AND CAUTIONS

1. Warm water should be used on the speculum instead of lubricant if cultures or other specimens are to be obtained.
2. Gloves should be changed before a rectal examination. This prevents the spread of infection from the vagina to the rectum.
3. When a multidose tube of water-soluble lubricant is used, the lubricant should be squirted onto a surface such as the speculum wrapper. This prevents cross-contamination between patients.
4. Institutional policy may require the presence of a chaperone, especially if the examiner is a man.

EQUIPMENT

Light source
Vaginal speculum (appropriate size for the patient)
Lubricating jelly (water based)
Gloves
Ring forceps and gauze dressings or long swab sticks
Specimen collection supplies—any or all of the following, depending the diagnostic test requested (Papanicolaou smear, potassium hydroxide, wet mount [normal saline], specimen slide with cover slips, gonorrhea or chlamydia transport media)
Drape or sheet
Damp wash cloth and towel

PATIENT PREPARATION

1. For a woman's first pelvic examination, time should be spent explaining what will occur. Models and illustrations may be used as adjuncts to the discussion.
2. Have the patient empty her bladder.
3. Assist the patient into the lithotomy position with her buttocks at the edge of the table and place a pillow under her head. Do not place the patient into this position until the examiner is ready to see her. Weak or dizzy patients may not be able to maintain this position without assistance.

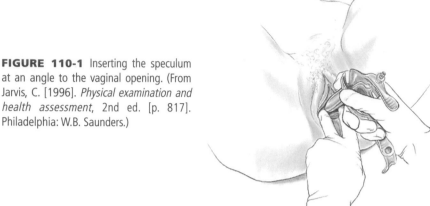

FIGURE 110-1 Inserting the speculum at an angle to the vaginal opening. (From Jarvis, C. [1996]. *Physical examination and health assessment,* 2nd ed. [p. 817]. Philadelphia: W.B. Saunders.)

PROCEDURAL STEPS

1. *To avoid startling the patient, advise her that she will feel you touching her. Touching the inner thigh first will let the woman know the examination is beginning and may place her at ease. Inspect the external genitalia for swelling, inflammation, bleeding, discharge (clear and odorless is normal), nodules, or skin changes.

2. *Insert one or two fingers into the introitus and press downward on the lower edge. Insert the appropriately sized speculum, moistened with warm water, into the introitus by passing it over your fingers. The speculum is inserted at an angle to the vaginal opening and gently rotated to avoid trauma and discomfort to the patient (Figure 110-1).

3. *Remove your fingers from the perineal body and make sure that the speculum is fully inserted into the vagina. Open the speculum and adjust it until the cervix is seen, and tighten the thumb screw to hold the blades open (Figure 110-2). If a plastic speculum is used, lock it into place by pressing down on the lever. Advise the patient that she will hear a clicking noise when the speculum is locked.

4. *If the os of the cervix is obscured, wipe the cervix with a dry gauze dressing held by a ring forceps or with a long swab stick.

5. *Inspect the cervix, noting color, lesions, bleeding, discharge (other than pale white secretions), and ulcerations, as well as the position of the uterus (see Figure 110-2).

6. *Obtain specimens as needed for the necessary diagnostic tests. These may include one or more of the following:
   a. Gonorrhea
   b. Chlamydia

---

*Indicates portions of the procedure usually performed by a physician or an advanced practice nurse.

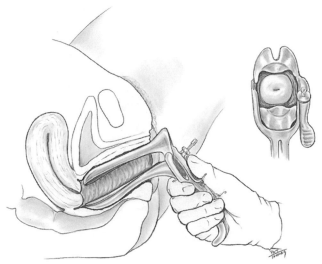

FIGURE 110-3 Opening the speculum to bring the cervix into view. (From Jarvis, C. [2000]. *Physical examination and health assessment*, 3rd ed. [p. 812]. Philadelphia: W.B. Saunders.)

    c. Gram's stain
    d. Potassium hydroxide slide to look for *Candida* (yeast) organisms
    e. Wet mount (normal saline) to look for trichomonas or clue cells for bacterial vaginosis

7. *View the vagina around the cervix by gently rotating the speculum. Gradually withdraw the speculum while rotating it to allow visualization of the vaginal walls and mucosa for color, lacerations, ulcers, discharge, or inflammation. When the cervix is cleared, release the lock on the speculum, being careful not to pinch the vagina.

8. *Perform a bimanual examination by first inserting the lubricated index and middle fingers of your dominant hand gently into the vagina. The fourth and fifth fingers are flexed on the palm, and the thumb is extended away from the perineum. Palpate the cervix, and note the position (anterior or posterior), consistency (soft or firm), mobility, and any tenderness of the cervix.

9. *Place your nondominant hand on the abdomen between the symphysis pubis and the umbilicus. Gently press down on the abdomen toward the fingers in the vagina, and elevate the cervix and the uterus with the other hand. This allows you to feel the uterus between the two hands and palpate to identify size, shape, tenderness, and masses (Figure 110-3).

10. *Continue to palpate with the hand on the abdomen in the right lower quadrant with the fingers in the vagina to the right of the cervix and again on the left. Palpate the ovary on each side (the ovaries may be difficult to palpate 4-5 years after menopause) and any masses that might be present.

---

*Indicates portions of the procedure usually performed by a physician or an advanced practice nurse.

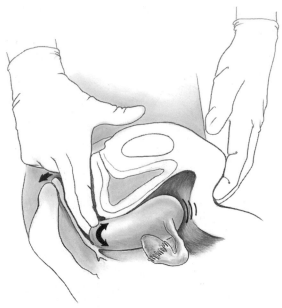

FIGURE 110-3 Palpating the uterus. (From Jarvis, C. [2000]. *Physical examination and health assessment*, 3rd ed. [p. 818]. Philadelphia: W.B. Saunders.)

11. *Change gloves and add lubrication. Reinsert the index finger into the vagina and the middle finger into the rectum. Assess the rectovaginal wall, the posterior surface of the uterus, and the area behind the cervix.

12. Assist the patient in removing her feet from the stirrups. Offer her a damp washcloth and towel to cleanse herself after the examination.

AGE-SPECIFIC CONSIDERATIONS

1. In the well child, a gynecologic examination need only be an external examination. This may be accomplished by having the young child or infant lie in the mother's lap in the frog-leg position. The older preadolescent child may position herself with her knees to her chest. An internal examination should be performed if there is bleeding, discharge, evidence of trauma, or suspected sexual abuse. This examination should be performed only by an examiner who is skilled and knowledgeable in pediatric gynecologic examination.

2. In virgins or those with a small introitus, the examination technique may need to be modified with the use of one finger instead of two. Use an appropriately sized speculum, such as a pediatric speculum or a nasal speculum.

3. Allow the adolescent to choose the person she would like as a chaperone during the examination.

4. An older woman may need assistance to get into the lithotomy position. She may need to hold her knees to support her legs, because they may tire quickly in this position. If she cannot assume this position, have her lie on her side with the upper leg held up to her chest.

5. When menopause occurs or in women 50 or older, the decreased estrogen results in a narrowing (atrophy) of the vagina and decreased lubrication.

These changes may result in some physical discomfort during the examination and a smaller speculum may be necessary.

COMPLICATIONS
1. Vaginal or labial laceration
2. Inaccurate results from an inaccurate specimen collection
3. Ruptured ovarian cyst or ectopic pregnancy from vigorous palpation
4. Spread of infection from one part of the body to another resulting from improper examination technique

PATIENT TEACHING
1. Instruct the patient on how to obtain her laboratory test results and designate the person with whom she should follow up.
2. Provide individualized instructions based on the final diagnosis.

PROCEDURE 111

Culdocentesis

Lucinda W. Rossoll, BSN, MS, CEN, CCRN, ARNP

INDICATIONS
Ultrasound and rapid beta-human chorionic gonadotropin testing have virtually replaced culdocentesis (Palmieri et al., 1998). If it is performed, it is for the following reasons:
1. To withdraw peritoneal fluid from the cul-de-sac to determine whether a female patient has free intraabdominal blood; this may be indicative of a ruptured ectopic pregnancy
2. To obtain fluid from the cul-de-sac to aid in the diagnosis of intraabdominal disease in female patients (e.g., ovulatory bleeding, ruptured ovarian cyst, acute salpingitis, pelvic abscess)
3. To help diagnose intraabdominal hemorrhage in blunt or penetrating trauma to the gravid female abdomen

CONTRAINDICATIONS AND CAUTIONS
1. Culdocentesis is not usually considered as accurate as ultrasonography but may be used when ultrasonography is not readily available.
2. Culdocentesis is contraindicated when a laparoscopy or an exploratory laparotomy is clearly indicated (e.g., in a hemodynamically unstable patient).

3. Culdocentesis is contraindicated in the presence of coagulopathy, a pelvic mass, or a nonmobile retroverted uterus diagnosed on a pelvic examination (Yip, 1992).
4. Culdocentesis should not be performed in late pregnancy to avoid perforating the uterus.

EQUIPMENT

Antiseptic solution
Sterile vaginal speculum (largest size possible)
Tenaculum
Ring forceps and gauze dressings or long swab sticks
20-ml syringe
Spinal needle (size varies from 10 G for aspirating thick or purulent drainage for the diagnosis of disease, to 18 G for aspiration of blood only, to 19 G, 1¼-inch butterfly)
IV extension tubing
Local anesthetic (1% lidocaine with epinephrine) (optional)
Syringe and needles for local anesthesia (optional)

PATIENT PREPARATION

1. Have the patient empty her bladder; insert a urinary bladder catheter (see Procedure 107) if she is unable to void.
2. If not contraindicated by the patient's condition, assist her in sitting up for 5-10 minutes to allow blood or fluid to pool in the cul-de-sac.
3. Assist the patient into the lithotomy position or have her hold her knees up to her chest while lying supine.
4. Administer analgesia or sedation as prescribed because this procedure is uncomfortable.
5. *Administer a local anesthetic (optional); if such an anesthetic is used, a paracervical block is usually chosen.

PROCEDURAL STEPS

1. *Gently insert the speculum into the vagina.
2. *Cleanse the vagina with gauze dressings soaked in antiseptic solution and held with the ring forceps (long swab sticks may be used instead).
3. *Place a tenaculum on the posterior lip of the cervix and elevate the cervix.
4. *Expose the posterior fornix and cleanse with antiseptic solution.
5. *Insert the needle with the attached extension tubing and syringe or the butterfly needle with or without 5 ml of anesthetic solution, 1 cm below the junction of the cervix and vaginal wall, into the posterior vaginal vault. Inject 1-2 ml of the anesthetic solution (if local anesthesia is to be used) (Figure 111-1).
6. *Insert the needle to a depth of approximately 2 cm or the length of the butterfly needle while maintaining aspiration. If fluid is aspirated freely into the syringe, correct placement is confirmed. Change the syringe to a new 10-ml syringe, and aspirate laboratory samples. If no blood or fluid is obtained, the procedure is repeated twice, once to the right and once to the left of the midline.
7. *Remove the needle, tenaculum, and speculum.

---

*Indicates portions of the procedure usually performed by a physician or an advanced practice nurse.

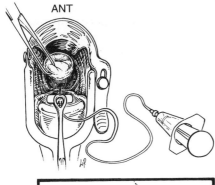

ANT

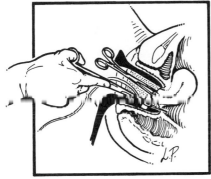

FIGURE 111-1 Performing a culdocentesis with a butterfly needle and syringe. (From Yip, L. [1992]. Culdocentesis [p. 111]. In Jastremski, M.S. Dumas, M., & Peñalver, L. (Eds.). *Emergency procedures.* Philadelphia: W.B. Saunders.)

INTERPRETATION OF RESULTS

1. Intraabdominal bleeding is diagnosed if more than 2 ml of nonclotting blood is obtained.
2. A dry tap should not be considered normal, only nondiagnostic. A positive tap should be considered in conjunction with other pertinent findings to make the final diagnosis.
3. Fresh vascular blood should clot in 5 minutes; true peritoneal blood should not clot unless there is active fresh bleeding.
4. More than 10 ml of clear fluid is suggestive of problems, such as a ruptured ovarian cyst, ascites, or carcinoma.
5. The aspirated blood should be sent for a hematocrit value; if it is greater than 10%, there is active intraperitoneal bleeding.
6. A diagnosis of ectopic pregnancy is favored if the culdocentesis sample has a hematocrit greater than 15; a hematocrit less than 10 is suggestive of a nonectopic cause (Yip, 1992).

COMPLICATIONS

1. Uterine perforation
2. Bowel perforation
3. Perforation of an artery or vein with resulting hemorrhage
4. Local infection at the puncture site (rare and late)
5. Damage to the fetus

PATIENT TEACHING

1. Report increasing abdominal pain, chills, fever, foul-smelling or purulent vaginal discharge, or decreased fetal movement.
2. The area heals quickly.

REFERENCES

Palmieri, A., Moore, J.G., & DeCherney, A.A. (1998). Ectopic pregnancy (pp. 493-494). In Hacker, N.F., & Moore, J.G. (Eds). *Essentials of obstetrics and gynecology*. Philadelphia: W.B. Saunders.
Yip, L. (1992). Culdocentesis (pp. 107-112). In Jastremski, M.S. & Dumas, M. (Eds.). *Emergency procedures*. Philadelphia: W.B. Saunders.

Assessing Fetal Heart Tones

Lucinda W. Rossoll, BSN, MS, CEN, CCRN, ARNP

Fetal heart tones (FHTs) are also known as heart tones or fetal heart rate (FHR).

INDICATIONS

1. To assess fetal status when the pregnant patient is ill or injured
2. To assess fetal status when the pregnant patient presents in labor or with a complication of pregnancy, such as abruptio placentae, placenta previa, or prolapsed umbilical cord
3. To assess FHR after spontaneous rupture of membranes because the umbilical cord may prolapse during the sudden release of fluid

CONTRAINDICATIONS AND CAUTIONS

1. To discriminate between the maternal heart rate and the FHR, the maternal pulse should be monitored simultaneously when the FHR is assessed.
2. A visibly pregnant patient should not remain in the supine position because hypotension may result from compression of the inferior vena cava and the aorta by the uterus, thus impeding venous return. If the patient must remain supine for a prolonged period of time, a folded sheet should be placed under the right hip. If the patient requires spinal immobilization, the backboard should be tilted approximately 15 to 20 degrees to the left to decrease compression of the vena cava. If this is not possible, then the uterus should be manually displaced to the left side (Emergency Nurses Association [ENA], 2000a).

3. FHTs may be heard with a regular stethoscope at 18-20 weeks' and with a Doppler at 10-12 weeks' gestation (Nettina, 2001).
4. The FHT is heard as a rapid ticking sound. A whooshing sound is the placental circulation being auscultated and is usually the same rate as the maternal pulse.
5. Anything that compromises the mother also compromises the fetus. If the condition of the mother is optimized, this helps optimize the condition of the fetus.
6. Consultation with an obstetrical nurse or physician is recommended to validate FHTs.
7. Obtain an obstetric consult early in the assessment of the pregnant patient.
8. If continuous fetal monitoring is needed, the ENA and the Association of Women's Health, Obstetric and Neonatal Nurses (AWHONN) believe that "when a fetal monitor is being used in the ED, the nurse responsible for monitoring will be appropriately educated and will meet institutional standards for fetal monitoring" (ENA, 2000b).

EQUIPMENT
Stethoscope
Doppler ultrasonic flowmeter (2.25-MHz frequency)
Conductive gel

PROCEDURAL STEPS
1. With the patient lying in a supine position, palpate to find the fetal position. Palpate the back of the fetus, which feels like a flat surface, and place the Doppler on the abdomen where the flat surface is palpated. The FHTs are usually located in the mother's right or left lower abdominal quadrant. The position of the fetus has an effect on where the FHTs are found (e.g., a fetus in the breech position has FHTs above the umbilicus). Before the third trimester, the fetal position is difficult to discern. During labor, as the fetus descends and rotates through the pelvis, the FHTs usually descend and move toward the midline.
2. Place the conductive gel on the abdomen or on the Doppler. If warmed gel is available, this is more comfortable for the patient.
3. Locate the heartbeat and listen at the point of maximal intensity. Changing the angle of the probe may intensify the sounds. Count the FHR for 30-60 seconds between contractions (if present) to obtain a baseline rate. A normal FHT ranges between 120 and 160 beats/min. A prolonged FHT less than 110 beats/minute (bradycardia) or greater than 160 beats/minute (tachycardia) may indicate fetal distress and should be immediately reported.
4. It is not unusual to have difficulty locating and auscultating the FHTs. This could be due to inexperience of the listener, excess noise from the surroundings, obesity, improper positioning of the stethoscope or Doppler, or fetal death. If the FHTs cannot be heard, reassure the mother that there are many possible reasons for this, and request assistance from an obstetrical nurse or obstetrician.
5. Check the FHTs each time the mother's vital signs are checked.

COMPLICATIONS
Supine hypotension

REFERENCES

Emergency Nurses Association (ENA). (2000a). *Trauma nursing core course*, 5th ed. Des Plaines, IL: Author.

Emergency Nurses Association (ENA). (2000b). *The obstetrical patient in the E.D. (joint position statement with AWHONN)*. Des Plaines, IL: Author. Retrieved June 13, 2003. Available at http://www.ena.org. Last updated September, 2000.

Nettina, S.M. (2001). *The Lippincott manual of nursing practice*, 7th ed. Philadelphia: Lippincott-Raven.

PROCEDURE 113

Emergency Childbirth

Lucinda W. Rossoll, BSN, MS, CEN, CCRN, ARNP

Emergency childbirth is also known as a precipitous ("precip") delivery or birth on arrival (BOA).

INDICATIONS
To deliver an infant when birth is imminent, as evidenced by the following:
1. The woman is pushing and has contractions.
2. The woman has the urge to defecate or bear down.
3. The woman tells you "the baby is coming."
4. The perineum is bulging (crowning), and the infant's head is seen at the vaginal opening, even between contractions. If you see the infant's head at any time in a woman who has had previous vaginal deliveries, birth is imminent.

CONTRAINDICATIONS AND CAUTIONS
1. It is important to remain calm and controlled. The delivery should not be delayed. An obstetrical nurse and an obstetrician should be contacted to come and assist.
2. The expulsion of the infant should be controlled to minimize perineal tearing, vaginal lacerations, or urethral damage to the mother.
3. If the mother is walking or in a wheelchair and there is not time to place her on a stretcher, she should be eased to the floor for the delivery.
4. The fingers should be kept out of the vagina to avoid infection.
5. This is a *clean* procedure. The umbilical cord should not be cut until sterile equipment is available.
6. The infant should not be stimulated to cry by holding it upside-down or slapping the buttocks. Suctioning, drying, rubbing the back, or flicking the soles of the feet should be enough stimulation to obtain respiratory effort in most infants.

7. The infant should be dried immediately and kept warm after delivery to avoid hypothermia and acidosis.

EQUIPMENT

Antiseptic solution
Gloves, preferably sterile
Basin or plastic bag
Sterile cloth towels
Baby blanket
Bulb syringe
Sterile scissors or scalpel
Two sterile cord clamps or Kelly forceps
Sterile perineal pad
(NOTE: Most emergency departments have a sterile obstetrics kit or "Precip Pack" available with all of the aforementioned items.)
Identification bands for both the mother and the infant
Resuscitation kit
Heated isolette (if available)
Warm blankets (if available)

PATIENT PREPARATION

1. Obtain a brief history to determine the presence of conditions that may complicate the birth or resuscitation of the neonate. Essential questions include expected due date, complications with this pregnancy, multiple birth anticipated, rupture of membranes, and color of amniotic fluid.
2. At this point, the mother is having intense contractions lasting 60-90 seconds every $1\frac{1}{2}$ to 2 minutes. She is not receptive to most teaching. Remain calm, and give instructions firmly and with confidence at important times in the delivery, such as when trying to control an explosive delivery of the head or when attempting to suction the infant's mouth and nose after delivery of the head.
3. Assist the mother with the breathing techniques she learned in prenatal classes. If she has not had prenatal classes, instruct her to inhale through her mouth and exhale slowly through pursed lips. You may need to breathe this way with her to gain her cooperation. Assisting the mother in using active breathing techniques helps her control the delivery.

PROCEDURAL STEPS

1. Position the mother in a dorsal recumbent position with her knees bent or in a side-lying (preferably left) position with her knees bent.
2. If time permits, cleanse the patient's perineum with soap and water or pour antiseptic solution over the area. Drape the perineal area with sterile towels.
3. If time permits, take vital signs, including fetal heart tones (see Procedure 112).
4. Place a clean towel, drape, or absorbent pad under the mother's buttocks.
5. Instruct the mother to pant as the head is being delivered, to help control the urge to bear down. This helps to control the rate of delivery.
6. Support the perineum just above the anus with a sterile towel or sterile gauze dressing. This prevents excess stretching of the perineum and helps to control the rate of delivery (Figure 113 1).

7. As the infant's head emerges, place gentle pressure on it with the palm of your hand (do not use the hand that is supporting the perineum) to avoid rapid expulsion of the infant (Figure 113-2). The head should never be pushed back to prevent delivery.

8. Support the head with both hands and allow it to rotate naturally. The infant turns and faces one of the mother's thighs.

9. If the membranes are still intact by the time the head is delivered, snip them at the nape of the neck and pull them away from the infant's face (Freishtat et al., 2001).

10. Check with your fingers to ascertain whether the umbilical cord is around the neck. If it is, attempt to slip it over the infant's head. If this is not possible because the cord is too tight, immediately clamp the cord in two places and cut the cord between the clamps.

11. Suction the infant's mouth and nose. Suction the mouth first because suctioning the nose often stimulates the infant to gasp and may cause aspiration of material in the oropharynx. Compress the bulb syringe, then place it in the infant's mouth and release the bulb. Squeeze the fluid out of the bulb between suctioning attempts. Repeat until most of the fluid is removed and then suction each naris. Remember, infants are obligate nose breathers so nasal suctioning is essential. A gauze dressing around your index finger may also be used to clear the oral secretions. If meconium is present in the amniotic fluid, the oropharynx and nares should be suctioned with a catheter or bulb syringe

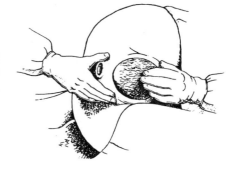

FIGURE 113-1 Placement of hands on perineum with the mother in the side lying position. (From Roberts, J., & McGowan, N. [1985]. Emergency birth. *Journal of Emergency Nursing, 11,* 127.)

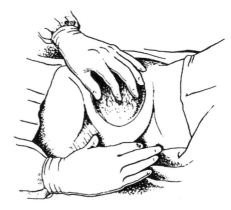

FIGURE 113-2 Placement of hands to control the emerging fetal head. (From Roberts, J., & McGowan, N. [1985]. Emergency birth. *Journal of Emergency Nursing, 11,* 128.)

before the shoulders are delivered (American Academy of Pediatrics [AAP] & American Heart Association [AHA], 2000).

12. Deliver the shoulders by placing the palms of your hands, one on each side of the infant's head, and applying gentle downward traction (Figure 113-3). This allows delivery of the anterior shoulder. If it is necessary to assist with delivery of the posterior shoulder, gently direct the infant's head upward (Figure 113-4).

13. The rest of the infant delivers rapidly. The infant is slippery, so support the body securely to prevent dropping of the infant.

14. Note the time of delivery.

15. Resuscitate the baby as indicated:
    a. Provide warmth in a preheated isolette or an infant resuscitation bed, if possible. Dry the infant immediately to prevent heat loss and to stimulate breathing.
    b. Position the baby's head to open the airway (head in "sniffing" position). Clear the airway, particularly if meconium is present. The method for clearing the airway after delivery depends on the presence of meconium and the baby's level of activity. If meconium is present and the baby is vigorous, use a bulb syringe or a large-bore suction catheter (12 or 14 Fr) to clear secretions from the mouth and nose. "Vigorous" is defined as strong

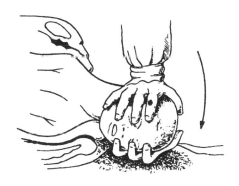

FIGURE 113-3 Delivery of the anterior shoulder. (From Roberts, J., & McGowan, N. [1985]. Emergency birth. *Journal of Emergency Nursing, 11,* 128.)

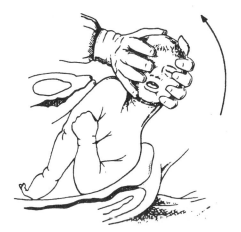

FIGURE 113-4 Delivery of the posterior shoulder. (From Roberts, J., & McGowan, N. [1985]. Emergency birth. *Journal of Emergency Nursing, 11,* 129.)

respiratory efforts, good muscle tone, and heart rate greater than 100 beats/min (AAP & AHA, 2000).

c. If the infant is apneic, exhibits signs of respiratory distress or central cyanosis after drying, positioning, and clearing of the airway, administer 100% oxygen via face mask or blow-by tubing for 30 seconds. If meconium is present and the baby is not vigorous, administer free-flow oxygen, intubate, and suction the trachea before performing positive-pressure ventilation.

d. After 30 seconds of 100% oxygen administration, if the baby is not breathing or has a heart rate of less than 100 beats/min, assist the baby's breathing by providing positive-pressure ventilation with a bag and mask at a rate of 40-60 times a minute for 30 seconds.

e. If the heart rate is less than 60 beats/min, after 30 seconds of positive-pressure ventilation, start chest compressions. Chest compressions are given at a rate that allows 90 compressions and 30 breaths a minute (3:1). Avoid giving a breath and a compression simultaneously. The two-thumb technique to depress the sternum, is preferred over the two-finger technique, in which where the middle finger and index or ring finger of one hand are used to compress the sternum. Chest compressions are performed over the lower third of the sternum and are given with enough pressure to depress the sternum to a depth approximately one third of the anterior-posterior diameter of the chest and deep enough to generate a palpable pulse. NOTE: The base of the umbilical cord can be palpated to determine heart rate. However, the umbilical stump may become constricted so that the pulse cannot be palpated, so listen for the heartbeat if in doubt.

f. Discontinue chest compressions when the heart rate is greater than 60 beats/min. Continue positive-pressure ventilation until the heart rate is greater than 100 beats/min and there are spontaneous respirations.

g. If the infant does not respond to ventilatory and circulatory support as outlined above, prepare to administer medications as prescribed.

16. Clamp the umbilical cord when it has stopped pulsating. Clamp the cord about 3 inches from the infant's abdomen and place a second clamp about 2-3 inches distal to the first clamp. Cut the umbilical cord between the clamps using the sterile scissors or a scalpel. If sterile equipment is not available, it is not necessary to cut the umbilical cord. Keep the infant at the level of the mother or below until the cord is cut.

17. Determine the Apgar score at 1 minute and again at 5 minutes (Figure 113-5). If the second Apgar score is less than 7, obtain an additional score every 5 minutes for a total of 20 minutes.

18. Keep the infant warm by wrapping in a heated blanket and placing in an isolette. If an isolette is not available, lay the infant on the mother's abdomen, skin to skin, and cover them both with a dry blanket. Make sure that the infant's head is covered to prevent heat loss.

19. Placing the infant to the mother's breast stimulates the release of oxytocin, causing the uterus to contract. This helps with placental separation and helps control bleeding. The placenta delivers within 20-30 minutes after the delivery of the infant. Watch for the signs of the separation and delivery of the placenta. You may see a lengthening of the umbilical cord from the vagina. The

	0	1	2
Heart rate	Absent	Less than 100	Over 100
Resp. effort	Absent	Slow, irregular	Good cry
Muscle tone	Limp	Some flexion	Active motion
Reflex irritability	No response	Grimace	Cry
Color	Pale	Body pink, extremities blue	All pink

FIGURE 113-5 Apgar score.

uterus becomes firm as it contracts and changes to a globular shape. Instruct the mother to bear down to deliver the placenta. You may apply gentle traction to the umbilical cord, but do not tug the cord, because this could tear the cord or placenta or invert the uterus. Do not apply pressure to the fundus to facilitate delivery of the placenta. Deliver the placenta into the basin. Once the placenta is delivered, check for intactness. Save the placenta in a basin or plastic bag and keep it with the mother.

20. Once the placenta has been delivered, oxytocin may be administered as per institutional protocol or by physician order. This may be given via IV infusion (not push) or intramuscularly. The oxytocin may be titrated on the basis of the firmness of the fundus. If the uterus is firm, the oxytocin drip may be decreased; if the uterus feels boggy, the drip is increased (Nettina, 2001).

21. Palpate the uterus. It should feel firm and about the size of a grapefruit. Massage is not necessary as long as the uterus is firm. Check the firmness of the fundus (top of the uterus) every 5 minutes to ensure that it is still firm. If the uterus does not feel firm, gently massage it by placing one hand above the symphysis pubis and the other on the top of the uterus. The palms of your hands should be facing each other. Gently massage the fundus of the uterus down toward your lower hand (Figure 113-6). This helps the uterus contract (you can feel it firm up) and prevents hemorrhage. When the uterus is firm, stop massaging. Do not overmassage the uterus.

22. Monitor the vital signs of the mother and the infant, the firmness of the uterus, and the cord stump for bleeding every 5 minutes or until the patient is stable.

23. Wash the mother's perineum and apply a sterile perineal pad.

24. Place identification bands on both the mother and the infant.

COMPLICATIONS
NOTE: For any complication, an obstetrician should be contacted immediately.

1. *Prolapsed cord:* the umbilical cord protrudes from the vagina. Instruct the mother not to push. Elevate the hips or place the mother in the knee-chest

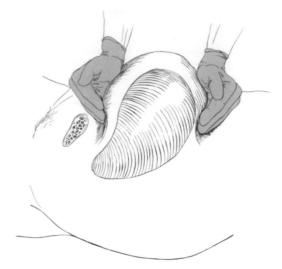

FIGURE 113-6 Uterine massage. One hand remains cupped against the uterus at the level of the symphysis pubis to support the uterus. The other hand is cupped and gently compresses the fundus toward the lower uterine segment. (From Gorrie, T., Murray, S.S., & McKinney, E.S., [2002]. *Foundations of maternal newborn nursing,* 3rd ed [p. 776]. Philadelphia: W.B. Saunders.)

position (kneeling with her face down and her chest to her knees) and place the bed in Trendelenberg position. Administer high-flow oxygen via nonrebreather face mask. Place a gloved hand into the vagina, and elevate the infant's head to relieve pressure on the cord. Do not remove your hand. Monitor the cord for pulsations. Do not try to place the cord back into the vagina. If this position is to be maintained for a prolonged period of time, keep the cord moist with towel moistened with normal saline solution. Prepare for an emergency cesarean section.

2. Fetal distress (hypothermia, aspiration).

3. *Shoulder dystocia:* the diameter of the shoulders is too wide to pass through the pelvis. This is an emergency, and an obstetrician needs to be called immediately.

4. *Breech birth:* the presenting part of the infant is the buttocks or lower limbs. If one or both feet are the presenting part, this is known as a footling birth. Support the legs and the buttocks of the infant after they have delivered, and apply gentle downward traction until the axillae are visible. Gently lift the body to deliver the posterior shoulder, then gently lower the body to deliver the anterior shoulder. Place your index finger in the infant's mouth and let the infant's chin rest on the palm of your hand (this will maintain the neck in a flexed position to help with delivery). Use your other hand to grasp the neck and shoulders posteriorly. Have someone apply downward pressure over the suprapubic region to push the infant's head under the symphysis. The head should then deliver. Allow the infant to attempt to deliver spontaneously. Do not pull on the infant, or the head may become lodged in the cervix.

5. Limb presentation (one of the infant's extremities is the presenting part). Elevate the mother's hips to slow the birth and contact an obstetrician immediately. Administer high-flow oxygen via nonrebreather mask to the mother.

6. Meconium aspiration leading to respiratory distress. The infant may need endotracheal suctioning to clear the airway of meconium.

7. Fetal death
8. Retained placenta
9. Perineal tearing or vaginal lacerations
10. Postpartum hemorrhage, as evidenced by a steady flow of bright red blood, greater than 750 ml; hypotension; tachycardia; and pale, cool, clammy skin. Administer high-flow oxygen via nonrebreather mask. Place the patient in a modified Trendelenburg position (see Procedure 51). Place the infant to the breast. Start two large-bore intravenous lines. Apply manual pressure to any external lacerations. Administer intravenous oxytocin as prescribed to contract the uterus.
11. Amniotic fluid embolism. The mother has sudden onset of respiratory distress and shock. Provide treatment to support airway, breathing, and circulation. Order a blood type and cross-match and have O-negative blood on hand, because disseminated intravascular coagulation may occur.

REFERENCES

American Academy of Pediatrics (AAP) & American Heart Association (AHA). (2000). *Textbook of neonatal resuscitation*, 4th ed. Elk Grove Village, IL: Author.
Freishtat, R.J., Vold, G.R., & Mallei, F.A. (2001). Emergency childbirth (pp. 662-665). In Goepp, J.G., & Hostetler, M.A. (Eds.). *Procedures for primary care pediatricians*. St. Louis: Mosby.
Nettina, S.M. (2001). *The Lippincott manual of nursing practice*, 7th ed. (pp. 691-696). Philadelphia: Lippincott-Raven.

PROCEDURE 114

Dilatation and Curettage

Maureen T. Quigley, MS, ARNP, CEN

Dilatation and curettage (D & C) is also known as suction curettage.

INDICATIONS

To empty the contents of the uterus after an incomplete or inevitable first-trimester abortion. Dilatation and uterine curettage provides a method for definitive diagnosis of completed miscarriage. When the cervix is closed, the uterus is contracted and all fetal and placental products have been expelled, a completed miscarriage has occurred. The confirmation of a completed miscarriage can be difficult unless an intact gestational sac is seen. In absence of an intact gestational sac, a dilatation and curettage should be performed. An ultrasound can be useful if retained tissue is in question. Only D & C performed during the first trimester of pregnancy is addressed in this procedure.

Dilatation and curettage should not be performed if ultrasound shows little or no tissue in the uterus, especially if the beta-human chorionic gonadotropin levels are low and decreasing.

CONTRAINDICATIONS AND CAUTIONS

1. Before the procedure, a thorough history should be taken, including last menstrual period, estimated gestational age, symptoms of pregnancy, degree of bleeding, duration of bleeding, presence of cramps, pain, or fever (Houry & Abbott, 2002).
2. A dilatation and curettage should always be preceded by a thorough pelvic examination to ascertain uterine position and size (see Procedure 110).
3. The patient should have stable vital signs and be afebrile. The patient is usually taken to the operating room if these criteria are not met.
4. The procedure should be discontinued if the patient is unable to cooperate because of anxiety or pain. An anesthesia consultation should be considered for sedation and pain management.
5. When the cervix is grasped with the tenaculum, the highly vascular area at 3 and 9 o'clock on the cervix should be avoided. A single tooth retractor can cause vascular injury, and a Bierer tenaculum is preferred (Guido & Stovall, 2002).
6. Perforation of the uterus is most likely to occur when the uterine sound or dilators are inserted.

EQUIPMENT (Figure 114-1)

    10-ml syringe
    Spinal needle (usually 20 or 22 G)
    Sterile vaginal speculum
    Tenaculum (Bierer tenaculum is preferred)
    Ring forceps
    Gauze sponges
    Cotton balls
    Uterine sound
    Curettes
    Hegar or Hank dilators
    Sterile drapes
    Antiseptic solution
    Pathology specimen container with preservative
    Paracervical anesthesia (optional)
    For suction curettage:
    Suction machine (Figure 114-2)
    Sterile tubing
    Sterile plastic suction cannulas (7-12 mm in diameter)
    Oxytocin infusion (optional)
    Sterile swivel handle

PATIENT PREPARATION

1. Teach the patient active relaxation techniques.

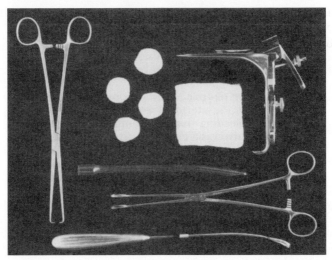

FIGURE 114-1 Suction curettage equipment. (From Farrell, R. [1991]. Abnormal vaginal bleeding, spontaneous abortion and post partum hemorrhage [p. 932]. In Roberts, J.R., & Hedges, J.R. [Eds.]. *Clinical procedures in emergency medicine*, 2nd ed. Philadelphia: W.B. Saunders.)

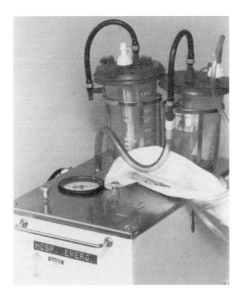

FIGURE 114-2 Vacuum pump and collecting apparatus. (From Farrell, R. [1991]. Abnormal vaginal bleeding, spontaneous abortion and post partum hemorrhage [p. 933]. In Roberts, J.R., & Hedges, J.R. [Eds.]. *Clinical procedures in emergency medicine*, 2nd ed. Philadelphia: W.B. Saunders.)

2. Prepare the patient for what to expect during the procedure, such as cramping and the noise of the vacuum machine.
3. Have the patient empty her bladder before the procedure. Insert an indwelling urinary catheter if she is unable to void (see Procedure 107).
4. Insert an intravenous catheter, preferably 18 G or larger (see Procedure 63).
5. Draw blood for ABO and Rh type and complete blood count if ordered.
6. Obtain baseline vital signs (heart rate, respiratory rate, blood pressure).

7. Administer analgesia or sedation as prescribed (see Procedure 181).
8. Start oxytocin infusion if prescribed.
9. Place the patient in the dorsal lithotomy position.

PROCEDURAL STEPS

1. *Perform a paracervical block (optional).
2. *Cleanse the vagina and the perineum with antiseptic solution.
3. *Drape the pubic area and the inner thighs. Place a sterile towel under the buttocks.
4. *Using a speculum, visualize the cervix.
5. *Grasp the anterior lip of the cervix with the tenaculum.
6. *Using gentle traction, bring the cervix down toward the vaginal opening.
7. *Visualize the cervix and examine it thoroughly.
8. *Gently insert the uterine sound into the cervix and advance it into the uterine cavity. This is accomplished using information about the size and position of the uterus found on pelvic examination. Avoid excessive pressure by holding the sound between the thumb and index finger.
9. *Note the depth of the uterine cavity.
10. *Beginning with the largest dilator the cervix can accommodate, insert progressively larger dilators until adequate dilatation is achieved.
11. *If performing a suction curettage, the diameter of the dilator in millimeters should be about 1 mm less than the estimated length of gestation in menstrual weeks. Then, a vacuum cannula of that same outside diameter should be inserted only to the level of the lower uterine segment and attached to the vacuum tubing. The suction machine is turned on, and the uterine contents are then evacuated by rotation of the cannula moving slowly in a side to side motion toward the cervix. Vigorous in-and-out motion of the cannula can cause uterine perforation. The curette is withdrawn under continuous suction once no additional tissues can be aspirated. To ensure that all products of conception have been evacuated, a metal curette may be used to gently scrape the endometrial cavity.
12. Save all the tissue obtained to be sent to pathology. The tissue should be placed in preservative as soon as possible.
13. Wash antiseptic and blood from the perineal area. Place a perineal pad and lower the patient's legs gently to the table.
14. Send the tissue to the pathology laboratory.
15. Assess the patient's vital signs in comparison to baseline findings.
16. Administer $Rh_o(D)$ immune globulin (RhoGAM) if prescribed.

COMPLICATIONS

1. Uterine perforation
2. Uterine hemorrhage
3. Sepsis
4. Infection
5. Incomplete curettage with retained products of conception

---

*Indicates portions of the procedure usually performed by a physician or an advanced practice nurse.

6. Cervical laceration or trauma
7. Intrauterine adhesions.

PATIENT TEACHING

1. Rest as needed. Do not perform strenuous work or exercise for 2-3 days or as directed by your physician.
2. Wipe from front to back after urinating and moving bowels.
3. Do not use tampons until reexamined by your physician.
4. Do not engage in intercourse or douching until your physician indicates that it is safe to do so.
5. Notify your physician of fever, chills, abdominal pain, severe cramping, vaginal bleeding that is heavier than a normal menstrual period, or foul-smelling vaginal drainage or if further tissue is passed.
6. Follow the instructions regarding $Rh_o(D)$ immune globulin (RhoGAM) (if prescribed and administered).
7. Schedule a recheck in your physician's office in 2 weeks.
8. The patient should be advised that she might experience a variety of emotions, including a sense of relief, guilt, sadness, or grief for the loss of the pregnancy. Referral to a grief support group or other community resources is appropriate.

REFERENCES

Guido, R.S., & Stovall, D.W. (2002). *Endometrial sampling and dilation and curettage.* 2002 Up to Date. Available at www.uptodate.com.

Houry, D., & Abbott, J. (2002). Acute complications of pregnancy (pp. 2413-2416). In Marx, J.A., Hockberger, R.S., Walls, R.M., et al. (Eds.). *Rosen's emergency medicine: concepts and clinical practice,* 5th ed. St. Louis: Mosby.

Musculoskeletal Procedures

Spinal Immobilization

Kyle Madigan, RN, CEN, BSN, CCRN, CFRN
and Jean A. Proehl, RN, MN, CEN, CCRN

INDICATIONS
A spinal injury should be suspected in all trauma victims with impaired consciousness; complaints of neck, back, or limb pain; evidence of significant head or facial trauma; localized spinal tenderness, deformity, or paravertebral muscle spasm; signs of a focal neurologic deficit; or unexplained hypotension. The mechanism of injury should be considered in the decision to immobilize patients. A high index of suspicion should accompany the following mechanisms and patient presentations:

Motor vehicle crashes

Falls

Head, neck, or facial trauma

Distracting injury

Multiple trauma

Trauma with history of loss of consciousness, altered level of consciousness, or intoxication

Unconsciousness or confusion with potential for unwitnessed trauma

If in doubt, immobilize.

CONTRAINDICATIONS AND CAUTIONS
1. Evacuation should precede immobilization in the presence of an environmental hazard, such as fire or noxious fumes.
2. Preexisting spinal deformities secondary to conditions as arthritis or ankylosing spondylitis may require modification of these procedures to align the head and neck in a normal position for the patient.
3. Realignment of the head to a neutral position is recommended and may improve neurologic function (Brunette & Rockwold, 1987). If realignment maneuvers cause additional pain or muscle spasm or compromise the airway, the maneuvers should be stopped immediately and the patient should be immobilized in the position found. If the patient holds the head rigidly angulated or is unable to move the head, realignment is contraindicated, and the patient should be immobilized in the position found.
4. Placing the patient on a backboard should be deferred until life-threatening problems (e.g., airway, breathing, circulation) are addressed and a secondary survey completed (Procedures 1 and 2). Manual stabilization of the head or temporary stabilization with adhesive tape and towel rolls or foam blocks should be used during initial resuscitative efforts.
5. Suction should be immediately available in the event that the immobilized or partially immobilized patient begins to vomit.

6. Immobilization of standing patients may be accomplished by placement of the cervical collar and backboard in a standing position before lowering the backboard and patient as a unit to a flat position. This procedure is not addressed here. A common hospital practice is to apply a cervical collar and assist the patient to lie down on a stretcher or backboard.

7. The following immobilization technique is not intended for patients in the prehospital setting or for interfacility transport. Further immobilization may be indicated for these patients.

EQUIPMENT
Stiff cervical collar of appropriate size for the patient
Long backboard
Straps or cravats
2- to 3-inch adhesive tape
Large-bore continuous oral suction
Towel rolls, foam blocks, or blankets to provide lateral head support
Four to five team members
NOTE: Vacuum mattresses are used in addition to backboards in some areas. They provide good immobilization but are not widely available in North America (Hamilton & Pons, 1996; Johnson et al., 1996). Consult the manufacturer's instructions for use.

PATIENT PREPARATION
1. Stabilize the head manually in the position found, and instruct the patient not to move. Large-bore oral suction should be immediately available in case the patient vomits.

2. Instruct the patient to remain as still as possible and to let the health care providers do all of the work.

3. Instruct the patient to alert you immediately if any of the maneuvers causes increased neck pain, numbness or tingling of the extremities, or difficulty breathing.

4. Assess and document neurologic status, including movement and sensation of all extremities both before and after the procedure.

5. If possible, remove the contents of the patient's back pants pockets to prevent pressure points.

PROCEDURAL STEPS
1. Return the patient's head to a neutral position with gentle in-line traction. The traction pull should be just enough to support the head. Place your thumbs under the mandible and your index and middle fingers on the occipital ridges to avoid soft tissue compression and secure a firm hold on the patient (Figure 115-1). This manual stabilization should be maintained until the patient is securely immobilized to a spine board with a cervical collar in place.

2. Apply a stiff cervical collar. Soft foam collars are inadequate for cervical spine immobilization. If possible, remove jewelry from the ears and neck before collar placement. A correctly sized collar should extend from the shoulders to the mandible. The StifNeck extrication collar should be sized by measuring the distance between the top of the shoulders and the bottom of the chin. This distance should be the same as the distance between the black sizing post and the

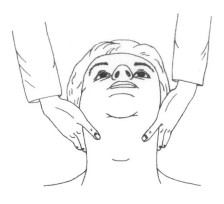

FIGURE 115-1 Manual stabilization of the head. The fingers are placed on the mandible and occipital ridges to avoid soft tissue compression and to secure a firm hold on the patient.

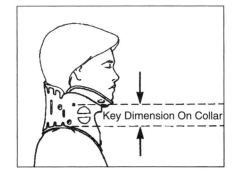

FIGURE 115-2 Key dimension for sizing a StifNeck collar. (Courtesy Laerdal Medical, 1989, Wappingers Falls, N.Y.)

Key Dimension On Collar

lower edge of the rigid plastic collar (Laerdal Medical, 1988) (Figure 115-2). Refer to the manufacturer's instructions for sizing other brands of collars.

3. Log roll the patient to a supine position on a long backboard. The team leader should maintain alignment of the head and coordinate the team's movements. A useful landmark for maintaining head position is to keep the nose aligned with the umbilicus. At least three additional people are preferred for this movement: one to roll the shoulders and hips, one to roll the hips and legs, and one to place the backboard under the patient.

4. Remove protective headgear if indicated (see Procedure 116).

5. Place a pad underneath the head if necessary to prevent hyperextension when the head is lowered to the board.

6. Secure the torso and legs to the board with straps or adhesive tape. Strap under the armpits at the level of the axilla, across the upper arms, abdomen, hips, distal thighs, and lower legs. One study demonstrated significant decreases in lateral movement with the addition of a strap around the abdomen but no improvement with cross-strapping (Mazolewski & Manix, 1994) (Figure 115-3).

7. Stabilize the head bilaterally with foam block or towel rolls, and place 3-inch adhesive tape directly on the skin across the patient's forehead and onto the board (Figure 115-4). The use of sandbags for lateral head stabilization is discouraged because the weight of the sandbags could increase head movement if the board is tipped to the side. Avoid taping across the hair or the eyebrows

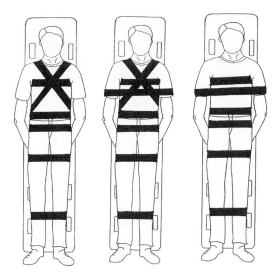

FIGURE 115-3 Acceptable strapping configurations. (From Mazolewski, P., & Manix, T.H. [1994]. The effectiveness of strapping techniques in spinal immobilization. *Annals of Emergency Medicine, 23,* 1292.)

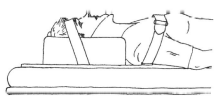

FIGURE 115-4 Head immobilization with adhesive tape and lateral head support.

to prevent patient discomfort and to optimize immobilization. Place the tape directly on the skin of the forehead to improve immobilization. Do not place tape or straps across the chin, because this could lead to aspiration if vomiting occurs (Emergency Nurses Association, 2000).

8. Discontinue manual stabilization of the head at this point.
9. Assess and document neurologic status, including movement and sensation of all extremities.
10. Maintain immobilization until the spine is cleared by radiographic studies or a physical examination.
11. Have suction available at all times, and be prepared to turn the patient on the board should vomiting occur.

AGE-SPECIFIC CONSIDERATIONS
1. Young children present challenges in the assessment of pain. Consider the mechanism of injury carefully to decide when to immobilize.
2. If a child is frightened and fighting, attempts at immobilization may increase movement. If possible, position a parent or caregiver at the top of the backboard in the child's direct line of vision; this can help calm the child and elicit cooperation. The parent can also assist with manual head immobilization.
3. The distinctive anatomic characteristics of infants and children up to 8 years include larger head-to-body ratio, underdeveloped cervical musculature, and incomplete vertebral ossification (Boswell et al., 2001). As a result, placement on a standard backboard may cause excess flexion. To achieve neutral

alignment, padding should be placed under the trunk or shoulders, or a back-board with a "cutout" for the head may be used. Optimal position results in the external auditory meatus in line with the shoulders (Mintz, 1994) (Figure 115-5).

4. Pediatric and infant stiff collars are available. If an appropriate-sized collar is not available, a folded towel around the neck may help prevent flexion. Tape across the forehead and head blocks are crucial in this instance. Care must be taken to ensure that the towel around the neck is not too tight.

5. Standard head blocks may be too large to be effective with small children. Rolled towels or blankets can be substituted.

6. Geriatric patients may be at increased risk for skin breakdown because of thinner skin, poor peripheral circulation, loss of subcutaneous padding, and concomitant disease processes.

7. Spinal immobilization restricts respiration by an average of 15% (Totten & Sugarman, 1999). Geriatric patients and patients who have cardiopulmonary disease may experience respiratory compromise when supine. Careful monitoring is essential to ensure that ventilatory status is adequate.

COMPLICATIONS

1. Further damage to the spine or the spinal cord as a result of movement. Incorrectly applied straps increase this risk.

2. Respiratory compromise secondary to tight straps across the chest, aspiration of vomitus, improperly sized or placed cervical collar, or excessive neck flexion in young children.

3. Pain related to backboard and collar. Using a vacuum mattress instead of a backboard is more comfortable for the patient (Chan et al., 1996; Hamilton & Pons, 1996; Johnson et al., 1996).

4. Tissue breakdown secondary to contact of bony prominences with the backboard or stiff cervical collar. Minimize the time spent on the backboard and pad any bony prominences to help decrease this risk.

5. Supine hypotension in pregnant patients (secondary to the pressure of the gravid uterus on the inferior vena cava). This can be minimized by tilting the backboard to the patient's left 15-20 degrees. Care must be taken to immobilize the patient in such a way that she does not slide to the side when the board is tilted.

PATIENT TEACHING

1. Do not move until spinal injury has been ruled out.

2. Immediately report any nausea, difficulty breathing, increased pain, numbness, or tingling.

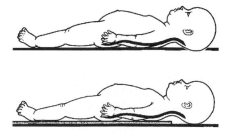

FIGURE 115-5 Immobilization of an infant with "cutout" to accommodate occiput or extra padding from shoulders down. Both techniques achieve optimal alignment (external auditory meatus in line with shoulders). (From Carruthers, G.N. [1997]. Spinal immobilization [p. 598]. In Dieckmann, R.A., Fiser, D.H., & Selbst, S.M. [Eds.]. *Pediatric emergency and critical care procedures.* St. Louis: Mosby.)

REFERENCES

Boswell, H.B., Dietrich, A., Sheils, W.E., King, D., Ginn-Pease, M., Bowman, M.J., & Cotton, W.H. (2001). Accuracy of visual determination of the immobilized pediatric cervical spine. *Pediatric Emergency Care, 17,* 10-14.

Brunette, D.D. & Rockwold, G.L. (1987). Neurologic recovery following rapid spinal realignment for complete cervical spinal cord injury. *Journal of Trauma, 27,* 445-447.

Chan, D., Goldberg, R.M., Mason, J., & Chan, L. (1996). Backboard versus mattress splint immobilization: a comparison of symptoms generated. *Journal of Emergency Medicine, 14,* 293-298.

Emergency Nurses Association. (2000). *Trauma nursing core course: provider manual,* 5th ed. Des Plaines, IL: Author.

Hamilton, R.S., & Pons, P.T. (1996). The efficacy and comfort of full-body vacuum splints for cervical-spine immobilization. *Journal of Emergency Medicine, 14,* 553-559.

Johnson, D.R., Hauswald, M., & Stockhoff, C. (1996). Comparison of a vacuum splint device to a rigid backboard for spinal immobilization. *American Journal of Emergency Medicine, 14,* 369-372.

Laerdal Medical. (1988). *Stifneck extrication collar* (package insert). Wappingers Falls, NY: Author.

Mazolewski, P., & Manix, T.H. (1994). The effectiveness of strapping techniques in spinal immobilization. *Annals of Emergency Medicine, 2,* 1290-1295.

Mintz, L.J. (1994). Traction (pp. 1241-1256). In Weinstein, S.L. (Ed.). *The pediatric spine: principles and practice.* New York: Raven Press.

Totten, V.Y., & Sugarman, D.S. (1999). Respiratory effects of spinal immobilization. *Prehospital Emergency Care, 3,* 347-352.

PROCEDURE 116

Helmet Removal

Kyle Madigan, RN, BSN, CEN, CCRN, CFRN and Jean A. Proehl, RN, MN, CEN, CCRN

INDICATION

To remove protective headgear (e.g., motorcycle or athletic helmets) from patients with potential cervical spine injuries.

CONTRAINDICATIONS AND CAUTIONS

1. Helmet removal may be deferred in a patient without airway compromise when cervical spine injury is strongly suspected. In this situation, a cast saw may be used to bivalve the helmet in the coronal plane (Koenig, 1997).

Leaving a helmet in place may require padding to elevate the patient's body from the shoulders down. Otherwise, flexion similar to that seen in a child may result (Procedure 115).

2. The presence of football shoulder pads after the removal of a football helmet results in significant cervical extension. Therefore football players should initially be immobilized with both helmet and shoulder pads left in place to maintain their neck in a position most closely approximating normal. Defer football helmet removal until both helmet and shoulder pads can be removed in a controlled setting (Swenson et al., 1997). This has not been studied in hockey players, but similar cautions should be considered because shoulder pads are also worn for hockey.

3. Remove the face mask before transport, regardless of current respiratory status (Kleiner et al., 2001).

4. Helmet removal should not be attempted without sufficient trained personnel.

EQUIPMENT
Two people skilled in this technique

NOTE: A one-person technique has been described; however, the two-person technique is the most widely endorsed.

PATIENT PREPARATION
1. Manually stabilize the patient's head.
2. Instruct the patient to remain as still as possible and let the health care providers do the work of removing the helmet.
3. Instruct the patient to alert you immediately if any of the maneuvers cause increased neck pain or numbness or tingling of the extremities.
4. If possible, remove the patient's glasses, necklaces, and earrings.
5. Assess and document neurologic status, including movement and sensation of all extremities both before and after removal.

PROCEDURAL STEPS
1. *Leader:* Stand at the patient's head and apply gentle in-line stabilization by placing your thumbs on the patient's mandibles and your index fingers on the occipital ridges.
   Assistant: Cut or remove any chin strap or face guard. If the helmet has snap-out ear protectors, remove them by prying them loose with a tongue blade.
2. *Assistant:* Assume in-line stabilization from the leader by cupping the mandible with the thumb and index finger of one hand and placing the other hand on the occipital ridge (Figure 116-1, *A*).
   Leader: Spread the helmet laterally and gently remove it (Figure 116-1, *B*). As the helmet comes over the occiput, it may be necessary to rotate the helmet anteriorly over the face, taking care to avoid the patient's nose.
   Assistant: Warning—the head drops as the helmet is removed unless adequate support is provided posteriorly to the occipital ridges.
3. *Leader:* Resume stabilization laterally with your fingers on the mandible and occipital ridges as described in Step 1 (Figure 116-1, *C* and *D*).
   Assistant: Place a folded towel or blanket under the patient's head if it is necessary to maintain alignment. Assemble equipment and personnel to immobilize the patient's spine definitively (see Procedure 115).

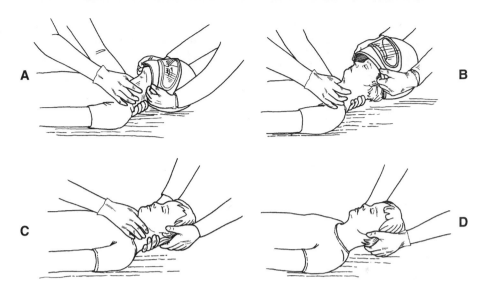

FIGURE 116-1 Technique of helmet removal. **A,** Assistant assumes in-line stabilization. **B,** Leader removes helmet. **C** and **D,** Leader resumes in-line stabilization. See text for explanations. (From Koenig, W.J. [1997]. Helmet removal [p. 603]. In Dieckmann, R.A., Fiser, D.H., & Selbst, S.M. (Eds.). *Pediatric emergency and critical care procedures.* St. Louis: Mosby.)

4. Assess and document the neurologic status, including movement and sensation of all extremities.

COMPLICATIONS

Further damage to the spine or the spinal cord as a result of movement

PATIENT TEACHING

Instruct the patient not to move until instructed to do so by the nurse or physician.

REFERENCES

Kleiner, D.M., Almquist, J.h., Bailes, J., et al. (2001). *Prehospital care of the spine injured athlete, Interassociation Task Force for Appropriate Care of the Spine Injured Athlete.* Dallas: National Athletic Trainers' Association.

Koenig, W.J. (1997). Helmet removal (pp. 602-603). In Dieckmann, R.A., Fiser, D.H., & Selbst, S.M. (Eds.). *Pediatric emergency and critical care procedures.* St. Louis: Mosby.

Swenson, T.M., Lauerman, W.C., Blanc, R.D., et al. (1997). Cervical spine alignment in the immobilized football player: radiographic analysis before and after helmet removal. *American Journal of Sports Medicine, 25,* 226-230.

General Principles of Splinting

Ruth L. Schaffler, PhD(c), CEN, ARNP

INDICATIONS

1. To immobilize and stabilize fractures, dislocations, or tendon ruptures as soon as possible after an injury in order to prevent further soft tissue, blood vessel, nerve, or bony damage.
2. To decrease pain from impaired neurologic function or muscle spasm.
3. To decrease swelling associated with injury by reducing blood and fluid loss into the soft tissues.
4. To immobilize injured areas after burns, bites, or stings.
5. To immobilize an area during the healing of infectious or inflammatory processes and after the surgical repair of muscles or tendons.

CONTRAINDICATIONS AND CAUTIONS

1. Injured extremities should be handled gently and movement of the affected area minimized to decrease pain and risk of complications (e.g., compartment syndrome, fat embolism, vascular or nerve damage, venous thrombosis).
2. Bony prominences should be padded to avoid undue pressure and skin breakdown.
3. The joints above and below the injury site should be immobilized.
4. Gentle longitudinal traction may be exerted while the splint is being applied, except when the injury site involves a joint, a dislocation, or an open fracture. In these cases, the injury should be splinted in the position found, unless circulatory compromise exists, in which case the injury site should be straightened only enough to restore distal pulses.
   NOTE: It is generally agreed that traction splints should be applied in cases of open femoral fractures; this is likely to cause the bone ends to slip beneath the skin. Open fractures are generally considered contaminated, and wound care becomes a high priority (Emergency Nurses Association, 2000).
5. Align a severely deformed limb with steady gentle traction so a splint can be applied. The extremity should not be forced into the splint. The splint may have to be improvised or altered to fit the limb in the position of deformity (Lucas, 2001).
6. No zippers, knots, or attachments of the splinting device should be placed directly over the injury site.
7. Neurovascular status should be assessed and documented before and after splinting. If sensation and circulation are diminished after splinting, the splint must be readjusted or removed and reapplied.
8. Rigid splints should be well padded to prevent local pressure.

9. If the limb is wrapped circumferentially, the wrapping material should be expandable and nonconstricting.
10. When doubt exists, a splint should be applied.
11. All open fractures should be considered contaminated (Emergency Nurses Association, 2000). Care should be taken to clean and cover open wounds with sterile dressings before splinting to minimize the potential for infection. Notify the physician of all open wounds and administer antibiotics promptly as prescribed.

EQUIPMENT

Splints are divided into four general categories: (1) soft (nonrigid), (2) hard (semi-rigid and rigid), (3) pneumatic (inflatable), and (4) traction. Table 117-1 lists indications. Plaster and fiberglass splinting are not addressed in this procedure (see Procedure 127).

Soft—nonrigid splints

   Bandaging material
   Blanket
   Cloth
   Cravat

TABLE 117–1
DEVICES FOR INITIAL IMMOBILIZATION OF ORTHOPEDIC INJURIES

Site	Type of Splint
Clavicle	Sling and swathe or figure-of-eight splint
Shoulder dislocation	
Anterior	Splint to the body with elastic bandage in the position found
Posterior	Sling and swathe
Scapula	Sling and swathe
Humerus	Rigid splint with sling and swathe
Elbow	Rigid splint with sling and swathe in position found
Forearm	Rigid splint with sling, air splint
Wrist	Rigid splint with sling
Hand, fingers	Rigid splint in position of function
Spine	Backboard, stiff cervical collar, lateral head support
Pelvis	Backboard, PASG, circumferential binding
Hip	Backboard, traction splint, or secure the injured leg to the uninjured leg with cravats or bandages
Femur	Traction splint, rigid splint, or PASG
Patella	Soft or padded rigid splint placed posteriorly in position found
Tibia/fibula	Air splint, rigid splint
Ankle	Air splint or pillow
Foot	Air splint or pillow
Toes	Tape to adjacent digit on medial side, rigid splint on great toe

PASG, Pneumatic antishock garment.

Foam rubber
Pillow
Clavicle strap
Sling and swathe
Binder

Hard—rigid and semirigid splints

Aluminum or other pliable metal
Cardboard
Fiberglass
Wire ladder splints
Leather
Molded plastic
Plaster
Vacuum
Wood, backboards
Cervical collar
Finger splint
Wrist splint
Knee immobilizer
Ankle support
Orthopedic shoe

Pneumatic—inflatable splints

Air splints
Pneumatic antishock garment

Traction—capable of maintaining longitudinal traction for lower extremity fractures

Sager (Minto Research & Development, Redding, CA)
Hare (Dynamed, Carlsbad, CA)
Kendrick traction device (Medix Choice, El Cajon, CA)
Thomas
Additional equipment may include:
    Padding material
    Elastic bandage
    Roller gauze bandage
    Tape
    Safety pins

PATIENT PREPARATION

1. Cut away clothing over the injury site and remove bulky material or sharp objects from pockets that may lie under the splint after application.
2. Assess and document the neurovascular status.
3. Measure the noninjured side to determine the correct size of the splint.
4. Pad bony prominences or soft tissue areas, such as the groin.
5. Remove jewelry from injured extremities (see Procedures 118 and 119).
6. Remove boots or shoes from lower extremity injuries to assess pulses and sensation. Footwear that is difficult to remove or that is supportive to the

ankle may be left on if some types of traction splint are used; however, the neurovascular status cannot be monitored.

7. Place a sterile dressing over all open wounds.
8. Pad areas of skin-to-skin contact under the splint to absorb perspiration and prevent tissue maceration.

PROCEDURAL STEPS

1. Remove clothing from the injured area to inspect for wounds, deformity, ecchymosis, and swelling.
2. Grasp the extremity with both hands, one hand below and one hand above the injury site, and exert gentle longitudinal traction to straighten any angulation. Maintain manual stabilization until the splint is secure. Fractures or dislocations of the joints should be splinted in the position found unless distal circulation is diminished or absent. In this situation, straighten the limb only enough to restore pulses. Do not attempt to realign fractures of the shoulder, elbow, wrist, or knee. Do not attempt to push protruding bone ends beneath the skin, but if bone ends slip back into the wound, document the existence of an open fracture, and notify the physician.
3. Immobilize the joints above and below the injury site.
4. The splint should fit snugly but not be constrictive. Leave fingers and toes exposed. If possible, elevate the injured part.
5. Assess and document distal neurovascular status. If sensation or circulation is diminished, the splint must be adjusted or removed and reapplied.
6. Use traction splints for fractures of the proximal tibia or femur. Use them with caution if fractures of the pelvis or ankle are also present (see Procedure 122).
7. Leave the splint intact until definitive treatment is determined. If it is necessary to remove or readjust the splint for diagnostic procedures, reassess and document the neurovascular status after splint removal and reapplication.

AGE-SPECIFIC CONSIDERATIONS

1. A child's bone structure is more elastic and malleable than an adult's. It takes significant force to result in a fracture. Many injuries in children younger than 5 years are related to abuse. Nonaccidental trauma should be suspected when a child under the age of 1 year presents with a long-bone fracture. Children who are abused may have multiple fractures in various stages of healing or may have repeated fractures (Burns & Brady, 2000).
2. The epiphyses (growth plates) at the ends of long articulating bones are more susceptible to trauma in preadolescent children. Fractures that involve the epiphysis (also known as Salter fractures) may interfere with normal bone growth and result in discrepancy of limb length (Burns & Brady, 2000).
3. Children's bones have a thicker periosteal covering, which enables faster and smoother recalcification after a fracture. Nonunion is rare.
4. Demineralization and loss of bone mass occur over the life span. The bones of older adults are more brittle and susceptible to fracture. The elderly have prolonged healing times, and complete healing may take 3 to 6 months (Maher, 2002).
5. Older adults have decreased mobility because of muscle weakness, joint stiffness, and unsteady gait, which make them vulnerable to falls and other

trauma. Additionally, pathologic fractures may occur as a result of chronic disease conditions.

6. The elderly have thinner skin and less soft tissue padding; therefore they are more prone to alterations in skin integrity.
7. Emergency nurses should be alert to the physical and behavioral signs of abuse in all age-groups, which may be covert and masked by the presenting injuries.

COMPLICATIONS

1. Decreased or absent pulses and sensation
2. Edema
3. Vascular or nerve damage
4. Compartment syndrome
5. Venous thrombosis
6. Fat embolism
7. Disruption of skin integrity and infection
8. Misalignment of bone ends
9. Increased pain

PATIENT TEACHING

1. Watch for changes in fingertips and toes—cool to touch, dusky color, swelling, altered or decreased sensation. If an elastic bandage is removed, rewrap it snugly but not too tightly.
2. Report pain that continues to increase in severity and does not respond to pain medications.
3. Elevate the limb above the level of the heart to decrease swelling and pain.
4. Use cold packs over the injured area to minimize bleeding and swelling.
5. Limit mobility and activity to allow healing of the injured site. Perform only approved activities (e.g., weightbearing, stretching, or bending of joints).
6. Do not use coat hangers or other sharp objects to scratch the skin inside the splint.
7. Review with the patient the length of time to wear the splinting or immobilization device and when to follow up with the physician or physical therapist.
8. Instruct the patient in crutch walking, if indicated, and have the patient give a return demonstration of the techniques (see Procedure 135).
9. Assess the patient's ability to continue activities of daily living and the possible need for family or professional assistance at home.
10. Discuss injury prevention strategies with patients and families.

REFERENCES

Burns, C.E. & Brady, M.A. (2000). Musculoskeletal disorders (pp. 1134-1171). In Burns, C.E., Brady, M.A., Dunn, A.M., Starr, N.B. (Eds.). *Pediatric primary care: a handbook for nurse practitioners*, 2nd ed. Philadelphia: W.B. Saunders.

Emergency Nurses Association. (2000). *Trauma nursing core course provider manual*, 5th ed. Des Plaines, IL: Author.

Lucas, G.L. (2001). General orthopaedics (pp. 81-87). In Greene, W.B. (Ed.). *Essentials of musculoskeletal care*, 2nd ed. Rosemont, IL: American Academy of Orthopaedic Surgeons.

Maher, A.D. (2002). Interventions for clients with musculoskeletal trauma (pp. 1125-1155). In Ignatavicius, D.D. & Workman, M.L. (Eds.). *Medical surgical nursing: critical thinking for collaborative care*, 4th ed. Philadelphia: Saunders.

PROCEDURE 118

Ring Removal

Kyle Madigan, RN, BSN, CEN, CCRN
and Jean A. Proehl, RN, MN, CEN, CCRN

INDICATIONS

To remove a ring when an upper extremity injury is present and when other methods, such as use of a lubricant and soap, have failed. In the presence of any upper extremity injury, all jewelry should be removed from the extremity as soon as possible.

CONTRAINDICATIONS AND CAUTIONS

1. If vascular compromise is present or imminent, the ring should be removed with a ring cutter as quickly as possible. A pulse oximeter applied to the tip of the finger can help evaluate perfusion to the digit (Jastremski, 1992).
2. The string method should not be used if there are lacerations, fractures, or dislocations to the involved finger; a ring cutter should be used.

PATIENT PREPARATION

1. Ring removal may not be possible without digital anesthesia if the finger is extremely painful. A digital or metacarpal block producing minimal tissue distention may be performed (see Procedure 139) (Stone & Koutouzis, 2004). Conscious sedation may also be indicated.
2. Before removal using the string method, attempt to decrease edema by using a Penrose drain wrapped distally to proximally along the finger (Stone & Koutouzis, 2004). Elevate the hand, apply an ice pack, and wait a few minutes.

STRING METHOD
Equipment for String Method

Penrose drain (optional)
2-3 ft of umbilical tape or heavy suture (1-0 or heavier silk)
Small, curved hemostat
Bar soap (optional)

Procedural Steps for String Method

1. Rub the bar soap along the length of the tape or suture. This step is optional, but it makes ring removal easier.
2. Pass the end of the string under the ring, using the hemostat if necessary.
3. Have the patient anchor the tape or suture against the palm with the thumb. Wrap the string tightly around the finger clockwise in close, concentric circles, starting next to the ring and moving toward the finger tip (Figure 118-1). Be especially careful to wrap firmly around the proximal interphalangeal joint, because this is the most difficult area of the ring removal process.
4. While pulling the proximal end of the string toward the finger tip and against the ring, unwrap the string in a clockwise direction from the finger. This moves the ring over the string-wrapped finger (see Figure 118-1).
5. Repeat the procedure until the ring is removed.

MANUAL RING CUTTER
Equipment for Manual Ring Cutter

Ring cutter
Hemostat
Pliers
Lubricant

Procedural Steps for Manual Ring Cutter

1. Insert the curved blade of the ring cutter under the narrowest part of the ring. Lubrication may be necessary (Figure 118-2).
2. Clamp the saw firmly down on the ring, and turn the blade manually until the ring is severed.
3. Pry the ends of the ring apart and away from the finger with a hemostat, pliers, or both.
4. Remove the ring carefully to prevent injury from the severed ring ends.

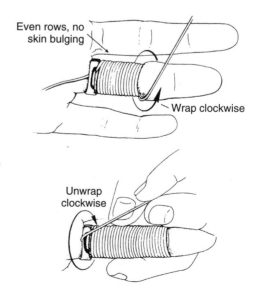

FIGURE 118-1 String method of ring removal. Wrap umbilical tape from proximal to distal in close concentric circles around the finger. Using the proximal tail of the tape, unwrap in a clockwise direction while maintaining slight traction. (From Stone, D.B., & Koutouzis, T.K. [2004]. Foreign body removal. In Roberts, J.R., & Hedges, J.R. (Eds.). *Clinical procedures in emergency medicine,* 4th ed. Philadelphia: W.B. Saunders.)

Even rows, no skin bulging

Wrap clockwise

Unwrap clockwise

BATTERY-POWERED RING CUTTER
Equipment for Battery-Powered Ring Cutter
Battery-powered ring cutter (Gem II [M.W. Mooney, Ashland, OR])
Water-soluble lubricating jelly
Hemostat or ring spreader
Pliers (optional)

Procedural Steps for Gem II Battery-Powered Ring Cutter
(M.W. Mooney, 1997)
1. Check to see that the correct blade is in place. Use the blue-coated carbide disk for gold, silver, aluminum, alloy, copper, and plastic. The diamond disk (red coated) is used for platinum, steel, iron, and brass.
2. Slide the finger guard completely under the ring (Figure 118-3). Liberally cover the area to be cut with water-soluble lubricating jelly. The cutting process generates heat, and the jelly helps dissipate the heat and prevents discomfort or burns. If the warmth becomes uncomfortable, pause and apply fresh lubricant. An ice cube placed against the ring during cutting also helps decrease heat.
3. Attach the cutter to the finger guard with the cutting disk on the ring. Disengage the lock.
4. Rest the blade on the surface of the ring.
5. Turn the ring cutter on by squeezing the contact switch.
6. Gently move the cutting disk backward and forward from one side of the ring to the other. The weight of the cutter head provides the necessary downward force. Do not press down on the blade. Rings made of high-tensile metal may require two cuts, one on each side of the ring. The first cut is made only about

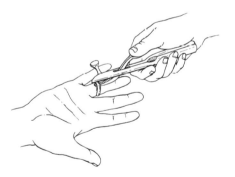

FIGURE 118-2 Use of a manual ring cutter. (From Rosen, P., & Sternbach, G.L. [1983]. *Atlas of emergency medicine*, 2nd ed. [p. 219]. Baltimore: William & Wilkins.)

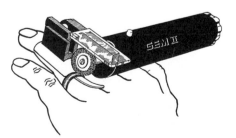

FIGURE 118-3 Gem II battery-powered ring cutter. (Courtesy M. W. Mooney & Co., Ashland, OR.)

halfway through the ring to relieve the tension of the metal. The second cut is made on the opposite side of the ring through the full thickness. If the patient plans to have the ring repaired, making two full-thickness cuts to remove a section of the band and gently spreading the ring apart with the ring spreader help preserve the geometry of the ring and facilitates repair.

7. A sudden increase in the rotating speed of the disk indicates that the ring is cut through.
8. Pry the ends of the ring apart and away from the finger with a ring spreader, a hemostat, or pliers.
9. Remove the ring carefully to prevent injury from the severed ring ends.

REMOVAL OF HARD METAL OR CERAMIC RINGS WITH VISE GRIP–PLIERS
Equipment for Removal of Hard Metal or Ceramic Rings
Vise-grip–style locking pliers

Procedural Steps for Removal of Hard Metal or Ceramic Rings
(Hadjuk, 2001)

1. Place Vice Grip–style locking pliers over ring and adjust the jaws to clamp lightly.
2. Release and adjust tightener one-third turn and then clamp again.
3. Repeat step 2 until a crack is heard; then continue clamping in different positions on the ring until the hard material breaks away.
4. If the ring contains an inlay of gold, the exposed gold can be cut in the usual fashion.

COMPLICATIONS
1. Abrasions (from the string method)
2. Laceration of the finger from the severed ring ends (if a ring cutter is used)
3. Minor burn if inadequate lubricant is used (battery-powered ring cutter)

PATIENT TEACHING
Instruct the patient to remove rings promptly if any future injuries to the upper extremity occur.

REFERENCES
Hajduk, S.V. (2001). Emergency removal of hard metal or ceramic finger rings (letter to the editor). *Annals of Emergency Medicine, 37,* 736
Jastremski, M.S. (1992). Ring removal (pp. 141–143). In Jastremski, M.S., Dumas, M., & Peñalaver, L. (Eds.). *Emergency procedures.* Philadelphia: W.B. Saunders.
M.W. Mooney & Co. (1997). *Gem II ring cutting system* (videotape). Ashland, OR: Author.
Rosen, P., & Sternbach, G.L. (1983). *Atlas of emergency medicine,* 2nd ed. Baltimore: Williams & Wilkins.
Stone, D.B., & Koutouzis, T.K. (2004). Foreign body removal. In Roberts, J.R., & Hedges, J.R. (Eds.). *Clinical procedures in emergency medicine,* 4th ed. Philadelphia: W.B. Saunders.

Body Jewelry Removal

Kyle Madigan, RN, BSN, CEN, CCRN, CFRN

INDICATIONS

To remove body jewelry in the presence of an injury or to facilitate diagnostic studies in which the jewelry would hinder or obstruct the ability to perform a necessary procedure or obtain a complete examination (e.g., surgical procedure, x-ray studies, magnetic resonance imaging). Removal of oral piercings should be attempted before intubation to decrease risk of trauma and subsequent hemorrhage, as well as aspiration of the jewelry.

NOTE: This procedure encompasses common, commercially available body jewelry inserted by professional piercers. Amateur piercings may involve other types of jewelry, including homemade items. If possible, ask the patient about the nature of the jewelry before attempting removal.

CONTRAINDICATIONS AND CAUTIONS

1. Health care providers may instruct patients with infected piercings to remove the jewelry; however, jewelry removal may allow healing and closure of the epidermis, while promoting abscess formation in deeper skin structures (Christiensen et al., 2000). Even momentary removal of jewelry from a healing piercing can result in amazingly rapid closure of the piercing and make reinsertion difficult or impossible (Association of Professional Piercers, 2001).
2. Electrical burns can occur if body jewelry is worn and exposure to a current, such as electrocauterization. Defibrillation during cardiac arrest could result in burns if a nipple ring is present (Christiensen et al., 2000).
3. Appropriate metal body jewelry is not magnetic and therefore does not need to be removed for magnetic resonance imaging procedures, unless it is located in the region being examined (Association of Professional Piercers, 2001). In emergency situations, it may be difficult to determine the type of metal used, and appropriate precautions should be taken.
4. Any jewelry that is removed should be treated as contaminated with body fluid and placed in a container with antiseptic solution (Leviton et al., 1997).

PATIENT PREPARATION

1. If possible, ask the patient to remove piercing.
2. Ascertain type of piercing to be removed (e.g., bead ring, captive bead ring, and circular barbell/barbell) (Figure 119-1).

CAPTIVE BEAD RING/BEAD RING REMOVAL
Equipment for Captive Bead/Bead Ring Removal

Two hemostats (smooth jaw preferred)
or
Two pairs of needle-nose pliers

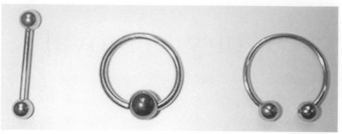

FIGURE 119-1 Barbell, captive bead ring, circular barbell. (Courtesy Association of Professional Piercers. Chamblee, GA, 2001).

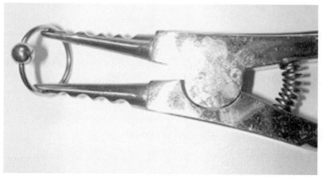

FIGURE 119-2 Ring expanding pliers with captive bead ring. (Courtesy Association of Professional Piercers. Chamblee, GA, 2001).

Ring-expanding pliers (optional)
External snap ring pliers (optional)

Procedural Steps for Captive Bead/Bead Ring Removal

1. Grasp the ring on each side of the bead with hemostats or pliers, pull gently in opposite directions; one end will be removed from the bead.
2. If using ring-expanding pliers or external snap ring pliers, place the head of the pliers inside the captive bead ring and squeeze handle to spread jaws to remove one end from the bead (Figure 119-2).
3. Grasp the jewelry with hemostats and rotate away from bead, out of the patient's tissue (Figure 119-3).

BARBELL/CIRCULAR BARBELL/LABRET REMOVAL
Equipment for Barbell/Circular Barbell/Labret Removal

Two hemostats (smooth jaw preferred) (optional)
or
Two pairs of needle-nose pliers (optional)

Procedural Steps for Barbell/Circular Barbell/Labret Removal

1. Using fingers or hemostats grasp both ends of the jewelry, usually in the shape of a bead (Figure 119-4).

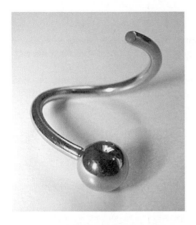

FIGURE 119-3 Captive bead ring removed with hemostats. (Courtesy Association of Professional Piercers. Chamblee, GA, 2001).

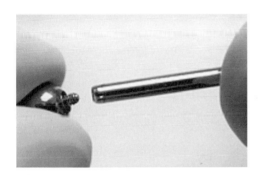

FIGURE 119-4 Removal of internally threaded barbell. (Courtesy Association of Professional Piercers. Chamblee, GA, 2001).

2. Unscrew the bead in a counterclockwise rotation. One or both ends may be threaded in this type of jewelry.
3. After removal of the threaded bead, slide jewelry from tissue.

COMPLICATIONS
1. Aspiration of jewelry during oral piercing removal.
2. Additional tissue trauma during removal of tongue piercing may result in edema, further complicating airway management.
3. Use of jewelry cutting methods may have limited success because of materials used (e.g., titanium). Cutting body jewelry may produce rough, burred edges that may further damage the tissue with its removal.
4. Jewelry may be slippery secondary to blood or body fluids; be careful not to cut yourself during removal.

PATIENT TEACHING
Instruct patient that unless the piercing is well established, the track closes quickly, and it can be difficult or even impossible to reinsert (Hatfield-Law, 2001).

REFERENCES

Association of Professional Piercers. (2001). *Body piercing: troubleshooting for you and your healthcare professional, 2001.* Available from the Association of Professional Piercers website, *http://www.safepiercing.org.*

Christiensen, M.H., Miller, K.H., Patsdaughter, C.A., & Dowd, L.J. (2000). To the point: the contemporary body piercing and tattooing renaissance. *Nursing Spectrum Online.* Retrieved December 29, 2002, from http://nsweb.nursingspectrum.com/ce/ce194.htm.

Leviton, R., Reilly J., & Storm B. (1997). Body piercing: EMS concerns. *Emergency, 2,* 18-20.

Hatfield-Law, L. (2001). Body piercing: issues for A&E nurses. *Accident and Emergency Nursing, 9,* 14-19.

PROCEDURE 120

Vacuum Splints

Ruth L. Schaffler, PhD(c), CEN, ARNP

The information in this chapter is specific to vacuum splints and should be used in conjunction with Procedure 117.

INDICATION

To temporarily immobilize injured extremities. Vacuum splints are particularly useful for immobilizing an extremity in the position found. They are lightweight and radiotranslucent.

CONTRAINDICATIONS AND CAUTIONS

1. Vacuum splints are bulky and nontransparent and may not allow access to the distal limb for reassessment after splint application.
2. The splint valve should be closed tightly to prevent loss of rigidity once the splint has been applied.

EQUIPMENT

Vacuum splint
Vacuum pump
Accessory straps or tape
Talcum power or cornstarch (optional)

PATIENT PREPARATION

1. Remove clothing, jewelry, or constrictive bulky material that may lie under the splint (Procedures 118 and 119).
2. Cover open wounds with sterile dressings.

3. Apply gentle traction to align the limb, if appropriate, or prepare to splint as found (Bergeron & Bizjak, 2001; Garcia, 2002).

PROCEDURAL STEPS

1. Lay the vacuum splint flat with all straps open and the inner surface facing up. Smooth the foam beads evenly throughout the splint to ensure uniform distribution.
2. Dust the splint with talcum powder or cornstarch (optional; contraindicated in the presence of open wounds).
3. Support the bone ends above and below the injury site as the splint is placed around the limb (Figure 120-1, *A*).

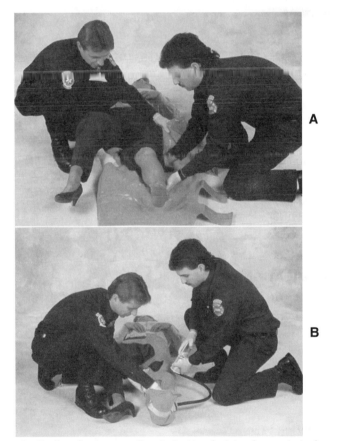

FIGURE 120-1 Application of a vacuum splint. **A,** Position the injured extremity in the center of the splint. **B,** Wrap the splint around the extremity and attach the vacuum pump. The splint forms to the extremity and becomes rigid after the air is evacuated. (From American Academy of Orthopedic Surgeons. [1993]. *Emergency care and transportation of the sick and injured,* 5th ed. [p. 279]. Rosemont, II : Author.)

4. Form or shape the splint over the sides and top of the limb.
5. Secure the splint with the attached straps or tape. Fold the distal portion of the splint outward as necessary to allow inspection of fingers or toes.
6. Attach the vacuum pump to the splint and evacuate the air until the splint converts from a soft, pliable device to castlike rigidity (Figure 120-1, *B*).
7. Twist the valve clockwise until it is tight before disconnecting the pump. Some models have a spring-loaded valve that is self-sealing when the pump is removed.
8. To remove the splint, open the splint valve by turning it in a counterclockwise motion. When the splint is pliable, open the straps, and carefully support the limb while the splint is removed.

AGE-SPECIFIC CONSIDERATIONS

1. Many vacuum splints are too large to fit on the smaller extremities of infants and children.
2. The skin of the elderly can be quite friable; a layer of padding may be necessary between the skin and the splint.

COMPLICATIONS

1. Accumulation of perspiration or moisture inside the splint may cause it to adhere to the skin and cause increased pain when removing or skin maceration. Dusting the interior of the splint with talcum powder or cornstarch before application may help decrease this.
2. The splint loses its rigidity if it is punctured or torn.
3. The splint may soften during significant changes in altitude and may need to be adjusted accordingly.
4. Vacuum is not maintained if the valve mechanism is not fully closed or if it is damaged.

REFERENCES

Bergeron, J.D., & Bizjak, G. (2001). *First responder*, 6th ed. Upper Saddle River, NJ: Prentice-Hall.

Garcia, B. (2002). Extremity trauma (pp. 315-349). In Hubble, M.W., & Hubble, J.P. (Eds.). *Principles of advanced trauma care*. Albany, NY: Delmar.

Air Splints

Ruth L. Schaffler, PhD(c), CEN, ARNP

The information in this chapter should be used in conjunction with the information in Procedure 117.

Air splints are also known as pneumatic splints.

INDICATIONS

1. To temporarily immobilize injuries of the distal extremities—arm, lower leg, and ankle (McSwain, 2001).
2. To decrease swelling and blood loss into the soft tissues, or to control external bleeding associated with distal extremity injuries (Limmer et al., 2001). A pneumatic antishock garment may also be used as an air splint for fractures of the pelvis or lower extremities (see Procedure 54).

CONTRAINDICATIONS AND CAUTIONS

1. Air splints are not suitable for angulated fractures or fractures involving joints. The design of the splint allows immobilization only in anatomic positions.
2. Air splints should not be applied over clothing because the pressure created by buckles, buttons, or wrinkles may injure the soft tissues.
3. Air splints should not be inflated with positive-pressure devices.
4. Overinflation of an air splint may cause circulatory compromise; underinflation may not provide enough support.
5. Air splints are not effective for fractures of the humerus or femur.
6. Air pressure within a pneumatic splint is subject to fluctuations with temperature and altitude variations. The pressure increases with warmth and ascent and decreases with cold and descent. Careful monitoring is required when this type of splint is used in a changing environment.
7. Air splints may not maintain adequate immobilization, because they have a tendency to leak (Garcia, 2002).

EQUIPMENT

Air splint (appropriate size and shape for area to be immobilized)
Talcum powder or cornstarch (optional)

PATIENT PREPARATION

1. Remove any clothing or jewelry that would lie under the splint (see Procedures 118 and 119).
2. Cover open wounds with sterile dressings.

PROCEDURAL STEPS

1. Open the zipper of the air splint. If the splint has no zipper, gather the distal portion of the splint over your arm (Figure 121-1, *A*).

551

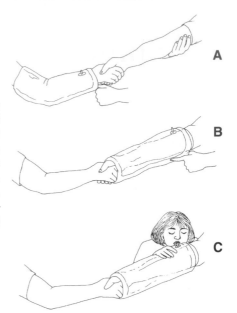

FIGURE 121-1 Application of an air splint. **A,** The rescuer supports the injured extremity with one hand and places the air splint on the other arm. **B,** An assistant slides the splint onto the patient's arm. **C,** The air splint is inflated until finger pressure makes a slight dent. (From Brabson, T.A., & Greenfield, B.S. [2004]. Prehospital Splinting [p. 90]. In Roberts, J.R., & Hedges, J.R. [Eds.]. *Clinical procedures in emergency medicine,* 4th ed. Philadelphia: W.B. Saunders.)

2. Dust the interior of the splint with talcum powder or cornstarch (optional; contraindicated in the presence of open wounds).
3. Grasp the patient's hand or foot and apply gentle longitudinal traction to straighten the limb slightly if necessary.
4. Place the splint, free of wrinkles, on the patient's extremity (Figure 121-1, *B*).
5. Twist the valve on the splint in a counterclockwise motion to open it.
6. Inflate the splint by mouth to a point where your finger makes a slight dent in the surface of the splint (Figure 121-1, *C*).
7. Twist the valve clockwise to close it and prevent air loss.
8. Monitor the air pressure within the splint frequently. You should be able to indent the splint wall with your finger.

AGE-SPECIFIC CONSIDERATIONS
1. Many air splints are an inappropriate size for children's extremities.
2. The skin of the elderly can be quite friable; a thin layer of smooth padding may be necessary between the skin and the splint.

COMPLICATIONS
1. Complications of air splinting can include constriction of blood supply and compression on nerves in the extremity (McSwain, 2001).
2. Excessive pressure variation within the splint may result in inadequate immobilization (decreased pressure) or compartment syndrome or soft tissue damage (increased pressure).
3. Accumulation of perspiration or moisture inside the splint may cause it to cling to the skin and make removal difficult or cause skin maceration.

Dusting the interior of the splint with talcum powder or cornstarch before application may help decrease this problem.
4. Some air splints are not transparent, and wounds under the splint cannot be visualized.

REFERENCES

Garcia, B. (2002). Extremity trauma (pp. 315-349). In Hubble, M.W., & Hubble, J.P. (Eds.). *Principles of advanced trauma care*. Albany, NY: Delmar.

Limmer, D., O'Keefe, M.F., Grant, H.D., Murray, R.H., & Bergeron, J.D. (2001). *Emergency care*, 9th ed. (pp. 564-611). Upper Saddle River, NJ: Prentice-Hall.

McSwain, M.J. (2001). Musculoskeletal trauma. In McSwain, N.E., & Paturas, J.L. (Eds.). *The basic EMT: comprehensive prehospital patient care*, 2nd ed. (pp 529-559.). St. Louis: Mosby.

PROCEDURE 122

Traction Splints

Ruth L. Schaffler, PhD(c), CEN, ARNP

The information in this chapter is specific to traction splints and should be used in conjunction with Procedure 117.

Traction splints are also known as Fernotrac, Hare, Kendrick, Sager, or Thomas splints.

INDICATION

To align and stabilize a fracture of the femur or proximal tibia. A traction splint is the preferred splint for a femur fracture.

CONTRAINDICATIONS AND CAUTIONS

1. Traction splints are not suitable for fractures of the distal fibula, distal tibia, ankle, foot, or upper extremity (Limmer et al., 2001; Prehospital Trauma Life Support Committee, 1999).
2. Bipolar traction splints, such as the Fernotrac, Hare, and Thomas splints, can displace the proximal third of a fractured femur because of the posterior

placement of the ischial pad. To reduce this problem, the ischial pad can be placed on the lateral aspect of the extremity fracture. Unipolar traction splints, such as the Sager and Kendrick splints, do not have this risk because they are designed differently (Garcia, 2002).

3. Traction splints should be used cautiously in patients who have concomitant pelvic fractures. If pelvic pain increases after splint application, the splint should be removed.

4. Traction splints may be used with open fractures of the femur. In this case, the bone ends usually slip back beneath the skin. Known or suspected open fractures are considered surgical emergencies, are potentially contaminated, and should be reported to the physician. Do not place straps directly over an open wound.

5. Two persons are needed to apply most traction splints; however, the Sager splint can be applied by one person.

6. In general, clothing and footwear should be removed before applying a traction splint. If a shoe or boot is difficult to remove or if it serves as a splint for the ankle, leave it on.

7. Blood loss from a femoral fracture can be as high as 2 L (Garcia, 2002). If early signs of shock are present in a patient with a femur fracture, a pneumatic antishock garment may be a better choice than a traction splint to stabilize the fracture.

EQUIPMENT
Splint

Hare traction splint (Dynamed, Carlsbad, CA) or Fernotrac traction splint (Rancho Cordova, CA)
  Metal frame with padded ischial bar and a heel stand
  Ratchet device
  Ankle hitch
  Elastic straps
Kendrick traction device (Medix Choice, El Cajon, CA) (The Kendrick traction device collapses into a compact package for easy storage and transport.)
  Snap-out traction pole
  Thigh strap with pole receptacle
  Ankle hitch
  Elastic straps
Sager traction splint (Minto Research & Development, Redding, CA) (The Sager splint is also available in a bilateral model.)
  Ankle harness
  Thigh strap
  Elastic leg straps
  Metal bar with padded arch support for groin
  Attached pulley-and-cable apparatus
Thomas splint
  Metal frame with padded ischial half-ring
  Spanish windlass for applying traction (A cravat and stick can be used to construct this.)

Other Equipment

Padding
Long backboard

PATIENT PREPARATION

1. Pad the anterior groin area (not necessary if a Sager splint is used).
2. Measure against the unaffected extremity to determine the needed length of the splint (not necessary if a Sager splint is used).
3. Place the patient on a backboard.
4. Assess and document the neurovascular status.

PROCEDURAL STEPS

Hare Traction Splint or Fernotrac Traction Splint

1. Adjust the splint to a length approximately 6-8 inches longer than the leg.
2. Place the ankle hitch under the heel of the foot, and cross the straps over the top of the foot (Figure 122-1).
3. Have an assistant exert longitudinal traction by placing one hand behind the patient's heel and the other hand over the dorsum of the foot and then pulling

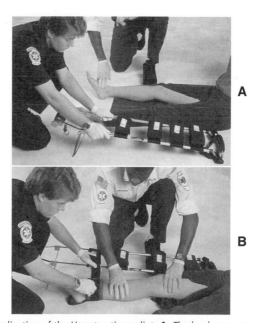

FIGURE 122-1 Application of the Hare traction splint. **A,** The leader assesses distal pulses and stabilizes the injury site while an assistant measures the splint against the unaffected side. **B,** The ankle strap is applied. (From American Academy of Orthopedic Surgeons. [1993]. *Emergency care and transportation of the sick and injured,* 5th ed. [pp. 280, 281]. Rosemont, IL: Author.)

(Continued)

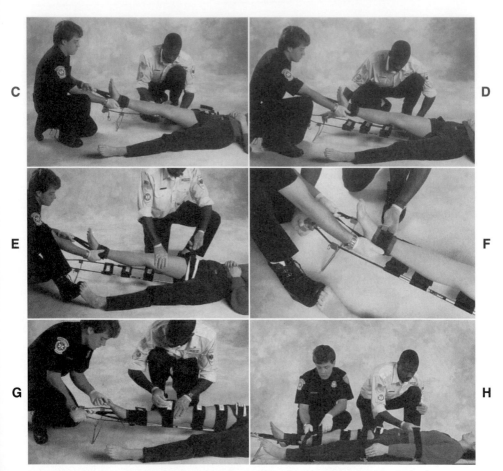

FIGURE 122-1, cont'd C, Manual traction is initiated by the assistant while the leader supports the fracture site. **D,** Position the splint under the extremity. **E,** Pad the groin area and secure the ischial strap. **F,** Attach the ankle strap to the ratchet and tighten it just enough to maintain limb alignment and relieve pain. **G,** Fasten the support straps after proper mechanical traction has been applied. **H,** Secure the patient and the traction splint to a backboard. (From American Academy of Orthopedic Surgeons. [1993]. *Emergency care and transportation of the sick and injured,* 5th ed. [pp. 280, 281]. Rosemont, IL: Author.)

firmly. The amount of traction required varies but is generally approximately 15 lb of pulling force.

4. Support the leg while lifting it just high enough to slide the splint under the extremity, and position the padded bar against the ischial tuberosity.
5. Fasten the attached groin strap around the leg over the padding.
6. Attach the S-ring of the ratchet to the D-rings of the ankle hitch, and twist the ratchet knob to tighten traction. Be careful not to overstretch the limb. The

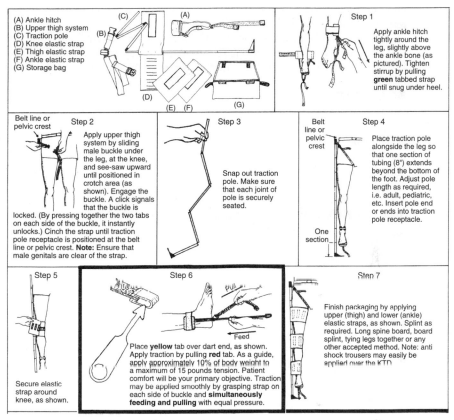

FIGURE 122-2 Application of the Kendrick traction device. (Courtesy Medix Choice. [1997]. *Instructional guide for Kendrick traction device.* El Cajon, CA: Author.)

amount of mechanical traction should equate the manual traction. Manual traction can be released when mechanical traction is established.

7. Secure the Velcro straps around the leg, two above and two below the knee, if possible. Do not place straps directly over the injury site.
8. Lower the heel stand into place to elevate the limb slightly.
9. Reassess distal neurovascular status.

Kendrick Traction Device

1. Adjust the plastic buckle on the thigh strap so it will be located on the anterior thigh when fastened (Figure 122-2).
2. Apply the ankle hitch slightly above the ankle and tighten the stirrup by pulling the green tab until the stirrup is snug under the patient's heel.
3. Slide the thigh strap under the leg and position it in the groin by using a see-saw motion. Fasten the buckle. Cinch the strap until the traction pole receptacle rests against the belt line or the pelvic crest.

4. Extend the folded traction pole, making sure that all joints are properly locked in position.
5. Place the traction pole beside the leg. Extend one end of the pole 8 inches beyond the bottom of the patient's foot. Adjust the opposite end to the patient's extremity length, and insert it into the traction pole receptacle on the groin strap.
6. Secure the elastic knee strap.
7. Place the yellow tab on the ankle strap over the dart end of the traction pole beyond the patient's heel.
8. Apply traction by simultaneously pulling and feeding the strap with both hands until 10% of the patient's body weight or a maximum of 15 lb of tension has been reached.
9. Apply the appropriate elastic thigh and ankle straps. Avoid placing straps directly over the injury site.
10. The legs may be wrapped together as needed to provide further stability.
11. Reassess distal neurovascular status.

Sager Traction Splint

1. Place the splint between the patient's legs (Figure 122-3). The cushioned arch should be seated against the ischial tuberosity. Tight-fitting clothing should be cut open or removed before the splint is applied. Cover the padded bar with a shoe cover turned inside out to help keep the splint clean.
2. Tighten the thigh strap until it fits snugly around the thigh of the injured leg.
3. Extend the shaft of the splint until the wheel of the pulley or the pulling handle is at the patient's heel level.
4. Prepare the ankle harness(es) to fit around the ankle(s) of the injured leg(s) just above the medial and lateral malleoli. Place the harness behind the ankle with one strap on either side of the ankle. Individual pads on the harness may be folded back so it fits snugly around the ankle.
5. Pull the tabs on the strap(s) to take up the slack.
6. Extend the shaft of the splint until the desired amount of traction is reached; usually 10% of the patient's body weight is adequate for a single femur fracture. More traction will be necessary if both femurs are fractured (approximately 20% of body weight).

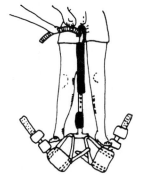 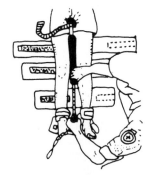 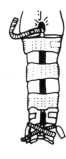

FIGURE 122-3 Application of the bilateral Sager splint. (Courtesy Minto Research & Development, Inc. [1996]. *Instructional guide.* Copyright 1992. Redding, CA: Author.)

7. Retighten the thigh strap if necessary.
8. Bind the patient's legs together with the three leg straps, the longest around the upper thighs, the middle-sized strap under the knees, and the shortest around the lower legs. This prevents rotation of the legs. If you cannot bind the patient's legs together, hip rotation can be minimized with towel rolls or sandbags placed along the lateral aspect of the legs.
9. Wrap the long strap in a figure-eight method around the forefeet to prevent external rotation of the legs.
10. Reassess distal neurovascular status.
    Figure 122-4 demonstrates application of the infant Sager splint.

Thomas Splint

1. Adjust the splint to the length of the patient's leg, and allow an extension of 6-8 inches beyond the foot.
2. Apply the traction strap over the patient's foot after padding the surfaces that lie under the strap.
3. Have an assistant exert longitudinal traction on the leg by placing one hand under the patient's heel and the other over the dorsum of the foot and pulling gently. Manual traction is maintained until the splinting process is complete.
4. Place the splint under the patient's leg by lifting the leg gently and moving the padded half-ring against the ischium. Be sure that the buckle on the splint faces outside and that the half-ring is turned downward.
5. Fasten the ischial strap over the thigh and padding.
6. Bring the long free end of the foot strap over and the under the top of the notched end of the splint.
7. Pass the strap through the link at the swivel in the stirrup under the patient's foot. Apply traction by pulling the strap toward the end of the splint. If no foot strap is available, create an improvised ankle hitch and a Spanish windlass (Figure 122-5) to maintain traction as illustrated.
8. Slide the footrest on the splint until it rests against the bottom of the patient's foot.
9. Apply four or five cravats around the splint to support the leg. Make sure that no fastening device is directly over the injury site. Apply two additional cravats to support the foot and secure it to the footrest.
10. Reassess distal neurovascular status.

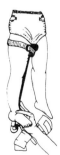

FIGURE 122-4 Application of the infant Sager Splint. (Courtesy Minto Research & Development. [1996]. *Instructional guide.* Copyright 1992. Redding, CA: Author.)

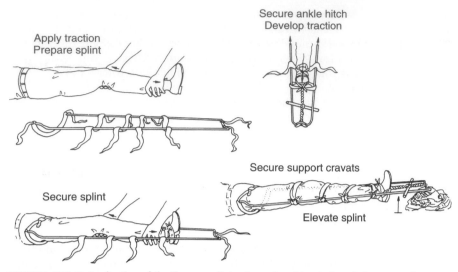

FIGURE 122-5 Application of the Thomas splint using a Spanish windlass (refer to text for procedural steps). Cravats lie over the splint to form a sling that supports the leg, and the Spanish windlass maintains traction. (From Caroline, N.L. [1995]. *Emergency care in the streets,* 5th ed. [p. 312]. Philadelphia Lippincott Williams & Wilkins)

AGE-SPECIFIC CONSIDERATIONS
1. The pediatric/infant Sager splint should always be used in a bilateral mode to provide the best stabilization (Minto Research & Development, 1997). It is appropriate for children from infancy to 6 years of age, depending on the child's height.
2. The Hare traction splint is also available in a pediatric size.
3. Frail elderly patients do not tolerate traction splints well. It may be preferable to use alternative splinting after the patient has been placed on a well-padded backboard.

COMPLICATIONS
1. Compression of the sciatic nerve or perineal tissues
2. Flexion and outward rotation of the proximal femur
3. Excessive traction and overstretching of the limb
4. Compromised neurovascular status in the distal limb(s)
5. Displacement of the proximal third of the fractured femur

PATIENT TEACHING
1. Report when muscle spasm subsides and pain in the injured leg decreases during traction application.
2. Report increased pain or discomfort while in the traction splint.

REFERENCES
Garcia, B. (2002). Extremity trauma (pp. 315-349). In Hubble, M.W., & Hubble, J.P. (Eds.). *Principles of advanced trauma care.* Albany, NY: Delmar.

Limmer, D., O'Keefe, M.F., Grant, H.D., Murray, R.H., & Bergeron, J.D. (2001). *Emergency care*, 9th ed. (pp. 564-611). Upper Saddle River, NJ: Prentice-Hall.

Minto Research & Development. (1997). *Instructional guide for Sager splint.* Redding, CA: Author.

Prehospital Trauma Life Support Committee, National Association of Emergency Medical Technicians. (1999). *PHTLS: basic and advanced prehospital trauma life support*, 4th ed. St. Louis: Mosby.

Sling Application

Ruth L. Schaffler, PhD(c), CEN, ARNP

The information in this procedure should be used in conjunction with the information in Procedure 117.

INDICATION
To support an injured shoulder, clavicle, or upper extremity

EQUIPMENT
Triangular bandage measuring $40 \times 40 \times 55$ inches (can be made by folding or cutting a 40 inch square of material in half)

or

Commercially prepared sling or collar and cuff

Safety pins or tape

PATIENT PREPARATION
1. Pad the axilla to absorb perspiration and prevent skin maceration if the sling is placed under the patient's clothing.
2. Splint the upper extremity as indicated before sling application.

PROCEDURAL STEPS
Sling
1. Place the longest edge of a triangular bandage vertically across the anterior chest with one tip over the uninjured shoulder. The apex of the bandage should lie under the elbow of the injured arm.
2. Place the humerus on the injured side next to the lateral chest wall, and bend the elbow so that the hand is positioned at the opposite fourth or fifth anterior rib (Figure 123-1). The weight of the arm should create an angle of slightly less than 90 degrees at the elbow while in the sling.

3. Bring the lower edge of the triangle over the injured arm, and tie a square knot to the other end of the bandage. The knot should be positioned at the side of the neck, not directly over the cervical spine. Place a pad under the knot.
4. Fold the apex of the triangle forward, and pin or tape it securely to the sling. The apex could also be twisted and knotted when it is snugly fitted against the elbow.

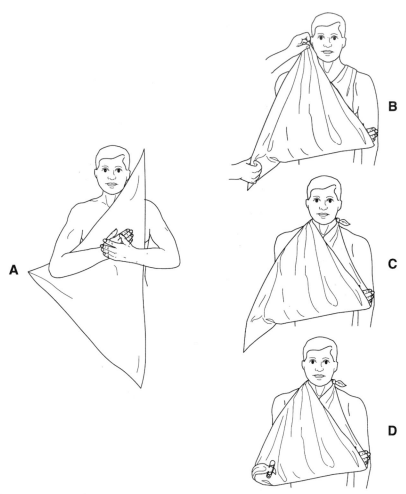

FIGURE 123-1 Applying a triangular bandage as a sling. **A,** The arm is placed across the chest and bandaged as shown. **B,** Bring the lower end of the bandage over the arm and behind the neck. **C,** Tie a square knot to the opposite end at the side of the neck. **D,** Secure the apex of the bandage with a knot or pin. The final position of the arm should create an angle of slightly less than 90 degrees at the elbow; fingers should be exposed.

5. Position the edge of the sling to expose the ends of the fingers.
6. The sling should stabilize the shoulder and upper arm and maintain elevation of the lower arm and hand (Bergeron & Bizjak, 2001; Limmer et al., 2001).

Collar and Cuff
1. Secure the cuff to the patient's wrist.
2. Place the collar around the patient's neck, making sure that it is secure but not restrictive.
3. Loop a strap through the cuff and collar to suspend the wrist. The final position of the elbow should be at slightly less than 90 degrees flexion (Figure 123-2).

Commercial Sling
1. Place the injured arm in the fabric holder with the elbow in the seamed corner.
2. Loop the attached strap across the chest toward the uninjured side, and loop it behind the neck, and then down the chest to the D-rings at the wrist end of the holder.
3. Pass the strap upward through the rings, and secure the Velcro edges together with the elbow flexed at slightly less than 90 degrees (Figure 123-3).

AGE-SPECIFIC CONSIDERATIONS
1. Slings are generally not suitable for children with fractures of the humerus or elbow. The preferred treatment is a sling and swathe, plaster casting, or surgical intervention.
2. Subluxation of the radial head in a child does not generally need immobilization after reduction, but a sling could be used (Garcia, 2002).
3. Additional padding behind the neck may be needed for an elderly patient to avoid excessive pressure over the spine from the weight of the arm in the sling.

COMPLICATIONS
1. Compression of the soft tissues in the neck
2. Increased edema of the distal limb as a result of greater than 90-degree elbow flexion in the sling

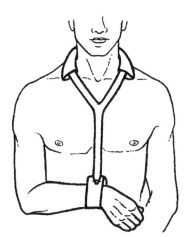

FIGURE 123-2 A collar and cuff. (From Connolly, J.F. [Ed.] [1981]. *de Palma's The management of fractures and dislocations: an atlas,* 3rd ed. [p. 695]. Philadelphia: W.B. Saunders.)

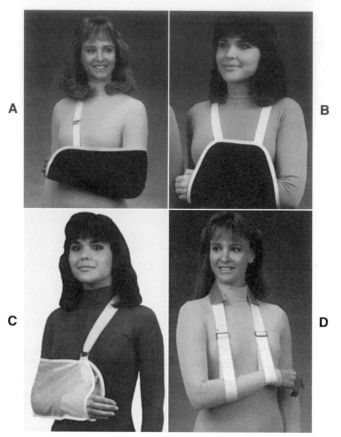

FIGURE 123-3 Examples of commercial slings. (Courtesy Tecnol, Inc. [1997]. *Orthopedic soft goods catalog.* Ft. Worth, TX.)

PATIENT TEACHING

1. Keep the knot positioned at the side of the neck and not directly over the spine to avoid excessive pressure on blood vessels, nerves, and spinous processes.
2. Keep the hand above elbow level, and open and close hand and wiggle fingers frequently to prevent or decrease swelling.

REFERENCES

Bergeron, J.D., & Bizjak, G. (2001). *First responder,* 6th ed. Upper Saddle River, NJ: Prentice-Hall.

Garcia, B. (2002). Extremity trauma (pp. 315-349). In Hubble, M.W., & Hubble, J.P. (Eds.). *Principles of advanced trauma care.* Albany, NY: Delmar.

Limmer, D., O'Keefe, M.F., Grant, H.D., Murray, R.H., & Bergeron, J.D. (2001). *Emergency care,* 9th ed. (pp. 564-611). Upper Saddle River, NJ: Prentice-Hall.

Shoulder Immobilization

Ruth L. Schaffler, PhD(c), CEN, ARNP

The information in this procedure should be used in conjunction with the information in Procedure 117.

Shoulder immobilization is also known as sling and swathe and Velpeau's bandage.

INDICATIONS

1. To immobilize the clavicle, acromioclavicular joint, shoulder, or proximal humerus. A sling and swath is also useful for anterior dislocations of the shoulder (Limmer et al., 2001; McSwain, 2001).
2. To immobilize unstable fractures of the proximal humerus to prevent recurrent dislocation as a result of contraction of the pectoralis major muscle (Velpeau's bandage).
3. To provide greater immobilization than a sling alone because the chest wall acts as a splint.

EQUIPMENT

Commercial sling and swathe
or
Two to three triangular bandages to create a sling and swathe
or
Three to four rolls of 6-inch-wide elastic bandage or a 3- to 4-m length of stockinette to create a Velpeau bandage
Safety pins
Axillary padding (i.e., gauze dressings, bandages, cast padding, pillows)

PATIENT PREPARATION

1. Pad the axilla on the affected side, across the chest where the arm will lie, and over the opposite shoulder where the bandaging material will lie.
2. Flex the elbow on the injured side and place the forearm across the chest.

PROCEDURAL STEPS
Sling and Swathe

1. Apply the cloth sling to the forearm with the elbow positioned in the seamed corner, the hand extending into the open end.
2. Pass the self-fastening strap behind the neck, and secure it to the sling at the wrist.
3. Place the fabric swath around the arm and chest to keep the extremity and shoulder immobilized (Figure 124-1).

Shoulder Immobilizer

1. Apply the elastic band around the chest, and secure with the Velcro fastener.
2. Fasten the arm strap around the humerus, and then fasten the wrist strap around the lower forearm (Figure 124-2).

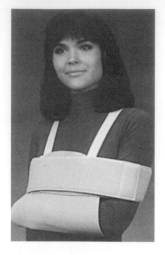

FIGURE 124-1 Example of a sling and swathe. (Courtesy Tecnol, Inc. [1997]. *Orthopedic soft goods catalog.* Forth Worth, TX.)

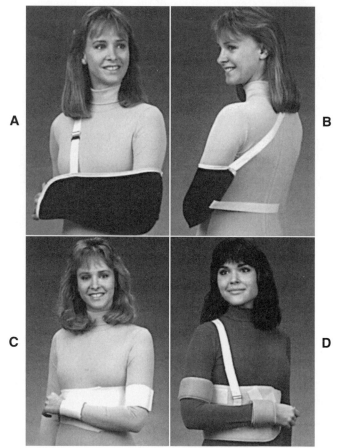

FIGURE 124-2 Examples of commercial shoulder immobilizers. (Courtesy Tecnol, Inc. [1997]. *Orthopedic soft goods catalog.* Fort Worth, TX.)

Velpeau's Bandage

1. Position the affected arm across the chest so that the hand rests on the opposite shoulder.
2. Roll the bandage away from the injury beginning underneath the crossed arm in the center of the chest, and pass the roll under the uninjured axilla.
3. Continue the roll diagonally behind the patient's back and over the top of the affected shoulder.
4. Roll downward diagonally over the folded arm and then loop the bandage behind the elbow, across the middle of the humerus, and through the axilla.
5. Repeat the diagonal roll over the shoulder on the affected side, covering the upper arm and supporting the elbow. Continue into the axilla.
6. Encircle the entire thorax and affected arm.
7. Continue the pattern of alternating the roll of the bandage over the shoulder and arm with a pass around the torso (Figure 124-3).

Gilchrist Stockinette-Velpeau Sleeve

1. Cut a piece of 4-inch-wide stockinette into a 3- to 4-m (approximately 10- to 12-ft) length. Make a horizontal slit halfway across the width of the stockinette approximately one third from one end.

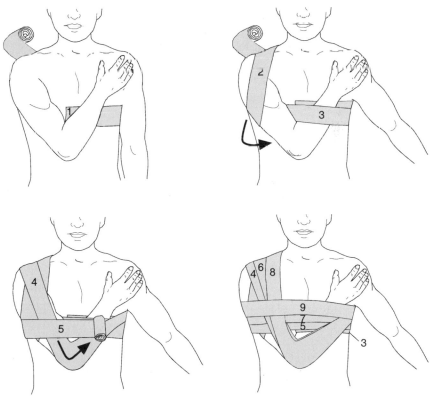

FIGURE 124-3 Application of a Velpeau bandage. Direction of the rolled bandage alternates between arm stabilization and chest encirclement.

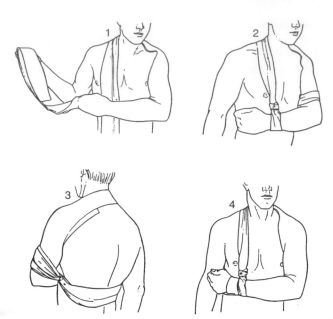

FIGURE 124-4 The stockinette Velpeau bandage encircles the neck and waist and is secured with safety pins or ties. (From Connolly, J.F. [Ed.] [1981]. *de Palma's The management of fractures and dislocations: an atlas,* 3rd ed. [pp. 603, 604]. Philadelphia: W.B. Saunders.)

2. Insert the patient's affected arm into the longer end of the stockinette until the axilla rests in the slot.
3. Place the injured arm across the chest. Pass the long end of the stockinette around the patient's back, through the space between the injured arm and chest, and loosely drape it over the patient's forearm.
4. Pass the shorter end of the stockinette around the patient's neck, loop it around the wrist, and secure it with a safety pin.
5. Pull the loose end of the stockinette tightly, wrap it around the affected arm, and secure it with a safety pin.
6. Make a slit in the stockinette over the patient's wrist to free the hand. Reinforce the slot with tape to prevent fraying or stretching (Figure 124-4).

AGE-SPECIFIC CONSIDERATION

For children under the age of 12 years, a sling and swath may be used for immobilization. Children older than 12 years old may need a hanging arm cast (Sanders et al., 1996).

COMPLICATIONS

1. Frozen shoulder or joint stiffness
2. Neurovascular compromise
3. Restriction of chest wall expansion
4. A sling and swath should not be used in the bedridden because of the loss of gravity needed for alignment and union of a fracture

PATIENT TEACHING
1. Loosen the swath and reapply if it becomes too tight or restricts breathing.
2. Report numbness, tingling, increased swelling, or pain in the distal extremity.
3. Do not lean on the elbow.

REFERENCES
Limmer, D., O'Keefe, M.F., Grant, H.D., Murray, R.H., & Bergeron, J.D. (2001). *Emergency care*, 9th ed. (pp. 564-611). Upper Saddle River, NJ: Prentice-Hall.

McSwain, M.J. (2001). Musculoskeletal trauma (pp. 529-559). In McSwain, N.E., & Paturas J.L. (Eds.). *The basic EMT: comprehensive prehospital patient care*, 2nd ed. St. Louis: Mosby.

Sanders, J.O., et al. (1996). Fractures and dislocations of the humeral shaft and shoulder (pp. 905-916). In Rockwood, C.A. Jr., Wilkins, K.E., & King, R.E. (Eds.). *Fractures in children*, 4th ed. Philadelphia: Lippincott-Raven.

PROCEDURE 125

Knee Immobilization

Ruth L. Schaffler, PhD, CEN, ARNP

The information in this procedure should be used in conjunction with the information in Procedure 117.

INDICATIONS
1. To immobilize a fracture, dislocation, or soft tissue injury of the knee or adjacent structures.
2. To immobilize an unstable knee joint.

CONTRAINDICATIONS AND CAUTIONS
1. The knee should be handled gently and movement of the injured area minimized to decrease pain and the risk of complications, such as damage to the popliteal artery or to the femoral and peroneal nerves (Garcia, 2002).
2. Bony prominences and body contours should be padded to avoid undue pressure or skin breakdown.
3. Realign the angulated limb into an anatomic position before splinting (Bergeron & Bizjak, 2001). The extremity should not be forced to fit the splint. The splint may need to be altered to fit the deformity.
4. Neurovascular status should be assessed and documented before and after the device is applied (Garcia, 2002; McSwain, 2001). If compromise exists, a

physician should be notified immediately. If deterioration occurs after splinting, the device must be readjusted or removed and reapplied.

5. Gross soft tissue swelling may make the application of an immobilizing device difficult or impossible. A plaster or fiberglass splint may have to be applied (see Procedure 127).

EQUIPMENT

Commercial knee immobilizer
or
Plaster or fiberglass splinting material
or
12 to 15 4- × 30-inch or 5- × 30-inch plaster strips
Stockinette or rolled cotton padding
Two to three rolls of 6-inch elastic bandage
Bucket of lukewarm water
Gloves
Absorbent pads
Pillows

PATIENT PREPARATION

1. Remove constrictive clothing that would lie under the immobilization device. If the immobilizer is to be removed occasionally and swelling is minimal, it may be applied over loose clothing.
2. Clean and dress all open wounds.
3. Measure the thigh circumference and the length of the leg to determine the correct size of the immobilizing device.
4. Assess and document neurovascular status.

PROCEDURAL STEPS
Commercial Knee Immobilizer

1. Position the immobilizer under the leg while the patient is supine. If the device has a cutout in the front, place it so that the open area is over the patella. If no cutout is present, place the splint with the upper end at midthigh and the lower end at midcalf. Splints are available in 16- and 22-inch lengths.
2. Secure the device with the attached buckles or Velcro fasteners (Figure 125-1).

Plaster Long Leg Posterior Splint

1. Splint fractures of the knee joint in the position found unless circulatory compromise is present. If circulatory compromise is present, gently apply longitudinal traction manually until circulation is restored.
2. If possible, place the patient in a prone position on a stretcher or examination table.
3. Measure the posterior surface of the unaffected leg from the ball of the foot to midthigh. This measurement determines the length of plaster or fiberglass splinting material needed.
4. Wrap the affected leg with rolled cotton bandage or put on a stockinette that is cut to the measured length.
5. Moisten the plaster or fiberglass material and gently pinch to remove excess water. Do not squeeze or twist (see Procedure 127).

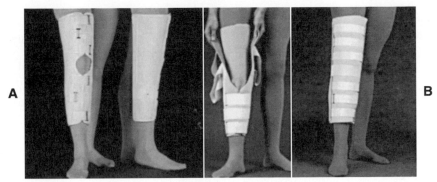

FIGURE 125-1 Examples of knee immobilizers. (Courtesy Tecnol, Inc. [1997]. *Orthopedic soft goods catalog.* Fort Worth, TX.)

6. Apply the plaster or fiberglass to the posterior surface of the limb from toes to midthigh. Keep the foot flexed at 90 degrees.
7. Wrap with elastic bandages to secure the splint in place.
8. Place limb on pillows for support while the splint dries. Extend the distal leg beyond the edge of the stretcher or table to allow the foot to remain in a neutral position.
9. Assess and document neurovascular status.

AGE-SPECIFIC CONSIDERATIONS
Commercial knee immobilizers are available in pediatric lengths (as small as 6 inches long).

COMPLICATIONS
1. Neurovascular compromise
2. Increased edema
3. Increased pain
4. Joint stiffness resulting from prolonged immobilization
5. Joint effusion
6. Compartmental syndrome

PATIENT TEACHING
1. Keep the splint clean and dry.
2. Apply ice packs to the affected area to minimize swelling and pain.
3. Elevate the lower extremity above the level of the heart to reduce swelling.
4. Follow crutch walking and weight-bearing limitations if indicated (see Procedure 135).
5. Notify your physician or return to the emergency department for any symptoms of numbness, tingling, increased swelling, increased pain, or discoloration of the foot.
6. Wear the immobilization device for the recommended length of time and keep your appointments with your physician or physical therapist. (Patients who have sustained a knee injury should be referred to an orthopedic specialist.)

REFERENCES

Bergeron, J.D., & Bizjak, G. (2001). *First responder*, 6th ed. Upper Saddle River, NJ: Prentice-Hall.

Garcia, B. (2002). Extremity trauma (pp. 315-349). In Hubble, M.W., & Hubble, J.P. (Eds.). *Principles of advanced trauma care*. Albany, NY: Delmar.

McSwain, M.J. (2001). Musculoskeletal injuries (pp. 529-559). In McSwain, N.E., & Paturas, J.L. (Eds.). *The basic EMT: comprehensive prehospital patient care*, 2nd ed. St. Louis: Mosby.

PROCEDURE 126

Finger Immobilization

Jean A. Proehl, RN, MN, CEN, CCRN

The information in this procedure should be used in conjunction with the information in Procedure 117.

INDICATIONS

1. To relieve pain, provide stability, promote healing, and prevent functional disability in the presence of finger fractures
2. To protect a repaired tendon, nerve, or vessel from tension
3. To protect soft tissue injuries from further trauma

    Specific splinting recommendations are based on fracture location and type:

    Dorsal splint: Distal phalanx only for mallet-type injury of the distal phalanx involving less than 25% of the articular surface or for avulsion of the profundus tendon at the attachment (Simon & Koenigsknecht, 2001). Dorsal splints may also be applied to the length of the digit for sprains, soft tissue injuries, or stable distal or middle phalangeal fractures.

    Plaster or fiberglass gutter splint: For stable fractures of the middle and proximal phalanx that do not involve articular surfaces (see Procedure 127).

    Volar splint (plaster, fiberglass, or aluminum splint): For uncomplicated extraarticular fractures, sprains, and dislocations and for temporary immobilization until operative reduction can be accomplished (see Procedure 127).

    Buddy taping (also known as dynamic splinting): For middle and proximal phalanx extraarticular fractures that are stable and nondisplaced.

Prong, hairpin, or cage splints: For protection of distal finger injuries such as tuft fractures, fingernail avulsions, or tip amputations.

Internal fixation (Kirschner wire or pin or K-wire, smooth wire, Riordan pin): For precise reduction with unstable or intraarticular fractures.

CONTRAINDICATIONS AND CAUTIONS

1. The fingers should not be immobilized in full extension; fingers should be immobilized in the position of function. Position of function for the hand is 20-degree wrist extension with the thumb in palmar abduction, 50- to 90-degree flexion of the metacarpophalangeal joints, and 15-degree flexion of the interphalangeal joints. The thumb is immobilized in the fist position with the interphalangeal joint extended (Simon & Koenigsknecht, 2001).

2. *Rotational malalignment and angulation should be assessed. With the fingers flexed, lines drawn through the fingernails meet at the scaphoid in the normal hand (Figures 126-1). Rotational malalignment is not acceptable in metacarpal and phalangeal fractures (Figure 126-2) (Simon & Koenigsknecht, 2001).

3. The hand performs many intricate maneuvers, and even small deficits may cause significant functional limitations. The history should include hand dominance and vocations and avocations that involve use of the injured hand (e.g., musical instruments, sports, crafts).

4. Open fractures require antibiotic administration. Clean, distal phalangeal fractures without significant soft tissue damage or crushing may be managed in the emergency department; all other open fractures of the hand are generally managed in the operating room (Simon & Koenigsknecht, 2001).

PATIENT PREPARATION

1. Remove all rings on the injured hand (see Procedure 118).
2. Assess and document neurovascular status.

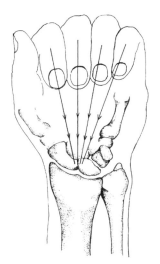

FIGURE 126-1 In a normal hand, lines drawn through the fingernails meet at the scaphoid. (From Simon, R.R. & Koenigsknecht, S.J. [2001]. *Emergency orthopedics: the extremities,* 4th ed. [p. 102]. New York: McGraw-Hill.)

---

*Indicates portions of the procedure usually performed by a physician or an advanced practice nurse.

DORSAL SPLINT
Equipment

$\frac{1}{2}$- to 1-inch tape
Dorsal splint (metal, plastic)

Procedural Steps

1. Extend the distal joint fully for a mallet finger; for other injuries, bend each interphalangeal joint 15 degrees.
2. Size the splint, apply it to the dorsum of the finger, and tape it to the middle phalanx. Place the splint over any necessary dressings or padding (Figures 126-3 and 126-4).

BUDDY TAPING
Equipment

$\frac{1}{2}$- to 1-inch tape
Cast padding or felt

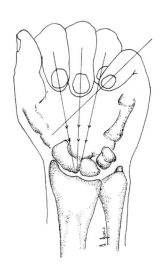

FIGURE 126-2 In the presence of a finger fracture with rotational malalignment, the fingernail of the fractured finger does not point to the scaphoid. (From Simon, R.R., & Koenigsknecht, S.J. [2001]. *Emergency orthopedics: the extremities,* 4th ed. [p. 102]. New York: McGraw-Hill.)

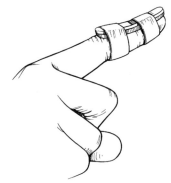

FIGURE 126-3 Dorsal splint of distal interphalangeal joint. (From Chudnofsky, C.R., & Byers, S. [2004]. Splinting techniques [p. 1001]. In Roberts, J.R., &. Hedges, J.R. [Eds.]. *Clinical procedures in emergency medicine,* 4th ed. Philadelphia: W.B. Saunders.)

Procedural Steps

1. Place a single layer of cast padding or felt between the injured finger and the adjacent finger. Use the adjacent finger that is longer than the injured finger. If the middle finger is the injured finger, use the adjacent ring finger.
2. Tape circumferentially around both fingers at the level of the proximal phalanx and the distal phalanx (Figure 126-5).

PRONG OR CAGE SPLINT
Equipment

Prong or cage splint
$1/2$- to 1-inch tape

Procedural Steps

1. Size splint and mold to fit over finger or dressing.
2. Leave a small gap between the distal end of the digit and the splint to prevent transfer of force if the splint is hit.

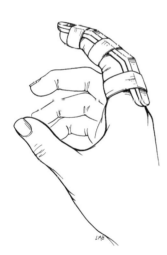

FIGURE 126-4 Dorsal splint of finger. (From Chudnotsky, C.R., & Byers, S, [2004]. Splinting techniques [p. 1000]. In Roberts, J.R., &. Hedges, J.R. [Eds.]. *Clinical procedures in emergency medicine*, 4th ed. Philadelphia: W.B. Saunders.)

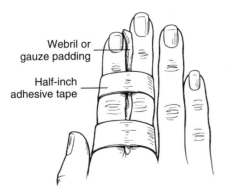

Webril or gauze padding

Half-inch adhesive tape

FIGURE 126-5 Buddy taping or dynamic splinting. (From Chudnofsky, C.R., & Byers, S. [2004]. Splinting techniques [p. 1000]. In Roberts, J.R., &. Hedges, J.R. [Eds.]. *Clinical procedures in emergency medicine*, 4th ed. Philadelphia: W.B. Saunders.)

K-WIRE/RIORDAN FIXATION PIN
Equipment
Antiseptic solution
Pin and drill
Dressing supplies

Procedural Steps
1. *Anesthetize the finger with a digital block before manipulation or reduction of the fracture (see Procedure 139). A regional block at the wrist or a Bier block may also be used (see Procedure 140).
2. Cleanse the affected hand with particular attention to the skin overlying the insertion site with antiseptic solution.
3. *Drill the wire through skin and into the bone.
4. *Test fracture site for stability.
5. Obtain an x-ray study to confirm reduction and pin placement.
6. *Cut the pin off below the skin line.
7. Apply a dressing.
8. Apply an external splint if indicated.

COMPLICATIONS
1. Fracture deformity or nonunion
2. Infection of soft tissue or bone if the skin was broken
3. Loss of mobility, function, or both if the fracture is inadequately reduced, splinted improperly, or the patient does not receive appropriate rehabilitation

PATIENT TEACHING
1. Elevate your arm with your hand above the level of the elbow and the heart.
2. Apply cold packs to fracture site.
3. Report signs of infection, such as redness, swelling, and draining pus (for open fractures or pin insertions).
4. Report increasing pain, numbness, or swelling.
5. Wear splint until directed to remove it.

REFERENCE
Simon, R.R., & Koenigsknecht, S.J. (2001). *Emergency orthopedics: the extremities*, 4th ed. New York: McGraw-Hill.

---

*Indicates portions of the procedure usually performed by a physician or an advanced practice nurse.

Plaster and Fiberglass Splinting

Jean A. Proehl, RN, MN, CEN, CCRN*

The information in this chapter is specific to plaster and fiberglass splints and should be used in conjunction with Procedure 117.

INDICATIONS
1. To immobilize extremities in order to
   a. Maintain bony alignment
   b. Rest ligamentous injuries
   c. Decrease pain
   d. Prevent further soft tissue injury from movement of fracture fragments
   e. Decrease risk of clinically significant fat embolism
2. To allow soft tissue swelling to occur without circulatory compromise, in contrast to circumferential plaster or fiberglass casts.

CONTRAINDICATIONS AND CAUTIONS
1. Bony prominences should be protected by using the appropriate size of splint and shaping it carefully. Patients with diabetes or who are long-term steroid users are also at high risk. Additional padding over bony prominences is recommended.
2. Hot water should never be used to wet the plaster or fiberglass. The chemical reaction that sets the agents into an active state is exothermic (heat producing). This heat, in combination with the heat of the water, may burn the patient. Hot water also accelerates hardening and makes the splint difficult to mold.
3. When using plaster splinting material, the desired position of the extremity should be maintained from the time the first layer of padding or splinting material is applied. Any movement during the splinting process may weaken the splint and may move the extremity out of acceptable alignment.
4. The plaster or fiberglass should never completely encircle an extremity because this does not allow for postinjury swelling.
5. Wear gloves to protect your skin when working with exposed fiberglass or plaster.
6. Fiberglass edges can be sharp and cause lacerations and abrasions; be sure to cover all exposed edges.

---

*The author would like to thank Vaner Smith and Scott Rodi for their expert review of this procedure.

EQUIPMENT

Cotton or synthetic cast padding (SoftRoll, Webril)
Plaster or fiberglass splints or roll
Scissors or knife (to cut plaster or fiberglass)
Measuring tape
Spray bottle or soaking bucket
Elastic bandages
Towels

NOTE: Preassembled plaster and fiberglass splinting material with incorporated padding is available in 1- (fiberglass only), 2-, 3-, 4-, 5-, and 6-inch widths in rolls or packaged lengths. Padding such as stockinette or sheet wadding (SoftRoll or Webril) is used with plain plaster splinting material to provide protection for friable skin or over bony prominences.

PATIENT PREPARATION

1. Assess and document neurovascular status and skin integrity before splint application. If there is a break in the skin at or near a fracture site, an open fracture must be considered. Notify the physician before applying the splint.
2. Dress all wounds before splint application.
3. Cleanse and dry the extremity before splint application.
4. Remove all jewelry from the injured extremity (see Procedure 118).

PROCEDURAL STEPS

1. Place the patient in a position of comfort. If the injury is an upper extremity, the position may be upright; if a lower extremity, the patient may be flat on the abdomen (for short leg posterior splint) or supine (for long leg splint). The prone (inverted) position should be avoided with unstable ankle fractures and obese patients who have trouble breathing when they lie on their abdomen. Also, in this position, the calf is flexed, and the splint may not fit as well when the patient returns to a supine or upright position.
2. For plaster, prepare bucket of tepid water, 70°-84° F or 21°-29° C. For fiberglass splints, only a small amount of water is used, and a water bottle or spray bottle is adequate.
3. If possible, measure for the splint on the unaffected extremity. Accuracy is increased and discomfort decreased by avoiding movement of the injured extremity.
4. Cut prepared splints, rolls, or loose sheets to measured length. Width is determined by the largest surface to be supported.
5. With loose plaster splint sheets, the number of layers required depends on the size of the extremity to be supported, with variance between eight and 20 sheets. When using loose sheets or plain plaster, pad the entire area to be splinted. One or two layers (some prefer three to four layers) of cast padding are sufficient, unless there is marked edema, friable skin, or bony prominences. These conditions require extra padding. Padding is wrapped in circular motion from distal to proximal, seeking conformity and uniform pressure. If padding is too loose, it wrinkles, and pressure sores can develop. If it is too tight, swelling causes constriction. Alternatively, the padding may be folded and placed directly under the splint. This avoids circumferential wrapping of the extremity.

6. When incorporating digits in splints (e.g., gutter splints), place a single layer of padding between them to prevent tissue maceration.

7. Activate preassembled fiberglass splint rolls with a minimum of water, a single line of water down the middle of splints ≤ 3 inches wide or a zig-zag of water down wider splints. Roll the moistened splint up inside a towel, and press it smooth to remove excess moisture (do not squeeze); repeat on the dry side of the towel (Figure 127-1). Immerse and maintain plaster splints in the soaking bucket until bubbling stops, take from the bucket, and gently squeeze to remove excess moisture, then smooth together to meld the layers.

8. Apply the now activated and smoothed splinting material and form and shape using the palmar surface of the hand and an elastic bandage (Figure 127-2). Apply the elastic bandage in a circular motion, wrapping from the distal to the proximal, seeking uniform pressure and conformity.

9. Assess and document the neurovascular status after splint application.

10. Elevate on a smooth surface, and allow 15 minutes drying time before dismissal. Do not place the splint on a plastic surface for drying, because plastic reflects the heat produced by the curing process of the plaster or fiberglass, and the splint may get too hot.

11. In the case of upper extremity injury, if a sling is appropriate, apply it after the splint has been cured to firmness.

   NOTE: See Figures 127-3 through 127-9 for information about specific types of splints.

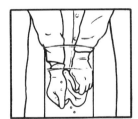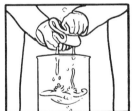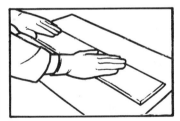

FIGURE 127-1 Submersion, water removal, and smoothing of plaster or fiberglass splint. (Courtesy Johnson & Johnson, Inc. Orthopedics. *Specialists J Splints.* New Brunswick, NJ.)

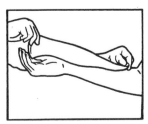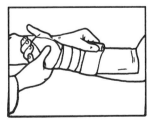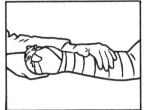

FIGURE 127-2 Application of a splint and an elastic bandage, and molding of the splint to the extremity. (Courtesy Johnson & Johnson, Inc., Orthopedics. *Specialists J Splints.* New Brunswick, NJ.)

Also known as:	Posterior boot, posterior slab
Indications:	Fracture or soft tissue injuries of the foot or ankle
Equipment:	4- to 5-in. cast padding
	4- to 6-in. plaster (10-15 layers) or fiberglass
	4- to 6-in. elastic bandage
Measure:	From the metatarsal 2 inches below the popliteal area to 2 inches beyond the toes.
Extremity position:	Foot should be at a 90-degree angle to the leg. The splint should not impede knee flexion. Fold the splint under 1 inch at the toes to provide reinforcement.

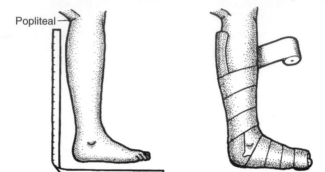

Popliteal

FIGURE 127-3 Posterior short leg splint. (Courtesy BSN Medical, Posterior ankle splint, 2001, Charlotte, NC.)

Also known as:	Anterior posterior splints, sandwich splints, reverse sugar tong
Indications:	Fractures or soft tissue injuries of the forearm/wrist
Equipment:	3- to 4-in. cast padding
	3- to 4-in. fiberglass or plaster splints (8-10 layers)
	3- to 4-in. elastic bandage
Measure:	From the fingertips, over the dorsum of the hand, over the flexed elbow, and on over the volar aspect of the forearm to the fingertips. Fold the splint in half and cut across the fold, leaving approximately ½ inch attached. Slide the splint over the patient's arm with the attached section in the web space between the thumb and index finger. Wrap with elastic bandage and fold excess splint around the elbow and overlap with the other side.
Extremity position:	Forearm with thumb up and 90-degree flexion of the elbow (consult with physician for prescribed position as other positions may be indicated).

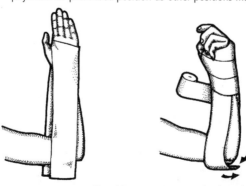

FIGURE 127-4 Forearm sugar tong splint. (Courtesy BSN Medical, Reverse sugar tong, 2001, Charlotte, NC.)

Also known as:	Hanging humeral splint
Indications:	Immobilization of a humeral shaft fracture
Equipment:	4- to 5-in. cast padding
	4- to 5-in. fiberglass or plaster (8-15 layers)
	4- to 5-in. elastic bandage
Measure:	From the acromioclavicular (AC) joint, over the humerus, around the elbow, and up the axillary crease.
Extremity position:	Forearm is either pronated or supinated with a 90-degree flexion of the elbow (consult with physician for prescribed position).

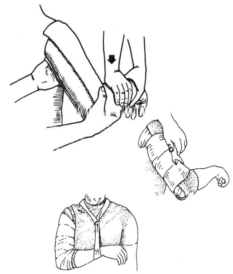

FIGURE 127-5 Humerus sugar tong. (From Simon, R., & Brenner, B. [2002]. *Emergency procedures and techniques,* 4th ed. [p. 269]. Baltimore: Williams & Wilkins.)

AGE-SPECIFIC CONSIDERATIONS

1. In pediatric or geriatric populations, splints and elastic bandage size should be in accordance with the width of the extremity to be splinted.
2. In both the pediatric and the geriatric population, the skin tends to be thinner and thereby at higher risk for maceration, pressure sores, and exothermic burns. Attention to the cautions and the procedural steps assists in minimizing the risks.

COMPLICATIONS

1. Pressure sores may develop because of wrinkling of the cotton padding or indentations of the plaster. When this pressure continues, compression of the skin and underlying fat can result in tissue necrosis.
2. Plaster burns can occur because of the chemical accelerators, the temperature of the water bath, the amount of water in the splinting material, the

Also known as:	Wrist gauntlet
Indications:	Soft tissue injury, metacarpal fracture of the thumb, or fracture of the navicular or scaphoid bone. If splinting for a scaphoid fracture, some authors advocate extension of the splint to above the elbow (Simon & Koenigsknecht, 2001).
Equipment:	2- to 3-in. cast padding 2- to 3-in. fiberglass or plaster splints (8-10 layers) 2- to 3-in. elastic bandage
Measure:	From the distal tip of the thumb to approximately two thirds of the way up the forearm. Splint should not impede flexion of the elbow, and the fingers should be free, allowing full motion of the metacarpophalangeal joints.
Extremity position:	The hand is positioned as if holding a beverage can, with the thumb curved toward the fingers and the wrist neutral or slightly dorsiflexed (Simon & Koenigsknecht, 2001).

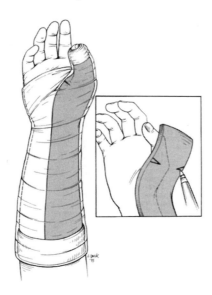

FIGURE 127-6 Thumb spica splint. (From Chudnofsky, C.R., & Byers, S. [2004]. Splinting techniques [p. 998]. In Roberts, J.R., & Hedges, J.R. [Eds.]. *Clinical procedures in emergency medicine,* 4th ed. Philadelphia: W.B. Saunders.)

thickness of the splint, and sensitivity to the product. To aid in prevention of burns, use cool to tepid water to activate the material, follow the manufacturer's suggestions for padding and protection of the skin, and allow adequate air circulation to aid in the drying process. If the patient complains that the splint is burning, remove it immediately.
3. Improper positioning of the splinted extremity can result in misalignment, neurovascular compromise, or both. Verify the desired position before splint

Also known as:	Anterior splint or radial slab
Indications:	Fracture or soft tissue injury to the wrist or carpal bones
Equipment:	3- to 4-in. cast padding
	3- to 4-in. fiberglass or plaster splint (8-10 layers)
	3- to 4-in. elastic bandage
Measure:	From palmar crease to approximately 3 cm proximal to the antecubital fossa
Extremity position:	Wrist in a neutral position, slightly extended, with the fingers at 10-20 degrees of flexion, with the thumb pointing up. Fold the splint at an angle across the palmar crease.

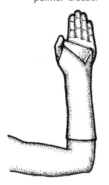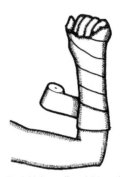

FIGURE 127-7 Volar forearm splint. (Courtesy BSN Medical, Volar splint, 2001, Charlotte, NC.)

Also known as:	Phalangeal or metacarpal gutter splint, boxer splint
Indications:	Fracture or soft tissue injury of the fourth and fifth metacarpals
Equipment:	2- to 3-in. cast padding
	2- to 3-in. fiberglass or plaster splints (6-8 layers)
	2- to 3-in. elastic bandage
Measure:	From the fingertips and up two thirds of the forearm
Extremity position:	Position the hand with the fingers held at 50-90 degrees of flexion at the metacarpophalangeal (MCP) joint and 20 degrees of flexion at the interphalangeal (IP) joint (Simon & Koenigsknecht, 2001). The wrist should be slightly extended. Place padding between the 4th and 5th fingers.

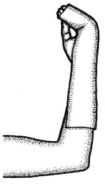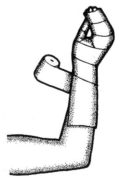

FIGURE 127-8 Ulnar gutter splint. (Courtesy BSN Medical, Boxer splint, 2001, Charlotte, NC.)

Also known as: Teardrop, phalangeal, or metacarpal gutter splint
Indications: Fractures or soft tissue injuries of the 1st-3rd metacarpals
Equipment: 2- to 3-in. cast padding
                      2- to 3-in. fiberglass or plaster splints (6-8 layers)
                      2- to 3-in. elastic bandage
Measure: From the fingertips and up two thirds of the forearm (Simon & Koenigsknecht,
                      2001). Cut a 2 ½-inch hole for the thumb and tape the edges.
Extremity position: Position the hand with the fingers held at 50-90 degrees of flexion at the
                      metacarpophalangeal (MCP) joint and 20 degrees of flexion at the inter-
                      phalangeal (IP) joint (Simon & Koenigsknecht, 2001). The wrist should be
                      slightly extended.

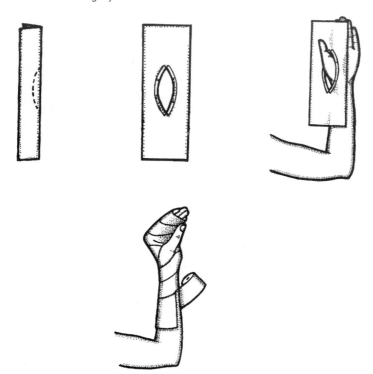

FIGURE 127-9 Radial gutter splint. (Courtesy BSN Medical, Teardrop splint, 2001, Charlotte, NC.)

application, and check pulses, sensation, and capillary refill before and after application of the splint.

4. Although it is less common with splint application than with full casts, compartmental syndrome can develop in conjunction with injury or as a result of splint application.

PATIENT TEACHING

1. Fiberglass activates in minutes and is cured when it is no longer warm. Plaster requires at least 12-24 hours' drying time. For both products, care

should be taken to prevent impression during the first 12-24 hours, which could result in misalignment or pressure sores.

2. Elevate and ice the injured extremity to minimize edema and increase comfort (see Procedure 132).

3. Watch for swelling, increasing pain, numbness, pale or blue fingers or toes, or tingling in the extremity. If any of these occur, loosen the elastic wrap and elevate the extremity above the level of the heart. If symptoms persist, contact your physician or return to the emergency department.

4. Splints should be kept dry. If a plaster splint gets wet, it crumbles, and it will not harden again. If the fiberglass product gets wet, it should be blotted with a towel, then fully dried with blow dryer (hair dryer). Do not wear a wet splint, because skin breakdown may occur.

5. Do not stick anything into the splint. If itching is a problem, use an ice pack over the area, or rearrange the splint and elastic bandage.

6. Do not use or walk on the injured extremity. Splints are not strong enough to support the body weight (see Procedures 134 and 135).

REFERENCES

Simon, R.R., & Brenner, B.E. (2002). *Emergency procedures and techniques*, 4th ed. Baltimore: Williams & Wilkins.

Simon, R.R., & Koenigsknecht, S.J. (1995). *Emergency orthopedics: the extremities*, 3rd ed. Norwalk, CT: Appleton & Lange.

PROCEDURE 128

Removal and Bivalving of Casts

Margo E. Layman, MSN, RN, RNC, CN-A

Bivalving is also known as a bilateral split or splitting a cast.

INDICATIONS
1. To relieve neurovascular impairment caused by pressure from the cast
2. To facilitate care and access when the circumferential strength is no longer required
3. To remove a cast when it is no longer required or when a new cast is indicated

CONTRAINDICATIONS AND CAUTIONS
1. Cutting directly over a bony prominence should be avoided.
2. Cast cutter blades vibrate instead of rotate. Therefore, skin injury is unlikely. If excessive pressure is used when the plaster or fiberglass is cut, however, lacerations or abrasions may occur.
3. When bivalving to relieve pressure, the inner wadding needs to be split all the way to the skin (Simon & Koenigsknecht, 2001).
4. Fiberglass is significantly more difficult to cut than plaster.

EQUIPMENT
Cover sheet
Cast cutter or saw
Cast spreader
Protective eyewear
Elastic bandages (for bivalving)
Scissors

PATIENT PREPARATION
1. Arrange a nonverbal signal so that the patient can communicate despite the noise when excessive heat or pressure is felt. Heat is generated with the movement of the cast blade. A brief pause relieves the sensation.
2. Demonstrate the safety of the cutter by touching the blade to your thumb or the stretcher mattress, which stops the motion of the blade.

PROCEDURAL STEPS
Bivalving
1. Place a sheet under the cast to collect plaster material and cover the patient's clothing.
2. Mark the cast lengthwise into two equal parts, avoiding bony prominences. Univalving the cast may be sufficient if neurovascular impairment resolves after one side of the cast is cut. Wedges are commercially to hold the cast open so that it does not have to be bivalved in all cases.
3. Cut with an even up-and-down motion, releasing when you feel the cutter break through the plaster or fiberglass material (Figure 128-1, *A*).
4. Separate the cast with the cast spreader, and cut the cotton wadding with scissors (see Figure 128-1, *A*).
5. Reassess neurovascular status, and notify the physician of residual deficits.
6. Wrap the cast with an elastic bandage to secure it in place (Figure 128-1, *B*).

Removal of Cast
1. Bivalve cast as directed previously.
2. Once the cast is split through to the skin surface, remove the anterior portion of the cast.

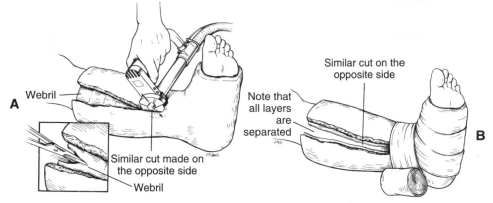

FIGURE 128-1 Bivalving a cast. See text for explanation. (From Chudnofsky, C.R., & Byers, S. [2004]. Splinting techniques [p. 1008]. In Roberts, J.R., & Hedges, J.R. [Eds.]. *Clinical procedures in emergency medicine,* 4th ed. Philadelphia: W.B. Saunders.)

3. With support to the extremity, remove the posterior portion. Clean and dry the skin gently.
4. Apply splints or other orthopedic adjuncts as prescribed.

AGE-SPECIFIC CONSIDERATIONS
1. The noise of the cast saw is intense and can be disturbing. Pediatric patients should be warned about the sounds and the process before the saw is turned on.
2. Elderly patients have thinner, more friable skin and are at increased risk for abrasions or lacerations.

COMPLICATIONS
1. Laceration or abrasion of the skin with the cast cutter
2. Displacement of an unhealed fracture

PATIENT TEACHING
1. Exercise and weight bearing are specified by the physician on the basis of the injury and the healing process.
2. It is normal to have peeling, dry skin where the cast was; this resolves within a few days. Moisturizing lotions may be applied.
3. If the extremity has atrophied because of lack of muscle activity, reassure the patient that with exercise the limb will eventually strengthen and normalize.

REFERENCE
Simon, R.R., & Koenigsknecht, S.J. (2001). *Emergency orthopedics: the extremities*, 4th ed. Norwalk, CT: Appleton & Lange.

Elastic Bandage Application

Margo E. Layman, MSN, RN, RNC, CN-A

Elastic bandages are also known as Ace wraps and crepe bandages.

INDICATIONS

1. To immobilize a fracture in conjunction with a splint
2. To provide a hemostatic dressing
3. To anchor dressings and decrease tension on sutures
4. To provide support, minimize swelling, and prevent further injury in the presence of soft tissue trauma

CONTRAINDICATIONS AND CAUTIONS

1. The patient may have an allergy to the sizing material in new fabrics or latex allergy (may use flannel or muslin bandage instead). Latex-free elastic bandages are available.
2. Elastic bandages may decrease peripheral circulation and should be used with caution in the presence of peripheral vascular disease or diabetes.

EQUIPMENT

Elastic bandage (for legs and knees, 3-4 inches wide; for hands, wrist, and elbows, 2-3 inches wide)
Tape or safety pins or clips
Dressings as indicated
Cast padding (optional)

PATIENT PREPARATION

1. Place extremity in the position of function. See Procedure 127 for information on positioning.
2. If possible, before application, elevate the extremity for 15-30 minutes to facilitate venous return and help decrease edema.
3. *Optional:* Apply three to four layers of cast padding under the area to be wrapped. The wrapping configuration is the same as that used for the overlying elastic bandage.

PROCEDURAL STEPS

1. Unroll 3-4 inches and hold the bandage with the roll facing up, and anchor the bandage by circling twice around the distal extremity (Figure 129-1).
2. To ensure uniform pressure, unroll the bandage as you wrap the body part. Stretch the bandage only slightly while wrapping.
3. Overlap each layer of the bandage by half to two thirds the width of the bandage.
4. Wrap firmly but not tightly. You should be able to insert a finger easily under the bandage.

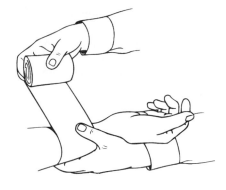

FIGURE 129-1 Elastic bandage application: anchor the bandage by circling twice around the extremity. (From Proehl, J.A., & Jones, L.M. [1998]. *Mosby's emergency department teaching guides.* [p. I-2]. St. Louis: Mosby.)

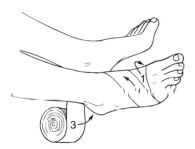 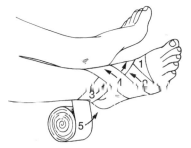

FIGURE 129-2 Figure-eight wrap around joint. (From Proehl, J.A., & Jones, L.M. [1998]. *Mosby's emergency department teaching guides.* [p. I-2]. St. Louis, Mosby.)

5. Include the wrist when wrapping the hand and the foot when wrapping the ankle.
6. Use a figure-eight wrap on joints (Figure 129-2). A spiral wrap is used if a joint is not involved. Toes and fingers should be visible for follow-up circulation assessment.
7. Secure the bandage with tape or pins or clips. Do not place pins or clips on posterior or medial surfaces because they may cause soft tissue injury if pressure is applied to them.

COMPLICATIONS
1. Neurovascular impairment or skin irritation may be caused by bandages that are too tight. Assess and document neurovascular status before and after bandage application.
2. Distal edema as a result of obstruction of venous return can occur. This edema can be decreased by including the hand or foot in distal extremity wraps and by elevating the wrapped extremity.

PATIENT TEACHING
1. Reapply the bandage if it loosens unless otherwise instructed.
2. Launder the bandage as needed.

3. Watch for numbness, tingling, coldness, swelling, or discoloration of the hand or foot. Loosen the bandage and elevate the extremity if any of these signs or symptoms occur. Report any symptoms not relieved by loosening the bandage or elevating the extremity.
4. Elevate the extremity and apply ice as directed to help prevent and decrease swelling.

PROCEDURE 130

Skeletal Traction

Jean A. Proehl, RN, MN, CEN, CCRN

Skeletal traction is also known as Steinmann pin, Kirschner wire, and K-wire.

INDICATIONS
To maintain alignment of fractured bone ends via continuous traction on a pin or wire through bone. Traction helps decrease muscle spasm and movement of bone ends. Skeletal traction may be used when heavier weights and longer periods of immobilization are required than are permitted by skin traction. It is most frequently used with fractures of the femur but is also used for fractures of the tibia and humerus. The cervical spine may also be immobilized with traction (see Procedure 97).

CONTRAINDICATIONS AND CAUTIONS
1. Aseptic technique must be maintained to prevent contamination of the pin sites during insertion.
2. Pins are not inserted through infected or abraded soft tissue.

EQUIPMENT
Antiseptic solution
Local anesthetic
Syringes and needles for local anesthesia administration
No. 11 scalpel

Steinmann pin or Kirschner wire set (assorted sizes) (NOTE: Kirschner wires [K-wires] are generally smaller in diameter than Steinmann pins. Either may be smooth or threaded.)

Drill to drive pin

Pin cutter

Cork, tape, or rubber stoppers (e.g., those from blood tubes) to place over the cut pin ends

Gauze dressings

Antibiotic ointment (optional)

Traction bow or caliper (Bohler-Steinmann pin holder or Kirschner wire tractor)

Hospital bed with traction setup as indicated

Rope

Weights, usually 15-25 lbs (7-12 kg) for extremity fractures

PATIENT PREPARATION

1. Move the patient onto the hospital bed before removal of the temporary splint.
2. Assess and document neurovascular status distal to the injury.

PROCEDURAL STEPS

1. Cleanse the skin at the pin insertion site with antiseptic solution.
2. *Anesthetize the skin, tissue, and periosteum along the intended tract of the pin on both sides (see Procedure 138).
3. *Make a small incision in the skin at the insertion site in the direction of the pull of traction.
4. *Attach the pin to the drill.
5. *Drive the pin through the bone perpendicular to the long axis of the bone. Drilling too quickly can generate heat and should be avoided for secure pin placement.
6. *Incise the skin over the exit site as it is tented by the exiting pin.
7. *Remove the drill when the pin is sufficiently through the bone to attach the traction bow.
8. *Apply the traction bow, and cut off the excess pin.
9. Place cork, tape, or rubber stoppers over the cut pin ends.
10. *Attach the rope to the traction bow, run it through the pulley, and attach the weights.
11. *Suspend the extremity as indicated. The most common and most versatile traction setup for femur fractures is balanced suspension with a Thomas splint and a Pearson attachment. The patient is able to move about in bed while the leg remains supported and traction is constant (Figure 130-1).
12. Assess and document neurovascular status.
13. Perform pin care per institutional protocol. Options include:
    a. Gauze dressing around the pin
    b. Antibiotic ointment around the pin entrance and exit
    c. No dressing or ointment to sites

---

*Indicates portions of the procedure usually performed by a physician or an advanced practice nurse.

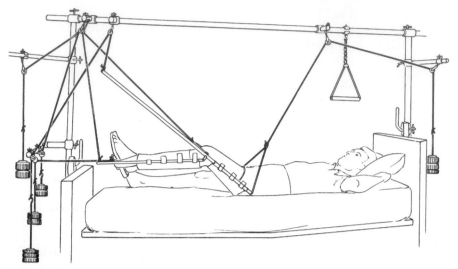

FIGURE 130-1 Thomas splint with Pearson attachment for balanced suspension. (From Smeltzer, S.C., & Bare, B.G. [2004]. *Brunner and Suddarth's textbook of medical-surgical nursing,* 10th ed. [p. 2027]. Philadelphia: Lippincott Williams & Wilkins.)

14. Obtain postreduction x-ray studies.
15. Secure all rope knots with tape.

COMPLICATIONS

1. Osteomyelitis at the pin insertion site
2. Skin necrosis at the pin site
3. Sudden loss of traction and motion of fractured bone ends caused by equipment failure. Be sure that traction weights hang freely at all times and that knots in the traction rope are not caught in the pulleys. Traction should not be interrupted.
4. Wire or pin migration during insertion or slips after insertion. Both are more common with smooth wires or pins.
5. Compartmental syndrome as a result of excessive traction.

PATIENT TEACHING

1. Do not attempt to adjust traction device. Request help to reposition yourself in bed.
2. Report any signs of infection immediately, including redness, swelling, increased pain, or pus.
3. Report any signs of compartmental syndrome immediately, including pain, swelling, numbness, or tingling.
4. Report any problems with the pin or traction.

Heat Therapy

Daun A. Smith, RN, MS, CEN

Heat therapy is also known as hot compress, hot pack, and warm moist pack.

INDICATIONS

1. To decrease the pain and stiffness associated with subacute and chronic injuries of soft tissues and joints. Heat increases blood flow, producing an inflammatory response that may be beneficial at some stages of a disease or injury process.
2. To assist in the treatment of dermatologic or infectious conditions and pain associated with muscle spasm in the patient with degenerative joint disease.

CONTRAINDICATION AND CAUTIONS

1. Heat therapy should be avoided in the presence of severe peripheral vascular disease, venous insufficiency, vasculitis, thromboangiitis obliterans, thrombophlebitis, vasospastic disorders (e.g., Raynaud's phenomenon), immature scar tissue, infected wounds, bleeding tendencies, and known sensitivity to heat. Use extreme caution with paralyzed or insensate areas.
2. Heat treatments should be instituted after the 48 hour acute phase. When the treatments are started prematurely, increased bleeding and swelling may result and prolong the inflammatory process.
3. Therapeutic benefit for the injured patient is seen only when applied heat is used in conjunction with passive range of motion and stretching (Earley, 1999).

EQUIPMENT

Dry towel or cloth
Hot moist pack or
Heat lamp or commercial hot pack
NOTE: Commercial products are available that offer temperature control and delivery of moist heat.

PROCEDURAL STEPS

1. Place a towel in warm water: 96°-103° F (36°-39° C).
2. Express excess water and place in a dry towel and apply to the injured area. You may also use a thin plastic wrap to contain the heat and excess moisture.
3. For appropriate penetration, the application must be left in place for 15-30 minutes (Earley, 1999).
4. Heat lamps can also be used in conjunction with wet packs (see Procedure 153).

AGE-SPECIFIC CONSIDERATIONS

1. Aging skin is less vascular, thinner, and therefore more easily injured. Care should be taken to ensure that water temperature or heat is within the stated

parameters and that the duration of the therapy be 20 minutes or less in the elderly patient (Simon & Koenigsknecht, 2001).
2. Infants and young children have thinner skin and are easily burned with temperatures that would not affect adult skin. Warm—not hot—water is recommended.

COMPLICATIONS
1. If applied acutely in the injured patient, heat increases tissue edema.
2. Excessive or prolonged heat can burn the skin.
3. Prolonged contact with a moist pack can result in skin maceration.

PATIENT TEACHING
1. Heat treatments applied for 20- to 30-minute intervals two to four times daily assist with healing and resumption of normal function.
2. Full trunk and extremity immersion may be used. Use caution to avoid prolonged direct pressure from air jets on the injured area because this may cause increased damage to the tissues.

REFERENCES
Earley, D. (1999). A hot topic: superficial heat agents. *OT Practice, 4* (1), 26-30.
Simon, R.R., & Koenigsknecht, S.J. (1995). *Emergency orthopedics: the extremities,* 3rd ed. Norwalk, CT: Appleton & Lange.

PROCEDURE 132

Cold Therapy

Daun A. Smith, RN, MS, CEN

Cold therapy is also known as cryotherapy, cold pack, or ice pack.

INDICATIONS
To control soft tissue pain and edema in the presence of fractures, soft tissue injuries, sprains, and strains. The initial physiologic response is constriction of the local cutaneous and subcutaneous vessels, which results in reduced blood volume to the affected site, which decreases edema.

CONTRAINDICATIONS AND CAUTIONS

1. Cold therapy should be avoided in patients with a history of severe peripheral vascular disease, venous insufficiency, vasculitis, thromboangiitis obliterans, thrombophlebitis, vasospastic disorders (e.g., Raynaud's phenomenon, Buerger's disease), anesthetized extremities, or known sensitivity to cold. Use extreme caution with paralyzed or insensate areas. In these conditions, the vasoconstriction caused by cold therapy may exacerbate underlying tissue perfusion problems.
2. Excessive or prolonged cold treatments can freeze the skin, resulting in frostnip, superficial frostbite, or deep frostbite and vascular damage. Ice bags should have a dry interface with the skin to decrease the risk of damage to the skin.
3. Cold should be discontinued if the skin blanches then turns red after application (Tittler & Rakel, 2001).

EQUIPMENT

Ice in waterproof bag
or
Commercial cold or gel pack
Small cloth or towel
NOTE. Chemical cold packs should not be used on the face because puncture of the bag may result in chemical injury to the eyes.

PROCEDURAL STEPS

1. Place cubed or crushed ice in a waterproof bag.
2. Wrap the bag in a dry cloth or towel before application to the skin.
3. If a commercial product is used, follow the instructions regarding insulation and application to the skin surface.
4. Complete extremity immersion can be performed for irregularly shaped areas. The mixture of water and ice should be at 55°-60° F (13°-16° C). Reassess distal circulation after 10-15 minutes.
5. Cold packs or ice water immersion is applied for a period of 20-30 minutes per exposure. To avoid skin and tissue damage, longer application is not recommended (Titler & Rakel, 2001).
6. Reapply cold every 1-2 hours for 24-72 hours after injury.

AGE-SPECIFIC CONSIDERATIONS

1. Cold therapy is recommended for all populations after acute injury or after orthopedic surgery. The application time should be shortened to 15-20 minutes on a 3- to 4-hour reapplication cycle in pediatric and geriatric patients who have thinner, more easily injured skin.
2. Monitoring for signs of frostnip or frostbite must be stressed during patient and family teaching for these populations.

COMPLICATIONS

Frostnip, superficial frostbite, or deep frostbite and vascular damage from excessive or prolonged cold treatment.

PATIENT TEACHING

1. Always put a dry cloth between the cold pack and the skin.

2. Apply cold for 20-30 minutes every 1-2 hours in conjunction with rest and elevation of the affected site to assist with lessening pain and edema. Small children and elderly patients have thinner skin. To prevent injury in the very young or very old, apply cold for 15-20 minutes every 3-4 hours.
3. The effective cycling period for this treatment in the acute phase is 24-72 hours.
4. Complete extremity immersion can be performed with caution, limiting the exposure time to 20-30 minutes and elevating the injury site after therapy.
5. Discontinue cold therapy if the skin blanches and turns red or if the area becomes completely numb.

REFERENCES

Titler, M.G., & Rakel, B.A. (2001). Nonpharmacological treatment of pain. *Critical Care Clinics of North America, 13*, 221-232.

PROCEDURE 133

Measuring Compartmental Pressure

Jean A. Proehl, RN, MN, CEN, CCRN

Compartmental pressure is also known as compartment pressure, intracompartmental pressure, and tissue pressure.

INDICATIONS

To measure tissue pressure when compartmental syndrome is suspected. Causes of compartmental syndrome include, but are not limited to, fractures, soft tissue or vascular trauma, crush injuries, exercise, envenomation, tight casts or circumferential dressings, pneumatic antishock garments, automatic blood pressure devices, massive fluid resuscitation, and burns.

Tissue pressure is normally 10 mm Hg or less (Hays, 2001). Follow-up monitoring is indicated if tissue pressures are between 20 and 30 mm Hg. Pressures in excess of 30-40 mm Hg in the presence of positive clinical findings suggest the need for decompression of the compartment via fasciotomy. Metabolically, the differential pressure between diastolic blood pressure and compartment pressure may be more important than absolute compartment pressure. A differential pressure of less than 30 mm Hg (diastolic blood pressure – compartmental pressure) was a safe indicator for fasciotomy in one study (McQueen & Court-Brown, 1996).

CONTRAINDICATIONS AND CAUTIONS

1. When compartmental syndrome is clinically evident, there is no need to measure compartmental pressures, and the patient should proceed immediately to the operating room for decompression via fasciotomy.
2. Inserting the needle or catheter through infected or contaminated tissue should be avoided.
3. The needle or catheter should be inserted as far away from fractured bone ends as possible to prevent conversion of a closed fracture to an open fracture. An open fracture does not rule out the possibility of a compartmental syndrome (McQueen & Court-Brown, 1996).
4. Application of cold packs to suspect extremities is controversial because further vasoconstriction may exacerbate the already decreased tissue perfusion. Consult with the physician before applying cold packs.
5. The techniques presented here are the most easily implemented in the emergency department setting but are not suitable for continuous pressure monitoring. Other equipment setups may include pressure monitoring systems of the type used for invasive lines, continuous infusion devices, and wick or slit catheters.

PATIENT PREPARATION

1. Remove circumferential dressings or casts (see Procedure 128).
2. Keep the extremity at the level of the heart (not elevated) to optimize blood flow to the tissues until compartmental syndrome has been ruled out.
3. Treat systemic hypotension with fluids, medications, or both to sustain tissue perfusion.
4. Cleanse the skin overlying the insertion site with antiseptic solution. Multiple insertion sites may be used to measure pressures in different compartments of the same extremity (Figure 133-1).
5. *Infiltrate the insertion site with local anesthetic (optional). If local anesthetic is used, care should be taken to infiltrate only the skin because injection of additional fluid into the compartment could increase the tissue pressure.
6. Instruct the patient to keep the extremity relaxed during pressure measurements because movement causes the pressure to change.

STRYKER INTRACOMPARTMENTAL PRESSURE MONITOR
Equipment

Antiseptic solution
Gauze dressings
Local anesthetic with needles and syringe (optional)
Intracompartmental pressure monitor (Stryker, Kalamazoo, MI)

---

*Indicates portions of the procedure usually performed by a physician or an advanced practice nurse.

Four compartments of the leg: the anterior compartment (AC), the lateral compartment (LC), the superficial posterior compartment (SPC), and the deep posterior compartment (DPC).

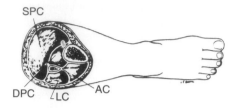

Two compartments of the forearm: the volar compartment (VC) and the dorsal compartment (DC).

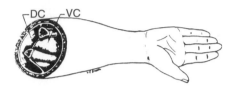

Five interosaeous compartments of the hand.

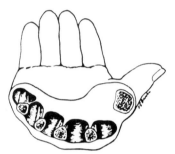

FIGURE 133-1 Compartments of the lower leg, forearm, and hand. (From Matsen, F. A., III. [1980]. *Compartmental syndromes* [p. 82]. New York: Grune & Stratton, with permission.)

Needle, transducer, and syringe assembly supplied by manufacturer
NOTE: Through-the-needle slit catheters are also available for continuous pressure monitoring with this unit.

Procedural Steps (Stryker, 1999)

1. Turn the pressure monitor on. The pressure should be between 0 and 9 mm Hg.
2. Assemble the needle, transducer, and syringe, and place into the pressure monitor with the black side of the transducer down (Figure 133-2).
3. Close the cover of the pressure monitor until the latch snaps.
4. Remove the clear end cap of the syringe, and attach the plunger to the syringe.
5. Hold the monitor at a 45-degree angle with the needle upright, and push on the plunger to purge the unit of air. Do not allow fluid to flow back into the transducer well.
6. *Hold the monitor at the intended angle of insertion into the skin, and press the zero button (Figure 133-3). The digital display should read 00 after a few seconds. The display must read 00 before continuing.
7. *Insert the needle into the compartment. Slowly inject less than 0.3 ml of saline into the compartment to equilibrate the monitor with the interstitial fluids.

---

*Indicates portions of the procedure usually performed by a physician or an advanced practice nurse.

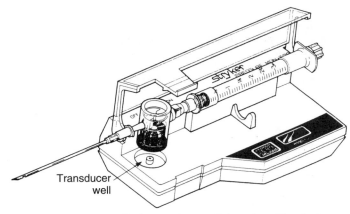

FIGURE 133-2 Assemble the needle, the transducer, and the syringe. Place in the pressure monitor with the black side of the transducer down. (Courtesy Stryker Surgical. [1996]. Intra-compartmental pressure monitor system: Maintenance manual and operating instructions. Kalamazoo, MI.)

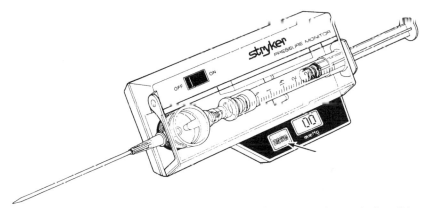

FIGURE 133-3 Hold the monitor at the intended angle of insertion and press the "zero" button. (Courtesy Stryker Surgical. [1996]. Intra-compartmental pressure monitor system: Maintenance manual and operating instructions. Kalamazoo, MI.)

8. Wait for the digital display to equilibrate, and note the pressure. For additional measurements, repeat steps 5-8.

WHITESIDES' TECHNIQUE
Equipment

Antiseptic solution
Gauze dressings
Local anesthetic with needles and syringe (optional)
Three-way stopcock
Two intravenous extension tubing sets
30-ml vial of sterile saline for injection

20-ml syringe

18- or 19-G needles

Mercury manometer (NOTE: an aneroid manometer is not accurate for this
   procedure.)

Procedural Steps (Whitesides et al., 1975; Milne, 2001)

1. Connect one intravenous extension set to a sideport of the stopcock.
   Connect an 18- or 19-G needle to the distal end of the tubing.
2. Aspirate 15 ml of air into the 20-ml syringe, and attach the syringe to the middle stopcock port.
3. Insert the needle into the vial, and inject 1-2 ml of air from the syringe into the
   vial. Withdraw saline until the extension tubing is approximately half-filled.
   The saline meniscus must be easily visible within the tubing (Figure 133-4).
4. Connect the other intravenous extension set to the remaining stopcock port.
   Connect the distal end of the tubing to the mercury manometer (Figure 133-5).
5. *Insert the needle into the compartment, and open the stopcock so that all
   ports are open.
6. *Push gently on the plunger of the syringe while watching the fluid meniscus
   and the manometer. It is helpful to have one person to watch the meniscus
   and another to watch the manometer.
7. Document the pressure at which the meniscus flattens. Repeat steps 5-7 as
   needed to verify the reading.
8. Change needles, and repeat steps 5-7 for additional readings.

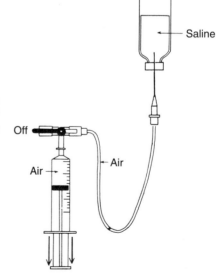

FIGURE 133-4 Fluid meniscus in IV extension
tubing. (From Kuska, B. M. [1982]. Acute onset of
compartment syndrome. *Journal of Emergency
Nursing, 8,* 77.)

---

*Indicates portions of the procedure usually performed by a physician or an advanced practice
nurse.

AGE-SPECIFIC CONSIDERATIONS

1. Needles as small as 25 G (without a sideport) can be used to measure compartmental pressure accurately (Mars et al., 1997).
2. Compartmental syndrome may develop more rapidly in children because the size of the compartment is relatively smaller and the fascial tissue is tighter.

COMPLICATIONS

1. Inaccurate pressures if the needle is inserted into a tendon or occluded with tissue. Needle function can be tested by squeezing the extremity; immediate pressure fluctuations should be noted if the needle is patent.
2. Infection (late).

PATIENT TEACHING

1. Report the following symptoms immediately: pain of increasing severity; pain that does not respond to prescribed pain medications; pain on passive movement; numbness or tingling; weakness; tenseness of the injured extremity in comparison to the noninjured extremity; pallor, mottling, cyanosis, or coldness of the extremity.
2. Position the injured extremity as instructed. (NOTE: If an early compartmental syndrome is suspected, the patient is instructed to keep the extremity at the level of the heart to optimize blood flow to the tissue.)

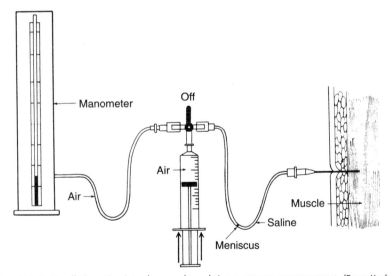

FIGURE 133-5 Needle insertion into the muscle and tissue pressure measurement. (From Kuska, B.M. [1982]. Acute onset of compartment syndrome. *Journal of Emergency Nursing 8*, 78.)

REFERENCES

Hays, E.P. (2001). Leg injuries: tibia and fibula (pp. 432-442). In Ferrera, P.C., Colucciello, S.A., Marx, J.A., Verdile, V.P., & Gibbs, M.A. (Eds.). *Trauma management: an emergency medicine approach*. St. Louis: Mosby.

Mars, M., Tufts, M.A., & Hadley, G.P. (1997). Towards reducing the trauma of direct intracompartmental pressure measurement for children: an in vitro assessment of small diameter needles. *Pediatric Surgery International, 12*, 172-176.

McQueen, M.M., & Court-Brown, C.M. (1996). Compartment monitoring in tibial fractures: the pressure threshold for decompression. *Journal of Bone and Joint Surgery, 78-B*, 99-104.

Milne, L.W. (2001). Fascial compartment pressure measurement (pp. 228-231). In Rosen, P., Chan, T.C., Vilke, G.M., & Sternbach, G. (Eds.). *Atlas of emergency procedures*. St. Louis: Mosby.

Stryker Instruments. (1999). *Intra-compartmental pressure monitor system*. Kalamazoo, MI: Author.

Whitesides, T.E., Jr., Haney, T.C., Morimotor, K., & Harada, H. et al. (1975). Tissue pressure measurements as a determinant for the need of fasciotomy. *Clinical Orthopedics and Related Research, 113*, 43-51.

PROCEDURE 134

Measuring and Fitting for Ambulation Aids

Margo E. Layman, MSN, RN, RNC, CN-A

Ambulation aids include crutches, canes, and walkers.

INDICATIONS
1. To provide support or stability when walking.
2. To compensate for impaired balance, decreased strength, pain during weight bearing, or injury of a lower extremity.

CONTRAINDICATIONS AND CAUTIONS
1. If initial measurement is performed with the patient in a position other than standing, the fit of the aid must be evaluated and adjusted accordingly when the patient is upright.
2. An improperly fitted aid adversely affects the patient's gait pattern and may result in unstable or unsafe ambulation, decreased function, and decreased safety for the patient. Improperly fitted crutches may pain or nerve damage if excessive pressure is exerted on the axillae.
3. The energy consumption associated with non–weight bearing is substantial. Elderly, debilitated, or sedentary patients could be a risk for severe exercise challenge and pronounced fatigue.
4. The patient should be instructed that the fit may need to be revised as the patient becomes stronger and more proficient with the ambulation aid.

EQUIPMENT

Measuring tape
Prescribed ambulation aid (crutches, cane, or walker)

PATIENT PREPARATION

1. Assess the patient's limitations and capabilities to determine which ambulation device is appropriate.
2. If at all possible, the patient should be fitted wearing the shoes he or she intends to wear when using the ambulation aid.

PROCEDURAL STEPS

Cane

1. Determine the length of the cane with the patient standing or supine.
2. The handgrip of the cane should be level with the greater trochanter or the ulnar side of the wrist when the arm is straight down at the side.
3. With the cane parallel to the femur and tibia, the foot (tip) of the cane should be on the floor or at the bottom of the heel of the shoe (Figure 134-1).
4. Confirm fit with the patient standing. There should be approximately 15-25 degrees of elbow flexion when the patient grasps the hand piece and positions the aid for ambulation. To position for ambulation, the tip of the cane is placed forward approximately 4-5 inches and laterally to the forefoot approximately 2-4 inches.

Crutches

1. If the patient's height is known, subtract 16 inches from the height; the resulting value approximates the length from the axillary pad to the crutch tip.

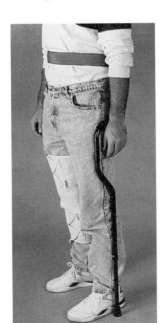

FIGURE 134-1 Confirming the fit of a cane. (From Pierson, F.M., and Fairchild, S.L, [2002]. *Principles and techniques of patient care,* 3rd ed. [p. 219]. Philadelphia: W.B. Saunders.)

2. If height is uncertain or unknown, measure the supine patient from the anterior axillary fold (crease of armpit) to a point approximately 6 to 8 inches lateral to the patient's heel. This value represents the overall crutch length.

3. To determine the hand piece height, with the patient's arm held close to his or her side, measure from the anterior axillary fold to the trochanter or lunar wrist crease (Figure 134-2). Use this value to position the hand piece by measuring down from the center of the axillary pad.

4. Confirm the fit with the patient standing with head and trunk erect, shoulders relaxed and level, feet flat on the floor, and knees slightly flexed. The crutch tips should be 2-4 inches lateral and 4-6 inches anterior to the toes of the forefoot. The elbows should be flexed approximately 15-25 degrees when the hand piece is grasped with the wrist in a neutral position (Figure 134-3).

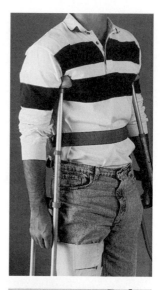

FIGURE 134-2 Determining hand piece height. (From Pierson, F.M., & Fairchild, S.L. [2002]. *Principles and techniques of patient care,* 3rd ed. [p. 222]. Philadelphia: W.B. Saunders.)

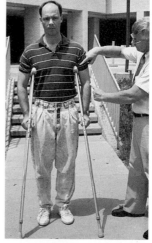

FIGURE 134-3 Confirming the fit of crutches. (From Pierson, F.M., & Fairchild, S.L. [2002]. *Principles and techniques of patient care,* 3rd ed., [p. 222]. Philadelphia: W.B. Saunders.)

Walker

1. Measurement can be accomplished with the patient either standing or supine.
2. The handgrip of the walker should be level with the ulnar wrist crease or greater trochanter with the walker in front of and along the patient's sides.
3. The feet of the walker should rest on the floor or be even with the heels of the shoes with the hips and knees straight (Figure 134-4).
4. Confirm the fit with the patient standing. There should be approximately 15-25 degrees of elbow flexion when the patient grasps the hand piece and positions the aid for ambulation. To position for ambulation, the tips of the aid are placed forward approximately 4-5 inches and laterally to the forefoot approximately 2-4 inches.

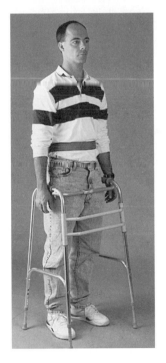

FIGURE 134-4 Confirming the fit of a walker. (From Pierson, F.M., & Fairchild, S.L. [2002]. *Principles and techniques of patient care,* 3rd ed., [p. 221]. Philadelphia: W.B. Saunders.)

Patient Teaching for Ambulation Aids

Margo E. Layman, MSN, RN, RNC, CN-A

INDICATION

To teach a patient how to walk with crutches, a cane, or a walker. The patient may need an ambulation aid to compensate for impaired balance, decreased strength, pain during weight bearing, or injury to a leg.

CONTRAINDICATIONS AND CAUTIONS

1. The energy consumption associated with non–weight-bearing crutch walking is considerable. Elderly, debilitated, or sedentary patients could be at risk for severe exercise challenge and pronounced fatigue. The three-point gait requires the most strength and balance.
2. Selection of the proper ambulation device and gait pattern is essential for the patient's safety and well-being.
3. Before discharge, the patient must be able to demonstrate use of the ambulation aid safely.

PATIENT PREPARATION

1. Measure and adjust the ambulation aid (see Procedure 134).
2. Ensure that the patient is wearing shoes. Free the area of potential hazards (equipment or furniture in the path or a wet floor surface).

PROCEDURAL STEPS

Three-Point Pattern (Two Crutches or a Walker)

1. This pattern is referred to as a step-to or step-through pattern and is used when the patient is able to bear weight fully on one leg but cannot bear weight on the opposite leg. This is the least stable pattern and requires balance, coordination, and good strength in the arms, trunk, and the unaffected leg. This pattern requires considerable energy expenditure while allowing for rapid ambulation.
2. The walker or crutches and the injured leg are advanced, and the patient steps up to the walker or slightly ahead of the crutches (Figure 135-1).

Modified Three-Point Pattern (Two Crutches or a Walker)

1. This pattern is used when the patient is permitted full weight bearing on one leg and partial weight bearing on the other. This is a more stable pattern than the three-point pattern and requires less strength and less energy expenditure.
2. The walker or crutches are advanced simultaneously with the partial weight-bearing leg (Figure 135-2, *A* and *B*).
3. The full weight-bearing leg is then advanced (Figure 135-2, *C* and *D*).

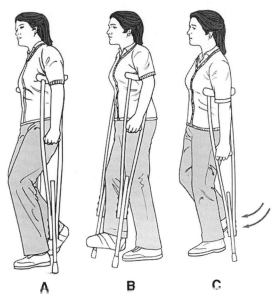

FIGURE 135-1 Three-point gait with crutches. **A,** Standing with crutches, all weight is on the good leg. **B,** Move crutches and injured leg forward simultaneously. **C,** Bearing weight on the palms of the hands, step forward onto the good leg. (From Proehl, J.A. & Jones, L.M. [1998]. *Mosby's emergency department patient teaching guides* [p. I-7]. St. Louis: Mosby.)

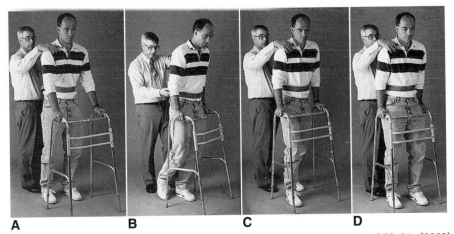

FIGURE 135-2 Modified three-point gait pattern. (From Pierson, F.M., & Fairchild, S.L. [2002]. *Principles and techniques of patient care,* 3rd ed. [p. 234]. Philadelphia: W.B. Saunders.)

Modified Two-Point Pattern (One Cane or Crutch)

1. This pattern requires one ambulation aid and is used when additional support, protection, or improved gait stability is needed.
2. Hold the ambulation aid in the arm opposite to the leg that requires protection or support (Figure 135-3, *A*).

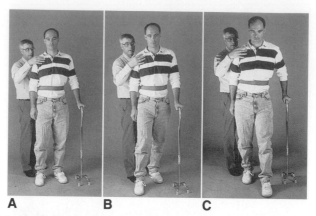

A   **B**   **C**

FIGURE 135-3 Modified two-point pattern. (From Pierson, F.M., & Fairchild, S.L. [2002]. *Principles and techniques of patient care,* 3rd ed., [p. 222]. Philadelphia: W.B. Saunders.)

3. From a stationary position, the ambulation aid comes forward simultaneously with the leg to be protected. This broadens the base of support and stabilizes the gait pattern (Figure 135-3, *B*).
4. The ambulation aid and protected leg maintain position while the unaffected leg steps forward (Figure 135-3, *C*).

Four-Point Pattern (Two Crutches or Canes)
1. This gait approximates a normal step pattern, is stable, and requires low energy expenditure. It uses alternate and reciprocal forward movement. The patient must be able to bear weight on both legs.
2. The right crutch or cane comes forward, then the left leg (Figure 135-4, *A*).
3. The left crutch or cane comes forward, then the right leg (Figure 135-4, *B*).

Sitting Down or Standing Up From a Chair
1. To sit down in a chair:
    a. Hold both crutches in one hand on the affected leg side.
    b. Place the unaffected leg close to the chair edge.
    c. Put the free hand on the seat bottom and lower to chair using crutches, the unaffected leg, and the free hand for balance and support (Figure 135-5).
2. To stand:
    a. Hold both crutches in one hand on the affected leg side.
    b. Push up using the free hand, the unaffected leg, and the hand that is holding the crutches.

Ascending and Descending Stairs
1. Going up and down stairs with crutches can be difficult and dangerous. A safer alternative may be to sit down and scoot up and down the stairs. An assistant may be necessary to help support an injured leg and carry the crutches.
2. Remember "up with the good, down with the bad" (Ogle, 2000).

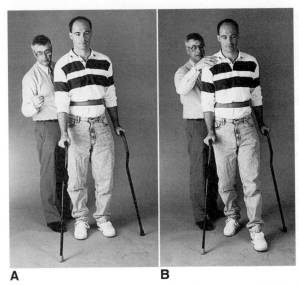

A   **B**

FIGURE 135-4 Four-point pattern. (From Pierson, F.M., & Fairchild, S.L. [2002]. *Principles and techniques of patient care*, 3rd ed., [p. 228]. Philadelphia: W.B. Saunders.)

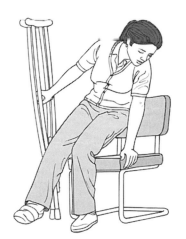

FIGURE 135-5 Sitting down or standing up from a chair. (From Proehl, J.A., & Jones, L.M. [1998]. *Mosby's emergency department patient teaching guides* [p. I-7]. St. Louis: Mosby.)

With a Handrail

1. To go up stairs with a handrail:
   a. Hold both crutches in the hand opposite the handrail.
   b. Push down on the crutches and the handrail while stepping up with the good leg.
   c. Straighten the back, and lift the crutches and injured leg up to the same step (Figure 135-6).
2. To go down stairs with a handrail:
   a. Hold both crutches in the hand opposite the handrail.

b. Bend the good leg (to assist with balance), and lower both crutches and the injured leg one step.
c. Leaning on the crutches and the handrail, step down to the same step with the good leg (Figure 135-7).

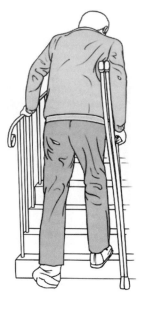

FIGURE 135-6 Ascending stairs with a handrail. (From Proehl, J.A., & Jones L.M. [1998]. *Mosby's emergency department patient teaching guides* [p. I-8]. St. Louis: Mosby.)

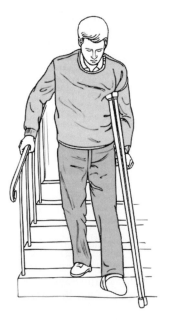

FIGURE 135-7 Descending stairs with a handrail. (From Proehl, J.A., & Jones, L.M. [1998]. *Mosby's emergency department patient teaching guides* [p. I-8]. St. Louis: Mosby.)

Without a Handrail

1. To go up stairs without a handrail:
   a. Use the three-point gait pattern.
   b. Advance the crutches and good leg, then step up.
   c. Extend the hip and flex the knee on the injured side to 90 degrees to assist with safely clearing the stair (Figure 135-8).
2. To go down stairs without a handrail:
   a. Bend the good leg (to assist with balance), and lower both of the crutches and the injured leg to the step.
   b. Lean on the crutches, and step down with the good leg (Figure 135-9).

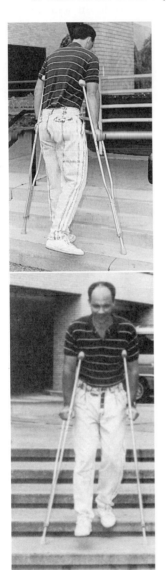

FIGURE 135-8 Ascending stairs without a handrail. (From Pierson, F.M., & Fairchild, S.L. [2002]. *Principles and techniques of patient care* 3rd ed., [p. 263]. Philadelphia: W.B. Saunders.)

FIGURE 135-9 Descending stairs without a handrail. (From Pierson, F.M., & Fairchild [2002]. *Principles and techniques of patient care* 3rd ed., [p. 263]. Philadelphia: W.B. Saunders.)

AGE-SPECIFIC CONSIDERATIONS

1. By the age of 4-6 years, children should be able to use ambulation aids. Their ability to do so depends on their growth, development, strength, and coordination.
2. The elderly patient may have difficulty using gaits such as the three-point pattern, which requires considerable energy expenditure, good balance, and arm strength. A walker, rather than crutches, and modified gait patterns may be needed.

COMPLICATIONS

1. If weight bearing is inappropriately placed with pressure to the axilla, damage to the brachial plexus and radial nerve can occur, causing pain and triceps weakness.
2. Falls, with the potential for additional injury

PATIENT TEACHING

1. Wear sturdy, low-heeled shoes.
2. Remove trip hazards, such as throw rugs and toys, from the walking environment. Be careful around pets and small children.
3. Be extremely careful when taking medications or alcohol because perception and judgment are affected.
4. Use caution on wet, icy, or snow-covered surfaces. Attachments are available to help prevent crutches from slipping on icy or snow-covered surfaces.
5. Do not rest on your armpits when using crutches; nerve damage may occur.
6. A backpack may be used to carry items, but be careful because it shifts the center of gravity and may alter your gait.

REFERENCE

Ogle, A. (2000). Canes, crutches, walkers, and other ambulation aids. *Physical Medicine and Rehabilitation: State of the Art Reviews, 14,* 485-492.

Arthrocentesis and Intraarticular Injection

Jean A. Proehl, RN, MN, CEN, CFRN, CCRN

Arthrocentesis is also known as joint aspiration and "joint tap."

INDICATIONS

1. To relieve the pain and distention associated with intraarticular fluid accumulation.
2. To determine the cause of acute joint swelling. Joint swelling may be due to trauma, gout, infection, or rheumatoid arthritis.
3. To inject medications, usually steroids, into the joint space.

CONTRAINDICATIONS AND CAUTIONS

1. Infection of the tissue at the puncture site (Milne, 2001).
2. Caution should be exercised with patients who have bleeding disorders or who are taking anticoagulant medications (Milne, 2001).
3. An orthopedic surgeon should be consulted for prosthetic joints (Milne, 2001).
4. Repeated steroid injections can cause tissue damage.

EQUIPMENT

Antiseptic solution
Gauze dressings
Elastic bandage (optional)
Local or topical anesthetic
Syringes and needles for infiltration of local anesthetic
Sample tubes for laboratory specimens
10- to 20-ml syringe (for knee aspiration, a 30- to 60-ml syringe may be necessary)
18- to 23-G 1½-inch needle
Medications for intra-articular injection
Sterile towels or drapes

PATIENT PREPARATION

The joint may be wrapped with an elastic bandage, leaving the puncture site exposed, to help compress the fluid into the puncture area (Simon & Brenner, 2002).

PROCEDURAL STEPS

1. Cleanse the skin at the puncture site with an antiseptic solution for 5 minutes. The needle is usually introduced on the extensor surface of the joint to

decrease the risk of neurovascular injury. Also, the synovial pouch is closer to the skin on the extensor surface (Simon & Brenner, 2002).

2. *Anesthetize the skin and soft tissue down to the level of the joint capsule. Topical application of ethyl chloride may provide adequate anesthesia in patients with markedly distended joint capsules (Simon & Brenner, 2002).

3. Position the joint. Placing the joint in 20-30 degrees of flexion and gently applying longitudinal traction to the bone distal to the joint helps to open the joint space (Simon & Brenner, 2002).

4. *Insert the needle into the joint space while aspirating, and advance until synovial fluid is obtained (Figure 136-1).

5. Removal of synovial fluid:
   a. Apply manual pressure to the opposite side of the joint to help force fluid over to the needle.
   b. *Aspirate all readily accessible fluid.
   c. Place fluid in appropriate specimen containers to send to the laboratory. Commonly performed laboratory tests include viscosity, cell count, protein, glucose, culture, and Gram's stain. Synovial fluid requires special handling; package it per laboratory protocol.

6. Injection of medications:
   a. *Taking care not to displace the needle, remove the syringe from the needle, and attach the syringe containing the medication.
   b. *Inject the medication into the joint space.

7. *Remove the needle.

8. Apply direct pressure to the puncture site for 2 minutes; then apply a sterile dressing.

9. Apply an elastic bandage to help stabilize the joint if a large amount of fluid was aspirated (see Procedure 129).

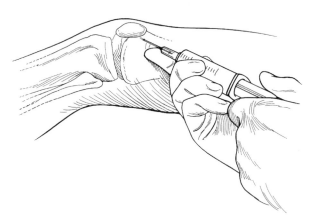

FIGURE 136-1 Arthrocentesis of the knee. (From Milne, L.W. [2001]. Arthrocentesis of the knee [pp. 233]. In Rosen, P., Chan, T.C., Vilke, G.M., & Sternbach, G. (Eds.). *Atlas of emergency procedures.* St. Louis: Mosby.)

---

*Indicates portions of the procedure usually performed by a physician or an advanced practice nurse.

AGE-SPECIFIC CONSIDERATION

Lidocaine infiltration for anesthesia is usually avoided in children because it increases the number of skin punctures necessary. Eutectic mixture of local anesthesia (EMLA) cream may be used instead (Hostetler & Weisman, 2001).

COMPLICATIONS

1. Joint infection, sepsis (rare if the site is adequately cleansed) (Milne, 2001; Simon & Brenner, 2002)
2. Hemarthrosis (Milne, 2001)
3. Dry tap
4. Trauma to intraarticular or neurovascular structures (Stahl & Kaufman, 1997; Milne, 2001)

PATIENT TEACHING

1. Report any fever, increased pain, redness, or recurrent swelling, which could indicate infection.
2. Avoid excessive use of the joint for the next few days. If the injection/aspiration was in the knee, ankle, or foot, crutches may be prescribed to prevent weight bearing
3. Apply ice to the joint and elevate it above the level of the heart to help prevent recurrent swelling.
4. Change dressings as indicated if the joint is draining.
5. Wear the elastic bandage as instructed to help stabilize the joint.
6. If steroids were injected, skin lightening and sun sensitivity may occur in the area (Hostetler & Weisman, 2001).

REFERENCES

Hostetler, M.A., & Weisman, D.S. (2001). Orthopedic procedures (pp. 152-184). In Goepp, J.G. & Hostetler, M.A. (Eds.). *Procedures for primary care pediatricians*. St. Louis: Mosby.

Milne, L.W. (2001). Arthrocentesis of the knee (pp. 232-233). In Rosen, P., Chan, T.C., Vilke, G.M., & Sternbach, G. (Eds.). *Atlas of emergency procedures*. St. Louis: Mosby.

Simon, R.R., & Brenner, B.E. (2002). *Emergency procedures and techniques*, 4th ed. Baltimore: Williams & Wilkins.

Stahl, S., & Kaufman, T. (1997). Ulnar nerve injury at the elbow after steroid injection for medial epicondylitis. *Journal of Hand Surgery (British)*, *22*, 69-70.

Integumentary Procedures

Wound Cleansing and Irrigation

Joni Hentzen Daniels, MSN, RN, CEN, CCRN, CFRN, CNS

Wound cleansing and irrigation is also known as wound preparation or "scrub." Cleansing and irrigation are the fundamentals of good wound care. Although these steps can be the most tedious and time consuming, it is essential that all contaminants and devitalized tissue be removed before wound closure (Trott, 1997). Infection or poor wound healing are both associated with inadequate cleaning techniques. Neither clever suturing technique nor use of prophylactic antibiotics can replace meticulous cleansing and irrigation (Trott, 1997).

INDICATIONS
1. To cleanse any disruption in skin integrity.
2. To cleanse the skin before suturing, incision and drainage, invasive procedures, and removal of foreign bodies.
3. To promote healing without infection.
4. To provide the best possible function and appearance for the patient.

CONTRAINDICATIONS AND CAUTIONS
1. Injuries that require special care include:
   a. *Eyelids:* The eye itself should be assessed for trauma and visual acuity checked (see Procedure 157). Suturing of the eyelid may require specialist consultation.
   b. *Neck:* Wounds of the neck can appear superficial. Care should be taken not to underestimate a penetrating injury that could quickly compromise the patient's airway.
   c. *Spray gun injuries:* Extensive tissue destruction may be present despite a benign-appearing entrance wound. Injected chemicals or embedded foreign bodies frequently require surgical exploration.
   d. *Scalp:* Lacerations may disguise skull fractures, and the patient may lose a significant amount of blood because of the scalp's extensive vascularity. The extent of a scalp laceration can be easily overlooked because of hair matting or the patient lying supine on a backboard.
   e. *Crush or avulsion injuries:* Wounds with extensive tissue damage or loss of tissue are at increased risk for infection and delayed healing.
   f. *Facial:* Meticulous care of facial wounds is required for optimal cosmetic results.
   g. *Hand:* Impairment of hand function, especially the dominant hand, may result in permanent disability.
   h. *Associated fractures:* Open fractures are at high risk for infection. Specialty consultation is indicated.

    i. *Puncture wounds:* The type and condition (e.g., rusty or dirty) of the penetrating object are important. If the puncture occurred through clothing or a shoe, the wound should be evaluated for the presence of a foreign body. Puncture wounds are at increased risk for infection.

    j. *Bite wounds:* The risk of rabies should be evaluated. Patients are frequently discharged with antibiotics and instructions to return in 24-48 hours for follow-up care. Obtaining skull films in bite wounds to the cranium in children should be considered because of possible penetration of the skull. Bites wounds, especially cat bites, are at increased risk for infection.

2. Soaking macerates the skin, and povidone-iodine causes tissue destruction. There is no evidence that soaking wounds in saline and povidone-iodine is of any benefit (Simon & Hern, 2002).

3. Excessive scrubbing and powerful irrigation can damage healthy tissue.

4. Wound cleansing agents:

    a. Hydrogen peroxide should be used with caution. It is a weak disinfectant and is ineffective against anaerobes, it absorbs oxygen in the wound, and it destroys cells. It is toxic to tissue in open wounds (Simon & Hern, 2002).

    b. Povidone-iodine solutions provide good antimicrobial activity and effectively kills gram positive and gram negative rods, fungi, and viruses with little toxicity or damage. Iodine compounds are less irritating to tissue than is tincture of iodine but may still cause cellular damage and allergic reactions (Simon & Hern, 2002).

    c. Nontoxic agents such as Pluronic F-68 (Shur-Clens) are nontoxic to open wounds and eyes. Although they have no antimicrobial activity, they appear to be safe and effective and cause minimal cellular damage (Simon & Hern, 2002).

    d. Baby shampoo provides gentle cleaning of fragile tissue but is nonsterile and is not antimicrobial. It is used for facial lacerations in some institutions.

EQUIPMENT

Wound cleansing agent (see discussion under Contraindications and
    Cautions)
Sterile sponges or gauze dressings
Cotton swabs
Sterile drapes or towels
Wound irrigation supplies:
    16- or 18-G blunt needle or plastic cannula
    30- to 35-ml syringe
    Splash shield (optional)
    Sterile basin
    Normal saline
NOTE: Preassembled irrigation kits with splash shields are also available.
For contaminated wounds and wounds embedded with foreign bodies:
    Sterile toothbrush or surgical brush
    No. 11 scalpel blade
For tar wounds:
    Petroleum jelly, topical antibiotic ointment, or mineral oil

PATIENT PREPARATION

1. Obtain a history, including time of injury, mechanism of injury, location and extent of injury, other injuries, and potential for the wound to be contaminated with soil or dirt. Assess the wound for foreign objects, such as clothing, grass, and glass. Also assess tetanus immunization status and potential for rabies (bite wounds).
2. Assess and document neurovascular status. Assess for adjacent bony injury or open fractures. Suspect damage to muscle and tendons if deep fascia is involved.
3. Obtain radiology studies as indicated to rule out presence of foreign bodies, fractures, and air in joint spaces.
4. Anesthetize the area as indicated (see Procedures 138, 139, and 140).
5. Drape or undress the patient to protect clothing if extensive wound preparation and irrigation is planned.

PROCEDURAL STEPS

1. Maintain hemostasis by direct pressure. *Clamp and ligate vessels if necessary. Use a pneumatic tourniquet or a blood pressure cuff to help control bleeding during wound cleansing and repair, if prescribed by a physician.
2. Shaving is seldom indicated. Shaving causes many small wounds and skin nicks and increases the chance of infection. If hair removal is necessary, clip the hair close to the wound edge or smooth hair out of the way with lubricant or antibiotic ointment. Never shave eyebrows because realignment is difficult to achieve without the landmark hair, and complete hair regrowth may not occur.
3. Begin wound cleansing using sponges or brushes and a cleansing agent. The preparation should begin at the wound site and should move distally, encompassing a large area of skin surrounding the wound. For example, with hand lacerations, clean the hand and arm to the elbow. Continue until the wound is clean.
4. Irrigate wounds that are contaminated or those containing foreign bodies. Wound irrigation helps remove foreign bodies and dilutes bacteria. Irrigation is particularly important in bite wounds. Use a 16- or 18-G needle or plastic cannula and a 35-ml syringe for high-pressure irrigation (Simon & Brenner, 2002) (Figure 137-1). Other options include a needle attached to a pressurized intravenous bag or tubing or a commercially available irrigation setup. Normal saline is most commonly used. Low-pressure irrigation (e.g., bulb syringe) is not effective.
   The following formula for determining volume of irrigant has been associated with less than 0.01% wound infection (Daniels, 2003):

   100 ml/inch of length of laceration/hours since injury

   Thus, a 3-inch laceration that was 6 hours old would be irrigated with 1800 ml ($100 \times 3 \times 6 = 1800$ ml).
5. Abrasions with embedded foreign bodies (except glass) require careful wound preparation to remove the foreign bodies and prevent traumatic tat-

---

*Indicates portions of the procedure usually performed by a physician or an advanced practice nurse.

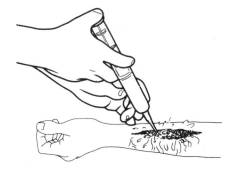

FIGURE 137-1 Irrigation of a wound. An 18-G needle or plastic cannula attached to a 35-ml syringe is ideal for providing proper irrigation pressure. (From Simon, R., & Brenner, B. [2002]. *Emergency procedures and techniques,* 4th ed. [p. 363]. Baltimore, Williams & Wilkins.)

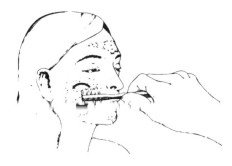

FIGURE 137-2 Removal of embedded particles from a traumatic abrasion with a sterile toothbrush. The tip of a no. 11 blade can be used to remove deeply embedded or larger particles. (From Simon, R., & Brenner, B. [2002]. *Emergency procedures and techniques,* 4th ed. [p. 363]. Baltimore: Williams & Wilkins.)

tooing. Use surgical scrub brushes, sterile toothbrushes, and the point of a No. 11 blade for foreign body removal (Simon & Brenner, 2002) (Figure 137-2). Wounds with glass embedded require special evaluation and management; radiographic imaging may be necessary. *Wound débridement may be necessary after anesthesia is completed.

6. Use petroleum jelly, antibiotic ointment, or mineral oil to facilitate tar removal. After application, allow tar to dissolve for 10-15 minutes before attempting removal. Repeat applications may be necessary.

AGE-SPECIFIC CONSIDERATIONS

1. Parents may not know the full details of the mechanism of injury; careful wound assessment is necessary in young children.
2. Patient age is an important factor in host resistance to infection; those individuals at extremes of age—young children and the elderly—are at greatest risk.

COMPLICATIONS

1. The chance of infection, including cellulitis, soft tissue abscess, and osteomyelitis, increases in wounds to the hands and feet because of their poor circulation. Infection is also more common in dirty or old wounds. Bacterial growth begins in wounds after 3 hours.

---

*Indicates portions of the procedure usually performed by a physician or an advanced practice nurse.

2. Medications such as steroids and hormones may impair wound healing.
3. Other medical conditions may impair wound healing. Patients with diabetes, immune diseases, associated trauma, hypoxia, uremia, circulatory impairment, and infection, as well as the elderly, are all at increased risk for infection and delayed healing.

PATIENT TEACHING

1. High-risk patients should return for wound evaluation and dressing change within 24-48 hours.
2. The wound should be kept dry for the first 24 hours. The patient may shower but should not soak in a tub. Wet dressings should be changed as soon as possible.
3. The wound should be cleaned four times a day with half-strength hydrogen peroxide or mild soapy water. Crusted material should be gently removed with cotton swabs. Keeping crusted material off allows for quicker epithelialization.
4. Apply a light layer of topical antibiotic ointment after wound cleansing. A gauze dressing may be applied, depending on the wound location, especially for the first 48 hours.
5. Watch for bleeding, a wound that reopens, signs of circulatory compromise, or signs of infection (wound tenderness, redness, swelling, draining pus, fever). A minor amount of wound redness is normal.
6. Elevate the injured area as much as possible.
7. New wounds should not be exposed to the sun for 6 months. Permanent hyperpigmentation may result. Sun block is advisable, especially for facial wounds.

REFERENCES

Daniels, J.H. (2003). Unpublished data. Sugarland, TX.
Simon, B., & Hern, H.G. (2002). Wound management principles (pp. 737-751). In Marx, J.A., Hockberger, R.S., Walls, R.M., et al. (Eds.), *Rosen's emergency medicine: concepts and clinical practice*, 5th ed. St. Louis: Mosby.
Simon, R.R., & Brenner, B.E. (2002). *Emergency procedures and techniques*, 4th ed. Baltimore: Williams & Wilkins.
Trott, A.T. (1997). Wound cleansing and irrigation (pp. 90-101). In Trott, A.T. (Ed.). *Wounds and lacerations*, 2nd ed. St Louis: Mosby.

Wound Anesthesia: Local Infiltration and Topical Agents

Maureen T. Quigley, MS, ARNP, CEN

INDICATIONS
To provide local and topical anesthesia before:
1. Suturing of a laceration
2. Removal of an imbedded foreign body
3. Incision and drainage of an abscess
4. Invasive procedures, such as lumbar puncture or chest tube insertion
5. Wound débridement and cleansing
6. Insertion of nasal packing or nasal tubes
7. Venous cannulation, venipuncture, or any needle insertion, including preinfiltration anesthesia

CONTRAINDICATIONS AND CAUTIONS
1. A known sensitivity or history of allergic reaction to a local anesthetic is a contraindication to its use. Patient-reported allergic reactions to amide preparations are rare (see Background Information).
2. The use of agents containing epinephrine may be contraindicated in patients with known peripheral vascular disease. Because of epinephrine's vasoconstrictive action, it may delay healing and increase the risk of infection.
3. The use of epinephrine may be helpful in vascular areas, such as the face and scalp, to slow absorption and lower peak blood levels of anesthesia. Epinephrine also decreases bleeding at the site.
4. The use of epinephrine preparations is contraindicated in cartilaginous areas of the ear and nares and in areas served by end arteries (fingers, toes, and the penis). Epinephrine also distorts and discolors the vermilion border of the lip and is contraindicated in lip lacerations that extend through the lip border.
5. Injection of anesthetic agents can distort wound margins, which may increase the complexity of plastics repair. Care should be used in flap-type lacerations to preserve vascularity of the flap by not injecting directly into the flap and avoiding the use of epinephrine-containing preparations.
6. Avoid rapid infiltration of the wound to decrease pain.
7. Amide preparations should be used cautiously in patients with liver disease (see Background Information).
8. Cocaine is vasoconstrictive, and absorption can continue for up to 4 hours. It should be used only topically and with caution in the pediatric and elderly population.
9. The use of tetracaine-adrenaline-cocaine (TAC) is no longer recommended because of safety concerns.

10. Lidocaine (5%), epinephrine (1:2000), and tetracaine (1%) solution (LET) is a safe and effective alternative to TAC for topical use (Schilling et al., 1995). LET should be not used on mucous membranes, noses, pinna of the ear, fingers, toes, and the penis.

11. Benzocaine is found in a wide variety of over-the-counter preparations for sunburn and abrasions. Toxic and allergic reactions are common.

12. Cetacaine spray has two principal ingredients: benzocaine and tetracaine. Tetracaine is rapidly absorbed by the pharynx and tracheobronchial tree and is long acting. Spray application greater than 2 seconds is contraindicated because of rapid mucosal absorption and potential toxicity of tetracaine.

13. EMLA is an effective topic anesthetic for intact skin in the pediatric population. Local skin reactions are relatively common but are generally mild and transient, resolving after cream is removed. Methemoglobinemia may be caused by EMLA because of the metabolites of prilocaine, but this is rare when the preparation is used properly. EMLA should not be used in any infant <3 months of age and in infants between 3 and 12 months of age who are being treated with methemoglobinemia-inducing drugs, such as acetaminophen, phenobarbital, nitrites, sulfonamides, and antimalarial agents (McGee, 2004). Patients with anemia, respiratory or cardiovascular disease, glucose-6-phosphate dehydrogenase (G-6-PD) or methemoglobin reductase deficiencies are at higher risk for untoward effects (McGee, 2004).

EQUIPMENT
Antiseptic wipes
3-, 5-, and 10-ml syringes (for infiltration)
18-, 25-, and 27-G needles (for infiltration)
Local or topical anesthetic as prescribed:
    1% lidocaine without epinephrine
    1% lidocaine with epinephrine
    2% lidocaine without epinephrine
    2% lidocaine with epinephrine
    0.25%-0.5% bupivacaine
    LET
    EMLA (2.5% lidocaine and 2.5% prilocaine)

BACKGROUND INFORMATION
1. There are two general types of local anesthetics: ester compounds (procaine, cocaine, and tetracaine) and amide compounds (bupivacaine, lidocaine, and mepivacaine).

2. Amide compounds are metabolized in the liver. Ester compounds are hydrolyzed by the pseudocholinesterase in the serum. The lone exception is cocaine, which is excreted unchanged in the urine. All ester agents except cocaine share a common degradation pathway via serum to para-aminobenzoic acid, which can produce allergic or sensitizing reactions. Amide-type agents are believed to be incapable of stimulating antibody formation and so are noteworthy for their low evidence of sensitivity reactions. Reactions probably are toxic rather than allergic. Patients may be allergic, however, to the preservatives found in multiple-dose vials. Care must be taken to administer safe doses to avoid systemic toxicity.

3. The mechanism of local anesthesia is to decrease the rate and degree of depolarization and repolarization, decrease the conduction velocity, and prolong the refractory period of the neural action potential.
4. Nerve fibers are classified by their conduction velocity. Smaller fibers responsible for pain, temperature, and autonomic activity are affected rapidly by anesthetic. Local infiltration provides pain reduction without blockage of motor function.
5. All local anesthetic agents are vasodilators because of the relaxant effect on smooth muscles, with the exception of cocaine, which produces an immediate vasoconstriction (Simon & Brenner, 2002). However, cocaine has toxicity and abuse potential and should not be given to patients who are sensitive to exogenous catecholamines (McGee, 2004).
6. Epinephrine added to the anesthetic solution helps with wound hemostasis and slows systemic absorption.
7. Similar to reactions to infiltration anesthesia, toxic reactions to topically applied anesthetics correlate with the peak blood levels that were achieved and not necessarily with the dose that was administered. Systemic absorption of a topical agent is more rapid and therefore achieves a higher peak blood level than the same dose given by infiltration.

PATIENT PREPARATION
Carefully question the patient about medication allergies. Patients may confuse vagal response with allergy history. True allergy is rare but does occur and may include urticaria, bronchospasm, changes in neurologic status, and fatal cardiac collapse. Allergic reaction is more common with ester preparations (Table 138-1).

PROCEDURAL STEPS
Topical Agents—Options
1. Apply a thick layer (1-2 g/10 cm^2) of EMLA to intact skin under an occlusive dressing for approximately 30 minutes to 1 hour before a procedure. For minor procedures such as needle insertions, apply 2.5 g of EMLA over 20-25 cm^2 for at least 1 hour. Preparation of two potential sites is recommended when an intravenous line is started, in the event of technical difficulties at the initial site. When a more painful procedure is anticipated, 2 g of EMLA per 10 cm^2 should be applied for at least 2 hours (McGee, 2004).
2. Apply lidocaine (Xylocaine) topically as a liquid, ointment, jelly, or viscous fluid (2%-10%). Absorption is rapid. Do not exceed recommended dosage (maximum safe dosage is 250-300 mg) because total absorption cannot be calculated (McGee, 2004).
3. Use Cetacaine spray primarily for oral procedures. Spray application should not exceed 2 seconds.
4. Anesthetic solutions: Use LET primarily for minor facial and scalp lacerations in lieu of injectable anesthetic, especially in children.
   a. Apply LET by saturating sterile gauze and applying it to the wound with firm pressure for 15-20 minutes with gloved hands to prevent skin absorption for the caregiver. The solutions may also be applied by dripping into a wound with a syringe or by applying to a wound with sterile cotton swabs. Clean the wound to remove debris and clots before using LET to increase its efficacy.

TABLE 138-1
LOCAL ANESTHETIC AGENTS: CONCENTRATIONS AND CLINICAL USES

Agent	Concentration and Clinical Use	Onset and Duration of Action	Maximal Single Dose (mg)	Comments
Lidocaine (Xylocaine)	0.5%-1.0% for infiltration or intravenous 1.0%-1.5% for peripheral nerve, 4.0% for topical	Rapid onset; short-to-intermediate duration (60-120 min)	300 plain 500 adrenaline	Excellent spreading ability. Wide range of applications.
Prilocaine	0.5%-1.0% for infiltration or intravenous block 1.0% for peripheral nerve	Slower onset; short-to-intermediate duration (60-120 min)	400 plain 600 adrenaline	0.5% is choice for intravenous block. Most rapidly metabolized and safest of all amide-type agents. Doses in excess of 600 mg produce significant amounts of methemoglobin. Therefore avoid doses above 600 mg and repeated doses. Good choice in out-patient block. Not suitable for obstetrics.
Mepivacaine (Carbocaine)	1.0% for infiltration 1.0%-1.5% for peripheral nerve	Slower onset; intermediate-to-longer duration (90-180 min)	300 plain 500 adrenaline	Duration slightly longer than equal dose of lidocaine, and blood levels not as sensitive to inclusion of adrenaline as lidocaine; thus may be useful if adrenaline not desirable.
Etidocaine	0.5% for infiltration 0.5%-1.0% for peripheral nerve	Rapid onset; long duration (4-8 hr)	200 plain 300 adrenaline	Capable of producing profound motor block. Useful in postoperative pain management by peripheral blocks.
Bupivacaine (Marcaine)	0.25%-0.5% for infiltration 0.25%-0.5% for peripheral nerve	Slow onset; long duration (4-8 hr)	175 plain 250 adrenaline	Favored for obstetric nerve blocks because of minimal fetal effects. Excellent for postoperative analgesia because of minimal motor block.

ESTERS

Procaine (Novocain)	1.0% for infiltration	Slow onset; short duration (30-45 min)	500 plain 600 adrenaline	Indicated with history of malignant hyperpyrexia (MH). Ideal for skin infiltration. Very rapidly metabolized.
Chlorprocaine	1.0%-2.0% as for procaine	Rapid onset; short duration	600 plain 750 adrenaline	Drug of choice for obstetric and outpatient neural blockade. Metabolized four times more rapidly than procaine.
Amethocaine (tetracaine)	0.5%-1.0% for topical 0.1%-0.2% for infiltration and peripheral nerve	Slow onset; long duration	100 approximately	May be useful alternative if amides contraindicated (e.g., MH). Metabolized four times more slowly than procaine.
Cocaine	4.0%-10.0% for topical	Slow onset; medium duration	150 approximately (1.5 ml of 10% or 4 ml of 4%)	Topical use only. Addictive. Indirect adrenoceptor stimulation. No evidence that 10% solution more effective than 4%. Patients sensitive to exogenous catecholamines should receive topical lidocaine rather than cocaine.
Benzocaine	0.4%-5.0% for topical only. Usually dispensed in admixture with other therapeutic ingredients related to site of application	Rapid onset; short duration	No information available	Occasionally dispensed in urethane solution. Urethane is a suspect carcinogen and should not be used.

From Simon, R., & Brenner, B. (2002). *Emergency procedures and techniques*, 4th ed., [pp. 110-111]. Philadelphia: Lippincott Williams & Wilkins.

b. Take care to ensure that LET does not run or drip into the eyes, nasal passages, or mouth. Observe the patient carefully during and after administration. If the first dose of LET is not effective, infiltrate the laceration with local anesthesia rather than repeating a dose of LET.
5. Assess adequacy of anesthesia by testing sharp-dull sensation and observing blanching before beginning the procedure.

Wound Infiltration
1. Several techniques can be used during wound infiltration to decrease pain. Slow administration of anesthetic intradermally through the inside margins of wound edges with small-gauge needles causes less pain.
2. Lidocaine is alkalinized by adding 1 ml of sodium bicarbonate (8.4% shelf life.) to every 10 ml of lidocaine solution. It remains effective after mixing for 1 week, and refrigeration may increase (Mc Gee, 2004).
3. Consider the anesthetic agent that most fits the patient's need. A longer-acting local anesthetic (bupivacaine) may prevent the wound from having to be reinfiltrated, especially in a busy emergency department. Lidocaine's onset is more rapid, but it has a short duration of action. Reinfiltration is a poor option, especially in children or in wounds in which tissue viability is already a problem, such as in the face. If prolonged postanesthesia pain is anticipated, bupivacaine is useful.
4. Use the smallest possible needle for infiltration. A 27-G needle is usually adequate except for digital blocks, the scalp, or callused areas; in these situations, a 25-G needle may be required.
5. *Infiltrate wound edges through the dermis and not through the skin. Approaching the dermal layer directly from the inside edges of the cut margin of the wound is less painful. Continue to infiltrate as the needle passes through the dermis, injecting as you go. Some clinicians recommend injection through surrounding intact skin if the wound is grossly contaminated (Figure 138-1).
6. *As additional needle entry is needed, reenter through areas already infiltrated with anesthetic to lessen the pain of infiltration.
7. Assess sharp-dull sensation to ensure adequate anesthesia before beginning the procedure. If epinephrine has been used, observe the wound edges for blanching.

AGE-SPECIFIC CONSIDERATIONS
1. Calculate dosages carefully when administering local and topical anesthesia with children. Incorrect dosage calculations can cause significant side effects.
2. For extensive wound repair in children, consider the use of sedation (see Procedure 181) in conjunction with local anesthesia. If necessary, consider repair in a surgery or minor procedure area.
3. Viscous lidocaine should not be used for infants who are teething or have oral irritation, because they cannot expectorate well.

---

*Indicates portions of the procedure usually performed by a physician or an advanced practice nurse.

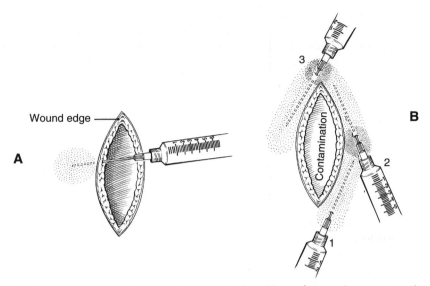

FIGURE 138-1 **A,** Injection of local anesthetic into the dermal layer of a wound margin. **B,** In the event of gross contamination, injection may be via surrounding intact skin. (McGee, D. [2004]. Local and topical anesthesia [p. 543]. In Roberts, J.R., & Hedges, J.R. (Eds.). *Clinical procedures in emergency medicine*, 4th ed. Philadelphia: W.B. Saunders.)

COMPLICATIONS

1. Local reactions may include local irritation, burning, erythema, and skin sloughing.
2. The major cause of systemic reactions is high serum levels. This is most common after topical applications to the trachea and upper airway passages because of rapid bronchial tree absorption.
3. Topical anesthesia of the nose, mouth, and pharynx may create an inadvertent suppression of the gag reflux, which may cause aspiration when combined with difficulty swallowing.
4. Resistance to injection or patient complaint of paresthesia may indicate intraneural injection. Withdraw the needle 1-2 mm, and reinject to avoid disruption of nerve fibers.
5. Signs of central nervous system toxicity include apprehension, nausea, vomiting tremor, lightheadedness, muscle twitching, incoherent speech, and seizures. As toxicity increases, the anesthesia may interfere with the electrical and mechanical function of the myocardium. Symptoms include a prolonged PR and QRS interval, bradycardia, hypotension, and asystole. Factors influencing toxicity include quantity, concentration of solution, presence or absence of epinephrine, vascularity of injection site, rate of absorption of drug, rate of destruction of drug, hypersensitivity of patient, patient age, and physical status, and weight of patient.
6. Methemoglobinemia can occur, related only to the use of prilocaine. Signs of toxicity include dyspnea, lethargy, dyspnea, cyanosis, and coma.

7. True allergic reactions are rare and may occur in response to the preservatives found in multiple-dose vials. Symptoms include bronchospasm and urticaria. If epinephrine has been used, the patient may experience pallor, anxiety, palpitations, tachycardia, hypertension, and tachypnea.

PATIENT TEACHING
1. Instruct the patient when to expect the return of sensation.
2. Protect the area until sensation returns.
3. Provide analgesia when local anesthesia wears off.
4. Use of oral topical anesthestic agents, such as viscous lidocaine and benzocaine (including over-the-counter preparations), can cause difficulty swallowing. The medication should be used at the appropriate interval, and patients should be cautioned to avoid using it more frequently. It should be swished and expectorated within 1-2 minutes, not swallowed. Food and drink should be avoided for 1 hour after application to prevent aspiration.

REFERENCES
McGee, D. (2004). Local and topical anesthesia [pp. 533-551]. In Roberts, J.R., & Hedges, J.R. (Eds.). *Clinical procedures in emergency medicine*, 4th ed. Philadelphia: W.B. Saunders.
Schilling, C.G., et al. (1995). Tetracaine, epinephrine (adrenalin), and cocaine (TAC) versus lidocaine, epinephrine, and tetracaine (LET) for anesthesia of lacerations in children. *Annals of Emergency Medicine, 25*, 203-208.
Simon, R.S., & Brenner, B.E. (2002). *Emergency procedures and techniques*, 4th ed. Philadelphia: Lippincott, Williams & Wilkins.

PROCEDURE 139

Digital Block

Joni Hentzen Daniels, MSN, RN, CEN, CCRN, CFRN, CNS

The digital nerve block is one of the most useful and most frequently performed blocks in the emergency department. It is considered superior to local infiltration in most circumstances (Kelly & Spektor, 2004). Wound infiltration may be difficult in the digit that has tight skin and can accept only a limited volume of anesthesia. Distortion of the anatomic landmarks or reduced capability for good wound approximation is also associated with local infiltration of a digit.

INDICATIONS
To provide digital anesthesia for patients
1. With isolated finger/toe lacerations or fingertip amputations
2. Requiring removal of a fingernail or repair of a nailbed
3. For reduction of interphalangeal joint dislocation
4. To obtain a satisfactory examination of the digit if pain prevents patient cooperation

CONTRAINDICATIONS AND CAUTIONS
1. Known sensitivity or history of allergic reaction to local anesthetics is a contraindication.
2. Digital blocks should not be performed on the stump of digits under consideration for replantation.
3. The vascular status of the finger should be monitored during and after injection.
4. Preparations containing epinephrine should never be used for digital blocks.
5. Circumferential ring block (placing a ring of anesthesia in a circle around a finger) is generally contraindicated because of the risk of vasospasm and ischemia, except in the thumb and great toe.

EQUIPMENT
Local anesthetic without epinephrine (usually, lidocaine 1.0%-2.0% or bupivacaine 0.25%-0.5%)
5-ml syringe
18- and 25-G or 27-G needles
Povidone-iodine or alcohol wipe

BACKGROUND INFORMATION
Before using local anesthetic agents, the practitioner must understand the principal agents and the mechanisms of their actions (see Procedure 138). Knowledge of the anatomy of the hand and foot is essential for successful digital blocks.
1. Hand and fingers (Fig. 139-1):
   a. The primary nerve supply of the hand is received from the radial, ulnar, and median nerves (Figure 139-2). Anatomic variation of the radial nerve can be significant, making the thumb difficult to block.
   b. Each digit is supplied by four nerve branches that are the terminal branches of the radial, ulnar, and median nerves (two dorsal and two palmar). Thus, the digital nerves lie in pairs on either side of the phalanges.
2. Foot and toes:
   a. Two dorsal and two volar nerves supply each toe. These nerves are branches of the major nerves of the ankle. In the toes, the nerves lie at the 2, 4, 8 and 10 o'clock positions in close relationship to the bone.
   b. The digital nerves can be blocked at the metatarsals, interdigital web spaces, or toes.

PATIENT PREPARATION
1. Place the patient in a supine position with the hand or foot extended on a firm surface.

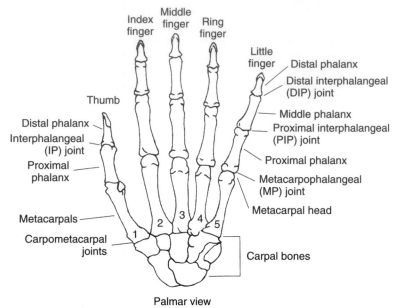

FIGURE 139-1 Bony anatomy of the hand.

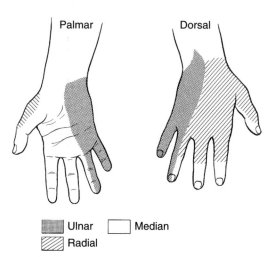

FIGURE 139-2 Sensory distribution in the hand. (From Dunmire, S.M., & Paris, P.M. [1994]. *Atlas of emergency procedures* [p. 47]. Philadelphia: W.B. Saunders.)

2. Assess and document sensation, circulation, and mobility distal to the wound. Mobility can be tested by testing grip, opposition of thumb and finger, and function of the interphalangeal and metacarpophalangeal joints. Sensation can be effectively evaluated by the use of two-point discrimination using two blunt ends of a paper clip. Assess for tendon damage by having the patient flex and extend the finger or toe against pressure.

3. Suspect nerve injury if a digital artery laceration is present because of the nerve's proximity to the artery. Do not attempt to clamp a digital artery because of the risk of damaging a digital nerve. Digital nerve laceration causes hemisensory loss to the finger.

PROCEDURAL STEPS
General Remarks for Any Technique
1. *Determine anesthetic of choice (see Table 138-1 in Procedure 138). Patients almost always benefit from the use of a longer-acting anesthetic, such as bupivacaine, especially if a lengthy repair is anticipated or the patient is expected to have pain after a shorter-acting anesthetic wears off. Consider using buffered lidocaine if a less lengthy repair is required. Digital blocks are less painful when buffered lidocaine is used.
2. *After infiltration of local anesthesia, gently massage the tissue to facilitate spread of anesthetic and increase absorption.
3. *Anesthesia is not effective if the periosteum has not been anesthetized. Introduce the needle down to the periosteum, and infiltrate closely to the bone.
4. *It is difficult to reach the nerves on both sides of a finger with a single injection. Separate injections on either side of the digit are usually needed.
5. *Several approaches may be used to block the common digital nerves. The metacarpal and dorsal approaches are described here.

Fingers: Metacarpal Approach
1. *Palpate the metacarpal head approximately at the level of the distal palmar crease.
2. *Cleanse the palmar surface at the injection site with an antiseptic wipe.
3. *On the palmar surface of the hand, insert a 25-G needle perpendicular to the skin just medial or lateral to the metacarpal head into the web space (Figure 139-3).
4. *After aspirating to ensure vascular penetration has not occurred, inject 1-2 ml (depending on size of the finger) as the needle is advanced to the periosteum.
5. *Repeat step 4 on the opposite side of the metacarpal head. In total, 3-4 ml of anesthetic are required for effective anesthesia for both sides of the digit.
6. *The radial nerve enervates the dorsal surface of the index and middle finger (see Figure 139-2). It may also be necessary to infiltrate locally the dorsal side of the finger at the metacarpal head if injury is present to either of these fingers on the dorsal side of the hand.

Fingers: Dorsal Approach
1. *Cleanse dorsal surface with an antiseptic wipe.
2. *Inject anesthetic with a 25-G needle to raise a wheal of anesthesia on the dorsum of the finger near the base (Figure 139-4).
3. *Inject a total of 3-5 ml anesthetic through the wheal by passing the needle downward until the needle is felt on the palmar surface (do not pierce the palmar skin).
4. *Subcutaneous infiltration is now accomplished at the base of the finger into the intraosseous spaces.

---

*Indicates portions of the procedure usually performed by a physician or an advanced practice nurse.

5. *For the index and little finger, the appropriate digital nerve is located in subcutaneous fatty tissue just anterior to the metacarpal head. Injection of anesthesia produces a half-ring wheal on the radial border of the index finger and on the ulnar border of the little finger.

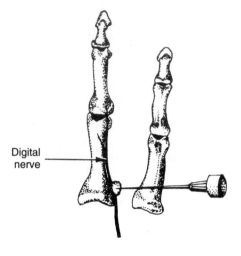

FIGURE 139-3 Digital nerve block. (From Simon, R., & Brenner, B.E. [2002]. *Emergency procedures and techniques,* 4th ed. [p. 133]. Baltimore: Williams & Wilkins.)

Digital nerve

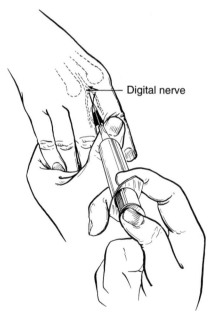

FIGURE 139-4 Dorsal approach for digital nerve block in the web space. (From Dunmire, S.M., & Paris, P.M. [1994]. *Atlas of emergency procedures* [p. 48]. Philadelphia: W.B. Saunders.)

Digital nerve

---

*Indicates portions of the procedure usually performed by a physician or an advanced practice nurse.

Thumb

1. *Circumferential block is completed by placing a ring of anesthetic around the thumb. Block of the thumb is more difficult to attain because it is supplied by multiple branches of the radial and medial nerves.
2. *Insert the needle at the base of the thumb on the dorsal surface, and angle it toward the web space while injecting the anesthetic. Then reverse the needle direction and inject toward the opposite side of the thumb. Inject close to the periosteum, as noted earlier.
3. *Next, inject on the palmar side at the base of the thumb while angling the needle toward the web space. Then reverse the needle direction while injecting toward the opposite side of the thumb, thus completing the ring.
4. Effective anesthesia can usually be accomplished by injecting a total of 4-5 ml of anesthetic.

Toes

1. *Anesthesia of the great toe requires a band of anesthesia introduced via three separate injections (Figures 139-5 and 139-6). This block usually takes 5-10 minutes to take effect.
2. *To perform digital nerve blocks of other toes, introduce the needle at the dorsal side at the base of the midpoint of the involved toe (Figure 139-7).

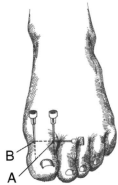

FIGURE 139-5 Digital block of the great toe. The needle is first inserted at point A and directly medially while injecting. Then, the needle is redirected posteriorly through the same puncture and anesthetic is injected in this direction. Then insert the needle at point *B* along the medial portion of the great toe and inject anesthetic posteriorly. (From Simon, R., & Brenner, B. [2002]. *Emergency procedures and techniques,* 4th ed. [p. 141]. Baltimore: Williams & Wilkins.)

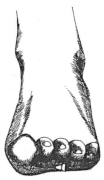

FIGURE 139-6 To complete a digital block of the great toe, the needle is inserted at the lateral, posterior aspect of the toe and directed medially while injecting anesthesia. (From Simon, R., & Brenner, B.E. [2002]. *Emergency procedures and techniques,* 4th ed. [p. 142]. Baltimore: Williams & Wilkins.)

---

*Indicates portions of the procedure usually performed by a physician or an advanced practice nurse.

3. *Angle the needle toward the bone, while slowly injecting anesthetic.
4. *Before withdrawing the needle, redirect the needle toward the opposite side of the toe, and infiltrate the second side of the toe.
5. Effective anesthesia can be achieved by injecting a total of 3 ml in the small toes and a total of 4-6 ml in the great toe.

AGE-SPECIFIC CONSIDERATIONS
1. Calculate anesthetic dosages and total anesthetic volume for the pediatric patient to avoid circulatory compromise of the digit.
2. The pediatric patient is not able to monitor return of sensation after digital block. Instruct the parents to assess circulation and limit activity until the return of expected normal sensation.

COMPLICATIONS
1. Avoid repeated jabbing while injecting to minimize hematoma formation and decrease postanesthesia neuritis.
2. Position the needle adjacent to the nerve. Intraneural infiltration should be suspected if excessive injection force is required. The patient may also complain of tingling or feeling a shock if the nerve is touched. Reposition the needle to avoid nerve injury.
3. Frequent aspiration helps avoid intravascular infiltration.
4. Vascular compromise may result if too large a volume of anesthesia is used. The amount required varies with each patient. An effective block can usually be accomplished with 3-4 ml in the digits, 4-5 ml in the thumb, and 4-6 ml in the great toe.
5. Digital block is used with finger injuries or infections. Local wound infiltration of the finger is contraindicated because of the risk of circulatory impairment.
6. Consider regional or general anesthesia if finger injury is severe or more than two fingers need digital blocks.

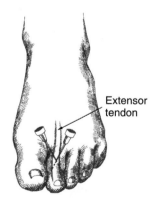

FIGURE 139-7 Digital block of toes other than the great toe. (From Simon, R., & Brenner, B.E. [2002]. *Emergency procedures and techniques,* 4th ed. [p. 142]. Baltimore: Williams & Wilkins.)

Extensor tendon

---

*Indicates portions of the procedure usually performed by a physician or an advanced practice nurse.

PATIENT TEACHING

1. Teach the patient how to assess circulatory compromise and motor or nerve impairment. Instruct the patient to return to the emergency department if compromise or impairment is suspected.
2. Adjacent fingers may also be numb because of the nerve pathways. When applying dressings to the digit, consider immobilizing the adjoining digit(s) depending on the severity of the injury.
3. Begin analgesia when anesthesia wears off, if needed. Instruct the patient when to expect return of sensation if lidocaine (1-2 hours) or bupivacaine (4-8 hours) is used (Simon & Brenner, 2002). If numbness persists longer than 24 hours, instruct the patient to contact a physician or return to the emergency department.
4. Provide wound or fracture care as indicated.

REFERENCES

Kelly, J.J., & Spektor, M. (2004). Nerve blocks of the thorax and extremities (pp. 567-590). In Roberts, J.R., & Hedges, J.R. (Eds.). *Clinical procedures in emergency medicine*, 4th ed. Philadelphia: W.B. Saunders.

Simon, R.R., & Brenner, B.E. (2002). *Emergency procedures and techniques*, 4th ed. Baltimore: Williams & Wilkins.

PROCEDURE 140

Bier Block

Joni Hentzen Daniels, MSN, RN, CEN, CCRN, CFRN, CNS

Bier block is also known as intravenous regional anesthesia.

The Bier block was invented in 1908 by August Bier and is a regional block that employs local anesthesia to cause a temporary block of nerve conduction. Venous blood of the extremity (usually upper extremity) is drained by gravity or bandaging and filled with local anesthetic held in place by a tourniquet. This type of regional anesthesia provides a bloodless field and anesthesia for injured extremities.

INDICATIONS

1. To provide regional anesthesia for patients who require evaluation of soft tissue injuries, for fracture reduction, for repair of nerves and tendons, and for complex suturing in an extremity. Bier block anesthesia is rapid, reliable, and low risk. It provides good muscle relaxation and a bloodless field.

2. This technique is best used for brief minor surgery (up to 60-90 minutes) of the hand, forearm, foot and ankle (Simon & Brenner, 2002).
3. To permit patient cooperation when constant evaluation of nerve and motor function is required. Bier block decreases the patient's pain and anxiety.
4. To provide regional anesthesia for extremities when systemic anesthesia is not an option because a patient has recently eaten or is compromised by alcohol or drug ingestion.

CONTRAINDICATIONS AND CAUTIONS

1. Sensitivity or history of allergic reaction to local anesthetics is a contraindication.
2. Bier block should not be used in patients with peripheral vascular disease or blood coagulation disorders.
3. Caution with extensive crush injury of the affected limb where tissue perfusion may already be compromised.
4. If the patient exhibits excessive fear or anxiety that prevents cooperation, a Bier block could still potentially be used with appropriate sedation and analgesia (see Procedure 181).
5. Close attention must be paid to proper maintenance of equipment with detailed check of equipment before use.
6. Bier block can be used only when adequate personnel and monitoring and resuscitation equipment are available.

EQUIPMENT

Local anesthetic without preservative
Antiseptic wipes
60-ml syringe
18- and 21-G needles for anesthesia
Equipment to start an intravenous saline or heparin lock
Cardiac monitor/defibrillator
Resuscitation equipment
3- to 4-inch elastic bandage
Cast padding
Cast or splinting material
Pneumatic tourniquet *(The use of a standard blood pressure cuff is not acceptable because of the risk of air leakage and systemic release of anesthesia.)*

PATIENT PREPARATION

1. Establish intravenous access distal to site of injury (see Procedure 63).
2. Establish a second intravenous site in an uninjured extremity for emergency access, if needed.
3. Place the patient on the cardiac monitor (see Procedure 58).
4. Apply two to three layers of cast padding at the tourniquet site to protect the skin.
5. Assess and document vital signs.
6. Place the patient in a supine position.
7. Consider sedation to decrease patient anxiety and analgesia to decrease cuff discomfort during the procedure (see Procedure 181).

PROCEDURAL STEPS

1. Test the pneumatic tourniquet by inflating it to 250 mm Hg, and ensure that there is no air leakage.
2. *Place the pneumatic tourniquet proximally on the injured extremity.
3. *Exsanguinate the extremity by either wrapping with an elastic bandage or elevating the extremity to allow gravity drainage. Gravity drainage alone is probably as effective as wrapping with an elastic wrap and can be less painful if the patient has fractures or significant injury (Bolte et al., 1994). Proper exsanguination allows even distribution of anesthesia, ensures a bloodless field, and decreases early tourniquet pain (Figure 140-1).
4. *Inflate the tourniquet to 250 mm Hg to ensure absence of radial artery pulsation. Patients who are hypotensive or hypertensive may require less or more tourniquet inflation. Inflate the cuff to 100 mm Hg above the patient's systolic blood pressure (Simon & Brenner, 2002).
5. *A double-tourniquet system may be used for procedures lasting longer than 30 minutes to decrease tourniquet pain. The proximal cuff is inflated first. When the patient begins to develop tourniquet pain, the distal cuff is inflated, and the proximal cuff is deflated. The area under the distal cuff is already anesthetized, and the patient does not experience tourniquet pain. A double-tourniquet system has narrower cuffs that require higher pressure to occlude arteries (Figure 140-2). If a single-cuff system is used, consider additional sedation and analgesia.
6. *With the tourniquet inflated, inject the anesthetic over a 60-second period into the intravenous line of the injured extremity. The anesthetic agent of choice depends on physician preference, rapidity of onset, duration and degree of motor block needed, relative toxicity of agent, and spreading power of agent. Dosage should be individualized by patient weight. Do not use anesthetic agents that contain preservatives. Lidocaine 1%, 3-5 mg/kg, without preservative is the most commonly used anesthetic (see Table 138-1 in Procedure

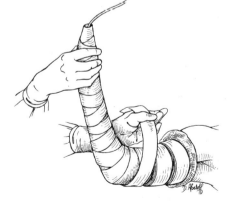

FIGURE 140-1 Exsanguinate the extremity by wrapping with an elastic bandage and/or elevating the extremity. (From Rosen, P., & Sternbach, G.L. [1983]. *Atlas of emergency medicine,* 2nd ed. [p. 209]. Baltimore: Williams & Wilkins.)

---

*Indicates portions of the procedure usually performed by a physician or an advanced practice nurse.

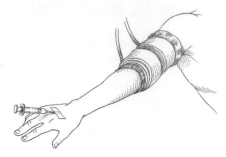

FIGURE 140-2 A double-tourniquet system. (From Rosen, P., & Sternbach, G.L. [1983]. *Atlas of emergency medicine,* 2nd ed. [p. 209]. Baltimore: Williams & Wilkins.)

138). If anesthesia is incomplete after 5 minutes, an additional 5-10 ml of anesthetic may be injected (Simon & Brenner, 2002).

7. After injection of anesthesia, continue to monitor the patient's vital signs, cardiac rhythm, and level of consciousness. Discontinue the intravenous line in the injured extremity.

8. If the patient has a fracture, casting or splint and postreduction films are performed before the tourniquet is released.

9. *At completion of the procedure, tourniquet release is begun. Do not release the tourniquet for at least 10 minutes after the last injection of anesthetic. If total tourniquet time is 20-30 minutes, use one of the following cycled deflation techniques:

   a. Deflate the tourniquet totally for 2-3 seconds, then reinflate the tourniquet for 1 minute. Deflate the tourniquet again for 2-3 seconds and reinflate for 1 minute, then deflate the tourniquet totally.

   b. Stage the release of the tourniquet in cycles by deflating and inflating the tourniquet for 20-second intervals for approximately 1 minute before the tourniquet's final release (Blasier & White, 1996).

   If total tourniquet time is longer than 40 minutes, deflate the tourniquet without cycling. If the tourniquet is inflated for longer than 30 minutes, 50% of the anesthetic is bound to tissue, and systemic reactions are rare.

10. During and after release of the tourniquet, continue to monitor the patient's vital signs, cardiac rhythm, and level of consciousness for symptoms of anesthetic toxicity. After the tourniquet release, the patient should be monitored for a minimum of 30-60 minutes. Circulation, sensation, and mobility of the patient's injured extremity should also be monitored during this time.

AGE-SPECIFIC CONSIDERATIONS

1. Lidocaine in a smaller dose (1.5 mg/kg) is often effective in children (Bolte et al., 1994).

2. Children may require additional sedation before the procedure.

COMPLICATIONS

1. Severe toxicity is rare and is usually due to a faulty tourniquet. High blood concentrations of anesthetic as a result of rapid release into the systemic circulation may be life-threatening.

---

*Indicates portions of the procedure usually performed by a physician or an advanced practice nurse.

2. Systemic toxicity is dose dependent and is related to the effects of anesthesia on the cardiovascular or central nervous systems. Cardiovascular effects may include hypotension and arrhythmias, such as conduction disturbances, bradycardia, tachycardia, and asystole. Central nervous system effects are more common and include perioral numbness, dizziness, visual disturbances (blurred vision), lightheadedness, near-syncope, seizure, and coma (Blasier & White, 1996).
3. Reactions are more common if the tourniquet is released within less than 30 minutes, if the tourniquet is released too rapidly, or if the anesthetic dosage is too high.
4. Tourniquet pain can be significant when a single cuff is used for procedures lasting longer than 30 minutes. Even with the use of a double cuff, tourniquet pain limits the length of use to 60-90 minutes.
5. True allergic reactions are rare and are usually caused by ester-derivative anesthetics not used in Bier block anesthesia (see Procedure 138).

PATIENT TEACHING

1. Teach the patient symptoms of circulatory compromise and nerve and motor impairment, and ask the patient to contact a physician or return to the emergency department if problems are suspected.
2. Instruct the patient when to expect return of sensation and to begin analgesia promptly.

REFERENCES

Blasier, R., & White R. (1996). Intravenous regional anesthesia for management of children's extremity fractures in the emergency department. *Pediatric Emergency Care, 12,* 404-406.
Bolte, R., Stevens, P.M., Scott, S.M., & Shunk, J.E. (1994). Mini-dose Bier block intravenous regional anesthesia in the emergency department treatment of pediatric upper-extremity injuries. *Journal of Pediatric Orthopaedics, 14,* 534-537.
Simon, R.R., & Brenner, B.E. (2002). *Emergency procedures and techniques,* 4th ed. Baltimore: Williams & Wilkins.

Fishhook Removal

Daun A. Smith, RN, MS, CEN

INDICATION
To remove fishhooks embedded in soft tissue

CONTRAINDICATIONS AND CAUTIONS
1. There are two types of fishhooks; both are curved with an extremely sharp tip, with the barb just distal to and on the inside of the curve. One has a barbed shaft, and the other has an unbarbed shaft.
2. Fishhooks embedded in or near the eye may need to be removed by an ophthalmologist. Emergency or field treatment should consist of covering the affected eye with a shield or cup (see Procedure 165). Patching the unaffected eye decreases movement in the injured eye (see Procedure 163).
3. Fishhooks embedded in bone or cartilage; in the oropharynx, nose, ear, or other orifice; or associated with neurovascular dysfunction distally may need to be surgically removed.

EQUIPMENT
Wound cleaning supplies
Local anesthetic
Other specific supplies depend on the removal method and may include the following:
Heavy silk suture material (00 or 1-0) or umbilical tape
Forceps (curved or straight) or needle holder
Wire cutters

PATIENT PREPARATION
1. Cleanse the wound (see Procedure 137).
2. Consider local anesthesia (see Procedures 138 and 139).
3. Consider radiographic studies to locate tip of fishhook and visualize barbs.
4. Administer tetanus immunization as indicated.
5. *Perform a neurovascular assessment of distal structures before attempting to manipulate the fishhook.

PROCEDURAL STEPS
Numerous methods exist for the removal of fishhooks, depending on the depth of fishhook penetration, the location of the fishhook, and the remover's preference.

---

*Indicates portions of the procedure usually performed by a physician or an advanced practice nurse.

Simple Retrograde Removal

1. *Gently press down on the shank of the fishhook (this releases the barb at the tip) (Figure 141-1).
2. *Remove the fishhook by backing it out, following the pathway of entry.

String Method

1. For this technique, wear eye protection because the fishhook exits from the skin in an uncontrolled manner.
2. *Wrap the middle of a piece of umbilical tape or heavy silk suture material (at least 10 inches long) around the bend of the fishhook, grasping both free ends in your dominant hand, holding the ends in the opposite direction from the direction of the fishhook entry (Figure 141-2).
3. *Gently press down on the shank of the fishhook, disengaging the barb.
4. *Tug or snap the ends of the tape or suture material in the direction away from the fishhook entry and parallel to the skin. This action removes the fishhook in a retrograde fashion.

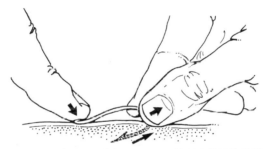

FIGURE 141-1 Simple retrograde removal. (From Jastremski, M.S. [1992]. Fishhook removal [p. 129]. In Jastremski, M.S., Dumas, M., & Peñalaver, L. [Eds.]. *Emergency procedures*. Philadelphia: W.B. Saunders.)

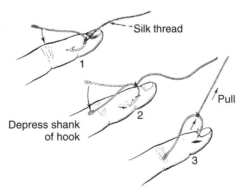

FIGURE 141-2 String removal method. (From Dunmire, S.M., & Paris, P.M. [1994]. *Atlas of emergency procedures* [p. 111]. Philadelphia: W.B. Saunders.)

---

*Indicates portions of the procedure usually performed by a physician or an advanced practice nurse.

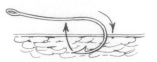

Advance hook through skin

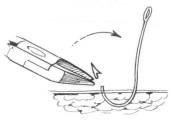

Cut off barb

FIGURE 141-3 Advance and cut method. (From Dunmire, S.M., & Paris, P.M. [1994]. *Atlas of emergency procedures* [p. 111]. Philadelphia, W.B. Saunders.)

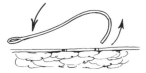

Reverse direction and extract hook

Advance and Cut

This method is used for deeper fishhook penetrations, when multiple barbs are embedded, or when other methods have failed.

1. *Advance the tip of the fishhook through the skin using the forceps or the needle holder (Figure 141-4).
2. *Cut the tip and barb from the fishhook with wire cutters.
3. *Remove the remainder of the fishhook in a retrograde manner.
4. *If the fishhook shaft is barbed, the eye of the fishhook is cut off with wire cutters and the fishhook is removed in an antegrade fashion.
5. Reassess the distal neurovascular function, and clean the wound according to institutional guidelines.

COMPLICATIONS

1. Infection
2. Distal neurovascular compromise

PATIENT TEACHING

1. Monitor for signs and symptoms of infection, including pain, swelling, drainage, tenderness, and redness.
2. Report any signs of infection to your primary care provider.

---

*Indicates portions of the procedure usually performed by a physician or an advanced practice nurse.

Wound Care for Amputations

Jean A. Proehl, RN, MN, CEN, CCRN

INDICATION

To preserve amputated or avulsed tissue or appendages for possible replantation or revascularization. Replantation is the correct term for complete amputations; partial amputations are revascularized. For simplicity, the term replantation is used for both situations in this procedure.

CONTRAINDICATIONS AND CAUTIONS

1. Replantation is attempted only after life-threatening problems are resolved.
2. The decision to attempt replantation is made by the surgeon after consideration of technical, esthetic, medical, and psychosocial factors. A promise should not be made to the patient that replantation will be attempted. The replantation team should be consulted as soon as possible to determine whether a replantation attempt is indicated.
3. Time is of the essence for successful replantation. Cooling the tissue prolongs its viability. The more muscle, the higher the metabolic needs, and the shorter the acceptable ischemic time frame. Fingers have relatively little muscle in comparison to extremities.
4. The amputated tissue should not be allowed to freeze. Freezing causes cell membrane rupture and irreversibly damages the tissue. A temperature of 4° C is optimal (Dagum & Mirza, 1997; Dalsey & Luk, 2004). Dry ice should not be used, because it results in temperatures that are too cold.
5. No tissue bridge should be severed, no matter how thin. It should be treated as a partial amputation and splinted to preserve the integrity of the skin bridge.
6. Tourniquets, tying, or clamping vessels in the stump should be avoided, because these maneuvers may damage the structures that will be reanastomosed during replantation. Bleeding should be controlled with direct pressure if possible. A blood pressure cuff on the proximal extremity inflated to 30 mm Hg above systolic blood pressure can be used to help control bleeding if necessary (Dalsey & Luk, 2004).
7. Digital block anesthesia of the stump should be avoided (O'Hara-Speert & Mullaly, 1996).
8. All avulsed or amputated tissue should be preserved; even if replantation is not attempted, the tissue may be used for grafting.

EQUIPMENT

Gauze dressings
Insulated container (for prolonged storage or transport to another facility)
Plastic bag or waterproof container

Ice
Sterile normal saline solution or lactated Ringer's solution
Antibiotic, if prescribed, for tissue preservation solution

PATIENT PREPARATION

1. Consult with your referral replantation team as soon as possible to determine the feasibility of replantation and to receive specific instructions regarding care of the amputated part and the patient.
2. Remove all jewelry from the injured extremity (see Procedure 118).
3. Obtain wound cultures before antibiotic administration. Send laboratory specimens for type and crossmatch if the amputation is proximal to the forearm because these patients tend to bleed more heavily (Goldberg et al., 1997).
4. Administer parenteral antibiotics, analgesia, and sedation as prescribed.
5. Administer tetanus prophylaxis as indicated.
6. Administer aspirin or low-molecular-weight dextran if prescribed by the replantation surgeon.
7. Obtain x-ray studies of the stump and the amputated part.
8. Prepare the patient for transport if indicated (see Procedure 195).

PROCEDURAL STEPS
Complete Amputation

1. Cleanse the stump and the amputated part by gently rinsing with normal saline solution or lactated Ringer's solution to remove gross contamination. Do not scrub or use antiseptic solution.
2. Apply a soft-pressure dressing and elevate the stump. Splint the stump as indicated.
3. Wrap the amputated part in gauze moistened with saline solution or lactated Ringer's solution, and seal it in a plastic bag (Dagum & Mirza, 1997; Dalsey & Luk, 2004; O'Hara-Speert & Mullaly, 1996; Yoshida, 1997). Be sure to wrap the part well so that it is protected from freezing. Some replantation teams prescribe antibiotics to be added to the solution used to moisten the dressings.
4. Place the plastic bag or container on an ice bath in an insulated container.
5. Label the bag or container containing the amputated part so that it is not inadvertently discarded.

Partial Amputation

1. Wrap the entire extremity in moist dressings per replantation team orders.
2. Splint and elevate the extremity.
3. Cooling the extremity may not be possible because it can be painful. If there is evidence of arterial insufficiency, attempt to cool the distal part with ice packs.

AGE-SPECIFIC CONSIDERATIONS
Children have better nerve regeneration capability and usually have better functional outcomes than adults. Replantation attempts are considered in children, even in the presence of relative contraindications (Yoshida, 1997).

COMPLICATIONS
1. Cellular damage or death as a result of freezing or inadequate cooling.

2. Cellular damage or death as a result of excess time between injury and replantation. Time limits vary with the type of injury, the body part involved, and how the part is stored. Every effort should be made to replant the part as soon as possible.

PATIENT TEACHING

1. Do not smoke, eat, or drink until after surgery. Caffeine and nicotine are not allowed for several months if replantation is attempted.
2. Keep the injured part elevated.
3. The replantation surgeon is the most qualified person to discuss your prognosis with you.

REFERENCES

Dagum, A.B., & Mirza, M.A. (1997). Replantation surgery in the upper extremity (pp. 1187-1192). In Dee, R., Hurst, L.C., Gruber, M.A., & Kottmeier, S.A. (Eds.). *Principles of orthopedic practice*, 2nd ed. New York: McGraw-Hill.
Dalsey, W.C., & Luk, J. (2004). Management of amputations (pp. 919-926). Roberts, J.R., & Hedges, J.R. (Eds.). *Clinical procedures in emergency medicine*, 4th ed. Philadelphia: W.B. Saunders.
Goldberg, J.A., Buncke, H.J., & Buncke, G.M. (1997). Replantation of amputated parts (pp. 971-977). In Georgiade, G.S., Riefkohl, R., & Levin, L.S. (Eds.). *Georgiade plastic, maxillofacial and reconstructive surgery*, 3rd ed. Baltimore: Williams & Wilkins.
O'Hara-Speert, M., & Mullaly, S.G. (1996). Nursing care of the patient with a complete scalp avulsion. *Journal of Emergency Nursing, 22*, 552-558.
Yoshida, D. (1997). Amputations (pp. 645-649). In Dieckmann, R.A., Fiser, D.H., & Selbst S.M. (Eds.). *Illustrated textbook of pediatric emergency and critical care procedures*. St. Louis: Mosby.

PROCEDURE 143

Surgical Tape Closures

Jean A. Proehl, RN, MN, CEN, CCRN

Surgical tape closures also known as tape closures, skin tapes, butterfly closures, Steri-Strips, Cover-Strips, Shur-Strips, Curi-Strips, Nichi-Strips, Cicagraf, and Suture Strips.

INDICATIONS

In appropriate wounds, surgical tape closures have the following advantages over suture or staple closure: No suture scars, less skin reaction, greater resistance to wound infection, less need for anesthesia, no return visit necessary for removal, may be used under casts and splints, less expensive than sutures or staples, and ease of application (Lammers & Trott, 2004; 3M Health Care, 1994). Surgical tape closures are indicated in the following situations:

1. To provide a noninvasive repair of a wound. Superficial, straight lacerations under little tension are the ideal wounds for surgical skin tapes.
2. To provide additional support to sutured or stapled wounds.
3. To provide wound stability and promote further healing after suture removal.
4. To approximate skin edges loosely on a wound too old to be sutured but gaping widely.
5. To hold skin flaps and grafts in place (Lammers & Trott, 1998).
6. To approximate wounds in skin that is compromised by long-term steroid use or peripheral vascular disease (Lammers & Trott, 2004).

CONTRAINDICATIONS AND CAUTIONS

1. Surgical skin tapes are not used in the following situations:
   a. Wounds under high skin stress, such as those over major joints
   b. Wounds that will become wet as a result of problems with hemostasis, perspiration, exudate, or ointment application
   c. Wounds that are infected
   d. Wounds that are surrounded by hair or skin abrasion
   e. Wounds that are irregular or over concave areas
2. Tapes should not be placed circumferentially around digits; digits should be wrapped in a semicircular or spiral fashion instead.
3. The tape should not be stretched during application; tape should be applied with only a small amount of tension to approximate wound edges.

EQUIPMENT

Surgical tape closures (available in widths from $1/8$ to $1/2$ inch)
Skin adhesive such as tincture of benzoin (optional)
Forceps
Scissors

PATIENT PREPARATION

1. Anesthetize the area as indicated (see Procedures 138 and 139).
2. Cleanse the wound (see Procedure 137).
3. Provide tetanus prophylaxis as indicated.

PROCEDURAL STEPS

1. Maintain hemostasis using direct pressure.
2. Ensure a dry field; surgical tape closures do not adhere to moist skin.
3. Apply a skin adhesive to the wound margins and the surrounding skin (optional). Do not allow the adhesive to enter the wound, and do not use adhesive near the eye. Even with local anesthesia, there may be a brief episode of discomfort as the alcohol fumes from the adhesive evaporate. Allow the adhesive to dry and become tacky.
4. Cut the tapes to the desired length; allow for a 2- to 3-cm overlap on each side of the wound (Lammers & Trott, 2004). Remove the end tab from the paper backing of the strips.

5. Remove a tape from the backing by pulling it straight back with forceps; do not curl the tape backward during removal because this curls the tape and makes it more difficult to work with (3M Health Care, 1994).
6. *Fresh wound (Figure 143-1):*
   a. Place the first tape at the middle of the wound on one side only, approximate the wound edges as closely as possible (a second person may be required to assist), and apply the second half of the tape. Run your finger along the strip to help set the adhesive.
   b. Place additional tapes halfway between the previous tape and the wound edges. Continue to apply tapes until the wound is sufficiently closed but not totally occluded.
   c. Place supporting tapes horizontally across the tapes, approximately 1 inch from the wound; this is known as the ladder technique. The supporting tapes help prevent the ends of the tapes from curling and decrease skin stress at the tape ends.

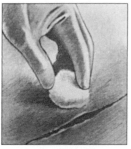

1. Clean and dry skin thoroughly, and remove any oils.

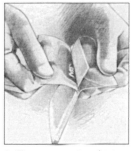

2. Remove card end tab from one end of card.

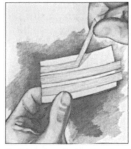

3. Grasp end of strip with fingers or fine forceps and lift straight forward from card using a slow motion.

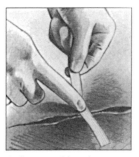

4. Appose skin edges with forceps.

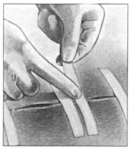

5. Place strips across wound, ensuring tension-less application. Divide the wound into sections, starting at the midpoint of the wound.

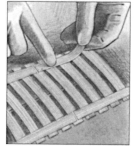

6. Set adhesive with light finger pressure by running along length of the strip.

7. Place strips about 1/8 inch apart until entire wound is covered.

FIGURE 143-1 Skin tape application technique. (Courtesy 3M Health Care. [1994]. *Professional adhesive closure education* [teacher's guide]. St. Paul, MN.)

7. *Healing wound (after suture removal):* Remove a few sutures at a time and replace them with tapes (apply tapes as described in steps 6a-c).
8. If a tape needs to be repositioned after application, remove it by peeling both ends toward the wound.

AGE-SPECIFIC CONSIDERATIONS

1. Surgical skin tapes are useful in frightened children with suitable wounds.
2. Cover the skin tapes with a dry dressing to prevent small children and confused adults from picking at them. Do not use occlusive or adhesive bandages that encourage moisture formation.

COMPLICATIONS

1. Wound infection.
2. Impaired wound healing. Medications, such as steroids and hormones, and medical conditions, such as diabetes, uremia, malnourishment, and poor skin perfusion, contribute to poor wound healing.
3. Wound dehiscence if the strips loosen, fall off too early, or are improperly applied, or if there is poor patient compliance with wound care.
4. Blisters under the ends of the tapes from excessive skin tension. This complication can be avoided by use of supporting horizontal tapes across the tape tails and by not stretching the tapes during application. Wound swelling after tape application can also cause excessive skin tension.

PATIENT TEACHING

1. The wound must remain clean and dry. After 24 hours, you may shower with surgical tape closures in place but limit exposure to water and gently pat dry as soon as possible. The strips adhere better if exposure to water is limited (3M Health Care, 2002).
2. Do not apply any ointments or petroleum-containing products on the strips. The adhesive dissolves, and the strips fall off.
3. Trim the edges of the strips as they loosen and curl to prevent inadvertent removal.
4. Elevate the injured area as much as possible for the next 24-48 hours.
5. Report any signs of infection (redness, swelling, draining pus, fever) to your health care provider or return to the emergency department.
6. Remove strips if they have not fallen off after the prescribed number of days. For fresh wounds, see Procedure 145 for the recommended number of days.

REFERENCES

Lammers, R.L., & Trott, A.T. (2004). Methods of wound closure (pp. 655-693). Roberts, J.R. & Hedges, J.R. (Eds.). *Clinical procedures in emergency medicine*, 4th ed. Philadelphia: W.B. Saunders.

3M Health Care. (1994). *Professional adhesive closure education* (teacher's guide). St. Paul, MN: Author.

3M Health Care. (2002). *3M Steri-Strip™ adhesive skin closures: commonly asked questions.* Available at http://products3.3m.com/catalog/us/en001/healthcare/professional/node_GS7K 20 M0LFbe/root_GST1T4S9TCgv/vroot_GS2PVC6H4Dge/gvel_GSTGM553HTgl/command_ AbcPageHandler/theme_us_professional_3_0. Accessed 5/9/03.

Skin Adhesive

Jean A. Proehl, RN, MN, CEN, CCRN

Skin adhesive is also known as tissue adhesive, wound glue, or DERMABOND topical skin adhesive (ETHICON, INC.).

INDICATION

Skin adhesive is used to close easily approximated, clean, traumatic, or surgical lacerations. It is faster and less painful than suturing and produces a similar or better cosmetic outcome (Osmond et al., 1999; Resch & Hick, 2000). It remains in place for 5-10 days before sloughing off. No removal is necessary.

CONTRAINDICATIONS AND CAUTIONS

1. Skin adhesive is not suitable for high tension wounds over joints unless they are immobilized.
2. Do not use in the presence of infection or contamination, on mucosal surfaces; on bites, jagged, stellate or puncture wounds; or in dense hair.
3. Skin adhesive is contraindicated for patients with hypersensitivity to cyanoacrylate or formaldehyde.
4. Do not use in areas subjected to repetitive rubbing or washing, such as the hands, because the top layer of epidermis may peel off before healing is complete.
5. Some skin adhesives are low viscosity and may run off of the wound and fuse unintended areas together, such as eyelids, the practitioner's gloves, and so on. High-viscosity formulations decrease this risk and are easier to control during application.

EQUIPMENT

Forceps (optional)
Gauze sponges
Skin adhesive in an applicator

PATIENT PREPARATION

1. If necessary, anesthetize the wound to facilitate cleansing (see Procedures 138 and 139).
2. Clean and irrigate the wound (see Procedure 137).
3. Establish hemostasis with direct pressure and dry the area completely. Water accelerates the polymerization process; thus skin adhesive should not be applied to wet wounds (ETHICON, 1998).
4. *For deeper wounds, place subcutaneous sutures to help approximate the skin.

---

*Indicates a portion of the procedure usually performed by a physician or an advanced practice nurse.

5. Position the area horizontally to prevent the skin adhesive from running onto adjacent tissue. If the wound is near the eye, position the wound slightly downhill from the eye and hold the eye closed with a gauze dressing.
6. Administer tetanus prophylaxis as indicated.

PROCEDURAL STEPS

1. Hold the applicator with the white tip up and squeeze to crush the inner glass ampule. Invert the applicator and squeeze gently to start the flow of adhesive through the tip.
2. Approximate the wound with forceps or gloved fingers and evert the wound edges slightly.
3. Gently apply a thin, even layer of adhesive to the wound edges and 0.5 cm beyond (Figure 144-1). Excessive pressure may force the wound open and allow the adhesive to enter the wound. The adhesive should not enter the wound, because it is not absorbed and can cause a foreign body reaction. Allow 15-30 seconds for the adhesive to dry between layers and apply three to four thin layers in this fashion. The patient may feel warmth as the adhesive polymerizes.
4. If the adhesive runs onto adjacent areas, it can be wiped off for the first 10 seconds. A petroleum-based ointment can be immediately applied to unintended areas of adhesive coverage to help promote dissolution.
5. Maintain manual wound approximation for at least 1 minute after the last layer. Full strength is attained about 2.5 minutes after the last layer is applied.
6. Do not apply ointment to the area. No dressing is necessary. If a dressing is preferred, wait at least 5 minutes to be sure that the adhesive is no longer sticky before applying a dry, sterile dressing. Do not apply skin tapes or adhesive tape directly to the skin adhesive.

AGE-SPECIFIC CONSIDERATION

Skin adhesive is particularly useful in children because it is quicker and less painful than suturing. Also, a return visit for suture removal is not necessary. A dressing may be helpful to keep children from picking at the adhesive.

COMPLICATIONS

Inadvertent adhesion to gloves, forceps, hair, or other skin surfaces. If this occurs, acetone or petroleum-based ointments can be used to loosen the adhesive. Peel off the film, but do not attempt to pull the skin apart.

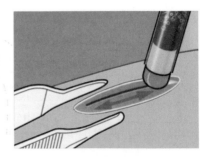

FIGURE 144-1 Apply the adhesive gently while approximating the wound edges. (Courtesy ETHICON, Inc., Somerville, NJ.)

PATIENT TEACHING

1. Report any signs of infection (e.g., redness, swelling, pus drainage, fever) or wound separation to your health care provider or return to the emergency department.
2. The skin adhesive will slough off the site in 5-10 days; no removal is necessary. Do not scratch, rub, or pick at the adhesive. Do not apply ointment, cream, or tape to the adhesive.
3. Do not expose the wound to sunlight or tanning lamps while the adhesive is in place.
4. Do not swim or soak the wound. Showering and brief wetting of the wound is allowed. To dry the wound, blot it with a towel instead of rubbing.

REFERENCES

ETHICON, INC. (1998). *A complete guide for using DERMABOND adhesive* (wall chart). Somerville, NJ: Author.

Osmond, M.H., Quinn, J.V., Sutcliffe, T., Jamuske, M., Klassen, T.P. (1999). *Academic Emergency Medicine, 6*(3), 171-177.

Resch, K.L., & Hick, J.L. (2000). Preliminary experience with 2-octylcyanoacrylate in a pediatric emergency department. *Pediatric Emergency Care, 16*, 328-331.

PROCEDURE 145

Suture Removal

Maureen T. Quigley, MS, ARNP, CEN

INDICATION

To remove nonabsorbable suture material inserted for the purpose of wound approximation and primary healing. Adequate epithelialization of the wound is evidenced by a sturdy wound appearance, approximated edges, and evidence of healing. Timely suture removal is important in minimizing scar formation. Removal of sutures is contingent on the integrity of the dermal closure and the degree of motion and healing properties of the particular area of the body. The dense vascularity and lack of tension on the face allows for quick, early healing and permits removal of sutures in only 3-5 days. Sutures on the trunk are left in place 6-7 days, and extremity sutures may remain for longer periods (Table 145-1).

CONTRAINDICATIONS AND CAUTIONS

1. To gain optimal cosmetic and functional results, sutures should be removed in a timely manner. The risk of infection at puncture sites and the difficulty of suture removal is increased when sutures are left in longer than necessary. Premature suture removal predisposes the patient to wound disruption, delayed healing, and widening of the scar.
2. When the suture line is located in an area exposed to tensile stretch (e.g., joints), the sutures may be kept in place for up to 14 days, and thereafter the wound may require superficial support with skin tapes for an additional 5-7 days. Skin tape closures provide support and protection and can minimize scar widening.
3. Sutures with short ends are more difficult to remove.
4. Certain conditions interfere with wound healing. Populations at risk for impaired healing include the elderly, smokers, and those with diabetes, obesity, vascular disease, and immunosuppression, as well as those who have used steroids long term. Deep wounds are at increased risk for infection.

EQUIPMENT

Scissors or suture removal scissors, no. 11 scalpel blade, or stitch cutter blade
Forceps
Gauze sponges
Normal saline solution
Antiseptic solution
Skin tape closures (optional)
NOTE: Prepackaged kits containing some of the listed items are available.

PROCEDURAL STEPS

1. The wound should be well visualized with proper lighting.
2. Cleanse sutures and the healed wound with antiseptic because it is impossible to avoid pulling a small portion of suture that has been outside the skin through the suture tract. Remove any crusting on the surrounding wound.
3. Grasp the knot of the suture with forceps with your nondominant hand and raise away from the skin.

TABLE 145-1
REMOVAL TIMES FOR SUTURES

Location	Time of Removal (Days)
Face	3-4 (adults)
	2-3 (children)
Scalp	5-7
Trunk	7
Lower extremity	8-10
Upper extremity	7-10
Extensor surface of joints	10-14
Delayed closure	8-12

4. Cut the suture distal to the knot and close to the skin surface on one side. This ensures that a contaminated suture is not drawn through the suture tract as the suture is withdrawn (Figure 145-1).
   a. If a vertical or horizontal mattress suture is in place, the suture must be cut on the side opposite the knot at a skin orifice (Figure 145-2).
   b. Running or continuous sutures (Figure 145-3) are removed by cutting every other loop. To determine that the ends are completely severed, gently lift the exposed ends away from skin (Perry & Potter, 2002).
5. Pull the suture out of the wound and discard.
6. Cleanse the wound with normal saline solution or an antiseptic solution.
7. Apply skin tape to wounds under tension or prone to separation (see Procedure 143).
8. Leave the suture line open to the air or apply a dressing as prescribed.

AGE-SPECIFIC CONSIDERATION
Because children heal and form suture marks faster than adults, they may require earlier suture removal.

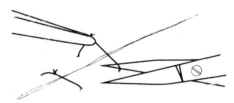

FIGURE 145-1 Correct method of removing a suture. The suture should be removed by cutting the end away from the knot near the skin to prevent passage of the contaminated outer portion of the stitch back through the skin. (From Simon, R., & Brenner, B. [2002]. *Emergency procedures and techniques,* 4th ed. [p. 413]. Baltimore: Williams & Wilkins.)

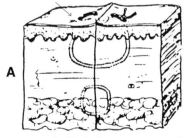 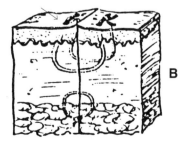

FIGURE 145-2 A, Vertical mattress suture. **B,** Horizontal mattress suture. Arrows indicate points where sutures should be cut. (From Schwartz, S. [1999]. *Principles of surgery,* 7th ed. [p. 2094]. New York: McGraw-Hill.)

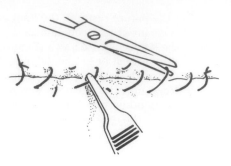

FIGURE 145-3 To remove a continuous suture, every other loop is cut. (From Mulliken, J.B. [1992]. Management of superficial wounds. In May, H., Aghababian, R., & Fleisher, G. [Eds.]. *Emergency medicine,* 2nd ed. [p. 639]. New York: Little, Brown.)

COMPLICATIONS
1. Wound infection
2. Widening of scar
3. Wound dehiscence
4. Retained suture

PATIENT TEACHING
1. Keep the wound clean and dry. Any crusted areas should simply be allowed to come off with usual soap and water cleansing. Do not pick at crusts or scabs.
2. Report any of the following signs and symptoms of wound infection: fever, increasing redness around the wound or on the extremity involved, swelling, drainage of pus, increased pain or tenderness, or opening of the wound.
3. If the wound is in an area exposed to the sun, a sunscreen containing para-aminobenzoic acid is recommended for application to wound area because scars in the first 4 months redden to a greater extent than the surrounding skin (Lammers, 2004).

REFERENCES
Lammers, R. (2004). Principles of wound management (pp. 623-654). In Roberts, J.R., & Hedges, J.R. (Eds.). *Clinical procedures in emergency medicine,* 4th ed. Philadelphia: W.B. Saunders.
Perry, A., & Potter, P. (2002). *Clinical nursing skills and techniques,* 5th ed. St. Louis: Mosby.

Staple Removal

Maureen T. Quigley, MS, ARNP, CEN

INDICATION

To remove skin staples inserted for the purpose of wound approximation and primary healing. Adequate epithelialization of the wound is evidenced by a sturdy wound appearance, approximated edges, and evidence of healing. Timely staple removal is important to minimize scar formation. Staple removal is performed under the same guidelines as skin sutures if healing is adequate.

CONTRAINDICATIONS AND CAUTIONS

1. To achieve optimal cosmetic and functional results, staples should be removed in a timely manner. There is a risk of infection at the puncture sites when staples are left in too long. Premature staple removal predisposes the patient to wound disruption, delayed healing, and widening of scar.
2. Generally, wound stapling and suturing have similar infection rates and wound healing. Staples should be removed promptly from patients who scar more easily, because in this population, the scar formed by staples may be more prominent than that formed by sutures (Lammers & Trott, 2004).
3. Some conditions interfere with wound healing. Populations at risk for impaired healing include the elderly, smokers, and those with diabetes, obesity, vascular disease, and immunosuppression, as well as those who have used steroids long term.

EQUIPMENT

Staple extractor (A variety of disposable skin stapler devices are on the market. Each stapler has its own specific staple extractor.)
Gauze sponges
Antiseptic solution
Normal saline solution

PROCEDURAL STEPS

1. Ensure adequate lighting on wound area.
2. Cleanse staples and healed wound with antiseptic solution. Remove any crusting on surrounding wound.
3. Place the lower tips of the extractor under the center of the staple (Figure 146-1).
4. Squeeze the extractor so that the center of the staple is depressed.
5. Lift the extractor and staple upward from the skin when both ends of the staple are visible.
6. After staple has been removed from skin, release handles of staple extractor, and dispose of staple in proper container.

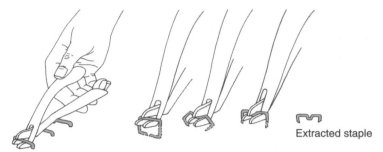

Extracted staple

FIGURE 146-1 Technique for removing staples. (From Earnest, V. [1993]. *Clinical skills in nursing practice,* 2nd ed. [p. 930]. Philadelphia: J.B. Lippincott.)

COMPLICATIONS
1. Wound infection
2. Scar widening
3. Wound dehiscence

PATIENT TEACHING
1. Keep your wound clean and dry. Any crusted areas should simply be allowed to come off with usual soap and water cleansing. Do not pick at crusts or scabs.
2. Report any of the following signs and symptoms of wound infection: fever, increasing redness around the wound or on the extremity involved, drainage of pus, increased pain or tenderness, or opening of the wound.

REFERENCE
Lammers, R. & Trott, A.T. (2004). Methods of wound closure (pp. 655-693). In Roberts, J.R., & Hedges, J.R. (Eds.). *Clinical procedures in emergency medicine,* 4th ed. Philadelphia: W.B. Saunders.

PROCEDURE 147

Minor Burn Care

Joni Hentzen Daniels, MSN, RN, CEN, CCRN, CFRN, CNS
and Margo E. Layman, MSN, RN, RNC, CN-A

This procedure discusses the débridement and dressing of minor burns only. Minor burns, as defined by the American Burn Association (Russell, 2001) guide-

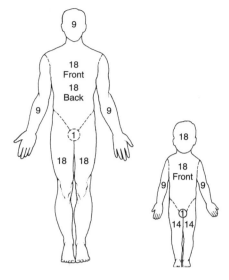

FIGURE 147-1 The rule of nines may be used to estimate body surface area burned. (From Bethel, C.A., & Krisanda, T.J. (2004). Burn care procedures [p. 757]. In Roberts, J.R., & Hedges, J.R. [Eds.]. *Clinical procedures in emergency medicine*, 4th ed. Philadelphia: W.B. Saunders.)

lines as well as the American College of Surgeons (1999), are burns that may be managed on an outpatient basis as follows:

1. Partial-thickness and full-thickness burns covering less than 10% of body surface area (BSA) in patients younger than10 years or older than 50 years.
2. Partial-thickness and full-thickness burns covering less than 20% BSA in other age-groups not involving the following:
   a. Face
   b. Hands
   c. Genitalia
   d. Feet
   e. Perineum
   f. Overlying joints
3. Full-thickness burns less than 5% BSA
4. No presence of electrical injury (including lightening)
5. No presence of chemical burns
6. No presence of inhalational injury
7. No presence of preexisting medical conditions that could complicate management, prolong recovery, or affect mortality
8. No presence of concomitant trauma
9. No question of the reliability of the caregiver or the home care environment.

Methods used to assess percentage of BSA involved with burn management include the rule of nines (Figure 147-1) and the Lund and Browder Burn chart (Figure 147-2). When small or irregular burns are being estimated, the patient's palmar surface is equal to about 1.25% BSA (Bethel & Krisanda , 2004).

INDICATION

Minor burns managed on an outpatient basis requiring débridement and dressing. Débridement and dressing serve the following purposes:
1. Minimize the potential for bacterial infection

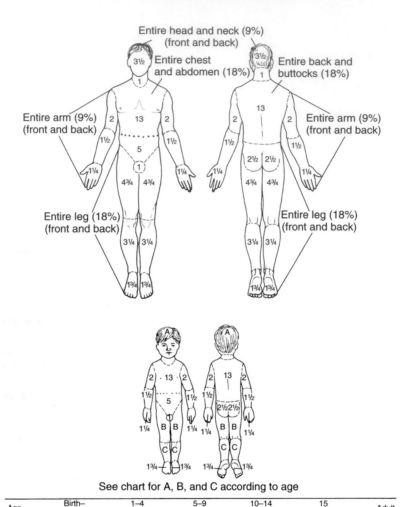

Entire head and neck (9%)
(front and back)

Entire chest
and abdomen (18%)

Entire back and
buttocks (18%)

Entire arm (9%)
(front and back)

Entire arm (9%)
(front and back)

Entire leg (18%)
(front and back)

Entire leg (18%)
(front and back)

See chart for A, B, and C according to age

Age	Birth–1 yr	1–4 yr	5–9 yr	10–14 yr	15 yr	Adult
Head	19	17	13	11	9	7
Neck	2					
Ant trunk	13					
Post trunk	13					
R buttock	2½					
L buttock	2½					
Genitalia	1					
R U arm	4					
L U arm	4					
R L arm	3					
L L arm	3					
R hand	2½					
L hand	2½					
R thigh	5½	6½	8	8½	9	9½
L thigh	5½	6½	8	8½	9	9½
R leg	5	5	5½	6	6½	7
L leg	5	5	5½	6	6½	7
R foot	3½					
L foot	3½					

FIGURE 147-2 The Lund and Browder chart is a more accurate way to estimate body surface area burned than the rule of nines. (From Bethel, C.A., & Krisanda, T.J. (2004). Burn care procedures [pg. 752]. In Roberts, J.R., & Hedges, J.R. [Eds.]. *Clinical procedures in emergency medicine*, 4th ed. Philadelphia: W.B. Saunders.)

2. Prevent the conversion of a partial-thickness burn to a full-thickness burn
3. Promote spontaneous healing
4. Maximize patient comfort
5. Minimize cosmetic changes
6. Maintain optimal range of joint motion

CONTRAINDICATIONS AND CAUTIONS

1. Most burn units request that in the case of major burns that require admission, no débridement of the wound is performed in the emergency department. During the transfer, a dry sterile gauze dressing should be applied to isolated burns. In the case of large BSA involvement, a dry sterile sheet is recommended.
2. Current recommendations are to reserve the use of sterile saline soaks to partial-thickness burns of less than 10% BSA. Moist dressings should not be used in any patient requiring transfer to a burn unit because of increased risk for both hypothermia and infection.
3. Cool saline may be used over the area initially to stop the burning process. Benefits of cooled fluids are:
   a. Inhibited lactate production and acidosis, thereby promoting catecholamine function and cardiovascular homeostasis
   b. Inhibited burn wound histamine release, which leads to blocked histamine-related increases in vascular permeability, minimizing edema formation
   c. Suppressed production of thromboxane (which has been implicated as the mediator of vascular occlusion and progressive dermal ischemia after burn injury)
4. Careful assessment must be made to determine whether, for any reason, admission of the patient is warranted.
5. The burn wound must be thoroughly cleaned and débrided before ointments or dressings are applied. If not, infection may be encouraged rather than avoided.
6. Ascertain that the patient or family has the financial, mental, and physical capabilities to follow aftercare instructions. If not, other arrangements or admission is required.

EQUIPMENT

Sterile gown, mask, and gloves
Sterile basin
Sterile towels
Sterile surgical instruments, such as fine-tipped scissors and forceps (with or without teeth)
Sterile normal saline solution for irrigation, warmed to body temperature, if possible (Many institutions use warm tap water.)
Mild soap, germicidal soap, chlorhexidine, or povidone-iodine
Mineral oil or petroleum ointments (for tar removal)
Sterile gauze dressings
Sterile (soft) surgical brush
Sterile gauze bandages
Adhesive tape
Burn dressing options:

Sterile fine-mesh gauze
1% silver sulfadiazine (Silvadene)
Antibiotic ointment (Bacitracin, Polysporin)
Nonadhering dressing (Adaptic)
Transparent wound dressing (Op-Site, Tegaderm)
Biobrane
Bismuth tribromophenate (Xeroform) gauze

PATIENT PREPARATION

1. Remove jewelry from affected extremity (see Procedure 118).
2. Apply moist sterile dressing to wound as soon as possible to stop the burning process. Do not apply ice to the wound.
3. If chemicals are involved, consult the Poison Control Center before initiating wound débridement. Most chemicals require a minimum of 20 minutes of fluid irrigation; additional therapy may be necessary.
4. Administer tetanus prophylaxis as indicated.
5. Administer analgesia as prescribed.

PROCEDURAL STEPS
Wound Débridement

1. Arrange and organize on a sterile towel all supplies, instruments, and medications before initiating wound care.
2. Don a sterile gown, mask, and gloves.
3. Using sterile saline and a cleansing solution, begin to wash the injured area gently. It may be less painful to begin in the center of the burn and work toward the margin. Use sterile gauze dressings or a soft, sterile surgical brush. Maintain a circular motion, and attempt to create a moderate amount of suds or foam.
4. Rinse with sterile saline, and repeat as often as necessary until the wound is thoroughly cleaned.
5. If a blister is ruptured, débride the tissue. Initial management of intact blisters remains controversial, and research is inconclusive. Intact blisters are associated with less pain than débrided blisters (Bethel & Krisanda, 2004). Consult with the attending physician regarding the management of blisters. Blisters may be managed in several ways:
   a. The blister may be left intact, allowing underlying wounds to heal spontaneously.
   b. The blister fluid may be aspirated with a needle and syringe, leaving the overlying tissue (roof) in place.
   c. Large blisters may be débrided, whereas small ones remain intact.
6. Do not shave the affected area (Bethel & Krisanda, 2004).
7. Using fine-tipped scissors and forceps, elevate loose, devitalized tissue and remove it.
8. Remove tar with mineral oil, petroleum ointments, 2%-3% lanolin, or 1% surfactant De-Solv-It (Hartford, 1996).
9. Continue the above-listed procedures until the area is clean, moist, and pink.

Wound Dressing

Wound dressings are designed to absorb drainage, provide protection, isolate the wound from the environment, and decrease pain. Wound dressings are used to cover the topical agents applied to the burn wound. In some cases, such as the face, the topical agent may be applied in an open fashion, and no dressing is placed over the top. The other method is the closed method, in which a dressing and bandage are placed over the topical agent. The open method is easy, decreases risk of infection, and avoids difficult dressing maneuvers. However, the open method may increase discomfort and heat loss and increase cross-contamination, and it may not be practical for a working or active individual. The closed method may be more practical and comfortable, aid in débridement, and help prevent infection. However, the closed method may require ingenious application of the dressing and bandage in awkward areas (Hartford, 1996).

Silver Sulfadiazine
1. Using a sterile gloved hand or a sterile tongue blade, apply a thin ($\frac{1}{8}$-inch, or the thickness of a nickel), smooth layer of cream over the area. Fine-mesh gauze may also be impregnated with the silver sulfadiazine, which is then cut to the appropriate size and placed over the wound. This may be less painful to the patient than rubbing the cream directly on the wound.
2. If using the closed method, cover with a sterile gauze dressing and bandage. When bandaging the hand, wrap each digit individually, or place a layer of dressing between adjacent skin surfaces. Anchor as necessary.
3. Silver sulfadiazine is not recommended for use on the face (Alson, 2002). Antibiotic ointment is usually used instead.

Antibiotic Ointment
1. Apply a thin layer of ointment to the wound, and place a piece of nonadhering dressing (Adaptic) over the area.
2. Cover with a sterile gauze dressing and bandage, and anchor as necessary.

Transparent Wound Dressing or Bismuth Tribromophenate Gauze
1. Using sterile technique, apply the appropriate size of dressing directly to the burn.
2. Leave a small, $\frac{1}{2}$-inch margin that can adhere to the nonburned skin.
3. Apply a gauze pressure dressing and bandage.

Biobrane
Biobrane is a synthetic skin substitute that consists of a flexible silicone-nylon membrane and bonded collagen peptides.
1. Apply Biobrane directly over the clean wound.
2. Use surgical tape closures (Steri-Strips) or a gauze bandage to hold the Biobrane in place.

AGE-SPECIFIC CONSIDERATION
Young children and debilitated elderly patients are at risk for nonaccidental burns; carefully evaluate the history of the burn incident for the possibility of abuse. The following injuries should be viewed suspiciously: cigarette burns, circumferential burns of the extremities or the perineum suggestive of immersion (splash marks are usually absent), and burns in the shape of an object, such as an

iron. Admission may be indicated to ensure a safe environment while the circumstances surrounding the injury are investigated.

COMPLICATIONS

1. Infection
2. Loss of function
3. Damage to newly formed epithelium and slowed healing as a result of removing a dressing too vigorously
4. Localized skin irritation, itching, or rash secondary to a topical agent

PATIENT TEACHING

1. Keep bandage clean and dry. Do not wash dishes, swim, or shower.
2. Elevate burned extremities above the level of the heart for 24-48 hours after the burn.
3. If the bandage requires changing, remove it carefully and reapply. If it sticks to the skin, soak it in lukewarm water. Remove and pat dry with a clean towel.
4. Do not break any blisters.
5. Clean the area once or twice a day with warm soapy water. Reapply a thin layer of the prescribed topical agent, cream, or ointment.
6. Dress and bandage as instructed.
7. If a clear dressing or Biobrane is used, trim the edges as they loosen.
8. Return for follow-up appointments as instructed (usually within 24 hours).
9. Increase fluid and protein intake to promote healing.
10. Gently move burned extremities through their range of motion several times a day.
11. Report the following signs or symptoms:
    a. Increased pain, swelling, redness, foul odor, or red streaks from the wound
    b. Fever greater than 38.0° C (100.4° F)
    c. Numbness or swelling distal to a joint or inability to move the joint
12. To prevent hyperpigmentation and repeat injury once the burn is healed, limit exposure to the sun and use sunscreen on the area for the next 6-12 months.

REFERENCES

Alson, R. (2002). Burns, thermal. *eMedicine Journal*, March 29, 2002. Retrieved July 26, 2002. *http://www.emedicine.com/emerg/topic72.htm*

American College of Surgeons, Committee on Trauma. (1999). *Resources for optimal care of the injured patient.* Chicago, Author.

Bethel, C.A., & Krisanda, T.J. (2004). Burn care procedures (pp. 749-772). In Roberts, J.R., & Hedges, J.R. (Eds.). *Clinical procedures in emergency medicine*, 4th ed. Philadelphia: W.B. Saunders.

Hartford, C.E. (1996). Care of out-patient burns (pp. 71-81). In Herndon, D.N. (Ed.). *Total burn care.* Philadelphia: W.B. Saunders.

Russell, T.J. (2001). The management of burns (pp. 549-565). In Ferrera, P.C., et al. (Eds.). *Trauma management: an emergency medicine approach.* St. Louis: Mosby.

Escharotomy

Joni Hentzen Daniels, MSN, RN, CEN, CCRN, CFRN, CNS

Escharotomies are not commonly performed in the emergency department but may be necessary in the critically burned patient before admission or transfer. Eschar is tough and rigid tissue that forms as a result of thermal or chemical burns. As edema forms in the injured extremity after the burn, the eschar restricts outward expansion of the tissue. The outcome is increased interstitial pressure that rises to the point that vascular flow is compromised (Alson, 2002). In short, the eschar behaves like a tourniquet. Incising the eschar allows return of flow and prevents further ischemic injury.

INDICATIONS
To decrease elevated intrathoracic or tissue pressure in the presence of:
1. Circumferential full-thickness burns to the chest, which mechanically constrict and compromise respirations.
2. Circumferential or electrical burns to the extremities causing loss of distal pulses, impaired capillary filling, paresthesias or motor weakness, cyanosis of distal uninjured skin, or tense edema with rigid muscle compartments (Edlich et al., 2002; Bethel & Krisanda, 2004) (Figure 148-1).
3. Loss of Doppler pulses (see Procedure 52) in the radial and ulnar arteries and digital vessels are indications for escharotomies of the upper extremity (Wald, 1998). Loss of dorsalis pedis or posterior tibialis artery signals indicates the need for escharotomy of the lower extremity (Wald, 1998).
4. Tissue pressure exceeding 30 mm Hg, which indicates a need for escharotomy or fasciotomy (Bethel & Krisanda, 2004) (see Procedure 133).

CONTRAINDICATIONS AND CAUTIONS
1. Failure to perform emergency escharotomy may result in the inability to ventilate lung parenchyma, loss of neuromuscular function, or ischemic tissue injury (Edlich et al., 2002).
2. This procedure may cause significant blood loss in the patient already predisposed to hypovolemic shock or altered coagulation.
3. These new open wounds further predispose the patient to infection and sepsis.
4. Underlying tissues may be damaged if procedures are incorrectly performed.
5. If compartmental pressures do not decrease after escharotomy, a fasciotomy must be performed in the operating room.
6. Improper technique or locations of the incisions may damage nerves (Bethel & Krisanda, 2004).
7. Prophylactic antibiotics are strongly discouraged to prevent the development of resistant bacterial strain (Lingnau et al., 1996).

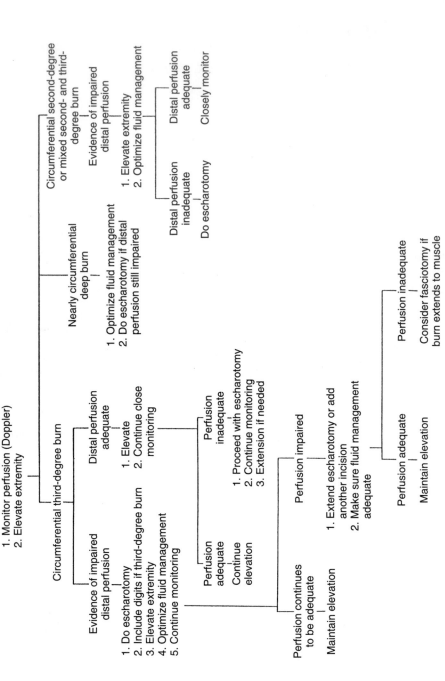

FIGURE 148-1 Algorithm for escharotomies of extremity burns. (From Demling, R.F., & Lalonde, C. [1989]. *Burn trauma* [p. 63]. New York: Thieme Medical Publishers.)

EQUIPMENT

Sterile gown, mask, and gloves for all team members
Local anesthetic infiltration (optional in deep, insensate burns)
Intracompartmental pressure monitor (may not be used in emergency
    situations)
Doppler to assess pulses
Sterile drapes
Sterile scalpel (coagulating or cutting device may be preferable)
Cautery, thrombin, hemostats
Sterile dressing and bandages
Antimicrobial creams

PATIENT PREPARATION

1. Remove all constricting clothing and jewelry (see Procedure 118).
2. Elevate the burned extremity slightly above the level of the heart.
3. Administer analgesics and sedatives as prescribed.
4. Administer tetanus prophylaxis as indicated.
5. Place the patient in a supine anatomic position, unless contraindicated by other injuries or conditions.

PROCEDURAL STEPS

1. Drape below and around the surgical area.
2. *Anesthetize with local anesthetic infiltration or regional nerve block (see Procedures 138 and 139).
3. *Incise indicated areas:
   a. *Chest:* Along the anterior axillary aspects of the chest extending from the clavicle to the costal margin (Figure 148-2). Make a second incision transverse across the chest at the level of the diaphragm. Cut through the eschar but not into the subcutaneous tissue (Bethel & Krisanda, 2004; Mlcak, 1996). The incision should cause the eschar to gap, thus releasing pressure.
   b. *Neck:* Posteriorly and laterally to avoid major vessels in the neck.
   c. *Upper extremities:* Medial and lateral aspects of arms avoiding the radial nerve (Figures 148-3 and 148-4).
   d. *Hands:* Dorsal aspect of the hands and along the palmar crease (Figure 148-4) and medial and lateral aspects of the digits (Figure 148-5).

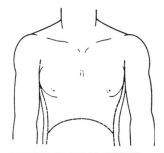

FIGURE 148-2 Chest escharotomy sites. (From Mlcak, R.P., & Buffalo, M.C. [2002]. Pre-hospital management, transportation and emergency care [p. 69]. In Herndon, D.N. (Ed.). *Total burn care.* Philadelphia: W.B. Saunders.)

---

*Indicates portions of the procedure usually performed by a physician or an advanced practice nurse.

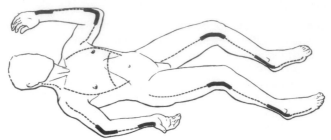

FIGURE 148-3 Extremity escharotomy sites. (From Davis, J.H., Foster, R.S., Drucker, W.K. [1995]. *Surgery: A problem-solving approach*, 2nd ed. [p. 651]. St. Louis: Mosby.)

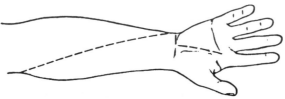

FIGURE 148-4 Arm and hand escharotomy sites. (From Edlich, R.F., Bailey, R.F., & Bill, T.J. [2002]. Thermal burns [p. 810]. In Marx, J.A., Hockberger, R.S., Walls, R.M. et al. (Eds.). *Rosen's emergency medicine: concepts and clinical practice,* 5th ed. St. Louis: Mosby.)

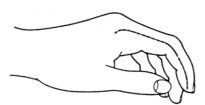

FIGURE 148-5 Escharotomy on a finger. (From Mlcak, R.P., & Buffalo, M.C. [2002]. Pre-hospital management, transportation and emergency care [p. 69]. In Herndon, D.N. [Ed.]. *Total burn care.* Philadelphia: W.B. Saunders.)

    e. *Legs:* Midmedial and midlateral incisions; toes in a similar manner to the fingers (Figure 148-3).
4. Reassess respiratory function and distal circulatory status.
5. *Apply direct pressure, cautery, clamps, or thrombin to all bleeding areas.
6. Reassess hematocrit, and consider blood administration if necessary.
7. Apply dressings impregnated with antimicrobial creams (e.g., silver sulfadiazine) to reduce the potential for infection (Hartford, 1996). See Procedure 147 for dressing technique.
8. Keep the affected extremities elevated, and monitor distal pulses frequently for 48 hours (Mlcak, 1996).

---

*Indicates portions of the procedure usually performed by a physician or an advanced practice nurse.

COMPLICATIONS
1. Wound infection
2. Sepsis
3. Blood loss
4. Nerve or vessel damage
5. Inadequate decompression may lead to tissue necrosis, myoglobinuria, renal failure, hyperkalemia, and acidosis (Bethel & Krisanda, 2004).

PATIENT TEACHING
1. This procedure will decrease the pain as it relieves the tissue pressure.
2. Care will be taken to help these wounds heal with as little scarring as possible.

REFERENCES
Alson, R. (2002). Burns, thermal. *eMedicine Journal*, March 29, 2002. Retrieved July 26, 2002. *http://www.emedicine.com/emerg/topic72.htm*

Bethel, C.A., & Krisanda, T.J. (2004). Burn care procedures (pp. 749-772). In Roberts, J.R., & Hedges, J.R. (Eds.). *Clinical procedures in emergency medicine*, 4th ed. Philadelphia: W.B. Saunders.

Edlich, R.F., Bailey, R.F., & Bill, T.J. [2002]. Thermal burns (pp. 801-813). In Marx, J.A., Hockberger, R.S., Walls, R.M., et al. (Eds.). *Rosen's emergency medicine: concepts and clinical practice*, 5th ed. St. Louis: Mosby.

Hartford, C.E. (1996). Care of out-patient burns (pp. 71-80). In Herndon, D.N. (Ed.). *Total burn care*. Philadelphia: W.B. Saunders.

Lingnan, W.W., et al. (1996). Anesthesia for burned patients (pp. 148-158). In Herndon, D.N. (Ed.). *Total burn care*. Philadelphia: W.B. Saunders.

Mlcak, R.P., Dimick, A.R., & Mlcak, G. (1996). Pre-hospital management, transportation and emergency care (pp. 33-43). In Herndon, D.N. (Ed.). *Total burn care*. Philadelphia: W.B. Saunders.

Wald, D.A. (1998). Burn management: systematic patient evaluation, fluid resuscitation and wound management. *Emergency Medicine Reports*, *19*, 45-52.

PROCEDURE 149

Incision and Drainage

Margo E. Layman, MSN, RN, RNC, CN-A

Incision and drainage is also known as I & D.

INDICATIONS
1. To drain localized infections, such as sebaceous cysts, subungual abscesses, and carbuncles.
2. To remove foreign objects from soft tissue.

CONTRAINDICATIONS AND CAUTIONS

1. Patients with poor hygiene, malnutrition, diabetes, and immune deficiencies require careful techniques and follow-up.
2. Patients with bleeding disorders should be referred to a surgeon.
3. Consultation with a specialist should be considered for deep or anatomically complex abscesses and those on the hands, feet, or face.
4. Abscesses in some areas are close to major vessels and should be aspirated with a needle and syringe to rule out mycotic aneurysm before any attempt at I & D. The high-risk body areas for this are (Simon and Brenner, 2002):

Peritonsillar and retropharyngeal region

Anterior triangle of the neck (bordered by the sternocleidomastoid muscle, the mandible, and the anterior midline of the neck.)

Supraclavicular fossa

Deep axilla

Antecubital space

Groin

Popliteal space

EQUIPMENT

Antiseptic solution

Local anesthetic

Syringes and needles for local anesthetic

$\frac{1}{4}$- or $\frac{1}{2}$-inch iodoform or plain sterile gauze packing

4 × 4-inch gauze dressings

Adhesive tape

Hydrogen peroxide (optional)

No. 11 scalpel

Hemostat (curved or straight)

Plain forceps

Surgical scissors

Cotton swabs

Culture collection supplies for aerobic and anaerobic specimens

PATIENT PREPARATION

1. Drape the area with waterproof drapes.
2. Clip the hair or shave the area as indicated.
3. Cleanse the area with antiseptic solution with firm, circular scrubbing motions from the abscess outward.
4. *Anesthetize the area with local anesthetic (see Procedure 138). Intravenous analgesia and sedation may be necessary for large or deep abscesses (see Procedure 181).

PROCEDURAL STEPS

1. *Incise the periphery of the abscess cavity with the scalpel; purulent material is expressed immediately (Figure 149-1).

---

*Indicates portions of the procedure usually performed by a physician or an advanced practice nurse.

2. *Disrupt adhesions with a hemostat.
3. Obtain anaerobic and aerobic cultures from the drainage.
4. Cleanse the cavity with cotton swabs and then irrigate with sterile saline solution (see Procedure 137).
5. *Pack the wound loosely with plain or iodoform gauze strip leaving 1 cm of gauze exiting from the cavity. This packing keeps the wound open and permits drainage (Figure 149-2).
6. Apply a sterile dressing, and secure with adhesive tape.

AGE-SPECIFIC CONSIDERATIONS
Children may require sedation in addition to local anesthesia (see Procedure 181).

COMPLICATIONS
1. Reoccurrence of the abscess
2. Spread of the infection, especially in the perineal and rectal areas
3. Systemic infection or sepsis
4. Injury to nearby vessels or nerves

PATIENT TEACHING
1. Leave dressing in place for 24 hours, unless it becomes soiled with excessive drainage; then it can be changed.
2. In 24 hours, remove the external dressing, and leave the packing in place.

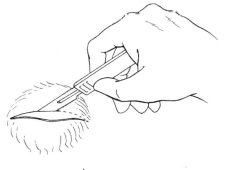

FIGURE 149-1 Incision of an abscess. (From Rosen, P., & Sternbach, G.L. [1983]. *Atlas of emergency medicine,* 2nd ed. [p. 185]. Baltimore: Williams & Wilkins.)

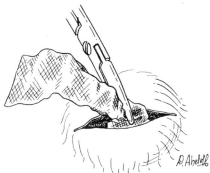

FIGURE 149-2 Gauze packing is packed loosely into the incised wound using a hemostat. (From Rosen, P., & Sternbach, G.L. [1983]. *Atlas of emergency medicine,* 2nd ed. [p. 185]. Baltimore: Williams & Wilkins.)

*Indicates portions of the procedure usually performed by a physician or an advanced practice nurse.

3. Follow-up with the physician in 2 days to have packing removed.
4. After packing is removed, soak the site 20-30 minutes in warm water three to four times a day.
5. Continue to soak for 5-7 days or until the incision has healed. Redress the incision with a clean dressing after each soaking.
6. Watch for signs of ongoing or worsening infection, such as redness, swelling, draining pus, and fever.

REFERENCE

Simon, R.R., & Brenner, B.E. (2002). *Emergency procedures & techniques*, 4th ed. Philadelphia: Lippincott Williams & Wilkins.

Thermoregulation

Measures to Reverse Hyperthermia

Daun A. Smith, RN, MS, CEN
and Jean A. Proehl, RN, MN, CEN, CCRN

INDICATION

To lower body temperature to 39° C (102° F) or less through rapid cooling in patients whose temperatures are greater than 40.5° C (105° F). Hyperthermia may result from fever, heatstroke, metabolic disorders, thermoregulatory dysfunction, or medications (e.g., malignant hyperthermia). The best treatment is prevention—providing proper clothing, administering fluid and salt replacement, or moving to a cool, shady environment.

CONTRAINDICATIONS AND CAUTIONS

1. Cooling must be initiated immediately on the discovery of a hyperthermic state and must proceed rapidly. For a successful outcome, temperatures must be decreased to 39° C (102° F) or below within 1 hour of initiating treatment.
2. Antipyretics are ineffective in lowering the body temperature and may result in additional complications, such as coagulopathy and hepatic damage (Yarbrough & Vicario, 2002).
3. Initial diagnosis is often difficult. Early symptoms of significant heat illness are usually nonspecific (drowsiness, confusion, headache) and may be overlooked or attributed to other causes (Yarbrough & Vicario, 2002).
4. Do not sponge the patient with alcohol because it may be absorbed transcutaneously with resultant toxicity (Yarbrough & Vicario, 2002).

EQUIPMENT

Ice packs
Ice water
Large circulating fans
Bathtub or wash basin
Cooling blanket
Peritoneal lavage equipment
Temperature probe for continuous monitoring (rectal, bladder, or esophageal)
Cooled intravenous fluids (place the bags in an ice water slurry for 15-20 minutes)

PATIENT PREPARATION

1. Place the patient on high-flow oxygen because oxygen demand is increased in the hyperthermic state.

2. Initiate an intravenous line to restore intravascular volume (see Procedure 63).
3. Initiate additional resuscitative efforts as indicated.
4. Place the patient on a cardiac monitor because nonspecific ST-segment changes, conduction disturbances, and ventricular arrhythmias have been reported during cooling (see Procedure 58).
5. Draw blood for complete blood count, potassium, sodium, phosphorus, calcium, magnesium, prothrombin time and partial thromboplastin time, blood urea nitrogen, glucose, creatinine, liver function tests, and creatine phosphokinase determinations (see Procedure 61).
6. Remove all clothing.
7. Establish continuous temperature monitoring. Urinary bladder, rectal, or esophageal probes are options. Check the rectum for stool before placement of a rectal probe; if the probe is placed in feces, the reading is inaccurate.
8. Obtain a baseline 12-lead electrocardiogram (see Procedure 59).
9. Insert a urinary bladder catheter to monitor fluid output (see Procedure 107).

PROCEDURAL STEPS
A variety of modalities may be used for rapid cooling, depending on the patient's condition, the availability of resources, and the institutional protocols. The most effective are evaporative cooling or immersion in ice water (Yarbrough & Vicario, 2002). Options include the following:
1. Evaporative cooling. Cover the patient with wet towels or spray the patient with water while circulating air around the patient with large fans to promote heat loss through evaporation. The latter method is preferred because of rapid heat loss, availability of supplies, and easy access to the patient.
2. Immersion in ice water is effective but logistically more difficult. Sponging the patient with ice water may be tried initially. If initial cooling efforts are not rapidly effective, ice water immersion should be undertaken.
3. Cover the patient with a cooling blanket (controversial and slow).
4. Apply ice packs to the neck, axilla, and inguinal area. Monitor the underlying skin for cold injury. This method is less effective than immersion in ice water.
5. Administer dantrolene as prescribed for malignant hyperthermia. Dantrolene is not effective in environmental hyperthermia.
6. Internal methods of cooling may be necessary in the patient with severe hyperthermia or who does not respond to external methods. Internal methods include cold peritoneal lavage (see Procedure 98) and cardiopulmonary bypass (Yarbrough & Vicario, 2002).
7. Stop cooling at $39°$ C ($102.2°$ F) because the body temperature continues to drift downward, and hypothermia may result if cooling measures are continued beyond this point.

AGE-SPECIFIC CONSIDERATIONS
1. Both the elderly and the very young are at risk for classic hyperthermia because of decreased thermoregulatory functioning. The elderly have a relative inability to adapt to environmental temperatures, a decreased ability to perspire, and other chronic medical conditions that affect their ability to acclimate to warmer temperatures; the very young have a shorter stature, placing them closer to radiated heat from asphalt or cement; have fewer sweat glands; and are more easily dehydrated.

2. Young adults (e.g., athletes, outdoor laborers, military personnel) are at risk for exertional hyperthermia.

COMPLICATIONS

1. Violent shivering with rapid cooling, which may result in further heat production. This can be controlled with chlorpromazine (Yarbrough & Vicario, 2002).
2. Hypotension
3. Acute renal failure
4. Metabolic acidosis
5. Increased serum potassium
6. Frostbite caused by ice packs
7. Rhabdomyolysis in severe exertional hyperthermia
8. Disseminated intravascular coagulation
9. Hypothermia from overly vigorous cooling

PATIENT TEACHING

Patients who have experienced hyperthermic episodes are predisposed to future recurrences. Instruct the patient on prevention strategies, as indicated by the cause of this episode (e.g., the importance of staying in a cool environment, drinking lots of fluids, and avoiding extreme exertion during the hottest times of the day or in extreme weather).

REFERENCE

Yarbrough, B., & Vicario, S. (2002). In Marx, J.A., Hockberger, R.S., Walls, R.M., et al. (Eds.). *Rosen's emergency medicine: concepts and clinical practice*, 5th ed. (pp. 1997-2009). St. Louis: Mosby.

PROCEDURE 151

Measures to Reverse Hypothermia

Daun A. Smith, RN, MS, CEN
and Jean A. Proehl, RN, MN, CEN, CCRN

INDICATION

To increase the core temperature in patients with temperatures less than 35° C (95° F) because of a decrease in heat production, an increase in heat loss, a combination of both, or an impaired thermoregulatory system. Rewarming should continue until the patient's core temperature is 35° C (95° F) (AHA/ILCOR, 2000).

CONTRAINDICATIONS AND CAUTIONS

1. Hypothermia creates myocardial irritability, so patients must be handled gently and procedures performed cautiously because stimulation may precipitate ventricular fibrillation. The risk is highest at temperatures below 29° C (85.2° F) (Danzl, 2002).
2. With active external rewarming, patients may experience rewarming shock, which is evidenced by a decrease in blood pressure resulting from vasodilation in previously vasoconstricted extremities.
3. With active external rewarming, patients may experience a temperature afterdrop, which results from the shunting of cold blood from extremities to the core, which further chills the myocardium and increases the potential for ventricular fibrillation.
4. Medications must be used judiciously because most drugs have little effect on the hypothermic patient and may cause complications on rewarming because of delayed metabolism of drugs (e.g., metabolic alkalosis with sodium bicarbonate, hypoglycemia with insulin).
5. Skin should not be massaged or rubbed, and alcohol should not be used on the skin of hypothermic patients; these techniques increase vasodilation and move cold blood from the extremities to the core.
6. Attempts at defibrillation are usually unsuccessful until core temperature is above 28°-30° C (82°-86° F).

EQUIPMENT

Cardiac monitor
Pulse oximeter
Warm intravenous (IV) solution (37.7° C) (100° F)
IV fluid warmers
IV tubing
Warm normal saline for irrigation
Radiant warming lights
Heating pads
Hot water bottles
Forced air warming blanket
Cascade nebulizer or similar equipment to administer heated, humidified oxygen
Peritoneal lavage equipment
Foley catheter
Hemodialysis equipment
Cardiac bypass equipment
Gastric lavage equipment
Pleural lavage equipment
Hypothermia thermometer (capability to measure temperatures <34.4° C (94° F)

PATIENT PREPARATION

1. Initiate resuscitation as indicated for the patient in cardiac arrest. Endotracheal intubation is necessary unless the patient is alert and has intact protective airway reflexes. Preoxygenate the patient before intubation to avoid dysrhythmias. Factors precipitating dysrhythmias during intubation are rough technique, hypoxia, and acid-base abnormalities (Danzl, 2002).
2. Establish continuous temperature monitoring. Urinary bladder, rectal, or esophageal probes are options. Check the rectum for stool before placement of a rectal probe; if the probe is placed in feces, the reading is inaccurate.
3. Apply the cardiac monitor for ongoing assessment during the rewarming procedures (see Procedure 58).
4. Obtain a baseline 12-lead electrocardiogram (see Procedure 59).
5. Perform a bedside blood glucose test (see Procedure 62). Obtain blood for complete blood count, arterial blood gases (uncorrected for temperature), potassium, glucose, calcium, magnesium, prothrombin time and partial thromboplastin time, fibrinogen, fibrin split products, amylase, lipase, blood urea nitrogen, and creatinine determinations (see Procedure 61).

PROCEDURAL STEPS

There are three methods of rewarming: Passive external rewarming (PER), active external rewarming (AER), and active core rewarming (ACR). The recommended rewarming methods are as follows (AHA/ILCOR, 2000):

Mild hypothermia	34°-36° C (93.2°-96.8° F)	PER, AER
Moderate hypothermia	30°-34° C (86°-93.2° F)	PER, AER (truncal areas only)
Severe hypothermia	<30° C (86° F)	ACR

Passive External Rewarming

1. Remove the patient from the cold or wet environment. Remove all clothing, dry the patient, and place the patient on a stretcher covered with sheets or blankets to prevent heat loss via conduction. Long hair should be dried or positioned away from the patient's head.
2. Cover the patient with blankets to prevent heat loss from radiation and convection. Be sure to cover the head because a significant amount of heat is lost from an uncovered head.
3. If IV fluids are indicated, they should be warmed before administration to assist with rewarming and prevent further heat loss.

Active External Rewarming

The current recommendation is to heat only the thorax during AER of the moderately hypothermic patient and leave the extremities unheated to allow for the maintenance of peripheral vasoconstriction, thus preventing temperature afterdrop and rewarming shock (Danzl, 2002).

1. Cover the patient with warm, electric blankets or a forced air warming blanket (see Procedures 154 and 155).
2. Place heated objects (e.g., heating pads, hot water bottles) in the groin or axilla or on the trunk.
3. Use overhead radiant warming lights (see Procedure 153).

Active Core Rewarming

1. Infuse IV fluid warmed to 37.7°-43° C (100°-109° F) (see Procedure 77) (AHA/ILCOR, 2000). Warmed IV fluid alone is not enough to rewarm the patient; it must be used in conjunction with other therapies.
2. Administer warm, humidified oxygen via a cascade nebulizer or similar device. Warmed oxygen alone is not enough to rewarm the patient; it must be used in conjunction with other therapies.
3. Perform peritoneal lavage with fluid warmed to 40°-45° C (105°-113° F) to conduct heat directly through the intraperitoneal structures, posterior parietal peritoneum to the kidneys, and diaphragm to the heart and lungs. Two catheters may be inserted to allow concomitant infusion and drainage (see Procedure 98). Two liters are infused, allowed to dwell for 20-30 minutes, and then drained. Peritoneal dialysis exacerbates hypokalemia, and potassium supplementation of the dialysis fluid may be necessary (Danzl, 2002).
4. Initiate extracorporeal blood warming via continuous arteriovenous rewarming with a Level One fluid warmer (see Procedure 156) or cardiac bypass equipment in the operating room.
5. Perform warmed mediastinal or pleural irrigation via thoracotomy (usually performed in the operating room) (see Procedure 57).
6. Initiate hemodialysis with 40°-45° C (104°-113° F) fluid.
7. Perform warmed lavage of the stomach or rectum (see Procedure 98). Both of these techniques result in limited heat gain because the surface area in contact with the fluid is minimal (Danzl, 2002). In addition, there is a risk of electrolyte imbalance and aspiration with gastric lavage.

AGE-SPECIFIC CONSIDERATIONS

1. Infants are particularly susceptible to the development of hypothermia because of their lack of subcutaneous fat and larger body surface area to mass ratio, which allows for greater heat loss, and because they are less able to regulate and generate their own heat.
2. Elderly individuals have a lower metabolic rate and reduced muscle mass and subcutaneous tissue and have difficulty maintaining a normal body temperature when ambient temperatures fall. The aging process also lowers the ability to sense temperature changes; therefore older individuals may not be aware of the need for countermeasures (i.e., warmer clothing, shelter).

COMPLICATIONS

1. Ventricular fibrillation from rough handling or stimulation associated with procedures
2. Rewarming shock and afterdrop associated with active external rewarming in severely hypothermic patients
3. Burns as a result of heating devices in direct contact with the skin (which is poorly perfused in hypothermia)
4. Complications of hypothermia include coagulopathies, pneumonia, pulmonary edema, thrombosis, decreased peripheral perfusion, and tissue ischemia.

PATIENT TEACHING

Patients who have experienced accidental hypothermia need to learn how to prevent future episodes: recognition of early symptoms (shivering, lethargy, confusion, loss of coordination), appropriate clothing for the environment (including the importance of wearing a hat), and the dangerous effects of alcohol and other intoxicants.

REFERENCES

American Heart Association/International Liaison Committee on Resuscitation (AHA/ILCOR) (2000). Guidelines 2000 for cardiopulmonary resuscitation and emergency cardiovascular care: an international consensus on science. *Circulation, 102*, I229-I251.

Danzl, D.F. (2002). Accidental hypothermia (pp. 1979-1996). In Marx, J.A., Hockberger, R.S., Walls, R.M., et al. (Eds.). *Rosen's emergency medicine: concepts and clinical practice*, 5th ed. St. Louis: Mosby.

PROCEDURE 152

Heat Shield

Daun A. Smith, RN, MS, CEN

INDICATIONS

1. To minimize heat dissipation through convection, conduction, and evaporation. Use of a heat shield combines active and passive rewarming techniques that may be especially useful when other sources of rewarming may not be appropriate.
2. Heat shields may be used on burn patients who cannot tolerate insulative material directly on the skin or on patients exposed to chemicals or chemotherapy resulting in skin sloughing.
3. See Procedure 151 for further information on management of hypothermia.

CONTRAINDICATIONS AND CAUTIONS

Frequent temperature assessment is necessary to identify advancing hypothermia or hyperthermia that adversely affects oxygen consumption and metabolic function.

EQUIPMENT

Heat shield

PROCEDURAL STEPS

1. Remove wet or heavy clothing from the patient.
2. Place a light blanket or sheet over the patient (if appropriate).

3. Place the heat shield over the patient, allowing enough space for continued patient assessment and intervention.

AGE-SPECIFIC CONSIDERATION

Heat shields may be used with any age-group and are often effective with pediatric patients.

PATIENT TEACHING

Explain to the patient the effect of the heat shield in reducing heat loss. Explain that when the air is stationary, less heat is lost to conduction, convection, and radiation.

Heat Lamp

Daun A. Smith, RN, MS, CEN

INDICATIONS

1. To provide direct transfer of exogenous heat (active external rewarming) to a patient who is hypothermic. See Procedure 151 for further information on management of hypothermia.
2. To maintain body temperature and prevent hypothermia in patients undergoing resuscitation who are at high risk for hypothermia.

CONTRAINDICATIONS AND CAUTIONS

1. Frequent temperature assessment is necessary to identify hypothermia or hyperthermia that adversely affects oxygen consumption and metabolic function.
2. Caution must be exercised to avoid thermal burns to poorly perfused and vasoconstricted skin when using heat lamps.
3. External rewarming measures (e.g., heat lamps, warmed blankets, forced warm air units, water bottles) should be used in conjunction with active core rewarming measures (e.g., peritoneal lavage, warm intravenous fluids) to help prevent afterdrop and rewarming shock in patients with core temperatures less than 30° C (86° F) (Danzl, 2002).

EQUIPMENT

Heat lamp
Light sheet or blanket
Yardstick

PATIENT PREPARATION

1. Remove any wet, frozen, or heavy clothing from the patient. Cover the patient with a light sheet or blanket for privacy.
2. Initiate cardiac monitoring because hypothermia may lower the threshold for dysrhythmias including ventricular fibrillation (see Procedure 58).

PROCEDURAL STEPS

1. Place the heat lamp over the thorax. If the heat lamp is focused only on the extremities, active external rewarming is not as effective.
2. Place the heat lamp at least 3 ft from the patient to avoid burns and skin irritation.
3. Duration of patient exposure to the heat lamp should be kept to a maximum of 5-minute intervals to avoid burns and skin irritation. Many lamps have a timer for this purpose.

AGE-SPECIFIC CONSIDERATIONS

1. Tables with thermostatically controlled overhead warming units are available for temperature resuscitation of the neonate.
2. Neonates, infants, and small children are at risk for iatrogenic hypothermia during resuscitative efforts; a heat lamp may be used prophylactically in these circumstances.

COMPLICATIONS

1. Temperature afterdrop (decreased core temperature when cold blood returns from the extremities)
2. Shock resulting from peripheral vasodilation with active external rewarming
3. Burns or skin irritation

PATIENT TEACHING

Patients who have experienced accidental hypothermia need to learn how to prevent future episodes: recognition of early symptoms (shivering, lethargy, confusion, loss of coordination), appropriate clothing for the environment (including the importance of wearing a hat), and the dangerous effects of alcohol and other intoxicants.

REFERENCE

Danzl, D.F. (2002). Accidental hypothermia (pp. 1979-1996). In Marx, J.A., Hockberger, R.S., Walls, R.M., et al. (Eds.). *Rosen's emergency medicine: concepts and clinical practice*, 5th ed. St. Louis: Mosby.

Forced Air Warming Blanket

Daun A. Smith, RN, MS, CEN

A forced air warming blanket is also known as a Bair Hugger.

INDICATION

To accomplish active external rewarming by passing heated air across the skin. Forced air rewarming has been shown to be the most effective method of active external rewarming (Giesbrecht et al., 1994; Giuffre et al., 1994; Krenzischak et al., 1995; Pathi et al., 1996). See Procedure 151 for further information on management of hypothermia.

CONTRAINDICATIONS AND CAUTIONS

1. The patient's temperature should be monitored continuously or at least every 10-20 minutes.
2. When desired temperature goal is reached (37° C [98.6° F]), air temperature should be reduced or use of the warming blanket discontinued.
3. Patients with poor perfusion should be monitored closely during prolonged warming therapy because thermal injury may occur if heat is applied to poorly perfused areas. High temperatures should be avoided in this setting.
4. Active external rewarming is not recommended for severely hypothermic patients. See Procedure 151 for alternative warming methods.

EQUIPMENT

Bath blanket
Forced air warming unit
Forced air warming blanket

PATIENT PREPARATION

Remove all clothing, sheets, and blankets from the top of the patient.

PROCEDURAL STEPS

1. Place the blanket with the perforated side toward the patient.
2. Insert the end of the hose of the forced air warming unit into the opening for the hose on the blanket, using a twisting motion to seat it securely (Figure 154-1).
3. Plug in the warming unit to a properly grounded power source.
4. Press the on button and select the appropriate temperature setting.
5. Place a bath blanket over the warming blanket to prevent warm air from escaping (Figure 154-2).
6. Assess the skin regularly for any sign of thermal injury.

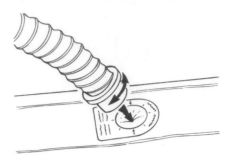

FIGURE 154-1 Insert the hose from the warming unit into the warming blanket. (Courtesy Mallinckrodt Medical Inc., Critical Care Division [1997], St. Louis, MO.)

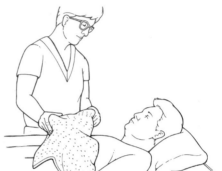

FIGURE 154-2 Cover the warming blanket with a bath blanket. (Courtesy Mallinckrodt Medical Inc., Critical Care Division [1997], St. Louis, MO.)

AGE-SPECIFIC CONSIDERATION

Do not leave infants or small children unattended while a warming blanket is in use because of the risk of suffocation.

COMPLICATIONS

1. Thermal burns
2. Hyperthermia
3. Rewarming shock or temperature afterdrop secondary to peripheral vasodilation (in severely hypothermic patients)

PATIENT TEACHING

1. Recognize early signs of hypothermia (lethargy, incoordination, confusion).
2. Wear adequate clothing for the weather.
3. Drugs and intoxicants predispose to heat loss by vasodilation and a decreased perception of cold.

REFERENCES

Giesbrecht, G.G., Ducharme, M.B., & McGuire, J.P. (1994). Comparison of forced air patient warming systems for perioperative use. *Anesthesiology, 80,* 671-679.

Giuffre, M., Heidenreich, T., & Pruitt, L. (1994). Rewarming cardiac surgery patients: radiant heat versus forced warm air. *Nursing Research, 43,* 174-178.

Krenzischak, D.A., Frank, S.M., & Kelly, S. (1995). Forced-air warming versus routine thermal care and core temperature measurement sites. *Journal of Postanesthesia Nursing, 10,* 69-78.

Pathi, V., Berg, G.A., Morrison, J., et al. (1996). The benefits of active rewarming after cardiac operations: a randomized prospective trial. *Journal of Thoracic and Cardiovascular Surgery, 111,* 637-641.

Warm Water–Circulating Blankets

Daun A. Smith, RN, MS, CEN

INDICATION

Warm water–circulating blankets are a method of active external rewarming for patients with hypothermia. Water is heated and pumped through coils in waterproof rubber or plastic mats that are placed under and/or over the patient. See Procedure 151 for further information about the management of hypothermia.

CONTRAINDICATIONS AND CAUTIONS

1. A physician's prescription is necessary for use of the blanket.
2. Do not place any other heating sources between the patient and the warm water–circulating blanket.
3. Prevent prolonged or excessive tissue pressure, especially over bony prominences, to prevent injury to hypothermic, poorly perfused skin.
4. The area between the patient and the blanket should be kept dry.

EQUIPMENT

Warming unit/console with blanket(s)
Sheets or bath blankets
Equipment to monitor temperature (rectal, skin, or esophageal probe for continuous monitoring is preferred)

PATIENT PREPARATION

1. Obtain baseline assessments of vital signs, level of consciousness, skin integrity and color, and initiate cardiac monitoring (see Procedure 58).
2. Moisturizing cream may be applied to the exposed skin.
3. Position the temperature probe (rectal, skin, or esophageal) per manufacturer's instructions if automatic mode will be used (see No. 6 below).

PROCEDURAL STEPS

1. Check blanket and tubing for leaks or kinks.
2. Check water level in the warming console. Add sterile or distilled water if necessary.
3. Place one warming blanket under the patient with a bath blanket or sheet between the patient and the warming blanket. The tubing should be positioned toward the warming console.
4. Cover the patient with a bath blanket or sheet and a second warming blanket (if prescribed).
5. Connect the blanket tubing to the warming console and turn it on.

685

6. Choose manual or automatic mode. Temperature choice is governed by the mode chosen. In the manual mode, the selected temperature regulates the warmth of the blanket. In automatic mode, the selected temperature is the desired patient temperature. Do not use a temperature probe when using the manual mode. In automatic mode, a temperature probe is required (Kelly, 2001).
7. Cover the patient's head with a warm towel or blanket to prevent heat loss.
8. Assess vital signs, cardiac rhythm, and level of consciousness frequently (every 15-30 minutes or more often, as indicated by the patient's condition).
9. Turn the patient for skin assessment and care hourly (Kelly, 2001).

AGE-SPECIFIC CONSIDERATIONS
1. Young children and the elderly may have impaired thermoregulation and should be monitored closely during rewarming.
2. These devices are somewhat heavy and may impede respiratory effort when placed on the chest/abdomen of an infant or small child.
3. The elderly are at increased risk for skin breakdown.

COMPLICATIONS
1. Inability to rewarm the patient to the desired temperature
2. Skin breakdown
3. Hemodynamic instability and cardiac arrhythmias related to hypothermia

REFERENCE
Kelly, E.M. (2001). External warming/cooling devices (pp. 591-597). In Lynn-McHale, D.J., & Carlson, K.K. (Eds.). *AACN procedure manual for critical care*, 4th ed. Philadelphia: W.B. Saunders.

PROCEDURE 156

Continuous Arteriovenous Rewarming

Daun A. Smith, RN, MS, CEN

Continuous arteriovenous rewarming (CAVR) is a method of active internal rewarming. CAVR is similar to cardiopulmonary bypass in that it reinfuses warmed blood to the central circulation, thereby decreasing the risk of rewarming arrhythmias. However, CAVR does not require a bypass pump or heparinization (Gentilello and Rifley, 1991). CAVR is accomplished by establishing a closed system in which blood flows from one of the patient's femoral arteries through an 8.5-Fr arterial catheter into a specially designed tubing, through the Level 1 fluid warmer (Level 1, Rockland, MA) and back into the patient's opposite femoral vein via another 8.5-Fr catheter. CAVR can return a patient's temperature to 36° C in 39-180 minutes (Schulman and Pierce, 1999). See Procedure 151 for additional information about the management of hypothermia.

INDICATION

1. To rewarm hypothermic patients with a core body temperature of 30° C (86° F) or less and a systolic blood pressure greater than 60-80 mm Hg. A blood pressure of 60 mm Hg systolic is necessary to push blood through the system at a rate of 150 ml/min, which will keep the system open (Level 1 Inc.). However, other sources recommend a blood pressure of at least 80 mm Hg (Andreoni and Massey, 2001; Schulman, 2001; Schulman and Pierce, 1999).
2. To rewarm hypothermic patients and reverse hypothermia-induced coagulopathies.

CONTRAINDICATIONS AND CAUTIONS

1. Profound hypotension. It may be possible to maintain an adequate systolic blood pressure with intravenous (IV) fluids, blood products, or vasopressors.
2. CAVR is contraindicated in patients less than 90 lb (41 kg) because of the possibility that the large femoral catheter may occlude the vessels in a smaller person (Schulman and Pierce, 1999).
3. CAVR should not be used in the presence of femoral occlusive disease or compartment syndrome of the lower extremities because the large catheters could impede circulation to and from the legs.
4. Patients requiring CAVR should have constant hemodynamic and temperature monitoring (Schulman and Pierce, 1999).
5. Remove all air from fluid bags and tubing before connecting them to the patient.
6. Use only the catheters provided in the rewarming kit. Other central catheters may be too small to sustain the flow rates needed (Schulman, 2001; Schulman and Pierce, 1999).
7. The maximum time for rewarming with CAVR is 3 hours to prevent clotting in the tubing (Level 1 Inc.).
8. Do not connect the Level 1 fluid warmer to the patient until the temperature of the device is at least 41° C (Schulman, 2001).
9. Do not add extensions, stopcocks, or other restrictive components to the tubing assembly because these may compromise blood flow (Schulman, 2001; Schulman and Pierce, 1999).
10. Do not close clamps in the system for more than 2-3 minutes because clotting may occur (Level 1 Inc.).

EQUIPMENT

Level 1 A/V rewarming kit (Figure 156-1)
Dressing materials for central venous and arterial line sites
1000 ml of normal saline IV fluid

AV-300 Disposable Set Components

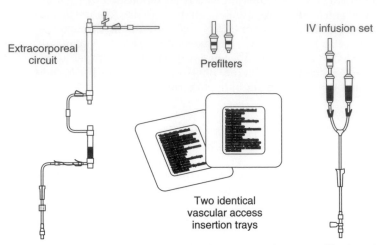

FIGURE 156-1 Level 1 A/V rewarming kit. (Courtesy Level 1, Inc., Rockland, MA.)

PATIENT PREPARATION

1. Obtain baseline vital signs. Initiate hemodynamic and core temperature monitoring.
2. Obtain baseline hemoglobin, hematocrit, coagulation studies, and arterial blood gases (see Procedures 21 and 61).
3. Place large-bore peripheral IV line for supplemental blood, IV fluid, or medication administration (see Procedure 63).
4. Minimize heat loss by using warm blankets, overhead heating lamps, or forced warm air heating blankets (see Procedures 153 and 154).

PROCEDURAL STEPS

Set Up the Level 1 Fluid Warmer (see Procedure 77 for more detailed information)

1. Push the bottom of the end of the heat exchanger into the socket labeled "1" (Figure 156-2).
2. Insert the heat exchanger into the guide. Slide the top socket, labeled "2," down over the top of the tube until it clicks.
3. Insert the filter/gas vent into its holder, labeled "3."
4. Plug in and press the "on" button. The green "system operational" indicator light on the display panel should be lit.
5. Ensure that all tubing connections are tight.

Prime Tubing

1. Attach the IV infusion set from the A/V rewarming procedural kit to the port just proximal to the heat exchanger.
2. Clamp the red arterial line off.

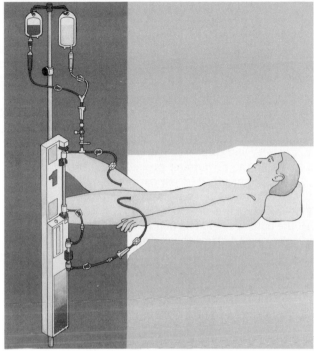

FIGURE 156-2 Assembly of tubing components for CAVR. See text for further details. (Courtesy Level 1, Inc., Rockland, MA.)

3. Spike the IV bag of saline and open the tubing clamp. Allow the infusion set, heat exchanger, filter assembly, and blue venous line to prime. Hold the filter/gas vent upside down until full. Gently tap the filter/gas vent against the chamber to dislodge any air bubbles. Return the filter to its holder, labeled "3."
4. Close the venous (blue) line clamp.
5. Open the arterial (red) line clamp. Allow saline to prime the arterial line, then close the arterial line clamp.

Establish Arterial and Venous Access
1. Use only the catheters included in the A/V rewarming kit.
2. See Procedure 68 for details.

Attach to the Patient
1. Ensure that the temperature of the Level 1 warmer has reached at least 41° C.
2. Close slide clamp to IV infusion set.
3. Connect arterial patient line (red tubing) to patient's arterial catheter and locate the ratchet clamp on the catheter.
4. Allow blood to flow completely through the tubing until it reaches the venous end of the line.
5. Close the venous patient line roller clamp A.

6. Gently tap filter/gas vent against cabinet to release any trapped air.
7. Attach the venous end of the line to the patient's venous catheter and open the roller clamp. Rewarming is now occurring.
8. Tape and anchor all catheters and lines to prevent kinking or dislodgement.
9. Dress catheter sites.
10. Monitor vital signs frequently during rewarming. Continuous temperature monitoring is recommended.

Transporting Patients During CAVR

CAVR must be interrupted during patient transport since the Level 1 fluid warmer does not have a battery and cannot function unless it is plugged in to an electrical outlet. Interrupting the rewarming procedure during transport prevents the patient's blood from being cooled by exposure to ambient temperature.

1. Clamp the CAVR tubing at the arterial side and back flush with saline IV solution until clear. Clamp the arterial catheter.
2. Flush all of the patient's blood through the venous side of the tubing with normal saline solution and clamp the venous side.
3. Remove the tubing from the fluid warmer and place it in bed beside the patient.
4. To reestablish warming on arrival, reinsert the tubing into the fluid warmer and turn the warmer on. When the warmer reaches $37°$ C, open the arterial and venous clamps to restart the blood flow.

Troubleshooting

Patency difficulties in CAVR are usually due to low patient blood flow (systolic blood pressure less than 60-80 mm Hg) or kinks/clots in the tubing.

1. Monitor the tubing for kinking. Tape the arterial and venous ends of the tubing to the patient at the insertion site to prevent kinking when the patient is moved.
2. If the filter becomes clogged, clamp both the arterial and venous ends of the tubing. Remove the old filter. Attach the new filter at the arterial end first. Slowly and partially open the arterial clamp and allow the filter to prime completely. Close the arterial clamp. Attach the venous end of the tubing to the filter and place the filter back in its holder (labeled "3"). Open both arterial and venous clamps to reestablish blood flow.
3. Maintain the patient's systolic blood pressure with IV fluids, blood products, and vasopressors as prescribed.
4. See Procedure 77 for troubleshooting Level 1 alarms.

Discontinuing CAVR

CAVR may be discontinued when the patient's temperature has been stable at $36.5°$ C for 2 hours (Schulman, 2001).

1. Backflush saline IV solution into the arterial end of the catheter until the tubing is clear. Clamp the arterial catheter.
2. Flush the venous end of the catheter with saline IV solution until clear. Clamp the venous catheter.
3. The catheters may be left in place until the patient is stable. Do not remove the catheters until any coagulopathy has resolved.

4. When the catheters are removed, apply direct pressure to the sites for at least 15 minutes. Dress the sites and monitor for hematoma formation.

AGE-SPECIFIC CONSIDERATION

CAVR is contraindicated in patients weighing less than 90 lb (41 kg) because the size of the catheters may occlude the smaller blood vessels of these individuals (Schulman and Pierce, 1999).

COMPLICATIONS (Schulman, 2001)

1. Hematoma formation at catheter insertion sites.
2. Impaired blood flow and loss of pulses to the lower extremities secondary to occlusion by vascular catheters.
3. Clotting and occlusion of the filter.
4. Kinking of tubing leading to decreased flow or clotting and occlusion.
5. Insufficient blood flow secondary to hypotension.
6. Persistent coagulopathy or hypothermia.

REFERENCES

Andreoni, C., & Massey, D. (2001). Continuous arteriovenous rewarming: rapid restoration of normothermia in the emergency department. *Journal of Emergency Nursing*, 27, 533-537.

Gentilello, L.M., & Rifley, W.J. (1991). Continuous arteriovenous rewarming: report of a new technique for treating hypothermia. *Journal of Trauma*, 3(8), 1151-1153.

Schulman, C.S., & Pierce, B. (1999). Continuous arteriovenous rewarming: a bedside technique. *Critical Care Nurse*, 19(5), 54-63.

Schulman, C. (2001). Continuous arteriovenous rewarming (pp. 768-776). In Lynn-McHale, D.J., & Carlson, K.C. (Eds.). *AACN procedure manual for critical care*, 4th ed. Philadelphia: W.B. Saunders.

SIMS Level 1, Inc. *A/V rewarming procedural kit: Gentilello technique* (product insert). Rockland, MA: Author.

Ophthalmic Procedures

Assessing Visual Acuity

Maureen T. Quigley, MS, ARNP, CEN

Assessing visual acuity is also known as the vision test, the Henry F. Allen Preschool Test, the Snellen test, the Rosenbaum pocket screen, and the eye test.

INDICATIONS
1. To assess the vision of patients presenting with ocular complaints
2. To document baseline visual acuity

CONTRAINDICATIONS AND CAUTIONS
Visual acuity testing should not precede treatment in patients whom have had chemical exposure to the eye. Copious saline irrigation should be performed immediately for all chemical exposures (see Procedure 159). Visual acuity testing is performed after irrigation when chemical exposure occurs.

EQUIPMENT
Snellen chart
or
Symbol chart such an "E" chart or a picture chart (for illiterate patients or preschool children)
or
Near-vision acuity chart (Figure 157-1)
Eye spoon, patch, or opaque card to cover the eye not being tested (optional)
Penlight (optional)
Marked distance of 20 or 10 ft for testing
Topical ophthalmic anesthetic (optional)

PATIENT PREPARATION
1. Instill a topical ophthalmic anesthetic (if prescribed) to increase the patient's comfort during the examination (optional).
2. Instruct the patient to occlude one eye during the vision test by using the eye spoon, patch, opaque card, or hand.
3. Instruct the patient not to apply excessive pressure on the eye being occluded because blurred vision may result.
4. Patients using a cupped hand should keep their fingers together to prevent a false reading caused by using binocular vision.
5. Leave glasses or contact lenses in place during the examination if not contraindicated by injury. When the patient's glasses or contact lenses are not available, testing should be documented as "uncorrected visual acuity."

PROCEDURAL STEPS
1. Each eye is tested separately, with and without glasses.

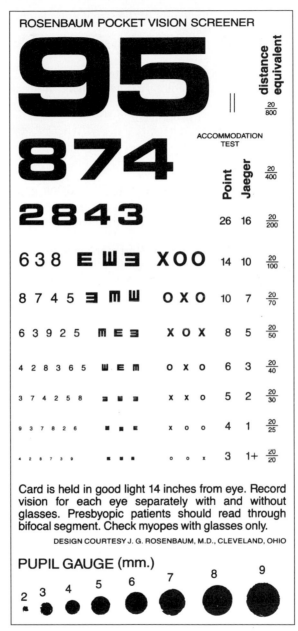

FIGURE 157-1 Rosenbaum pocket version screener for near-vision screening. This illustration is to scale and it, or a copy of it, may be used for assessment of visual acuity. (Courtesy Chiron Vision [1996], Claremont, CA.)

2. Letters and objects are of a size that can be seen by the normal eye at a distance of 6 m (20 ft) from the chart.

3. Letters appear in rows and are arranged so the normal eye can see them at distances of 9, 12, 15 meters (30, 40, 50 feet), and so forth.

4. A person who can identify letters of the size 6 at 6 meters (20 at 20 feet) is said to have 6/6 (20/20) vision.
5. Additionally, if vision is less than 6/60 (20/200), tests may be recorded as follows:
   a. Counting fingers (CF) at ___ meters (feet)
   b. Hand motion (HM) ___ ability to detect hand movement at a certain distance
   c. Light perception and projection (LP & P)
   d. Light perception only (LP)
   e. No light perception (NLP)

Standard Method

1. Sit or stand the patient at a marked distance of 20 ft from the standard Snellen chart with the chart positioned at eye level.
2. Test the vision of one eye at a time. Test the unaffected eye first to serve as a control.
3. Ask the patient to read the Snellen chart starting with the top line and working down until the letters are no longer legible.
4. Record the lowest line the patient is able to read, including the number of mistakes made on that line. For example, oculus dexter (O.D.), or right eye, 20/20 means the patient can read the 20/20 line with no mistakes. Oculus sinister (O.S.), or left eye, 20/25-1 means the patient can read the 20/25 line with one mistake. Visual acuity is recorded as a fraction. The numerator represents the distance to the chart, and the denominator represents the distance from which a normal eye can read the lines. For example, 20/50 means that the patient can read at 20 ft what a person with 20/20 vision can read at 50 ft. If the patient is unable to read the first line of the Snellen chart at 20 ft, he or she may be placed at a distance of 10 ft from the chart and asked to read the lines. The acuity is then recorded as 10/50.
5. Repeat steps 3 and 4 for the opposite eye and for both eyes together (documented as O.U.).

Alternative Methods

1. Hand-held near-vision testing cards are commercially available when distance testing is not possible, such as the Rosenbaum near-vision chart. This is used for patients who are unable to stand (see Figure 157-1). The card is held 14 inches away from the patient. Attaching a 14-inch string to the card facilitates correct usage; however, patients may choose their own distance. The same procedure is used as for the Snellen chart testing.
2. If commercially prepared charts are unavailable, have the patient read a newspaper or another document with similarly sized print. Record the distance at which the patient is able to read the print.
3. Occasionally, patients who wear glasses or contact lenses carry the prescription in their wallet. This may serve as a gross baseline of visual acuity.
4. The pinhole method may be used to assess a refractive error when the patient's glasses or contact lenses are not available. The patient reads the Snellen chart while looking through pinholes in an opaque card. If the visual acuity improves, the decreased visual acuity may be attributed to a refractive

error. When there is no improvement, causes other than refractive error should be considered.

5. If the patient is unable to read the top line of the Snellen chart (vision is less than 20/200 [6/60]), the following visual tests may be performed and recorded as follows:

   a. The patient can count the correct number of fingers at a measured distance. Counting fingers (CF) at ___ meters (___ feet).

   b. The patient can recognize hand motions at a measured distance and in a designated direction. Hand motion (HM) at ___ meters (___ feet).

   c. If the patient is unable to recognize hand motions, light perception is tested. Use a penlight and record whether the patient can determine the direction from which the light is coming. Light perception and projection (LP & P).

   d. If the patient cannot determine which direction the light is coming from, record it as light perception (LP).

   e. If the patient is unable to recognize perceive light, record the visual acuity as "no light perception" (NLP).

AGE-SPECIFIC CONSIDERATIONS

1. Use a symbol chart for illiterate patients or preschool children. Two symbol charts are available either as pictures or with the letter E turned in four different directions. The patient is asked either to point a finger in the direction of the E bars or to identify the picture symbol printed on the chart. Follow the same procedure as for the Snellen chart.

2. Infants and young children can best be evaluated while sitting upright in the arms of their parents or caregivers.

3. Visual acuity testing for the preschool child may be inaccurate and is dependent on the cognitive development of the child. Generally, visual acuity reaches the adult level of 20/20 vision between 3 and 5 years of age.

4. To measure vision in infants over 6 weeks of age, assess their ability to fixate and follow a target. The human face works well as a target; in addition, brightly colored toys may be used (Behrman, 2000).

5. Snellen charts do not accurately test vision in older patients with complaints of faded objects and decreased vision with bright light (Miller, 1999).

COMPLICATIONS

1. Injury causing edema or blepharospasm may prevent the patient from keeping the eyes open without manual assistance or medications to decrease pain or spasm.

2. Excessive tearing may blur the vision and affect the test results.

REFERENCES

Behrman, R.E. (2000). Disorders of the eye (pp. 1896-1897). In Behrman, R.E. (Ed). *Nelson textbook of pediatrics*, 16th ed. Philadelphia: W.B. Saunders.

Miller, D. (1999). Optics of the normal human eye. In Yanoff, M. (Ed.). *Ophthalmology*, 1st ed. (Section 2, 2.7-4.5). St. Louis: Mosby.

Contact Lens Removal

Margo E. Layman, MSN, RN, RNC, CN-A

INDICATIONS
1. To assist a patient who is unable to remove lenses
2. To remove contact lenses in the presence of chemical irritants or foreign bodies
3. To remove contact lenses from a patient with an altered level of consciousness

CONTRAINDICATIONS AND CAUTIONS
1. Never use force to remove a lens. If you have difficulty, slide the lens onto the sclera and notify the physician.
2. Look for "lost" lenses in the upper cul-de-sac of the eye. This is their most common hiding place.
3. Do not replace the lens until a physician examines the patient's eyes.
4. If you suspect that your patient has a penetrating injury to the eye, do not manipulate the eye in any way.
5. If the eyes appear dry, instill several drops of sterile saline solution and wait a few minutes before removing the lens to help prevent corneal damage.
6. Do not instill medications while the patient is wearing contact lenses. Contact lenses can combine chemically with the medication and cause eye irritation or lens damage.
7. Do not use saline solution with preservatives or tap water because they may damage the lenses.

EQUIPMENT
Contact lens storage case or two plastic specimen containers with lids
Contact lens soaking solution or sterile saline solution without preservative
Suction cup (optional)
Cotton balls
Towel

PATIENT PREPARATION
1. Place the patient in a supine or semi-Fowler's position.
2. Place a clean towel around the neck and across the chest.
3. Remove any glass particles with cellophane tape. Roll the tape so the adhesive is on the outside and gently touch it against the patient's closed eye to remove glass particles.
4. Gently remove blood, dirt, or makeup from the eyelids with a cotton ball moistened with saline solution.

5. Place several milliliters of sterile saline solution in each specimen container and label the containers "left" and "right." If a contact lens case is used, place a few drops of saline solution in each compartment.

PROCEDURAL STEPS
Hard Lenses
1. Use one thumb to pull the patient's upper eyelid toward the orbital rim.
2. Place your other thumb on the lower lid, gently move the lids toward each other to trap the lens edge, and break the suction (Figure 158-1).
3. Cup your hand below the eye to catch the lens when it pops out.
4. Place the lens in an appropriate specimen container or contact lens case compartment.
5. Remove and care for the other lens by use of the same technique.
6. Examine the patient's eyes for redness or irritation.

Soft Lenses
1. Raise the upper eyelid with your index finger and hold it against the orbital rim.
2. Lightly place your thumb on the lower lid and pull it down.
3. Have the patient look up and slide the lens down gently with the index finger of your other hand.
4. Pinch the lens together with your thumb and index finger and lift it out of the patient's eye (Figure 158-2).

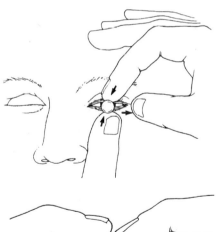

FIGURE 158-1 Removal of hard contact lenses. (From Novotny-Dinsdale, V. [1995]. Ocular emergencies. In Kitt, S., et al. [Eds.]. *Emergency nursing: a physiologic and clinical perspective,* 2nd ed. [p. 124]. Philadelphia: W.B. Saunders.)

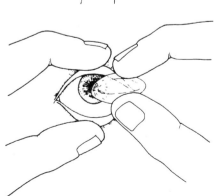

FIGURE 158-2 Removal of soft contact lenses. (From Novotny-Dinsdale, V. [1995]. Ocular emergencies. In Kitt, S., et al. [Eds.]. *Emergency nursing: a physiologic and clinical perspective,* 2nd ed. [p. 124]. Philadelphia: W.B. Saunders.)

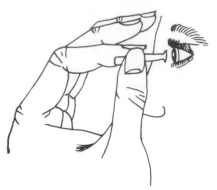

FIGURE 158-3 Removal of a contact lens with a suction cup.

5. Place the lens in the appropriate specimen container or the contact lens case compartment.
6. Remove and care for the other lens using the same technique.
7. Examine the patient's eyes for redness or irritation.

Suction Cup Removal of Hard and Soft Lenses

1. Wet the suction cup with a drop of sterile saline solution.
2. Gently pull up the patient's upper eyelid with your index finger and pull the lower lid down with your thumb.
3. Press the suction cup gently to the center of the lens (Figure 158-3).
4. Pull the suction cup and the lens away from the eye in a straight line.
5. Place the lens in the appropriate specimen container or the contact lens case compartment.
6. Remove and care for the other lens using the same technique.
7. Examine the patient's eyes for redness or irritation.

COMPLICATIONS

1. Corneal damage can result from touching the cornea with the suction cup or attempting to remove dry lenses.
2. Corneal damage can occur if the lens is replaced in the wrong eye. Always label the containers and place the lenses in the proper containers or compartments.

PATIENT TEACHING

1. Watch for signs of eye irritation, such as purulent drainage, redness, or swelling.
2. Follow the usual cleaning procedures for lenses.

Eye Irrigation

Maureen T. Quigley, MS, ARNP, CEN

Eye irrigation is also known as eye flushing.

INDICATIONS
1. To dilute or remove chemicals from the eye and restore a normal pH
2. To remove foreign objects from the eye and help prevent ocular damage and vision loss after an eye injury
3. To relieve pain or burning that is usually associated with a foreign body or a chemical injury to the eye

CONTRAINDICATIONS AND CAUTIONS
1. Do not delay irrigation when a chemical exposure occurs. Irrigation should be initiated immediately and should be continued by caregivers before arrival at the emergency department. Until the causative agent is known, exposures should be presumed to be acid or alkaline substances (Brunette, 2002).
2. It is critical to identify the causative agent and to obtain an initial pH. In general, alkaline substances have a pH less than 12 and acidic substances have a pH greater than 2 (Brunette, 2002).
3. Lactated Ringer's solution is preferred over normal saline. The pH of lactated Ringer's is 6.0-7.5, which is closer to the pH of tears (7.1) than that of normal saline, which may range from 4.5-7.0 (MorTan, Inc., 1996).
4. Use caution when a penetrating injury is present or suspected, and irrigate gently.
5. Paper clips sometimes used as modified lid retractors may chip after twisting, causing metal fragments to enter the eye (Knoop, Dennis, & Hedges, 2004).
6. If a patient has contaminated his or her eye with a cyanoacrylate adhesive (e.g., Super Glue), do not force the eyelids open. Irrigation is not the first line of treatment. Consider using gauze pads soaked with mineral oil to loosen the bond. For more definitive information, consult your local Poison Control Center.
7. An ophthalmology consultation may be necessary, depending on the type and the duration of the exposure as well as the clinical findings.

EQUIPMENT
Topical ophthalmic anesthetic
Sterile lactated Ringer's solution (1000-ml intravenous [IV] bag)
IV macrodrip tubing
18- or 20-G over-the-needle catheter with the stylet removed
or
Irrigation (Morgan) lens
or

Syringe irrigating device
Basin
Tape (optional)
Gauze dressings or a commercially prepared eye patch
Towels or a patient gown
Tissues
Cotton-tipped applicators
Shampoo board or sink area (optional)
Desmarres retractor (Figure 159-1)
pH paper

PATIENT PREPARATION

1. Instill the prescribed topical ophthalmic anesthetic into the affected eye.
2. If a chemical exposure has occurred, obtain a baseline pH measurement of the eye by placing pH paper in the conjunctival sac.
3. Another person may need to hold the eyelids open manually or with a retractor if an irrigating lens is not used.
4. Inform the patient that the eye irrigation may cause postnasal drip. Offer tissues for use as needed.
5. Use a gown or draped towels to protect the patient from excessive dampness during the procedure.
6. Position a basin or a large bag to catch the irrigant or position the patient over a sink. Using a shampoo board under the patient's head is another method to facilitate collection of the irrigant. Place the patient in a supine position. Place towels under the patient's neck to increase comfort.

PROCEDURAL STEPS
Manual Irrigation

1. Spike the IV tubing into the IV fluid and attach the catheter or irrigating syringe device.
2. Use gauze pads to hold the eyelids open for irrigation if the patient is unable to do so. A lid retractor may be used to separate the eyelids and allow irrigation.

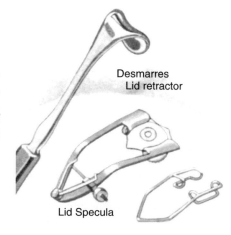

FIGURE 159-1 Devices for separating the eyelids. (From Fogle, J.A., Spyker, D.A. [1990]. Management of chemical and drug injury to the eye. In Haddad, L.M., & Winchester, J.F. [Eds.]. *Clinical management of poisoning and drug overdose* 2nd ed. [p, 372]. Philadelphia: W. B. Saunders.)

Desmarres
Lid retractor

Lid Specula

3. Direct the flow of the irrigant onto the conjunctiva from the inner to the outer canthus, avoid directing the stream directly onto the cornea, which can be harmful (Figure 159-2).
4. Instruct the patient to roll the eyes in all directions to ensure total eye irrigation.
5. For acidic exposure, irrigate with a minimum of 1000 ml of normal saline solution per eye. Acids (except hydrofluoric and heavy metal acids) are quickly neutralized by the proteins of the eye surface. After the eye is irrigated, acids cause no further damage (Knoop, Dennis, & Hedges, 2004).
6. Irrigate alkaline injuries with a minimum of 2 L of lactated Ringer's or normal saline solution per eye over 1 hour. Extensive irrigation is required because alkaline substances, hydrofluoric acid, and heavy-metal acids can penetrate the cornea rapidly and continue to produce damage for days (Knoop, Dennis, & Hedges, 2004).
7. Measure the pH of the eye at intervals during the irrigation by placing pH paper in the conjunctival sac. Continue irrigation is needed until the pH of the tear film is neutral. The normal conjunctival pH is 7.1. If the pH remains alkaline, irrigation should be continued.
8. *Evert the eyelid and remove traces of alkali by using a wet cotton-tipped applicator to swab the fornices (Figure 159-3).
9. Check the patient's comfort level periodically. Instill additional ophthalmic anesthetic as necessary.

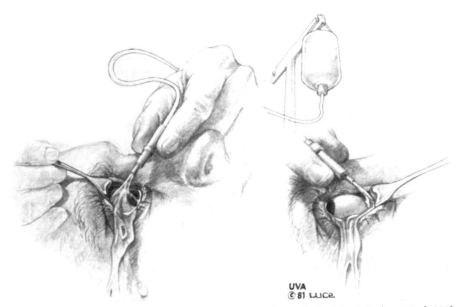

UVA
© 81 LUCE

FIGURE 159-2 Irrigation using a Desmarres retractor. (From Fogle, J.A., & Spyker, D.A. [1990]. Management of chemical and drug injury to the eye. In Haddad, L.M. & Winchester, J.F. [Eds.]. *Clinical management of poisoning and drug overdose,* 2nd ed. [p. 373]. Philadelphia: W.B. Saunders.)

---

*Indicates portions of the procedure usually performed by a physician or an advanced practice nurse.

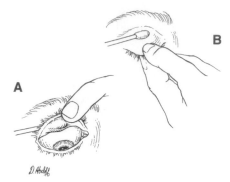

FIGURE 159-3 Eyelid eversion. **A,** Have patient look downward and grasp eyelashes and pull downward. **B,** Place cotton-tipped applicator at the midpoint of the eyelid and pull the eyelid over the applicator to complete the lid eversion. (From Rosen, P., & Sternbach, G.L. [1983]. *Atlas of emergency medicine*, 2nd ed. [p. 157]. Baltimore: Williams & Wilkins.)

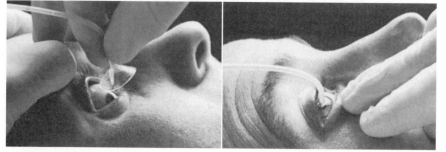

FIGURE 159-4 Placement of the Morgan lens for eye irrigation. **A,** Have the patient look downward, and then insert the lens under the upper lid. Have the patient look upward, and then retract the lower lid. **B,** For removal, have the patient look upward and then retract the lower lid, hold the position, and slide the lens out. (Courtesy of MorTan, Inc., [1996]. *Instructional chart for Morgan lens.* Copyright, 1996 by MorTan, Inc., Missoula, MT.)

10. Recheck the conjunctival pH approximately 20 minutes after completion of irrigation and periodically as indicated to ensure that it remains in the normal range. Delayed pH changes often result from inadequate irrigation techniques (Samples and Hedges, 1998).
11. Obtain a baseline visual acuity level (see Procedure 157).
12. Prepare the patient for a corneal examination to determine the extent of the injury (see Procedure 160).

Irrigating or Morgan Therapeutic Lens

1. The irrigating lens fits onto the cornea like a soft contact lens and provides optimal continuous irrigation of the corneal surface while increasing patient comfort. The lens allows the patient to close the eyelids and decreases the risk of iatrogenic trauma often encountered during a difficult irrigation (Figure 159-4).
2. Apply normal saline solution to the surface of the continuous irrigation lens to assist with insertion. Ask the patient to look downward. Grasp the upper

eyelid and retract it upward. Holding the lens between the thumb and fore-finger of your dominant hand, insert the upper portion of the lens under the upper eyelid. Ask the patient to look down. Retract the lower eyelid and place the lower portion of the lens onto the cornea. The insertion process is similar to that used to insert a contact lens.

3. Attach the IV tubing to the lens device, open the clamp, adjust the flow to a level tolerated well by the patient, and proceed with the continuous irrigation. A wide-open flow may create too much pressure and actually create more discomfort for the patient. Remind the patient to keep the eyes closed to ensure that the lenses stay in the eyes.

4. Tape the irrigation tubing to the patient's forehead to prevent accidental dislodgement of the lens (optional).

5. See steps 4-10 in the Manual Irrigation section of this procedure.

6. Remove the irrigation lens by asking the patient to look upward. Retract the lower lid, lift one side of the lens to break the suction, and gently slide the lens from the cornea.

AGE-SPECIFIC CONSIDERATIONS

1. Patients with chronic diseases, such as congestive heart failure or chronic obstructive lung disease, may need accommodations for positioning during irrigation. A supine position may not be tolerated.

2. The irrigating lens (Morgan lens) has been used for a child as young as 6 months of age with successful results and no complications (MorTan, Inc., personal communication, June 24, 1997).

COMPLICATIONS

1. Corneal or conjunctival abrasions may result from holding the eyelids open during the irrigation process.

2. Swelling or periorbital edema may occur after irrigation.

3. A fine punctate keratitis may result from direct irrigation onto the cornea (Knoop, Dennis, & Hedges, 2004).

PATIENT TEACHING

1. Following irrigation, the patient may experience a burning sensation in the eyes similar to that which occurs after prolonged exposure to chlorinated water in a swimming pool. The sensation is self-limiting and usually subsides about an hour after tear production resumes.

2. Take analgesic as directed.

3. Follow-up with emergency department if you are not better, or with an ophthalmologist as directed.

REFERENCES

Brunette, R. (2002). Ophthalmology. In Marx, J.A., et al. (Eds.). *Rosen's emergency medicine: concepts and clinical practice*, 5th ed. (pp. 909-929). St. Louis: Mosby.

MorTan, Inc. (1996). Instructional Chart for Morgan Lens. Missoula, MT: Author.

Knoop, K.J., Dennis, W.R., & Hedges, J.R. (2004). Ophthalmologic procedures (pp. 1241–1279). In Roberts, J.R., & Hedges, J.R. (Eds.). *Clinical procedures in emergency medicine*, 4th ed. Philadelphia: W.B. Saunders.

Fluorescein Staining of Eyes

Maureen T. Quigley, MS, ARNP, CEN

Fluorescein staining of the eye is also known as an ultraviolet examination, a Woods lamp examination, or a black light examination, all of which enhance visualization. Fluorescein reveals the area of epithelial defect by staining basement membrane, which may appear as yellow to the naked eye.

INDICATIONS

1. To diagnose blunt or penetrating eye injuries.
2. To evaluate suspected corneal abrasions, foreign bodies, or infections of the eye. The exposed edge of epithelium created by the edge of a foreign body usually stains, rather than the entire foreign body.
3. To test for epiphora, a condition characterized by the overflow of tears due to blockage of the lacrimal drainage system. If the drainage system is patent, traces of fluorescein are present in the oral and nasal secretions (Newell, 1996).
4. To detect perforation of the eye with the Seidel test (Knoop, Dennis, & Hedges, 2004). A large amount of fluorescein is instilled into the eye, and the globe is examined for a stream of fluid leaking from the globe. The stream appears fluorescent blue or green, whereas the rest of the globe appears orange.

CONTRAINDICATIONS AND CAUTIONS

1. Penlight and funduscopic examination of the eye, as well as a presumptive diagnosis of corneal abrasion based on history, physical examination, and exclusion of other disorders should be done before fluorescein examination (Jacobs, 2001). Confirmation of the problem, rather than diagnosis, is made after fluorescein staining.
2. Measurement of visual acuity and visualization of the anterior segment and fundus may be impaired by prior use of fluorescein.
3. Soft contact lens should be removed because the fluorescein stain may cause permanent tinting of the lens (see Procedure 158). Hard contact lenses are not affected by the dye.
4. With deep corneal disruption, the dye may enter the anterior chamber of the eye (Knoop, Dennis, & Hedges, 2004). The dye is nontoxic, but it is difficult to flush out completely.
5. Multiple-dose bottles of fluorescein stain are easily contaminated, and *Pseudomonas aeruginosa* flourishes in fluorescein solution. Sterile fluorescein-impregnated strips are safer (Newell, 1996). If fluorescein solution is used, individual dosettes are preferred.
6. Some patients may develop a superficial punctuate keratitis after use of a topical anesthetic, but for many patients, examination is difficult without prior use of an anesthetic (Knoop, Dennis, & Hedges, 2004).

EQUIPMENT

Normal saline solution, artificial tears, or dextrose solution for the irrigant
Sterile fluorescein-impregnated strips
Light source: Cobalt blue penlight, blue filter on slit lamp, or Woods lamp
Patient gown or towel
Tissues
Emesis basin
Topical ophthalmic anesthetic (optional)

PATIENT PREPARATION

1. Remove glasses or contact lens (see Procedure 158).
2. Cover the patient's clothing with a gown or towel. Fluorescein is a dye and may permanently stain clothing.
3. Place the patient in either a seated or a supine position.
4. Provide tissues and instruct the patient to gently blot tears. This is especially important if the physician uses a topical anesthetic for the procedure, because additional corneal irritation may result.

PROCEDURAL STEPS

1. Instill two drops of the prescribed topical anesthetic into the affected eye or eyes if needed (optional).
2. Moisten the appropriate end of the fluorescein strip with saline or artificial tears.
3. After depressing the lower eyelid, gently place the moistened fluorescein impregnated paper strip into the conjunctival sac. Placement of a nonmoistened fluorescein strip may cause additional epithelial damage (Figure 160-1).
4. Instruct the patient to blink once, which distributes the dye over the ocular surface. An alternative method is to touch the moistened fluorescein strip to the conjunctival sac and observe the flow of dye into the sac until an adequate amount is present to coat the corneal surface. Remove the strip and discard.
5. Instruct the patient to close the eyes for approximately 30-60 seconds. This promotes maximal distribution of the dye over the cornea by retaining tears within the eyelids.
6. Use the irrigant to remove excessive fluorescein dye. This enhances the contrast between the injured and the normal areas.
7. Dim the lights in the examination room.
8. *Use a cobalt blue penlight or black light source to inspect the corneal surface for epithelial defects, foreign bodies, or abrasions. Disrupted corneal surfaces are visualized as bright green under the blue light.
9. After the examination, irrigate the eye with saline solution or other irrigant to remove the fluorescein dye and prevent staining of either the clothing or the face. An emesis basin can be held close to the patient's cheek to catch the irrigant solution. This is optional and performed for aesthetic reasons only.

---

*Indicates portions of the procedure usually performed by a physician or an advanced practice nurse.

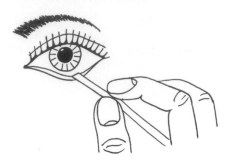

FIGURE 160-1 Placement of fluorescein strip into the conjunctival sac.

COMPLICATIONS

Although topical fluorescein is considered nontoxic, rare reactions, such as redness or swelling, have been reported when fluorescein solution was used. These reactions are usually caused by contaminants in the solution rather than the solution itself (Newell, 1996). Use of fluorescein-impregnated strips removes this risk.

PATIENT TEACHING

1. Yellowish-orange fluid may drain from your eyes or nose following the procedure.
2. Do not wear soft contact lenses for 3-5 hours after fluorescein staining to prevent permanent staining of the lens.
3. No special directions are needed if you wear hard contact lenses.

REFERENCES

Jacobs, D.S. (2001). *Corneal abrasions and corneal foreign bodies.* In 2002 UpToDate, online version 10.2. www.uptodate.com.

Newell, F.W. (1996). *Ophthalmology principles and concepts,* 8th ed. St. Louis: Mosby.

Knoop, K.J., Dennis, W.R., & Hedges, J.R. (2004). Ophthalmologic procedures (pp. 1241-1279). In Roberts, J.R., & Hedges, J.R. (Eds.). *Clinical procedures in emergency medicine,* 4th ed. Philadelphia: W.B. Saunders.

Ophthalmic Foreign Body Removal

Maureen T. Quigley, MS, ARNP, CEN

INDICATIONS

1. To remove a foreign body from the cornea or conjunctiva.
2. To prevent ocular damage or vision loss from a foreign body. Foreign bodies usually result from trauma or acts of nature, such as wind-blown objects or insects.

CONTRAINDICATIONS AND CAUTIONS

1. It is important to obtain a detailed description of the mechanism and circumstances of the injury. Find out the exact time of injury, the events leading to the injury, the description and composition of the foreign body, the distance it traveled to the eye, whether it was blown by the wind or propelled into the eye, the direction of travel, and the direction in which the eye was looking at the time of the injury.
2. A history providing material content of the foreign body is significant in management because some nonmagnetic foreign bodies may not be removed unless they are easily accessible. Siderosis (a rust brown or yellowish discoloration of the cornea, iris, or lens) may develop from steel and iron foreign bodies and may lead to chronic degenerative changes, such as visual field loss, cataracts, or open angle glaucoma (Mester and Kuhn, 2002). Copper, bronze, and brass foreign bodies may cause chalcosis. Nonmetallic foreign bodies can be inert or toxic: glass, stone, and plastic can be tolerated for many years, with a rare reaction, as opposed to vegetable matter, which often results in a severe inflammatory reaction. Trauma involving vegetable matter (lash, thorn, wood, or soil) increases the possibility of infection, particularly fungal infection (Gaudio et al., 1994) (see Table 165-1 from Procedure 165).
3. Plain film, computed tomography, or magnetic resonance imaging may localize intraorbital foreign bodies. Plain films are helpful in the identification of opaque foreign bodies. Computed tomography is considered to be the gold standard for most foreign bodies, with the exception of dry wood. Magnetic resonance imaging is helpful in the identification of dry wood foreign bodies (Mester and Kuhn, 2002). If an object is felt to be of metallic origin, magnetic resonance imaging is contraindicated.
4. It is possible that patients may not remember the precipitating event, because the symptoms can be delayed or could be intermittent.
5. Obtain previous ophthalmic history: previously existing eye disease, surgery, and trauma, as well as vision before the presenting injury.

6. Do not apply pressure to the eye. Direct pressure should not be used to stop bleeding from or around the eye when a penetrating object is suspected or evident. Instruct the patient not to touch or rub the eye.

7. Unless contraindicated by other injuries, elevate the head of the bed to decrease intraocular pressure. Limit patient movement as much as possible.

8. If a foreign body is impaled in the eye, immobilize the object and patch both eyes to decrease ocular movement (see Procedures 163 and 165).

9. Contact lenses should be removed immediately in the presence of a foreign body (see Procedure 158).

10. Chemical injuries are considered penetrating and require immediate copious irrigation to prevent irreversible damage (see Procedure 159).

11. Abrasions or actinic injuries often mimic the sensation of an ocular foreign body, but they are easily diagnosed by the fluorescein examination (see Procedure 160).

12. If you are unable to locate an external foreign body despite patient complaints, consider the possibility of an intraocular or intraorbital foreign body. Symptoms suggestive of a penetrating injury include an irregular pupil, hyphema, lens opacification, hemorrhage, or prolapsed iris. Some intraocular foreign objects are toxic (see Table 165-1).

13. Paper clips are frequently used as emergency lid retractors because of their ready availability in patient-care areas. This is not a safe practice, however, because bending a paper clip into a shape suitable for a lid retractor may produce metal fragments that may be introduced into the patient's eye (Vesser and O'Connor, 1995).

14. Only those with formalized training should do removal of ophthalmic foreign bodies with sharp instruments.

15. Ascertain tetanus status and immunize as indicated.

16. Maintain nothing per mouth (NPO) status in light of a possible operative intervention and ascertain when the patient had his or her last meal.

EQUIPMENT

Topical ophthalmic anesthetic
Sterile fluorescein strip
Irrigation solution
Sterile cotton swabs
25- or 27-G needle or eye spud
3-ml syringe (or any size that is comfortable to hold)
Ophthalmoscope
Ultraviolet light
Penlight
Magnification source: loupe or slit lamp
Cycloplegic ophthalmic drops
Antibiotic ophthalmic drops or ointment
Lid retractor
Eye drill with bits (optional)

PATIENT PREPARATION

1. Place the patient in a seated or high Fowler's position.
2. Assess and document visual acuity (see Procedure 157).

3. Remove contact lens or lenses if present (see Procedure 158).
4. Anesthetize the affected eye with 1 or 2 drops of a topical ophthalmic anesthetic, as prescribed.
5. Apply the fluorescein stain (see Procedure 160).

PROCEDURAL STEPS

1. The head, scalp, face, periorbital tissues, and eyelids should be inspected and palpated for occult subcutaneous foreign bodies, crepitus, and step-off deformities. If there is significant swelling involving the lids or the patient is unable to cooperate, an imaging study should be performed, if indicated (Harlan and Pieramici, 2002).
2. A full eye examination should be performed. Use a penlight to examine the anesthetized corneal surface lower fornix, conjunctiva, and upper-lid conjunctiva. Ask the patient to look in all directions. Vertical scratches suggest a foreign body trapped under the lid.
3. *Use a cotton swab to evert the upper eyelid (Figure 161-1). Place the applicator in the middle of the upper lid and instruct the patient to gaze downward. Grasp the patient's eyelashes, pull downward, and then fold upward over the swab. Laying the swab shaft across the bridge of the nose adds support when everting the eyelid. While the eyelid is everted, use a moist cotton swab to sweep the upper fornix area and remove any debris.
4. Removal techniques vary once the foreign body is located. Options include the following:
   a. Gently irrigate the eye to dislodge the foreign body into the lower conjunctival sac. Remove the foreign body with a moist cotton swab. This is helpful when there are multiple superficial foreign bodies.
   b. *Attempt to remove the foreign body by touching it gently with a moist cotton swab. Do not use a dry applicator or attempt prolonged dislodgment of the object, because additional epithelial damage may result.
   c. *Under a slit lamp or loupe magnification, embedded foreign bodies may be removed with a 27- or 25-G needle attached to a syringe, an eye spud, or a cotton swab. The syringe or cotton swab acts as a handle (Figures 161-2 and 161-3).

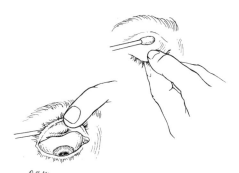

FIGURE 161-1 Eyelid eversion. (From Rosen, P., & Sternbach, G.L. [1983]. *Atlas of emergency medicine*, 2nd ed. [p. 157]. Baltimore: Williams & Wilkins.)

D. Adolff

---

*Indicates portions of the procedure usually performed by a physician or an advanced practice nurse.

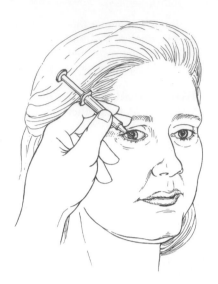

FIGURE 161-2 Removal of a foreign body using a syringe as a handle and a small gauge needle. (From Rosen, P. & Sternbach, G.L. [1983]. *Atlas of emergency medicine,* 2nd ed. [p. 157]. Baltimore: Williams & Wilkins.)

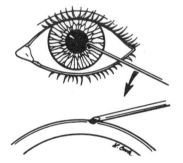

FIGURE 161-3 Removal of a foreign body from the cornea. Hold the syringe tangential to the foreign body and scrape gently away from the cornea. The side view demonstrates the thickness of the cornea relative to the beveled needle edge. (From Pavan-Langston, D. [2002]. *Manual of ocular diagnosis and therapy,* 5th ed. [p. 38]. Boston: Lippincott, Williams & Wilkins.)

Ideally, use a slit lamp that has a chin rest to secure the head. The slit lamp provides adequate illumination, magnification, and a light focus point. The patient may also be asked to focus on the practitioner's ear to steady the eye. If a slit lamp is unavailable, instruct the patient to fix his or her gaze on a stationary object. Secure the patient's head against the examination chair headrest with your fingers, steadying your hand against the patient's face. Dim the room lights. Use a penlight to provide increased illumination to the eye. Magnification loupes may also be used.

    d. *When these methods are unsuccessful, an eye drill may be used to remove a visible foreign body.

5. *To prevent rust rings, completely remove any metallic foreign body particles. If removal is incomplete, the rust ring softens within 24-48 hours, facilitating easy removal (Knoop, Dennis, & Hedges, 2004). Patients may be referred to an ophthalmologist for rust-ring removal.

6. *Magnetic removal is another method of extracting ferromagnetic foreign bodies. A magnet is placed on the handle of a sterile jeweler's forceps. The magnet attracts the foreign body, which is lifted or grasped from the cornea.

---

*Indicates portions of the procedure usually performed by a physician or an advanced practice nurse.

7. After removal of the foreign body, irrigate the eye with at least 10 ml of saline solution to remove any remaining traces of fluorescein or other particulate matter.
8. Instill prophylactic antibiotic ophthalmic drops or ointment as prescribed. Cycloplegics may also be prescribed to decrease ciliary muscle spasms and increase patient comfort.
9. Patch the affected eye (optional) (see Procedure 163).

AGE-SPECIFIC CONSIDERATIONS

1. Young children may require an immobilization device, such as a child restraint board to be evaluated effectively (see Procedure 193). An alternative method of examination is to have an assistant and parent sit facing each other, with the child positioned supine, with legs straddling the parent's waist. With the parent holding the child's extremities, the child's head is directed onto the assistant's lap, and the physician performs the examination. If these approaches fail, the evaluation should be performed under sedation in a monitored setting (see Procedure 181) or under general anesthesia.
2. In the elderly, eye and orbital trauma is frequently caused by falls, which may also cause other injuries, such as hip fractures. A fall could represent underlying cardiovascular disease, such as an arrhythmia or hypotension, which would necessitate further evaluation.
3. A child may be reluctant to provide a history of the injury if involved in behavior that was inappropriate.

COMPLICATIONS

1. Incomplete removal of a foreign body results in inflammation and delayed healing. Owing to the oxidation of iron, metallic foreign bodies create rust rings within hours. Rust rings cause continuing irritation of the eye.
2. Conjunctivitis may occur after the removal of a foreign body.
3. Use of a cotton swab, especially a dry one, may cause additional epithelial damage.
4. Pain after foreign object removal is common. Because topical anesthetics are contraindicated for ongoing use, a prescription for oral analgesia is often indicated.

PATIENT TEACHING

1. Do not touch or rub the injured eye.
2. Rest the uninjured eye, thus preventing involuntary movement of the injured eye.
3. Avoid reading or computer work. Television viewing is permitted at a distance of 10 feet or more. Fixed-gaze television watching limits the movement of the eye, as opposed to reading, which necessitates eye movement (Knoop, Dennis, & Hedges, 2004).
4. The sensation of having a foreign body in the eye may return after the topical anesthetic wears off. A topical anesthetic cannot be used at home, because continued use prevents healing and may mask pain related to complications.
5. Use protective eyewear when appropriate to prevent future injuries.
6. A safe home environment/living arrangement is important after a serious eye injury.

REFERENCES

Gaudio, A., et al. (1994). Intraocular foreign bodies (pp. 1169-1179). In Albert, D., & Jakobiec, F. (Eds.). *Principles and practice of ophthalmology.* Philadelphia: W.B. Saunders.

Harlan, J.B. Jr., & Pieramici, D.J. (2002). Evaluation of patients with ocular trauma. *Ophthalmology Clinics of North America, 15,* 153-161.

Mester, V., & Kuhn, F. (2002). Intraocular foreign bodies. *Ophthalmology Clinics of North America, 15,* 235-242.

Knoop, K.J., Dennis, W.R., & Hedges, J.R. (2004). Ophthalmologic procedures (pp. 1241-1279). In Roberts, J.R., & Hedges, J.R. (Eds.). *Clinical procedures in emergency medicine,* 4th ed. Philadelphia: W.B. Saunders.

Vesser, F.R., & O'Connor, R.E. (1995). Corneal abrasion during eyelid retraction. *Annals of Emergency Medicine, 24,* 756-758.

PROCEDURE 162

Instillation of Eye Medications

Maureen T. Quigley, MS, ARNP, CEN

INDICATIONS

1. To reduce the potential for secondary infection related to eye injury
2. To decrease pain related to eye irritation or injury
3. To provide treatment for an existing problem or infection
4. To assist in the examination of the eyes by anesthetizing the cornea or paralyzing the ciliary muscles, or both
5. To promote corneal reepithelialization

CONTRAINDICATIONS AND CAUTIONS

1. In the presence of penetrating injuries to the globe, do not instill medications without a physician's prescription.
2. Topical ocular steroids are usually used only on the order of an ophthalmologist because use of these medications can retard corneal epithelial wound healing and increase the risk of infection. They can also accelerate the activity of herpes simplex virus and should not be used if the diagnosis is uncertain (Brunette, 2002).
3. Caution should be used in instilling mydriatic, cycloplegic, or steroid drops in the elderly because angle-closure glaucoma can be induced.

4. With its rich supply of nerve fibers, the eye is very sensitive, and direct application of medication on the cornea should be avoided. Medication should be instilled in the less sensitive conjunctival sac (Perry and Potter, 2002).
5. If medication is refrigerated, warm it in your hands and instill at room temperature.

EQUIPMENT
Sterile gauze or tissues (if sterility is not indicated)
Prescribed ophthalmic medication

PATIENT PREPARATION
1. Assess visual acuity (see Procedure 157) before instilling myrdiatic medications. From a medicolegal standpoint, this documents that any decrease in vision is not a result of the medications (Knoop, Dennis, & Hedges, 2004).
2. Determine the patient's medication and significant ocular history, as well as history of allergies.
3. Place the patient in a supine position or in a sitting position with the head tilted back in a position of comfort.
4. Evaluate the eye for retained foreign matter.
5. Irrigate or remove the foreign matter from the eye (see Procedures 159 and 161).

PROCEDURAL STEPS
Instillation of Eye Drops
1. Instruct the patient to look up toward the top of his or her head.
2. Gently pull the lower eyelid down or evert the lower lid by using a piece of gauze, a cotton swab, or a clean gloved finger with thumb or forefinger against the orbit. Never apply pressure on the eyeball.
3. Instill a single drop into the conjunctival sac at the center of the lower lid (Figure 162-1). More than one drop at a time is not recommended because this increases tearing and decreases the concentration of the medication (Knoop, Dennis, & Hedges, 2004).
4. Have the patient close or blink the eyes gently to spread the medication.
5. Repeat steps 1-4 if additional drops of medication are prescribed.

Instillation of Eye Ointment
1. Instruct the patient to look up toward the top of his or her head.

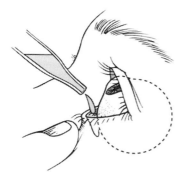

FIGURE 162-1 Instilling eye drops. (From Proehl, J.A., & Jones, L.M. [1998]. *Mosby's emergency department patient teaching guidelines* [p. J-3]. St. Louis: Mosby.)

2. Gently pull the lower eyelid down or evert the lower lid by using a piece of gauze or a cotton swab.
3. Spread a thin ribbon of ointment along lower eyelid on conjunctiva from the inner to the outer canthus.
4. Have the patient close or blink the eyes gently a few times to spread the medication.
5. The eyes should remain closed if an eye patch needs to be applied (see Procedure 163).

AGE-SPECIFIC CONSIDERATIONS
1. Have parent restrain infant or young child's head held in parent's lap when instilling eye medication.
2. Instill eye medication when child or infant is sleeping.
3. Instill eye medication in restrained supine position at nasal aspect of eye(s) of young child or infant with tightly clenched eyes, so that medication flows into eyes when opened (Perry and Potter, 2002).

COMPLICATIONS
1. Introduction of contaminated medication may result in an infection. Single-patient use of eye medications is recommended to prevent cross-contamination.
2. Trauma to the eye may result from movement of the patient's head during instillation.
3. Prolonged use of topical anesthetics can result in epithelial damage to the cornea.
4. Temporary blurred vision may be a side effect of the medication or may result from the presence of ointment in the eye.

PATIENT TEACHING
1. Do not rub your eyes or squeeze the lids together.
2. Some medications may make your eyes sensitive to light, so you may need to wear sunglasses.
3. If you experience any increase in eye pain, purulent drainage, or visual problems, report it immediately.
4. If you wear contact lenses, do not wear them until their use if approved by your physician.
5. Topical anesthetics are not prescribed for ongoing use, because they may retard healing.
6. Some medications may affect vision, and you should not drive or perform activities that require acute vision.

REFERENCES
Brunette, R. (2002). Ophthalmology (pp. 909-929). In Marx, J.A., et al. (Eds.). *Rosen's emergency medicine: concepts and clinical practice*, 5th ed. St. Louis: Mosby.
Knoop, K.J., Dennis, W.R., & Hedges, J.R. (2004). Ophthalmologic procedures (pp. 1241-1279). Roberts, J.R., & Hedges, J.R. (Eds.). *Clinical procedures in emergency medicine*, 4th ed. Philadelphia: W.B. Saunders.
Perry, A.G., Knoop, K.J., Dennis, W.R., & Potter, P.A. (2002). *Clinical nursing skills and techniques*, 5th ed. St. Louis: Mosby.

Eye Patching

Maureen T. Quigley, MS, ARNP, CEN

The routine use of eye patches after simple corneal abrasions has occurred previously under the assumption that it hastens healing and reduces pain; this has been proved false in multiple studies (Knoop, Dennis, & Hedges, 2004). Typically, hard patches or eye shields are used when the globe or cornea has been disrupted. Collagen shields and bandage contact lenses containing a topical nonsteroidal anti-inflammatory drug have been used for corneal abrasions, although these have not been incorporated into emergency department practice (Macsai, 2000). This procedure addresses soft patches and eye shields or hard patches; collagen shields and bandage contact lenses are beyond the scope of this procedure.

INDICATIONS
Hard and Soft Patches
1. To avoid further injury after trauma to the eye(s), such as occurs in corneal abrasion, chemical damage, or ultraviolet light injuries. It may be useful to patch patients with large abrasions occupying more than half of the corneal surface for pain relief (Jacobs, 2001).
2. To protect the eye after administration of an anesthetic
3. To protect a dilated eye from bright light
4. To aid in resting the eye(s)
5. To protect an injured globe without applying any pressure to the eye, a metal eye shield or paper cup may be used. Injuries that require this type of protection include hyphema, globe perforation, and protruding foreign objects imbedded in the globe, such as fishhooks or knives.
6. Pressure patching is used to hold the eyelid closed to facilitate healing of corneal defects to limit eyelid movement in an injured eye.

CONTRAINDICATIONS AND CAUTIONS
1. A visual acuity (see Procedure 157) and *complete eye examination should be completed before patching.
2. Patching is contraindicated when corneal epithelial loss is the result of an infection. Patching an infected eye provides a dark, moist environment for bacterial growth (Knoop, Dennis, & Hedges, 2004).
3. A pressure patch should never be applied to a patient who has a penetrating injury. Pressure applied to a globe that has anterior or posterior penetration can cause extrusion of the aqueous or vitreous humor, resulting in further injury to the eye. A protective cup should be used.

---

*Indicates portions of the procedure usually performed by a physician or an advanced practice nurse.

4. A pressure patch must be firm enough to keep the eyelid closed. A corneal abrasion may result if the patient is able to open the eye(s) under the patch, thereby scraping off new cells and further irritating the abraded area.
5. A patch should remain in place for no more than 24 hours; if it is left on too long, it may interfere with a diagnosis of infection, because while wearing a patch, the patient cannot monitor vision or discharge from the eye. If needed, a new patch can be placed to reduce the risk of infection.
6. Avoid placing tape directly onto the eyebrow.

EQUIPMENT

Eye patches (minimum of two per affected eye)
Metal eye shield (for selected injuries as noted above)
Tapeless eye shield (for long-term use)
Tape (1-inch paper tape, or nonallergenic tape)
Eye medications as prescribed

PATIENT PREPARATION

1. Place the patient in a supine position or seated with the head tilted back.
2. Cleanse the skin around the eye to remove dirt, fluids, drainage, or residual eye medications.
3. Facial hairs may interfere with taping the patch and may need to be trimmed to anchor the tape securely.
4. Consider instillation of a dilating eye drop, per physician or advanced registered nurse practitioner order, to relax ciliary muscle spasm. Consider also the use of a prophylactic antibiotic ointment before patching (Knoop, Dennis, & Hedges, 2004).

PROCEDURAL STEPS
Soft Patches

1. Determine the number of eye pads needed according to the depth of the patient's eye socket:
   a. Ask the patient to close both eyes gently, and to keep them closed during entire procedure.
   b. Fold the first eye patch in half vertically and place it horizontally over the closed lid.
   c. Cover that patch with one or more flat eye patches to fill the eye socket.
2. Tape the patches, starting from the mid-forehead to the cheek and apply firm pressure to the lid. Several strips of tape are necessary. Avoid placing tape near angle of the mandible to avoid loosening with jaw movement. Benzoin can be used to help the tape adhere to skin provided it is not used too close to the eye.
3. The tape should cover the entire eye patch to prevent slipping of the patch and movement of the eyelid (Figure 163-1). If the patient can blink, the patch should be reapplied.

Metal Eye Shield

1. Stabilize any protruding objects with gauze dressings and tape.
2. Place a metal shield or a paper cup over the affected eye. The shield should contact the superior and inferior orbital rims but not touch the eyelid. The

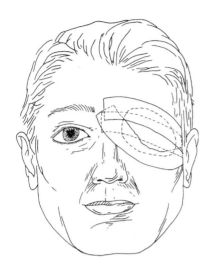

FIGURE 163-1 Eye patch taped in place.

eye shield or cup may need to be cut to accommodate a protruding object (see Procedure 165).
3. Apply strips of tape to secure the shield so that movement or irritation from a foreign object is eliminated.
4. The uninjured eye is often patched with soft patches to minimize movement of the injured eye; patching one eye doesn't totally immobilize the globe because of conjugate eye movement.

AGE-SPECIFIC CONSIDERATIONS
1. Pediatric patients may be more receptive to eye patching if you tell them the patch is like what a pirate wears.
2. Elderly patients may benefit from assistance with routine ambulation after eye patch application.

COMPLICATIONS
1. Eye patches applied too tightly can result in increased ocular damage (e.g., central retinal artery occlusion).
2. Further trauma may occur to the injured eye from excessive lid motion under a loose eye patch.
3. Eyelashes trapped between the lids can cause corneal abrasion.

PATIENT TEACHING
1. Emphasize need for follow-up.
2. Report any increase in eye pain or signs of infection, such as redness, swelling, or drainage.
3. Limit reading and computer work to help rest the injured eye because both eyes move together. Television viewing from a distance of 10 feet or more is acceptable because it promotes eye fixation (Knoop, Dennis, & Hedges, 2004).
4. Patching affects depth perception. Driving or operating dangerous machinery should be avoided. You may have difficulty walking up and down stairs.
5. Patching does not affect distance vision.

REFERENCES

Jacobs, D.S. (2001). *Corneal abrasions and corneal foreign bodies.* In 2002 UpToDate, version 10.2. www.uptodate.com.

Macsai, M.S. (2000). The management of corneal trauma: advances in the past 25 years. *Cornea, 9,* 617-624.

Knoop, K.J., Dennis, W.R., & Hedges, J.R. (2004). Ophthalmologic procedures (pp. 1241-1279). Roberts, J.R., & Hedges, J.R. (Eds.). *Clinical procedures in emergency medicine,* 4th ed. Philadelphia: W.B. Saunders.

PROCEDURE 164

Tonometry

Maureen T. Quigley, MS, ARNP, CEN

INDICATIONS

To assess intraocular pressure (IOP) under certain conditions:

1. Patients at risk of increased IOP, including hypertensive elderly patients who have glaucoma, normotensive children, adult patients who have glaucoma, and patients who have diabetes or a history of retinal detachment.

2. Patients suspected of having acute angle-closure glaucoma. When a patient complains of acute aching pain in one eye, blurred vision (including "halos" around lights), and a red eye with a smoky cornea, and a fixed midposition pupil, IOP should be determined (Knoop, Dennis, & Hedges, 2004). Sometimes the only complaints may be nausea, vomiting, and headache, suggesting a flu rather than an eye disorder (Knoop, Dennis, & Hedges, 2004).

3. Patients who have sustained blunt ocular injury. Acute increases in IOP are often seen in patients with hyphema (Knoop, Dennis, & Hedges, 2004).

4. Patients who have iritis can develop both open- and closed-angle glaucoma, as well as steroid-induced glaucoma (Knoop, Dennis, & Hedges, 2004).

CONTRAINDICATIONS AND CAUTIONS

1. Tonometry should not be performed if there is any question about the integrity of the globe. Application of pressure to the eye may lead to extrusion of contents and loss of vision.

2. For accurate determination of pressure, the patient must be completely relaxed. Patients who are unable to sustain a relaxed position because of anxiety, blepharospasm, uncontrolled coughing, or nystagmus cannot toler-

ate a satisfactory examination, and corneal injury may result when sudden movements occur during an examination (Knoop, Dennis, & Hedges, 2004).

3. When corneal defects are present, tonometry is relatively contraindicated. An abraded cornea may suffer further injury if a tonometer is used (Knoop, Dennis, & Hedges, 2004).

4. In the presence of eye infection, tonometry is relatively contraindicated. When possible, tonometry should be avoided in patients with active ocular and facial herpetic lesions as well as in those with acquired immune deficiency syndrome (Knoop, Dennis, & Hedges, 2004). A tonometer with a covered tip, such as Tono-Pen XL or Schiøtz with a sterile, disposable covering, should be used to measure IOP in infected eyes.

5. There are multiple limitations with the use and accurate interpretation of the Schiøtz tonometer, which are beyond the scope of this discussion. Potential inaccuracies occur with differences in ocular rigidity between eyes, scleral rigidity, or extremes in corneal shapes or thickness (Smith and Doyle, 1999).

6. The Tono-Pen XL is useful in measurement of IOP in patients with scarred or irregular corneas. It is believed that readings in the normal range are accurate, but they may not be accurate in readings that are in high and low ranges, underestimating high range IOPs, and overestimating IOPs in the low range (Smith and Doyle, 1999).

EQUIPMENT

Topical ophthalmic anesthetic

Tonometer (several types available) (Table 164-1). Tonometers work on the physical principle that the force needed to deform a globe is directly related to the pressure within the globe. There are three basic types:

1. Indentation or high displacement tonometers determine IOP with a plunger that changes the shape of the cornea, making a measurable indentation, which displaces a significant volume of intraocular fluid. Conversion tables are used to estimate the original IOP from the indentation tonometric read-

TABLE 164-1

COMPARISON OF DIFFERENT TONOMETRY DEVICES

	Devices			
	Schiøtz	**Goldmann**	**Tono-Pen**	**Pulsair**
Accuracy	Good	Excellent	Good	Good
Training	Minimal	Extensive	Minimal	Minimal
Difficulty	Simple	Complex	Simple	Simple
Cost	Low	Moderate	High	High
Position	Supine	Seated	Any	Any
Cross-contamination potential	Yes	Yes	No	No
Pediatric use	Difficult	Difficult	Simple	Simple
Portability	Yes	No	Yes	No

From Dieckmann, R., Fiser, D., & Selbst, S. (1997). Illustrated textbook of *pediatric emergency and critical care procedures* (p. 486). St. Louis: Mosby.

ing. An example is the Schiøtz tonometer, which is likely to be found in many emergency departments because of familiarity and relatively low cost.

2. Low-displacement or applanation tonometers measure IOP by using a force necessary to only flatten the cornea, which is converted to an IOP value. Examples include Goldmann, Perkins (portable), Draeger (portable), Maklakov, MacKay-Marg, and Tono-Pen XL (portable). The Goldmann applantation tonometer is considered the "gold standard" for IOP measurement (Smith and Doyle, 1999).

3. The noncontact tonometer applanates the cornea through a puff of air, measuring IOP without contact with the cornea. An example is the Keeler Pulsair device. The time needed to flatten the cornea is correlated with an estimated IOP. Noncontact tonometers are not useful when accurate readings are indicated; they are more helpful for screening purposes.

PATIENT PREPARATION
1. Place the patient in a darkened room to help decrease ocular pain.
2. Place the patient in a supine position or in a reclining chair.
3. Instruct the patient not to blink or touch the eyes during the procedure.

PROCEDURAL STEPS
Schiøtz and Tono-Pen XL tonometers are discussed in this section. Review complete instructions provided by manufacturer.

Schiøtz Tonometer (Figure 164-1)
1. Instill topical anesthetics or cycloplegics as prescribed. Anesthetics should be administered before cycloplegics.
2. Place the patient in a supine or semirecumbent position.
3. Ask the patient to gaze at a fixed spot directly above the eyes.
4. *While the patient keeps both eyes wide open and fixed on an object, separate the eyelids. Be careful to apply direct pressure to the orbital rims instead of into the orbit to avoid obtaining an IOP reading that is falsely raised with pressure into the orbit (Knoop, Dennis, & Hedges, 2004).
5. *Gently place the footplate of the tonometer onto the middle portion of the cornea in a position that allows free vertical movement of the plunger.
6. Fine movements on the scale indicate response to the ocular pulsations. The scale reading should be taken as the average between the extremes of these excursions. Extra weight should be added to the plunger when the scale reading is 5 or less (Knoop, Dennis, & Hedges, 2004). The IOP is derived from the scale reading and the plunger weight using a conversion table (Figure 164-2). The same procedure is repeated in the other eye. Normal IOP values are 12-21 mm Hg.

Tono-Pen XL (Figure 164-3)
1. Follow steps 1 and 2 of the procedure used for the Schiøtz tonometer.
2. The patient can be in any position that permits the Tono-Pen XL to be applied perpendicular to the corneal surface.

---

*Indicates portions of the procedure usually performed by a physician or an advanced practice nurse.

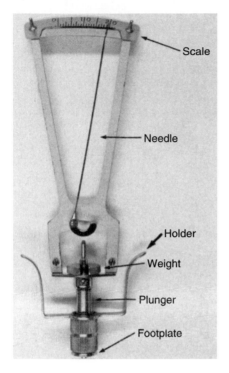

Scale

Needle

Holder

Weight

Plunger

Footplate

FIGURE 164-1 Schiøtz tonometer. (From Albert, D., & Jakobiec, F. [2000]. *Principles and practice of ophthalmology,* 2nd ed. [p. 2627]. Philadelphia: W.B. Saunders.)

3. Cover the probe tip of the calibrated Tono-Pen XL with a new Mentor Ocu-Film tip cover.
4. *Holding the Tono-Pen XL like a pencil, depress the activation switch briefly and then release.
5. When the Tono-Pen XL is available to take a measurement, a beep sounds, and a pattern (= = =) appears on the liquid crystal display.
6. *Touch the Tono-Pen XL unit to the cornea lightly and momentarily, and repeat several times.
7. When a valid reading is obtained, a click sounds, and a digital IOP measurement is exhibited.
8. A final beep is heard after four correct readings have been obtained. The average measurement with variability percentages appears on the liquid crystal display.

AGE-SPECIFIC CONSIDERATIONS

1. Hand-held applanation tonometers and the Tono-Pen are helpful in assessment of children. The normal intraocular pressure in young children is underestimated by applanation tonometry, especially in children under 3 years of age under general anesthesia. The Tono-Pen correlates relatively well with applanation tonometry in children with IOP in the normal range, but it may underestimate elevated IOP.

---

*Indicates portions of the procedure usually performed by a physician or an advanced practice nurse.

Scale Reading	Plunger Load (g)			
	5.5	7.5	10.0	15.0
0	41	59	82	127
.5	38	54	75	118
1.0	35	50	70	109
1.5	32	46	64	101
2.0	29	42	59	94
2.5	27	39	55	88
3.0	24	36	51	82
3.5	22	33	47	76
4.0	21	30	43	71
4.5	19	28	40	66
5.0	17	26	37	62
5.5	16	24	34	58
6.0	15	22	32	54
6.5	13	20	29	50
7.0	12	19	27	46
7.5	11	17	25	43
8.0	10	16	23	40
8.5	9	14	21	38
9.0	9	13	20	35
9.5	8	12	18	32
10.0	7	11	16	30
10.5	6	10	15	27
11.0	6	9	14	25
11.5	5	8	13	23
12.0		8	11	21
12.5		7	10	20
13.0		6	10	18
13.5		6	9	17
14.0		5	8	15
14.5			7	14
15.0			6	13
15.5			6	11
16.0			5	10
16.5				9
17.0				8
17.5				8
18.0				7

FIGURE 164-2 Intraocular pressure table for use with the Schiøtz tonometer. (Courtesy J. Sklar Manufacturing Co., Inc., Long Island City, NY.)

2. Infants and young children often require examination under sedation (see Procedure 181) or general anesthesia for definitive evaluation of IOP (Beck, 2001).

COMPLICATIONS

1. Extrusion of the globe contents can occur during the examination if there is a penetrating injury to the globe.
2. Contaminated tonometers transmit infection. In addition to the more ordinary bacteria and viruses that can cause ocular infection, hepatitis B surface antigen can be detected from the tonometer tip after use on infected patients (Albert and Jakobiec, 1994). To inactivate infectious human immunodeficiency virus, herpes, or adenovirus, the Centers for Disease Control and Prevention recommends wiping the tip of the tonometer clean and then disinfecting it with bleach. The entire prism should be removed from the tonometer and submerged for 5 minutes in a container that holds a 1:10 dilution of household bleach. The container should hold the applanating surface and the adjacent 2-3 mm of the tonometer. The tip should then be washed

TOP VIEW   SIDE VIEW

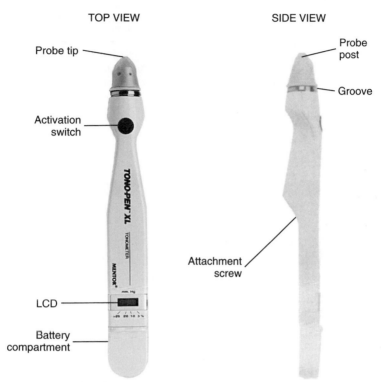

FIGURE 164-3 Iono-Pen diagram. (Courtesy Mentor O & O, Inc. [1993]. *Mentor Tono-Pen XL tonometer instruction manual* [p. 4]. Norwell, MA: Author.)

under running water and dried. Another option proposed by the Centers for Disease Control and Prevention calls for soaking the tip in 3% hydrogen peroxide (Schottenstein, 1996). This process is not necessary with the Tono-Pen because a new Ocu-Film tip cover is used for each patient.

3. Corneal abrasions can be caused by movement of the eye during measurement of IOP with contact tonometers.

PATIENT TEACHING

1. Do not blink or touch your eyes during the examination.
2. Do not rub your eyes for at least 30 minutes after the examination.
3. Do not bend over, cough, blow your nose, or strain at stool (if IOP is elevated).

REFERENCES

Albert, D., & Jakobiec, F. (1994). *Principles and practice of ophthalmology.* Philadelphia: W.B. Saunders.

Beck, A.D. (2001). Diagnosis and management of pediatric glaucoma. *Ophthalmology Clinics of North America, 14,* 501-12.

Dieckmann, R., Fiser, D., Selbst, S. (1997). *Pediatric emergency and critical care procedures* (p. 486). St. Louis: Mosby.

Knoop, K.J., Dennis, W.R., & Hedges, J.R. (2004). Ophthalmologic procedures (pp. 1241-1279). Roberts, J.R., & Hedges, J.R. (Eds.). *Clinical procedures in emergency medicine*, 4th ed. Philadelphia: W.B. Saunders.

Schottenstein, E. (1996). Intraocular pressure and tonometry (pp. 407-421). In Ritch, R., Shields, M., & Krupin, T. (Eds.). *The glaucomas*, 2nd ed. St. Louis: Mosby.

Smith, M.F., & Doyle, J.W. (1999). Clinical examination of glaucoma (section 12.4-1.3). In Yanoff, M. (Ed.). *Ophthalmology*. St. Louis: Mosby.

PROCEDURE 165

Immobilization of an Ophthalmic Foreign Body

Maureen T. Quigley, MS, ARNP, CEN

INDICATION
To immobilize a foreign object penetrating the eye or periorbital region

CONTRAINDICATIONS AND CAUTIONS
1. Ophthalmic injuries are treated immediately after life-threatening conditions are stabilized.
2. Do not apply pressure to the eye. Direct pressure should not be used to stop bleeding from or around the eye when a penetrating object is suspected or evident.
3. The use of ophthalmic ointments is contraindicated because they may enter the globe and, in the case of anesthetic ointments, may have a prolonged effect.
4. Uncooperative patients should be examined under sedation or general anesthesia (Harlan and Pieramici, 2002).

EQUIPMENT
Rigid eye shields
Gauze eye patches
4 × 4 gauze dressings
Fluffs
Roller bandages
Paper cups
Adhesive tape
Skin preparation material, such as alcohol or acetone

PATIENT PREPARATION

1. Instruct the patient not to touch or rub the eye.
2. Unless contraindicated by other injuries, elevate the head of the bed to decrease intraocular pressure.
3. Administer an antiemetic as prescribed to decrease nausea and vomiting if needed.
4. Administer tetanus immunization as indicated.
5. Maintain nothing per mouth (NPO) status in light of a possible operative intervention and ascertain when the patient had his or her last meal.
6. Obtain previous ophthalmic history: previous surgery and trauma, as well as vision before the presenting injury.
7. Key components of the history include the exact time of injury and events leading to the injury. Other important information include a description and composition of the foreign body (Table 165-1), the distance it traveled to the eye, whether it was blown by the wind or propelled into the eye, the direction of travel, and the direction in which the eye was looking at the time of the injury.

PROCEDURAL STEPS

1. Use a thick dressing to immobilize the foreign object. A variety of materials can be used, including a gauze dressing, fluffs, a paper drinking cup, or a paper cone.
2. Place the dressing around the foreign object to immobilize it and prevent further injury to the eye and surrounding structures. A hole may be cut in the center of the dressing, or the dressing can be arranged around the penetrating object to further immobilize it; the penetrating object should be in the center of the bandage.

TABLE 165-1

MOST COMMONLY SEEN INTRAOCULAR METALLIC AND NONMETALLIC FOREIGN BODIES

Metallic		Nonmetallic	
Toxic	Nontoxic	Toxic	Nontoxic
Aluminum	Gold	Cilia	Carbon
Brass	Platinum	Cloth particles	Glass
Bronze	Silver	Eyelid particle	Plastic (some types)
Copper		Plant matter	Porcelain
Iron		Sawdust	Stone
Lead		Wood	
Mercury			
Nickel			
Steel			
Zinc			

Data from Larson, S., & Rossi, J. (1992). In Schwartz, G. et al. (Eds.) *Principles and practice of emergency medicine,* 3rd ed. (pp. 765-770). Philadelphia: Lea & Febiger; Janda, A.M. (1996). Ocular emergencies. In Tintinalli, J. et al. (Eds.). *A comprehensive study guide,* 4th ed. (pp. 1059-1068). New York: McGraw-Hill.

3. Place a paper cup or other solid, lightweight object over the penetrating object. The paper cup should rest on the dressing. It should not place pressure on the eye or touch the penetrating object. With larger penetrating objects, it may be difficult or impossible to cover the end of the penetrating object with this type of protective bandage.
4. Patch or shield the uninjured eye to prevent movement in the injured eye (see Procedure 163). If rupture of the globe is suspected, be careful to apply a metal or plastic eye shield resting on the forehead and bony arch of the orbit.

AGE-SPECIFIC CONSIDERATIONS

1. Young children may require an immobilization device, such as a child restraint board, or sedation/anesthesia to be evaluated effectively (see Procedures 181 and 193).
2. In the elderly, eye and orbital trauma are frequently caused by falls, which may also cause other injuries, such as hip fractures. A fall could represent underlying cardiovascular disease, such as an arrhythmia or hypotension, which would necessitate further evaluation.
3. A child may be reluctant to provide a history of the injury if it involved behavior that was inappropriate.
4. A provider should consider abuse or neglect in the child or elder when a caregiver or parent seems unwilling to provide information about the injury.

COMPLICATIONS

1. Bacterial or fungal infection
2. Loss of vision or visual acuity
3. Penetration of sinuses or brain with concurrent risk of meningitis

PATIENT TEACHING

1. Do not touch or rub the injured eye.
2. Do not strain, cough, bend over, or lift heavy objects because pressure within the eye will be increased.
3. In some situations, both eyes may be patched to decrease eye movement.
4. Use protective eyewear when appropriate to prevent future injuries.
5. A safe home environment/living arrangement is crucial after a serious eye injury.

REFERENCES

Harlan, J.B. Jr., & Pieramici, D.J. (2002). Evaluation of patients with ocular trauma. *Ophthalmology Clinics of North America, 15,* 153-61.
Janda, A.M. (1996). Ocular emergencies (pp. 1059-1068). In Tintinalli, J., Krome, R., & Ruiz, E. (Eds.). *Emergency medicine: a comprehensive study guide,* 4th ed. New York: McGraw-Hill.
Larson, S., & Rossi, J. [1992]. In Schwartz, G., Cayten, C.G., Mangelsen, M.A., et al. (Eds.) *Principles and practice of emergency medicine,* 3rd ed. (pp. 765-770). Philadelphia: Lea & Febiger.

Otic Procedures

Instillation of Ear Medications

Daun A. Smith, RN, MS, CEN

INDICATION

To apply medicated solutions or suspensions (antibiotics, steroids, analgesics, or ceruminolytic agents) into the external auditory canal for otitis externa (swimmer's ear), otitis media, or cerumen accumulation.

CONTRAINDICATIONS AND CAUTIONS

1. Caution should be exercised to identify perforation of the tympanic membrane before instilling medications into the external auditory canal, because inadvertent introduction of foreign material into the middle ear may result in a bacterial infection.
2. Medications in suspension (oil based) do not absorb into ear wicks. Use ear wicks with medication in solution form only.
3. Ear medications should be single-patient use only.

EQUIPMENT

Otoscope
Ear wicks or cotton balls
Ear medication (antibiotic, analgesic, or ceruminolytic agent) as prescribed

PROCEDURAL STEPS

1. Place the patient on his or her side with the affected ear up.
2. Straighten and examine the external auditory canal. For an infant, gently pull the pinna down and back. For a child older than 3 years of age or an adult, pull the pinna up and backward.
3. Clear any debris from the ear canal (see Procedures 168 and 169).
4. Warm the ear medication container by holding it in your hand or placing it in warm water for a short time.
5. Draw up only the amount of medication needed into the ear dropper. Do not return excess medication to the bottle.
6. Instill the correct number of drops along the side of the ear canal. To prevent contamination, do not allow the tip of the ear dropper to touch any part of the ear. Hold it about $1/2$ inch above the ear canal.
7. Press firmly but gently on the tragus of the ear a few times. This helps the medication reach all portions of the canal.
8. Have the patient remain in the same position (with the affected ear up) for a few minutes.

9. Place a small piece of a cotton ball at the external auditory meatus for 15 minutes to help retain the medication when the patient is up. Do not press the cotton into the canal.

10. If an ear wick is to be used, see Procedure 167. Saturate the wick with a topical otic solution.

AGE-SPECIFIC CONSIDERATION

To straighten the external auditory canal of an infant, gently pull the pinna down and back; for a child older than 3 years of age or an adult, pull the pinna up and backward.

COMPLICATIONS

1. If cotton balls are used instead of an ear wick, disintegration may occur, and removal may be difficult. To avoid retention of pieces of cotton balls, place them only at the meatus.

2. Without an ear wick or cotton ball, solutions or suspensions may extravasate from the ear canal.

3. Otic solutions frequently cause a burning or stinging sensation; suspensions are less painful.

PATIENT TEACHING

1. Report immediately ear pain, an edematous canal, tender ear cartilage, purulent drainage, or hearing loss.

2. Leave the ear wick in place for 48-72 hours. Repeat instillation of medication onto the ear wick three to four times daily or as directed.

3. Continuation of medication may be necessary after ear wick removal (approximately 10 days for antibiotics).

4. If an ear wick is not used, you may place a cotton ball at the external auditory meatus to prevent extravasation of the medication.

PROCEDURE 167

Ear Wick Insertion

Margo E. Layman, MSN, RN, RNC, CN-A

INDICATION

An ear wick assists in keeping medication in the external ear canal to treat otitis externa.

CONTRAINDICATIONS AND CAUTIONS
1. If there are lacerations of the ear canal, an ear wick should not be inserted.
2. An ear wick could slip into the hole of a ruptured tympanic membrane.
3. Alcohol or acidic medications may cause a burning or stinging sensation.
4. If the ear canal is swollen shut, a wick cannot be inserted.

EQUIPMENT
Cotton, ½-inch × ½-inch selvedged gauze, or 2 × 10-mm compressed hydroxy-
cellulose manufactured ear wick
Prescribed ear drops
Cerumen spoon
Small metal suction tip
Small alligator forceps
Otoscope

PATIENT PREPARATION
Place the patient in semi-Fowler's position.

PROCEDURAL STEPS
1. Using an otoscope, check the external ear for redness or drainage.
2. Examine the internal ear with an otoscope.
3. Suction debris from the ear with the small metal suction tip, or remove debris gently with a cerumen spoon.
4. Irrigation may necessary before placement of ear wick to allow effective dispersal of medications to inflamed tissue.
5. Use a small alligator forceps to twist the ear wick in place in the canal. Follow the accompanying directions to insert a commercially prepared wick, or make a wick by wrapping cotton or selvedged gauze tightly around the tip of an alligator forceps, grasping the cotton or gauze with the forceps, and placing it in the ear canal.
6. Place the prescribed ear drops in the ear canal, taking care not to touch the dropper to the ear canal. Place drops along the side of the canal so that air is displaced as they flow. Cold drops may cause vertigo; this can be avoided by warming the medication slightly in your hands or by immersing the bottle in a cup of warm water for several minutes.
7. Place 1 or 2 additional drops on the ear wick to saturate it.

AGE-SPECIFIC CONSIDERATION
Place a small child in the supine position, restraining the knees, and holding the arms firmly against the head with the face turned left or right.

COMPLICATIONS
1. The ear wick may adhere to the ear canal if it is not kept moist.
2. The ear wick may slip deeper into the canal. This could cause irritation of the tympanic membrane.

PATIENT TEACHING
1. Return in 48 hours to have ear wick removed or follow up with your physician to have removed. Make sure the wick is moist before removing it.

2. Instill ear drops as instructed. Cold ear drops may cause dizziness. Warm the bottle between your hands or in a cup of warm water before instilling the drops.
3. Symptoms should subside in 1 or 2 days. If no improvement occurs or if symptoms worsen, contact your physician.
4. To prevent the ear wick from slipping, do not touch the ear, and do not place cotton in ear canal over wick, because the cotton will absorb all the drops.
5. Take oral pain medications as prescribed and apply a warm moist compress to ear for pain.
6. To prevent future infections, do not put foreign objects in the ear. Ear rinses used after swimming may be helpful. Avoid strong jets from shower heads.

PROCEDURE 168

Ear Irrigation

Lucinda W. Rossoll, BSN, MS, CEN, CCRN, ARNP

INDICATIONS
1. To remove drainage, cerumen, or foreign bodies from the external auditory canal
2. To irrigate the external auditory canal with an antiseptic solution
3. To apply heat or cold to the external auditory canal

CONTRAINDICATIONS AND CAUTIONS
1. Irrigation is contraindicated if the tympanic membrane is perforated or potentially not intact (secondary to injury, myringotomy tubes, or surgery).
2. If complications occurred during previous ear irrigations, caution should be used.
3. Avoid extreme temperatures, which may cause dizziness, nausea, and vomiting.
4. If there is water-absorbent material in the ear, such as vegetable matter (e.g., beans), do not irrigate, because the material may swell and make removal more difficult (see Procedure 169).
5. Be careful not to abrade the ear canal with the intravenous catheter.

EQUIPMENT
Otologic ear syringe (metal ear syringe)
or
60-ml syringe with an 18- or 20-G intravenous catheter sheath attached, or a butterfly that is cut about 1½ inches from the hub end

or
Dental irrigating device (WaterPik) on low setting
Irrigant—warm water, warm normal saline, or half strength hydrogen
  peroxide
Basin to hold irrigant
Towels or waterproof pad
Emesis basin
Otoscope
Gloves
Thermometer (optional)
Cotton balls or gauze dressings
Cotton-tipped applicators

PATIENT PREPARATION
1. Position the patient with the head tilted toward the affected ear.
2. Protect the patient's clothing with towels or a waterproof pad.

PROCEDURAL STEPS
1. Cleanse the outer ear of any discharge with a cotton-tipped applicator.
2. Examine the ear with an otoscope before starting the irrigation. To examine the ear, pull the auricle of the ear up and outward to straighten the ear canal.
3. Draw up the irrigation solution into the syringe and expel the air from the syringe. The solution may be water alone or water and hydrogen peroxide mixed 1:1. The solution should be at body temperature. If you drip some of the solution onto your inner wrist, it should be a comfortable temperature, or you can check the temperature with a thermometer.
4. Ask the patient to hold the emesis basin under the ear and against the neck.
5. Pull the auricle of the ear up and backward (Figure 168-1, *A*). Place the tip of the irrigating syringe at the opening of the ear canal. Do not occlude the opening of the ear canal, because this can cause excessive pressure, which could in turn lead to rupture of the tympanic membrane. Direct the fluid toward the posterior wall of the canal (Figure 168-1, *C*). Visualize the perimeter of the canal as a clock face. For the left ear, direct the fluid toward 1 o'clock; for the right ear, direct the fluid toward 11 o'clock (Zivic & King, 1993).
6. Irrigate slowly to prevent build-up of pressure inside the canal.
7. After each irrigation, inspect the ear canal to assess the progress being made, or check the irrigation solution as it returns to the basin for cerumen or foreign bodies.
8. Repeat the irrigation as needed, allowing the patient to rest between each irrigation if necessary.
9. If irrigation does not remove the cerumen, instill several drops of glycerin, carbamide peroxide (Debrox) or other solutions as prescribed 2-3 times a day to soften and dislodge cerumen (Nettina, 2001). Irrigation may be reattempted if cerumen impaction does not spontaneously resolve.
10. Dry the outer ear with a cotton ball. The cotton ball may be left loosely in place for 5-10 minutes to absorb any excess moisture.

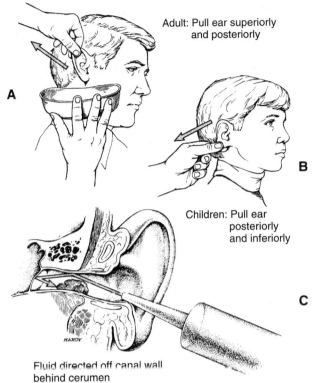

Adult: Pull ear superiorly
and posteriorly

A

B

Children: Pull ear
posteriorly
and inferiorly

C

HARDY

Fluid directed off canal wall
behind cerumen

FIGURE 168-1 Straightening the ear canal in an adult, **A,** in a child, **B,** and where to direct the irrigating fluid, **C.** (From Nettina, S.M. [2001]. *The Lippincott manual of nursing practice,* 7th ed. [p. 554]. Philadelphia: Lippincott Williams & Wilkins.)

AGE-SPECIFIC CONSIDERATIONS

1. The ear canal in a child is small. Caution should be exercised to avoid totally occluding the canal during irrigation, thus avoiding excessive pressure within the ear canal.
2. To straighten the ear canal in a child younger than 3 years of age, pull the ear down and outward (Figure 168-1, *B*).
3. Place the child in the supine position. If the child is uncooperative and all other appropriate control measures have failed, a child restraint board may be used to prevent movement (see Procedure 193).
4. A dental irrigation device should be used with caution in children because the jet stream is forceful. Use the lowest setting and aim toward the posterior wall of the ear canal. To decrease the child's fear, explain the procedure and demonstrate the device, allowing the child to feel the water on his or her hand and listen to the noise.
5. Do not use cool irrigant because dizziness or discomfort may result, especially in the older patient (Ernst et al., 1999).

COMPLICATIONS

1. Vertigo, nausea, or pain during or after the procedure. Stop immediately if any of these symptoms occur. Allow the patient to rest until the symptoms resolve and then restart. Be sure gentle pressure is used. Aim at the posterior portion of the ear canal and use the proper irrigant temperature to help prevent recurrence of symptoms.
2. Rupture of the tympanic membrane.
3. Loss of hearing.
4. Trauma or injury to the ear canal.

PATIENT TEACHING

1. Report any pain, nausea, dizziness, or loss of hearing as it occurs during or after the procedure.
2. Cleanse the outer ears daily with a washcloth, soap, and water.
3. Do not place objects in your ears.

REFERENCES

Ernst, A.A., Takakuwa, K.M., Letner, C., & Weiss, S. (1999) Warmed versus room temperature saline solution for ear irrigation: a randomized clinical trial. *Annals of Emergency Medicine, 34,* 347-350.

Nettina, S.M. (2001). *The Lippincott manual of nursing practice,* 7th ed. (pp. 552-554). Philadelphia: Lippincott Williams & Wilkins.

Zivic, R.C., & King, S. (1993). Cerumen-impaction: management for clients of all ages. *Nurse Practitioner, 18*(3), 29-36.

PROCEDURE 169

Otic Foreign Body Removal

Daun A. Smith, RN, MS, CEN

INDICATION

To remove a foreign body from the ear by means of water irrigation, suction, direct instrumentation, or magnet when digital removal has failed

CONTRAINDICATIONS AND CAUTIONS

1. Anatomic narrowing occurs at two separate points in the external auditory canal. Many objects can become lodged at these points. Avoid pushing a

foreign body beyond these narrowings during extrication attempts because damage to the ear may result (Figure 169-1).

2. The ear canal is sensitive, and instrumentation can be very painful. Conscious sedation or general anesthesia may be necessary.
3. If the patient's history or physical examination suggests a tympanic membrane disruption, irrigation is contraindicated for foreign body removal.
4. Irrigation of foreign bodies that have the potential to swell and become more firmly impacted when hydrated (e.g., vegetable matter) is contraindicated.
5. Live insects should be killed before removal is attempted. Instill mineral oil or alcohol into the ear to kill the insect. Another method is to irrigate with 2% lidocaine solution, which quickly kills the insect (Tami et al., 1992).
6. Miniature batteries lodged in the ear canal pose a special problem. In addition to a potential mechanical trauma, a chemical reaction may occur as a result of leakage of the battery contents. Tympanic membrane perforation, facial paralysis, or ossicular chain damage may result. Prompt removal of the battery using a right-angle hook followed by water irrigation is imperative to avoid these complications (Cannon, 1988).
7. Contralateral ear examination should be performed to rule out bilateral ear foreign bodies.
8. Instrumentation or direct irrigation onto the foreign body may cause it to move deeper into the canal toward the tympanic membrane.
9. If the foreign body cannot be easily removed, referral to an ear, nose, and throat specialist is warranted. Repeated unsuccessful attempts at removal may injure the auditory canal.

EQUIPMENT

Various procedures may be used for removal of a foreign body from the ear. Some or all of the following equipment may be needed:

Adequate light source (otoscope or headlamp)

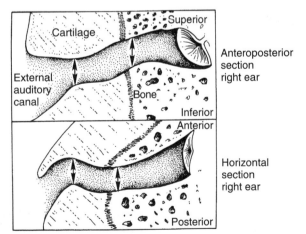

FIGURE 169-1 Horizontal and vertical cross-sections of external ear canal showing points of anatomic narrowing. (From Thomas, S.H., & Brown, D.F.M. [2002]. Foreign bodies [p. 754]. In Marx, J.A., Hockberger, R.S., Walls, R.M., et al. (Eds.), *Rosen's emergency medicine: concepts and clinical practice,* 5th ed. St. Louis: Mosby.)

Ear speculum

Magnetized speculum (used for removal of metallic batteries)

Blunt right-angle hook, wire loops, cerumen curette, alligator or bayonet forceps (Figure 169-2)

Suction catheter (Frazier)

Suction setup

Schuknecht foreign body remover (a suction catheter that works well on smooth, round foreign bodies)

Irrigation equipment (20-ml syringe with flexible 18-G intravenous catheter or the tubing of a butterfly catheter with the needle removed) (Figure 169-3)

Fogarty biliary catheter

PATIENT PREPARATION

1. Sedate or restrain the patient as indicated (see Procedures 181 and 193).
2. Emphasize the importance of not moving during the procedure.
3. For irrigation, drape the patient with towels and place an emesis basin nearby for collection of the irrigation fluid.

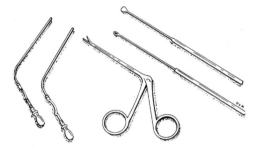

FIGURE 169-2 Instruments used for removal of foreign bodies from the external auditory canal (left to right): Frazier suction catheters, alligator forceps, wire loop, and ear curette. (From Votey, S., & Dudley, J.P. [1989]. Emergency ear, nose, and throat procedures. *Emergency Medicine Clinics of North America, 7,* 124.)

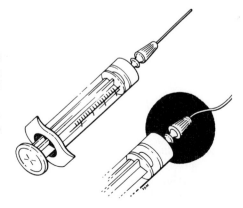

FIGURE 169-3 A flexible 18-G intravenous catheter attached to a 20-ml syringe (left) and a butterfly catheter with the needle cut off attached to a 20-ml syringe (right). (From Votey, S., & Dudley, J.P. [1989]. Emergency ear, nose, and throat procedures. *Emergency Medicine Clinics of North America, 7,* 124.)

PROCEDURAL STEPS

One or more of the following procedures may be necessary to remove a foreign body from the external auditory canal:

1. *Place the tip of the suction catheter on the foreign body and gently retract (Figure 169-4). If using a Schuknecht foreign body remover, apply suction only after the catheter has conformed to the shape of the foreign body.
2. Irrigate the ear canal with lukewarm water to avoid stimulating the labyrinths. Direct the stream of fluid to the edge of the foreign body and attempt to force the fluid gently behind the foreign body and out the ear canal (see Procedure 168).
3. *Pass a right-angle hook (blunt ended) beyond the foreign body and gently retract.
4. *If removing a battery, observe the battery directly and insert a solid ferro-magnetic metallic speculum into the external auditory meatus. The object should move toward the speculum and can then be withdrawn.
5. *Insert a Fogarty biliary catheter past the foreign body, inflate the balloon, and retract the catheter, thus dislodging the foreign body.
6. *Once the foreign body can be seen in the external ear canal, it can be removed with a forceps, a curette, or a loop.
7. *If removing a smooth round object, place a small drop of cyanoacrylate glue on the blunt end of a cotton-tipped swab. Straighten the ear canal with a slight traction (see Age-Specific Considerations number 4) to visualize the foreign object. Gently insert the blunt end of the swab into the ear canal to contact the object. The glue dries in 15 seconds, and the swab and object can both be removed. Mineral oil, alcohol, or acetone may be used to separate adherent edges if the glue comes in contact with the ear canal.

AGE-SPECIFIC CONSIDERATIONS

1. Otic foreign bodies are found most commonly in the younger pediatric population.
2. Toddlers consider any attempt to look into their ears as intrusive and threatening.

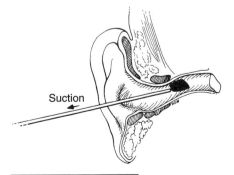

Suction

FIGURE 169-4 Use of Frazier suction catheter for removal of a foreign body in the external auditory canal. (From Votey, S., & Dudley, J.P. [1989]. Emergency ear, nose, and throat procedures. *Emergency Medicine Clinics of North America, 7,* 124.)

---

*Indicates portions of the procedure usually performed by a physician or an advanced practice nurse.

3. Occasionally, because of their age and inability to cooperate with the examination, young children may need conscious sedation or general anesthesia. For their safety, infants and toddlers should be restrained for otoscopic examination and foreign body removal. The small child can be held in the parent's lap. The parent can secure the child's arms by "hugging" the child. The child's head can then be turned with the ear to be examined tilted upward. If the child cannot be held securely in that manner, a mummy restraint or infant restraint board may be used (see Procedure 193).

4. In children who are younger than 3 years of age, the pinna should be pulled down to straighten the ear canal. In children older than 3 years, the ear canal is straightened in the same manner as an adult, by pulling up and back on the pinna.

COMPLICATIONS

1. Blind attempts at foreign body removal may lead to complications, such as tissue trauma or pushing the foreign body further into the ear canal. Direct visualization should always be used to remove foreign bodies from the ear.

2. Perforation of the tympanic membrane may occur as a complication of instrument use in the ear canal.

3. Topical antimicrobial therapy may be indicated if trauma is sustained to the epithelial tissue of the external canal during the procedure.

4. Part of the foreign body may be retained. Repeat direct observation after the foreign body has been removed.

PATIENT TEACHING

1. Do not attempt to remove foreign objects that are not readily visible or capable of being grasped easily.

2. Uncomplicated foreign body removal does not routinely require follow-up care unless there is evidence of otitis externa, injury to the external auditory canal or tympanic membrane, or retained foreign body. If drainage, fever, pain, or swelling occurs, seek medical attention.

3. Bleeding may occur as a result of damage caused by instrumentation.

4. Keep small objects away from small children to prevent recurrences.

REFERENCES

Cannon, C.R. (1988). The miniature battery: a new foreign body hazard. *Journal of Mississippi State Medical Association, 29,* 41-42.

Tami, T.A., Crumley, R.L., & Mills, J. (1992). ENT emergencies: disorders of the ears, nose, sinuses, oropharynx, and teeth (pp. 429-444). In Saunders, C.E., & Ho, M.T. (Eds.). *Current emergency diagnosis and treatment.* Norwalk, CT: Appleton & Lange.

Cerumen Removal

Daun A. Smith, RN, MS, CEN

INDICATION

To remove cerumen accumulation (partial occlusion of the ear canal) or impaction (complete occlusion of the ear canal with the tympanic membrane unable to be visualized) from the external auditory canal

CONTRAINDICATIONS AND CAUTIONS

1. An accurate history should be taken to identify signs of infection or past problems with the ears that may indicate perforation of the tympanic membrane.
2. Irrigation is contraindicated in the presence of tympanic membrane perforation, tympanotomy tubes, or an intact tympanic membrane that has an atrophic region after perforation and suboptimal spontaneous healing.
3. Otitis externa is a relative contraindication to the removal of cerumen because irrigation may aggravate the condition. Otitis externa should be treated with antibiotic eardrops, and cerumen removal should be accomplished after the condition is resolved (Fox and Bartlett, 2001).
4. Hearing loss, tinnitus, and head noise have been linked to impacted cerumen, along with the potential for psychosocial disturbances. Conductive hearing loss may be caused by cerumen impaction and is frequently overlooked (Fox and Bartlett, 2001).
5. Use of a high-pressure irrigating device may result in tympanic membrane injury.

EQUIPMENT

Otoscope
Ceruminolytic agent (optional) (triethanolamine polypeptide [Cerumenex], or docusate sodium [Colace]) (Singer et al., 2000)
Low-pressure water irrigation equipment (including ear syringe, tubing, and basin)
or
High-pressure water irrigation equipment (including WaterPik instrument, tubing, and basin)
Cerumen loop (metal or plastic)
Suction tip (optional)
Suction setup (optional)

PATIENT PREPARATION

1. Drape the patient with towels or absorbent padding to absorb excess irrigation fluid.
2. Advise the patient that sensations of dizziness are commonly experienced during irrigation.

3. The patient should be placed in a sitting or semi-Fowler's position with the head tilted toward the affected ear.

PROCEDURAL STEPS

1. Perform an otoscopic examination before and after cerumen removal. Gently pull the pinna up and back in adults (down and back in children younger than 3 years of age) before inserting the otoscope. Identify the cerumen plug and assess the integrity of the tympanic membrane.
2. If the tympanic membrane is intact, ceruminolytic agents may be used to penetrate the accumulation of cerumen and loosen the plug (see Procedure 166).
3. For irrigation, tilt the head 15 degrees toward the affected ear and position a basin to collect the fluid as it drains. Use lukewarm water to prevent dizziness and nystagmus. Direct the flow of water to the edge of the cerumen, not directly onto the tympanic membrane (see Procedure 168).
4. *Removal of cerumen can also be performed with various sizes and shapes of suction tips (Figure 170-1). Wall or portable suction can then be applied through the suction tip, which is placed directly on the cerumen plug.
5. *A cerumen loop or curette (either metal or plastic) may be used to scrape and remove cerumen gently from the external auditory canal (Figure 170-2). Curettage should never be performed blindly (Kemp, 1999).
6. If irrigation is used during the cerumen removal, gently dry the canal with a cotton-tipped applicator.

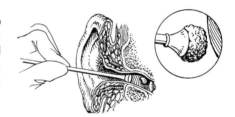

FIGURE 170-1 A suction tip can be used to remove cerumen from the ear canal. (From Harley, J.R. [1997]. Otic foreign body and cerumen removal [p. 351]. In Walsh-Sukys, M.C., & Krug, S.E. [Eds.]. *Procedures in infants and children.* Philadelphia: W.B. Saunders.)

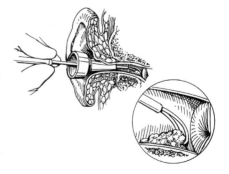

FIGURE 170-2 A curette or wire loop can be used to remove cerumen under visualization with an otoscope. (From Harley, J.R. [1997]. Otic foreign body and cerumen removal [p. 351]. In Walsh-Sukys, M.C., & Krug, S.E. [Eds.]. *Procedures in infants and children.* Philadelphia: W.B. Saunders.)

---

*Indicates portions of the procedure usually performed by a physician or an advanced practice nurse.

AGE-SPECIFIC CONSIDERATIONS

1. Cerumen impaction, accumulation, or both are common but often over-looked causes of conductive hearing loss in the elderly. Risk factors include hearing aids, overabundance of ear canal hairs, dry cerumen, and benign bony growths, such as osteophytes.
2. Small children are apprehensive about an otoscopic examination. If necessary, the small child may be positioned in the parent's lap with the child's arms secured. The parent can accomplish this by "hugging" the child. The child's head can then be turned and held with the ear to be examined turned upward (see Procedure 193).

COMPLICATIONS

1. Otitis media may result from irrigation in the presence of a tympanic membrane perforation.
2. If cold water is used with irrigation, dizziness, nystagmus, and nausea may result.
3. Damage to the external canal can occur if the lining of the canal is scratched by the instruments used for cerumen removal.
4. Perforation of the tympanic membrane can result from blind instrumentation or from sudden movements of the patient.
5. Otitis externa may result if the ear canal is not dried after irrigation (Fox and Bartlett, 2001).

PATIENT TEACHING

1. Cerumen accumulation may cause hearing loss. Hearing loss may also be caused by sensorineural problems that result from damage to the eighth cranial nerve. A combination of conductive and sensorineural hearing loss may occur. Seek medical care promptly in the presence of hearing loss.
2. Cerumen impaction, dermatitis, and skin infections may result from self-treatment with cotton swabs or other objects. Avoid introducing objects into your ears.
3. Excessive ear hair may cause difficulty in manual removal of earwax and may require special attention to prevent cerumen buildup.
4. Hearing aids may increase wax production and impede the normal propulsive action of the ear cilia.

REFERENCES

Fox, A. & Bartlett, P. (2001). Nurse-led ear care: training needs and the latest techniques. *Professional Nurse, 17*, 256-258.
Kemp, B. (1999). A practical guide to cerumen removal tools. *The Hearing Journal, 52*(4), 58-59.
Singer, A.J., Sauris, E., & Viccellio, A.W. (2000). Ceruminolytic effect of docusate sodium: a randomized controlled trial. *Annals of Emergency Medicine, 36*, 228-232.

Nasal Procedures

Topical Vasoconstrictors for Epistaxis

Margo E. Layman, MSN, RN, RNC, CN-A

INDICATION

To stop or slow anterior or posterior epistaxis. If topical vasoconstrictor therapy does not stop the bleeding, it may at least slow it and help provide a dry field for chemical or electrical cautery.

CONTRAINDICATIONS AND CAUTIONS

Topical vasoconstrictors may elevate the blood pressure and heart rate. Patients with cardiopulmonary problems or hypertension should be treated with caution.

EQUIPMENT

Headlamp
Nasal speculum
Atomizer (for medications not packaged in a spray bottle)
Topical vasoconstrictor, anesthetic, or both (phenylephrine hydrochloride, ephedrine, epinephrine, cocaine, oxymetazoline)
Cotton swabs
Tissues

PATIENT PREPARATION

1. Place the patient in semi-Fowler's position or in a seated position in a dental chair.
2. Have patient blow his or her nose to expel clots and apply firm, direct pressure by pinching the nares for a full 10 minutes.

PROCEDURAL STEPS

1. Place cotton swabs soaked with the topical vasoconstrictor in the nose for 5-10 minutes. Alternatively, have the patient spray the medication into each naris twice while inhaling through the nose. The spray application may be repeated if the bleeding does not stop within a few minutes. Do not exceed the maximum safe dose of the medication.
2. *Examine both nares using a headlamp and a nasal speculum to verify that the bleeding has stopped.
3. Reassess heart rate and blood pressure after medication administration as indicated, especially for patients with cardiac disease.

---

*Indicates portions of the procedure usually performed by a physician or an advanced practice nurse.

AGE-SPECIFIC CONSIDERATIONS

1. Anterior nosebleeds are the most common among children. These usually result from cracks in the nasal lining because of exposure to abrupt temperature changes, dry heat, and nose picking.
2. In adults, anterior nosebleeds result from hypertension, coagulopathy, sinus disease, respiratory infections, and allergies.

COMPLICATIONS

1. Dizziness, tachycardia, dysrhythmia, nausea/vomiting, or hypertension
2. Topical therapy may fail to control bleeding.
3. Continued blood loss may result in hypovolemia and shock.

PATIENT TEACHING

1. For the next few days, avoid anything that may lead to more bleeding, such as heavy exercise or lifting, alcoholic beverages, hot drinks, aspirin, ibuprofen, blowing your nose, sneezing, or coughing. If you must sneeze, open your mouth to relieve the pressure.
2. Apply petroleum jelly or antibiotic ointment to the nares to decrease drying and scab formation.
3. Use a humidifier at home, especially in your bedroom at night.
4. Return to the emergency department or call your physician for any recurrence of bleeding that does not stop after 10 minutes of firmly pinching your nose.

PROCEDURE 172

Electrical and Chemical Cautery for Epistaxis

Margo E. Layman, MSN, RN, RNC, CN-A

INDICATION

To stop anterior epistaxis.

CONTRAINDICATIONS AND CAUTIONS

1. Silver nitrate will not cauterize an actively bleeding area; hemostasis must be achieved first.
2. Septal damage or perforation may occur with overaggressive electrocautery.

3. Silver nitrate reduces the blood supply to the area; bilateral use may cause septal necrosis.
4. If cautery is unsuccessful or rebleeding occurs within 72 hours, anterior packing is usually placed (see Procedures 173 and 175) (Riviello, 2004).
5. Electrocautery may be performed with a small battery-operated cautery unit or a larger electrosurgical unit. If the electrosurgical unit is used, a practitioner appropriately trained in the safe use of this modality should be responsible for ensuring that the patient is grounded and that other necessary safety precautions are taken.

EQUIPMENT
Headlamp
Nasal speculum
Frazier nasal suction tip
Silver nitrate sticks
Electrocautery
Cotton swabs
Antibiotic ointment
Topical or local anesthetic

PATIENT PREPARATION
1. Place the patient in a dental chair or in semi-Fowler's position on a stretcher.
2. Have the patient blow his or her nose to clear it of clots.
3. Attach grounding pad to the patient and take other appropriate electrical safety precautions if using a large electrosurgery unit.

PROCEDURAL STEPS
1. *Using headlamp and nasal speculum, locate the bleeding site.
2. Suction the area until the site is visualized and dry. The bleeding site must be dry for silver nitrate sticks to be effective.
3. *Anesthetize the nasal mucosa with a topical anesthetic for electrocautery (see Procedure 138).
4. *Coagulate the bleeding site with the silver nitrate sticks or electrocautery.
   a. Silver nitrate: Hold the stick in place for only 20-30 seconds.
   b. Electrocautery: Coagulate only a 1-mm area. The cautery damages and weakens tissue and may cause additional bleeding.
5. *After application of silver nitrate, dry the cautery site with cotton swabs to prevent the silver nitrate from spreading.
6. Apply antibiotic ointment to the cautery site to soften the crust formed by the cautery.

AGE-SPECIFIC CONSIDERATIONS
1. Anterior nosebleeds are the most common among children. These usually result from cracks in the nasal lining because of exposure to abrupt temperature changes, dry heat, and nose picking.

---

*Indicates portions of the procedure usually performed by a physician or an advanced practice nurse.

2. In adults, anterior nosebleeds result from hypertension, coagulopathy, sinus disease, respiratory infections, and allergies.

COMPLICATIONS
1. Cauterization can weaken the tissue and make future cauterization more harmful.
2. Continued blood loss may result in hypovolemia and shock.

PATIENT TEACHING
1. Avoid the following activities and substances for the next few days because they may lead to more bleeding: heavy exercise or lifting, alcoholic beverages, hot drinks, aspirin, ibuprofen, blowing your nose, sneezing, or coughing. If you must sneeze, open your mouth to relieve pressure.
2. Apply petroleum jelly or antibiotic ointment to the nares to decrease drying and scab formation.
3. Use a humidifier at home, especially in your bedroom at night.
4. Return to the emergency department or call your physician for any recurrence of bleeding that does not stop after 10 minutes of firmly pinching your nose.

REFERENCE
Riviello, R.J. (2004). Otolaryngologic procedures (pp. 1280-1316). In Roberts, J.R., & Hedges, J.R. (Eds.). *Clinical procedures in emergency medicine*, 4th ed. Philadelphia: W.B. Saunders.

PROCEDURE 173

Anterior Packing for Epistaxis

Margo E. Layman, MSN, RN, RNC, CN-A
and Jean A. Proehl, RN, MN, CEN, CCRN

INDICATION
To tamponade bleeding from the anterior nasal cavity

CONTRAINDICATIONS AND CAUTIONS

1. Nasal packing in sedated patients may lead to hypoxia (Riviello, 2004); monitoring of oxygen saturation is recommended.
2. Antibiotics may be prescribed because of the risk of toxic shock syndrome and sinvsitis (Riviello, 2004; Sparacino, 2000).

EQUIPMENT

Headlamp
Swimmer's nose clip (optional)
Topical anesthetic agent (e.g., lidocaine, Pontocaine, cocaine)
Topical vasoconstricting agent (e.g., oxymetazoline, cocaine, phenylephrine)
Silver nitrate sticks
Atomizer (for medications not packaged in a spray bottle)
1-inch-wide strips of plain gauze impregnated with antibiotic ointment or petroleum jelly
or
Hemostatic mesh (Gelfoam, Surgicel)
or
Commercially prepared nasal tampon (a variety of sizes and shapes are available)
Frazier nasal suction tip
Long bayonet forceps
Nasal speculum
Pharyngeal mirror
2 × 2-inch gauze pads
4 × 4-inch gauze pads
Tape
Cotton-tipped applicators

PATIENT PREPARATION

1. Place the patient in a dental chair or in semi-Fowler's position on a stretcher.
2. Cover the patient's clothing with a gown or towel and provide a basin.
3. Administer sedation as prescribed (see Procedure 181).

PROCEDURAL STEPS

1. Have the patient blow his or her nose to dislodge clots.
2. Apply swimmer's nose clip or have the patient pinch the nose for minimum of 5 minutes.
3. *With a headlamp, introduce a nasal speculum into the naris, and suction clotted blood from nose to assess if an anterior or posterior bleed is present (Figure 173-1).
4. *Anesthetize the area with cotton-tipped applicators soaked in a topical anesthetic or vasoconstrictive agent.
5. *Apply silver nitrate to cauterize the bleeding site (see Procedure 172).
6. *Pack the anterior nose.

---

*Indicates portions of the procedure usually performed by a physician or an advanced practice nurse.

a. *Vaseline gauze or hemostatic mesh:* Pack the gauze/mesh loosely in accordion manner using bayonet forceps and allowing both ends to protrude anteriorly (Figure 173-2). Use a pharyngeal mirror to check for loose threads dangling into the nasopharynx and gagging the patient. The pack can then be held in place with a gauze dressing taped under the nose (a "mustache dressing") (Figure 173-3).

b. *Commercially prepared nasal tampon:* If necessary, trim the tampon before insertion. Lubricate the tampon with antibiotic ointment or lubricant. Using

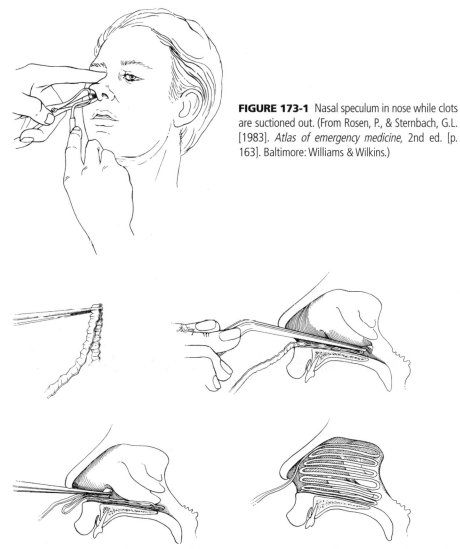

FIGURE 173-1 Nasal speculum in nose while clots are suctioned out. (From Rosen, P., & Sternbach, G.L. [1983]. *Atlas of emergency medicine,* 2nd ed. [p. 163]. Baltimore: Williams & Wilkins.)

FIGURE 173-2 Accordion packing of the anterior nasal cavity with Vaseline gauze. (Riviello, R.J. [2004]. Otolaryngologic procedures [p. 1305]. Roberts, J.R., & Hedges, J.R. [Eds.]. *Clinical procedures in emergency medicine,* 4th ed. Philadelphia: W.B. Saunders.)

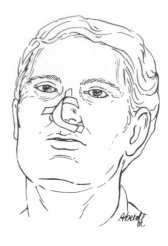

FIGURE 173-3 Packing taped in place with gauze under the nose. (From Rosen, P., & Sternbach, G.L. [1983]. *Atlas of emergency medicine,* 2nd ed. [p. 163]. Baltimore: Williams & Wilkins.)

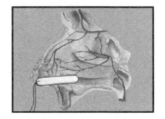

FIGURE 173-4 Merocel nasal tampon (compressed) inserted into the nose. (Courtesy Xomed Surgical Products, Jacksonville, FL.)

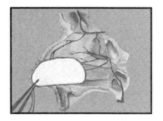

FIGURE 173-5 Merocel nasal tampon fully expanded after absorbing blood and/or saline. (Courtesy Xomed Surgical Products, Jacksonville, FL.)

forceps or gloved fingers, insert the tampon along the floor of the anterior cavity (Figure 173-4). Two tampons may be necessary; they should be inserted side by side (Riviello, 2004). The packing expands as it absorbs blood from the epistaxis, or it can be hydrated with sterile saline (Figure 173-5). The packing may be left in place for up to 3 days and should be rehydrated with 10 ml of saline or water and wait 5 minutes before removal.

AGE-SPECIFIC CONSIDERATIONS

1. Anterior nosebleeds are the most common among children. These usually result from cracks in the nasal lining because of exposure to abrupt temperature changes, dry heat, and nose picking (Sparacino, 2000).
2. In adults, anterior nosebleeds result from hypertension, coagulopathy, sinus disease, respiratory infections, and allergies.

COMPLICATIONS

1. Hypovolemia from blood loss
2. Inadequate hemostasis with recurrent hemorrhage
3. Airway obstruction from swelling or dislodgment of the packing
4. Hypoxia
5. Sinusitis
6. Toxic shock syndrome
7. Ethmoid fracture (Riviello, 2004)

PATIENT TEACHING

1. Do not remove the packing; see your physician or otolaryngologist for removal in 48-72 hours.
2. Avoid the following activities or substances for the next few days because they may lead to more bleeding: heavy exercise or lifting, alcoholic beverages, hot drinks, aspirin, ibuprofen, blowing your nose, sneezing, or coughing. If you must sneeze, open your mouth to relieve pressure.
3. Return to the emergency department or call your physician for recurrent bleeding, difficulty breathing, blood draining down the back of your throat, fever, malaise, or rash.

REFERENCES

Riviello, R.J. (2004). Otolaryngologic procedures (pp. 1280-1316). Roberts, J.R., & Hedges, J.R. (Eds.). *Clinical procedures in emergency medicine*, 4th ed. Philadelphia: W.B. Saunders.
Sparacino, L.L. (2000). Epistaxis management: what's new and what's noteworthy. *Lippincott's Primary Care Practice*, 4, 498-507.

PROCEDURE 174

Posterior Packing for Epistaxis

Margo E. Layman, MSN, RN, RNC, CN-A
and Jean A. Proehl, RN, MN, CEN, CCRN

INDICATION

To tamponade bleeding from the posterior nasal cavity. The most common site of posterior nosebleeds is from the lateral nasal branch of the sphenopalatine artery, which enters the nasal cavity behind the middle turbinate (Sparacino, 2000).

CONTRAINDICATIONS AND CAUTIONS

1. People aged 50 to 80 years with histories of cardiac and pulmonary disorders may develop problems (hyperventilation, hypoxia, and arrhythmias) because of compromised cardiac and pulmonary systems.
2. Baseline oxygenation with pulse oximetry should be established for patients with cardiopulmonary disease because hypoxia may result from nasal packing.
3. Patients with posterior packs should be admitted to the hospital (Riviello, 2004; Sparacino, 2000).
4. Antibiotics are usually prescribed because of the risk of toxic shock syndrome (Riviello, 2004; Sparacino, 2000).
5. Posterior nasal gauze packs are rarely used because balloons (see Procedure 175) or commercially prepared nasal tampons are easier to use and are less distressing to the patient.

EQUIPMENT

Headlamp
Topical anesthetic agent (e.g., lidocaine, Pontocane, cocaine)
Topical vasoconstricting agent (e.g., oxymetazoline, cocaine, phenylephrine)
Silver nitrate sticks
Frazier nasal suction tip
Long bayonet forceps
Nasal speculum
Pharyngeal mirror
Tongue blades
Cotton-tipped applicators
Pulse oximeter
Commercially prepared nasal tampon (a variety of sizes and shapes are available) coated with antibiotic ointment or lubricant
or
Posterior gauze pack supplies:
    2 × 2-inch gauze pads
    4 × 4-inch gauze pads
    Dental roll
    1-inch-wide strips of plain gauze impregnated with antibiotic ointment or petroleum jelly
    0 silk suture
    Red rubber catheter size 8-10
    Straight medium hemostat or ring forceps
    Tape
    Umbilical clamp or 2-0 silk ties

PATIENT PREPARATION

1. Place the patient in a dental chair or in semi-Fowler's position on a stretcher.
2. Cover the patient's clothing and provide a basin.
3. Administer sedation as prescribed (see Procedure 181).
4. Monitor the patient during procedure by pulse oximetry, cardiac monitor and vital signs (see Procedures 23 and 58).

PROCEDURAL STEPS
Commercial Nasal Tampon

1. *If necessary, trim the nasal tampon before insertion. Lubricate the tampon with antibiotic ointment or lubricant.
2. *Insert the nasal tampon along the floor of the nose (Figure 174-1). The packing expands as it absorbs blood from the epistaxis, or it can be hydrated with sterile saline (Figure 174-2). The packing may be left in place for up to 3 days and should be rehydrated with 10-15 ml water for at least 5 minutes before removal.

Posterior Nasal Gauze Pack

1. Roll and cut to 1¾-inch length a 4- × 4-inch gauze and tie silk suture around the pack.
2. Using cotton-tipped applicators, apply topical anesthetic or vasoconstrictor to the interior of the nose for 5-10 minutes.
3. *With a headlamp, introduce a nasal speculum into the naris, and suction clotted blood from the nose.
4. *Insert a red rubber catheter through the nose into the nasopharynx. Then, with a hemostat, pull it out through the mouth (Figure 174-3).
5. *Tie two ties to the postnasal pack. Tie one to the end of the catheter, and pull the pack with the catheter through the mouth into the posterior nasopharynx. A bulge of the postnasal pack should be visible above the soft palate (Figure 174-4).
6. *If necessary, push the postnasal pack into place manually. A tongue blade or bite block can help prevent the uncooperative patient from biting you.
7. *Remove the catheter, and tie the suture ends protruding from the nose to a dental roll at the base of the nose with two ties applying traction. One tie protrudes through the mouth and should be taped to the cheek for use in removing the pack (Sigler, 1993).

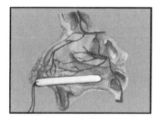

FIGURE 174-1 Merocel nasal tampon (compressed) for posterior epistaxis inserted into the nose. (Courtesy Xomed Surgical Products, Jacksonville, FL.)

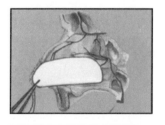

FIGURE 174-2 Merocel nasal tampon fully expanded after absorbing blood and/or saline. (Courtesy Xomed Surgical Products, Jacksonville, FL.)

---

*Indicates portions of the procedure usually performed by a physician or an advanced practice nurse.

FIGURE 174-3 Foley catheter threaded through the nose and gauze packing anchored to the end of the catheter and ready to pull into place. (From Rosen, P., & Sternbach, G.L. [1983]. *Atlas of emergency medicine,* 2nd ed. [p. 165]. Baltimore: Williams & Wilkins.)

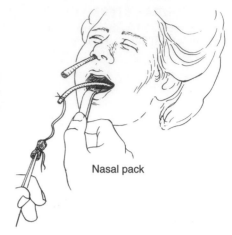

Nasal pack

FIGURE 174-4 Posterior gauze nasal packing in place. (From Rosen, P., & Sternbach, G.L. [1983]. *Atlas of emergency medicine,* 2nd ed. [p. 165]. Baltimore: Williams & Wilkins.)

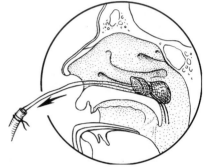

8. *Pack the anterior nose with gauze coated with antibiotic ointment or petroleum jelly using bayonet forceps and allowing both ends to protrude (see Procedure 173).
9. Place the patient on low-flow humidified oxygen by face mask until packing is removed (Viducich et al., 1995).

AGE-SPECIFIC CONSIDERATION

Posterior nosebleeds occur most often in the elderly and are associated with hypertension, atherosclerosis, and conditions that decrease platelets and clotting functions (Sparacino, 2000).

COMPLICATIONS

1. Hypovolemia from blood loss
2. Inadequate hemostasis with recurrent hemorrhage
3. Airway obstruction from swelling or dislodgment of postnasal pack
4. Hypoxia
5. Cardiac arrhythmias
6. Toxic shock syndrome
7. Ethmoid fracture (Riviello, 2004)

---

*Indicates portions of the procedure usually performed by a physician or an advanced practice nurse.

8. Hypertension as a result of the discomfort associated with posterior packing (Sparacino, 2000)
9. Requirement of a replacement pack or surgical intervention if nasal packing fails (occurs in 25% of posterior epistaxis cases) (Smith, 1996)

PATIENT TEACHING

1. Do not remove the packing; your physician or otolaryngologist will remove it in 48-72 hours.
2. Avoid the following activities and substances for the next few days because they may lead to more bleeding: heavy exercise or lifting, alcoholic beverages, hot drinks, aspirin, ibuprofen, blowing your nose, sneezing, or coughing. If you must sneeze, open your mouth to relieve pressure.
3. Immediately report recurrent bleeding, difficulty breathing, blood draining down the back of your throat, fever, malaise, or rash.

REFERENCES

Riviello, R.J. (2004). Otolaryngologic procedures (pp. 1280-1316). In Roberts, J.R., & Hedges, J.R. (Eds.). *Clinical procedures in emergency medicine*, 4th ed. Philadelphia: W.B. Saunders.

Sigler, B.A. (1993). *Ear, nose and throat disorders*. St. Louis: Mosby-Year Book.

Sparacino, L.L. (2000). Epistaxis management: what's new and what's noteworthy. *Lippincott's primary care practioner*, 4, (pp. 498-507). Philadelphia: Lippincott.

Viducich, R.A., Blanda, M.P., & Gerson, L.W. (1995). Posterior epistaxis: clinical features and acute complications. *Annals of Emergency Medicine*, 25, 592-596.

PROCEDURE 175

Balloon Catheters for Epistaxis

Margo E. Layman, MSN, RN, RNC, CN-A
and Jean A. Proehl, RN, MN, CEN, CCRN

INDICATION

To tamponade anterior or posterior epistaxis

CONTRAINDICATIONS AND CAUTIONS

1. People aged 50 to 80 years with histories of cardiac and pulmonary disorders may develop problems (hyperventilation, hypoxia, and arrhythmias) because of compromised cardiac and pulmonary systems.
2. Baseline oxygenation should be established with pulse oximetry for patients with cardiopulmonary disease because hypoxia may result from balloon catheter packing (Rothehaus & Paul, 2001).
3. Some balloons are filled with air and others with fluid, consult the manufacturer's directions for amount and substance to instill.

EQUIPMENT

Headlamp
Topical anesthetic (e.g., phenylephrine)
Silver nitrate sticks
Antibiotic ointment or petroleum jelly
Frazier nasal suction tip
Long bayonet forceps
Nasal speculum
4- × 4-inch gauze dressings
Cotton-tipped applicators
Intranasal balloon and syringe
Sterile water (for some products)
Note: A 12-French Foley catheter may also be used instead of a commercial balloon. If a Foley catheter is used, an umbilical clamp is used to clamp off the catheter and hold it in place (Rothehaus & Paul, 2001).
Pulse oximeter

PATIENT PREPARATION

1. Place the patient in a dental chair or in semi-Fowler's position on a stretcher.
2. Administer sedation as prescribed (see Procedure 181).
3. Monitor the patient during the procedure by pulse oximetry (see Procedure 23).

PROCEDURAL STEPS

1. *With a headlamp, introduce a nasal speculum into the naris, and suction clotted blood from the nose.
2. *Apply local anesthetic with cotton-tipped applicators.
3. *Coat the intranasal balloon per manufacturer's directions. Plain balloons are coated with antibiotic ointment or petroleum jelly; some balloons have a gel/mesh exterior that is premoistened by dipping in sterile water prior to insertion.
4. *Insert the intranasal balloon under direct vision with a headlamp.
5. *Instill air/fluid to about half of the posterior balloon's capacity (consult manufacturer's recommendations), and pull the balloon taut. Complete the inflation of the posterior balloon slowly while monitoring for pain. If the pain or downward deviation of the soft palate results, deflate the balloon until symptoms resolve (Riviello, 2004).

---

*Indicates portions of the procedure usually performed by a physician or an advanced practice nurse.

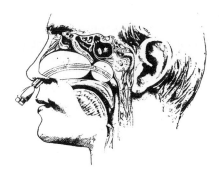

FIGURE 175-1 Epistaxis balloon in place. (Courtesy Xomed Surgical products, Jacksonville, FL.)

6. *Inflate the anterior balloon slowly with air/fluid as recommended by the manufacturer. Deflate for adverse effects as described in step 5 (Figure 175-1).
7. Place a small piece of gauze between the catheter hub and the nose to help prevent skin breakdown (Rothehaus & Paul, 2001).

COMPLICATIONS
1. Hypovolemia from blood loss
2. Inadequate hemostasis with recurrent hemorrhage
3. Airway obstruction from swelling, balloon dislodgment, or balloon overinflation
4. Hypoxia. Nasal balloons can cause a decreased PaO_2 as a result of nasopulmonary reflexes.
5. Sinusitis
6. Pressure necrosis of nasopharyngeal structures
7. Ethmoid fracture (Riviello, 2004)

PATIENT TEACHING
1. Do not remove or manipulate the balloon; see your physician or otolaryngologist for removal in 48-72 hours.
2. Avoid the following activities and substances for the next few days because they may lead to more bleeding: heavy exercise or lifting, alcoholic beverages, hot drinks, aspirin, ibuprofen, blowing your nose, sneezing, or coughing. If you must sneeze, open your mouth to relieve pressure.
3. Return to the emergency department or call your physician for recurrent bleeding, difficult breathing, blood draining down the back of your throat, fever, malaise, or rash.

REFERENCES
Riviello, R.J. (2004). Otolaryngologic procedures (pp. 1280-1316). Roberts, J.R., & Hedges, J.R. (Eds.). *Clinical procedures in emergency medicine*, 4th ed. Philadelphia: W.B. Saunders.
Rothehaus, T.C., & Paul, J.D. (2001). Nasal hemorrhage. In Harwood-Nuss, A. (Ed.). *The clinical practice of emergency medicine*. Philadelphia: Lippincott Williams & Wilkins.

---

*Indicates portions of the procedure usually performed by a physician or an advanced practice nurse.

Nasal Foreign Body Removal

Margo E. Layman, MSN, RN, RNC, CN-A

INDICATIONS
1. To remove a known nasal foreign body.
2. To rule out a foreign body in children or mentally compromised patients with foul, purulent nasal discharge or epistaxis. Unilateral nasal drainage is especially suggestive of a foreign body.

CONTRAINDICATIONS AND CAUTIONS
1. Beans or other vegetable matter should be removed as rapidly as possible because they swell as they absorb fluid.
2. If pushed further into the nose, the object can be aspirated.

EQUIPMENT
Headlamp
Nasal speculum
Topical vasoconstrictor (e.g., cocaine, phenylephrine)
Topical anesthetic (e.g., lidocaine, Pontocaine)
Cotton-tipped applicators
Miniature alligator forceps
Suction with no. 5 or no. 7 Frazier suction tip
Nasal packing
Hooked forceps

PATIENT PREPARATION
1. Place the patient in the Trendelenburg position.
2. Restrain the patient or use sedation if indicated (see Procedures 181 and 193).

PROCEDURAL STEPS
1. Anesthetize and decrease the swelling of the mucosa by spraying the nasal cavity with a nasal decongestant mixed with an anesthetic solution.
2. *Using a headlamp and nasal speculum, attempt to visualize the foreign body.
3. If nasal swelling prevents visualization, spray the turbinates with topical vasoconstrictor (or use cotton-tipped applicators to apply the vasoconstrictor).
4. *Attempt to reach the foreign object with the tip of the suction catheter, hooked forceps, or miniature alligator forceps.

---

*Indicates portions of the procedure usually performed by a physician or an advanced practice nurse.

5. *Remove mucus and debris to facilitate visualization with a small suction tip.
6. *After the swelling has decreased and the nasal debris is removed, use the hooked forceps, the miniature alligator forceps, or suction to retrieve the foreign body.
7. *Apply nasal packing to control bleeding caused by irritation or manipulation if needed (see Procedure 173).
8. Apply an antibiotic ointment or petroleum jelly to the interior of the nose with cotton-tipped applicators.

COMPLICATIONS

1. Irritations and infection (including sinus infections) as a result of prolonged retention of a nasal foreign body
2. Perforation of the nasal canal as a result of manipulation of the foreign object
3. Airway obstruction if the foreign body is aspirated
4. Epistaxis

PATIENT TEACHING

1. Use a humidifier in your bedroom at night.
2. Do not place foreign objects in the nose, and keep items small enough to swallow, aspirate, or insert into body orifices away from children.
3. Use an antibiotic ointment or petroleum jelly in the interior of the nose for 2-3 days after foreign body removal.

---

*Indicates portions of the procedure usually performed by a physician or an advanced practice nurse.

Dental and Throat Procedures

Indirect Laryngoscopy

Donna York Clark, RN, MS, CFRN, CCRN

INDICATIONS
1. To evaluate laryngeal or pharyngeal foreign body sensation
2. To evaluate hoarseness
3. To evaluate dysphagia

CONTRAINDICATIONS AND CAUTIONS
1. If possible, epiglottitis should be ruled out before attempting indirect laryngoscopy.
2. Indirect laryngoscopy has been almost replaced by the use of flexible fiberoptic laryngoscopes.

EQUIPMENT
Laryngeal mirror (size 3-6)
Gauze to grip tongue
Light source, such as a headlamp or head mirror
A method to prevent fogging (i.e., warming the mirror with warm water, an alcohol lamp, or an electric light bulb)
or
Antifogging solution (commercially available solution or soapy water can be used)
Topical anesthetic (e.g., lidocaine, Cetacaine, or aerosolized tetracaine)
Sedation (rarely needed)

PATIENT PREPARATION
1. Position the patient sitting upright with feet on the floor. Have the patient lean forward with the head in the sniffing position.
2. Place an emesis basin in the patient's hands.
3. *Anesthetize the pharynx as indicated by patient response and cooperation (see Procedure 138).

PROCEDURAL STEPS
1. Have the patient protrude the tongue from the mouth as far as possible.
2. *Lay gauze over the tongue and then wrap it under the tongue.
3. *Grip the gauze-wrapped tongue between the thumb and the index finger of the nondominant hand and brace the middle finger against the teeth; then elevate the upper lip (Figure 177-1).

---

*Indicates portions of the procedure usually performed by a physician or an advanced practice nurse.

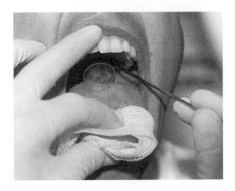

FIGURE 177-1 Grasp the tongue with a gauze dressing while elevating the upper lip with the middle finger. To prevent stimulation of the gag reflex, avoid touching the posterior pharynx or the tongue with the mirror. (From Riviello, R.J. [2004] Otolaryngologic procedures [p. 1281]. Roberts, J.R., & Hedges, J.R. (Eds.). *Clinical procedures in emergency medicine,* 4th ed. Philadelphia: W.B. Saunders.)

4. *Warm the mirror and test the temperature on your hand.
5. *Slide the mirror base down carefully, keeping it parallel to the tongue and without touching any tissue.
6. *Place the mirror with the back side against the uvula.
7. *Elevate the uvula and soft palate using one motion.
8. *Avoid touching the posterior tongue; this stimulation may result in gagging.
9. Instruct the patient to concentrate on breathing normally through the mouth with eyes open and focused on a distant fixed object.
10. *Direct the light onto the mirror.
11. *Examine the structures; look for pathology or a foreign body.
12. *Ask the patient to say E. Observe the vocal cords as the epiglottis is displaced.

AGE-SPECIFIC CONSIDERATION
This procedure may not be possible in children, because full cooperation and the ability to follow instructions are required for successful observation of the laryngeal structures.

COMPLICATIONS
1. Inability to perform the examination because of uncontrollable gagging
2. Burns from the laryngeal mirror if a warming method is used; nausea if soapy water is used.
3. Contusions on the lips or the underside of the tongue from pressure application during the procedure

PATIENT TEACHING
1. Have nothing to eat or drink until the topical anesthetic is no longer active (approximately 1 hour).
2. Use caution when resuming oral intake. Begin slowly with sips of water.

---

*Indicates portions of the procedure usually performed by a physician or an advanced practice nurse.

Esophageal Foreign Body Removal

Joni Hentzen Daniels, MSN, RN, CEN, CCRN, CFRN, CNS and Jean A. Proehl, RN, MN, CEN, CCRN

The esophagus has three areas of narrowing: upper esophageal sphincter, which consists of the cricopharyngeus muscle; crossover of the aorta; and lower esophageal sphincter. These areas are where most esophageal foreign bodies become entrapped (Munter, 2001). Structural abnormalities, including strictures, diverticula, and malignancies, increase the risk of foreign body entrapment, as do motor disturbances, such as scleroderma and achalasia. The oropharynx is well innervated, and patients can typically localize oropharyngeal foreign bodies; however, foreign bodies in the lower two thirds of the esophagus are poorly localized.

Two methods of removing a documented foreign body from the esophagus are described in this procedure: esophagoscopy and balloon-tipped catheter removal. Medications such as glucagon, nitroglycerin, nifedipine, and gas-forming agents are also used to remove esophageal foreign bodies in some cases.

ESOPHAGOSCOPY
Indications
1. This method provides direct visualization of the foreign body and the ability to evaluate the esophagus for pathology and allows control of the object during removal. Esophagoscopy is the preferred method of removal for sharp objects (e.g., bones, safety pins, and razor blades) and button batteries that may rapidly cause esophageal injury.
2. Esophagoscopy may also be used to rule out predisposing pathology or resultant complications (Munter & Heffner, 2004). An emergency physician does not usually perform esophagoscopy; a specialist is consulted.

Contraindications and Cautions
Sharp, pointed objects (e.g., toothpicks, bones) may require removal in the operating room.

Equipment
Endoscopic equipment
Suction setup
Pulse oximeter
Topical anesthetic
Emergency airway and resuscitative equipment

Patient Preparation

1. Establish venous access for medication administration (see Procedure 63).
2. If the object poses a high risk for esophageal perforation, prophylactic antibiotics should be administered intravenously before the endoscopy (Munter & Heffner, 2004).
3. Consider endotracheal intubation if the airway is at risk for compromise (see Procedures 9 through 12).
4. Place the patient in a Trendelenburg, lateral decubitus position.
5. Assess vital signs and oxygen saturation, and continue to monitor them frequently throughout the procedure (see Procedure 23).
6. *Administer a topical anesthetic as prescribed to control gagging (see Procedure 138).
7. Administer sedatives and analgesics as prescribed.
8. Have suction assembled and turned on at the patient's head.

Procedural Steps

1. *Intubate the esophagus with the endoscope.
2. *Visualize the foreign body.
3. *Push the foreign body into the stomach; grasp it and remove it through the scope; or grasp it and remove it with the scope as a unit.
4. *Evaluate the esophagus for preexisting pathology or trauma induced by the foreign body.
5. *Dilate the esophagus as necessary.

BALLOON-TIPPED CATHETER
Indications

This technique is used for removal of coins and other nonobstructing, smooth, blunt foreign bodies in cooperative patients who have ingestions of a short (24- to 48-hour) duration (Munter & Heffner, 2004; Thomas & Brown, 2002). This technique has a high success rate in pediatric patients who have ingested coins—96% in one series of 337 patients (Harned et al., 1997).

Contraindications and Cautions

1. Esophageal perforation or aspiration may occur.
2. There is no direct visualization of either the object or the esophagus and no direct control of the object.
3. This procedure cannot be used in the presence of a total obstruction because the catheter must be able to pass distal to the foreign body.
4. This procedure should not be used with sharp, irregularly shaped objects, because damage to the esophagus or balloon rupture may occur (Munter & Heffner, 2004).
5. The patient must be cooperative during this procedure; sedation may be necessary.
6. This procedure is not suitable for patients in respiratory distress or with symptoms of perforation (Thomas & Brown, 2002).

---

*Indicates portions of the procedure usually performed by a physician or an advanced practice nurse.

Equipment

Fluoroscopy equipment (optional)
Suction setup
Foley or Fogarty catheter, 8 to 26 French
Water-soluble lubricant
5-10 ml of normal saline solution or a contrast agent to inject into the
 balloon.
10-ml syringe
Laryngoscope
Magill forceps
Emergency airway and resuscitative equipment

Patient Preparation

1. Place the patient in the deep Trendelenburg (30-degree) position on a fluoroscopy table (if fluoroscopy is to be used).
2. Assess vital signs and oxygen saturation, and continue to monitor them frequently throughout the procedure.
3. Administer a local anesthetic as prescribed to control gagging.
4. Administer sedatives and analgesics as prescribed.
5. Have suction assembled and turned on at the patient's head.

Procedural Steps

1. Sedate the patient as indicated (see Procedure 181).
2. Inflate the catheter balloon to ensure that it expands evenly. Lubricate the
 catheter with a water-soluble lubricant.
3. *Insert the catheter through the nose or mouth until the balloon is distal to
 the foreign body.
4. Slowly inflate the balloon with saline solution or a contrast agent (fluid is
 preferred because it is less compressible than air). Stop the inflation immediately if the patient complains of increased pain; reposition the balloon and
 attempt inflation again.
5. *With smooth, steady traction, withdraw the catheter until the foreign body
 enters the patient's mouth. If significant resistance is encountered, stop and
 consider another modality.
6. *Grasp the object with forceps if the patient does not expel it.
7. Repeat radiographic assessment to rule out multiple foreign bodies.
8. If the foreign object is not retrieved, the object may have passed into the
 stomach; assess foreign body location with fluoroscopy or radiography.

AGE-SPECIFIC CONSIDERATIONS

1. The balloon-tipped catheter technique is frequently used for small children
 who have swallowed coins. A patient restraint board may be necessary to
 hold the child still during the procedure (see Procedure 193).
2. No more than 5 ml of fluid should be used to inflate a catheter in children
 (Munter & Heffner, 2004).

---

*Indicates portions of the procedure usually performed by a physician or an advanced practice
nurse.

COMPLICATIONS

1. Esophageal rupture may be caused by erosion of the foreign body, puncture by the foreign body, or iatrogenic trauma from the procedures used to remove the foreign body.
2. Esophageal fistula may develop.
3. Button batteries may lead to esophageal necrosis and death if not removed promptly.
4. Aspiration of saliva, vomit, or the foreign body may occur during removal.
5. If the foreign object cannot be removed in the emergency department, surgical intervention may be necessary.

PATIENT TEACHING

1. Immediately report fever, difficulty swallowing, and shortness of breath, swelling of the neck, chest pain, abdominal pain, vomiting, or blood in the stool or vomit.
2. Advance the diet slowly as tolerated or as directed.
3. If the object was pushed into the stomach, return for follow-up radiographs if the object does not pass in the stool within 4-7 days.
4. Prevention tips:
   a. Avoid alcohol while eating.
   b. Take small bites and chew food well.
   c. Place nothing but food in the mouth.
   d. Check meat for bones, especially if you have dentures.
   e. Small toys and hard candy should be out of the reach of children younger than 3 years of age
   f. Do not talk, laugh, or run with food in your mouth.

REFERENCES

Harned, R.K., II, Strain, J.D., Hay, T.C., & Douglas, M.R. (1997). Esophageal foreign bodies: safety and efficacy of Foley catheter extraction of coins. *American Journal of Roentgenology, 168,* 443-446.

Munter, D.W., (2001). Foreign bodies, gastrointestinal. *eMedicine Journal,* May 25, 2001. Retrieved July 26, 2002. *http:www.emedicine.com/emerg/topic897.htm.*

Munter, D.W., & Heffner, A.C. (2004). Esophageal foreign bodies (pp. 775-993). In Roberts, J.R., & Hedges, J.R. (Eds.). *Clinical procedures in emergency medicine,* 4th ed. Philadelphia: W.B. Saunders.

Thomas, S.H., & Brown, D.F.M. (2002). Foreign bodies. In Marx, J.A., Hockberger, R.S., Wall, R.M. et al. (Eds.). *Rosen's emergency medicine: concepts and clinical practice,* 5th ed. (pp. 752-774). St. Louis: Mosby.

Tooth Preservation and Replantation

Maureen T. Quigley, MS, ARNP, CEN

INDICATION

To preserve and replant a tooth that has been avulsed from the socket (Figure 179-1)

CONTRAINDICATIONS AND CAUTIONS

1. Patients who are unresponsive, combative, or have compromised airways are unable to facilitate preservation of teeth by replacing them in the socket. Replantation should not be attempted because of risk of aspiration.
2. If the bone and soft tissue are too traumatized to support the tooth, replantation should not be attempted.
3. If the location of the avulsed tooth is not known, there should be an attempt to locate it in the mouth and pharynx. Radiographs should be considered if there is a possibility that a tooth could have been forced into the bone, swallowed, or aspirated.
4. The treatment of an avulsed tooth is divided into 10 categories, depending on the specific clinical conditions associated with that particular avulsed tooth, which include the physiologic status of the periodontal ligament (PDL) fibers, the stage of development of the root apex, the type of storage environment, and the length of extraoral time (Table 179-1). Maintenance of the

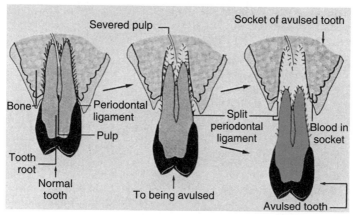

FIGURE 179-1 Anatomy of tooth avulsion. (From Krasner, P. [1990]. Treatment of tooth avulsion by nurses. *Journal of Emergency Nursing, 16,* 31.)

TABLE 179-1

TREATMENT CATEGORIES OF AVULSED TEETH

Category 1	Mature apex, <15 min extraoral time
Category 2	Mature apex, 15 min-24 hr extraoral time, reconstituting storage media
Category 3	Mature apex, 15-360 min extraoral time, nonreconstituting but wet storage media
Category 4	Mature apex, ≤120 min extraoral time, dry storage
Category 5	Mature apex, ≥120 min extraoral time, dry storage
Category 6	Immature apex, <15 min extraoral time
Category 7	Immature apex, 15 min-24 hr extraoral time, reconstituting storage media
Category 8	Immature apex, 15-360 min extraoral time, nonreconstituting but wet storage media
Category 9	Immature apex, ≤120 min extraoral time, dry storage
Category 10	Immature apex, ≥120 min extraoral time, dry storage

From Krasner, P. (1995). New philosophy for the treatment of avulsed teeth. *Oral Surgery, Oral Medicine, Oral Pathology, and Oral Radiology Endodontics, 79,* 619.

PDL fibers' vitality, rather than the length of extraoral time, is key to the success of the replanted tooth (Krasner, 1995).

5. The critical links in the pre-replantation stage are (Krasner, 1995):
   a. Storage of the avulsed tooth in a physiologic medium until replantation.
   b. Replenishment of the depleted cellular nutrients of the PDL cells.
   c. Protection of the root PDL cells from trauma, especially crushing.
6. Avulsed teeth should be placed in a pH-balanced cell preservative that reconstitutes PDL cells in a cushioned container (e.g., the basket device found in commercial preparations of Hank's solution, such as Save-A-Tooth) that permits atraumatic tooth retrieval. Before reimplantation, teeth that have been avulsed for more than 20 minutes need to remain in a cell preservative for at least 30 minutes to rehydrate the periodontal ligament cells.
7. Storage in media such as gauze or hard containers is contraindicated.
8. If the patient has other, more serious injuries, the tooth can remain in Hank's solution until reimplantation can be accomplished.
9. When a cell preservative is not available, cold milk is the best alternative storage medium. The osmolality and availability of milk are more conducive to maintaining the vitality of the periodontal ligament than is saline solution or tap water. Ideally, the avulsed tooth is placed in a container of milk that is packed in ice (McTigue, 2002).
10. If milk or cell culture media are not available immediately, saliva is an acceptable alternative (McTigue, 2002).
11. The neurovascular supply to the tooth is disrupted during avulsion of a tooth. Timely reimplantation may enable some return of the neurovascular supply. Often, avulsions lead to hypoxia, which causes pulpal necrosis. As a result, the pulp of most replanted teeth needs to be removed (root canal therapy) immediately or within 1 week of replantation.

EQUIPMENT

Solution for tooth storage—Hank's solution (commercially available as Save-A-Tooth emergency tooth-preserving system, made by Biological Rescue Producers, Inc., Pottstown, Pa)

Sterile normal saline
2×2 gauze or dental pads
Emesis basin
Tonsil-tip suction
Dental mirror (optional)
Coe-pak periodontal dressing *(optional)*

PATIENT PREPARATION

1. Cleanse the mouth with a gentle rinse of normal saline to remove debris, blood, and dirt.
2. Elevate the head of the stretcher, unless contraindicated, to help prevent the patient from swallowing blood, which may precipitate nausea.
3. Administer tetanus prophylaxis as indicated.

PROCEDURAL STEPS

1. Control hemorrhage in the mouth.
2. Inspect socket for blood clots or bone fragments. Gently suction as needed, avoiding sharp scraping, which can result in injury to the periodontal ligament or attachment fibers.
3. If the tooth is obviously dirty, gentle soaking in the preservation fluid helps loosen particles. Do not scrub the tooth, which damages remaining periodontal ligament fibers, which would make successful reattachment less likely.
4. The tooth should be gently removed by lifting the basket out of the container without using forceps, which could damage the PDL cells.
5. The tooth should be carefully held by the crown and not by the root so that the periodontal ligament cells are not damaged further.
6. *Application of a local anesthesia may be needed before replantation can be accomplished.
7. *If the avulsed tooth is classified in treatment category 1 (mature apex, less than 15 minutes extraoral time), flush the socket with a physiologic solution. For avulsed teeth in all other categories, consult a dentist.
8. *The tooth should be placed in the socket with the clinician's thumb slowly, with firm pressure. If position of the replanted tooth does not seem certain, the tooth should be removed and placed in a balanced solution, and the patient should be referred to a dentist.
9. *The replanted tooth should be splinted in place to adjacent teeth for a maximum of 2 weeks. A variety of methods can be used for stabilization, including Erich arch bars, stainless steel wire that is affixed to the teeth with an enamel bonding acrylic agent, an acrylic by itself, or a periodontal surgical splint, such as Coe-pak, which is a zinc oxide–eugenol preparation. (Benko, 2004). Application of an arch bar is not recommended by the nondentist.
10. A dentist should see the patient within 24 hours.
11. Antibiotic administration following tooth replantation is generally recommended, although efficacy has not been proved (Dale, 2000).

---

*Indicates portions of the procedure usually performed by a physician or an advanced practice nurse.

AGE-SPECIFIC CONSIDERATIONS
1. Avulsed primary teeth in children replanted because they may fuse to alveolar bone, causing craniofacial abnormalities or infection or they may interfere with eruption of secondary teeth (Benko, 2004).
2. Generally, immature permanent teeth have a better chance for survival than do older teeth (Benko, 2004).
3. When no satisfactory history of trauma is reported, child or elder abuse should be considered.

COMPLICATIONS
1. Pain from reinsertion of tooth
2. Infection
3. Loss of tooth
4. Improper alignment of replanted tooth
5. Ankylosis of replanted tooth to the bone. In children, this can cause facial deformity.

PATIENT TEACHING
1. Mouth protection during recreation and sports activities is recommended.
2. Consume a liquid or soft diet for the duration indicated by the dentist.
3. Loss of the replanted tooth is possible not only early after reimplantation but also several years later.

REFERENCES
Benko, K. (2004). Emergency dental procedures (pp. 1317-1340). In Roberts, J.R., & Hedges, J.R. (Eds.). *Clinical procedures in emergency medicine*, 4th ed. Philadelphia: W.B. Saunders.

Dale, R.A. (2000). Oral-facial emergencies. *Emergency Medicine Clinics of North America, 18*, 521-538.

Krasner, P. (1995). New philosophy for the treatment of avulsed teeth. *Oral Surgery, Oral Medicine, Oral Pathology, and Oral Radiology Endodontics, 79*, 616-623.

McTigue, D.J. (2002). Evaluation and management of dental injuries in children. In *UpToDate*, version 10.3. *http://uptodateonline.com* Information retrieved November 20, 2002. Last update October 16, 2001.

Medication Administration

Nitrous Oxide Administration

Jean A. Proehl, RN, MN, CEN, CCRN

Nitrous oxide combined with oxygen is also known as laughing gas, Nitronox, and Entonox.

NOTE: The use of nitrous oxide in the manner described herein is usually considered analgesia and anxiolysis, not sedation. Consult your institutional protocols to determine whether sedation guidelines apply to nitrous oxide use in your setting.

INDICATIONS

1. To provide rapid-onset (2-6 minutes), quickly reversible (2-5 minutes) analgesia for 30 minutes or less. Nitrous oxide may be used to relieve the pain associated with trauma, renal colic, myocardial infarction, minor surgical procedures, wound care, diagnostic procedures, and reduction of fractures and dislocations.
2. To relieve the anxiety associated with painful conditions and procedures.

CONTRAINDICATIONS AND CAUTIONS

1. When used for analgesia in the emergency setting (versus anesthesia in the operative setting), the gas mixture should be fixed at 50% nitrous oxide to 50% oxygen. For altitudes above 3500 feet, a 65% nitrous oxide to 35% oxygen mixture is recommended because the lower partial pressure of the nitrous oxide at higher altitudes does not provide adequate analgesia.
2. The patient should always self-administer the gas to prevent oversedation. Therefore, the patient must be cooperative and able to follow instructions. The mask or mouthpiece should never be strapped to or held on the patient's face.
3. Nitrous oxide causes drowsiness and should not be used in patients with altered levels of consciousness or head injuries, or those who are heavily sedated or intoxicated. Patients who have received narcotics should be individually evaluated for suitability before receiving nitrous oxide.
4. Nitrous oxide occasionally causes nausea and vomiting, so caution is indicated with recent ingestion of food or fluids.
5. The gas mixture contains 50% oxygen (35% at high altitude); therefore, it does not supply enough oxygen for patients who have pulmonary edema and may suppress the hypoxic respiratory drive in a patient who has chronic obstructive pulmonary disease.
6. Nitrous oxide collects in dead air spaces and can expand the preexisting pockets of air associated with pneumothorax, otitis media, perforated viscus, bowel obstruction, air embolism, and decompression sickness.
7. Nitrous oxide should not be used during early pregnancy, because it has been associated with fetal defects and spontaneous abortion.

8. A scavenger system to dispose of exhaled gas protects health care providers who administer nitrous oxide. Studies involving operating room and dental personnel have associated long-term exposure to nitrous oxide with psychomotor impairment and congenital malformations, as well as spontaneous abortion in exposed women and sexual partners of exposed men. Possible association with bone marrow suppression, cancer, liver disease, and renal disease has also been reported.

9. A mask is preferred to facilitate disposal of exhaled gas. If the patient is unable to use a mask because of facial trauma or other conditions, a mouthpiece may be used in place of a mask.

10. Nitrous oxide has abuse potential. The unit should be kept in a secure area. A pop-off demand valve is available; the valve can then be locked up with the narcotics.

11. A fail-safe valve should be incorporated into the system to prevent administration of 100% nitrous oxide if the oxygen supply is interrupted.

12. A nurse or physician should be present at all times during nitrous oxide administration in the hospital setting unless institutional policies are in place specifying other qualified personnel who may monitor the patient.

EQUIPMENT

Nitrous oxide and oxygen tanks connected to a blender preset to deliver 50% nitrous oxide and 50% oxygen (65% nitrous oxide and 35% oxygen at altitudes above 3500 feet) with demand valve and scavenger (Figure 180-1). (NOTE: Units are also available for use with nitrous oxide supplied by pipeline.)

Mask or mouthpiece

Wall suction and suction connection tubing

Pulse oximeter

NOTE: In countries other than the United States, nitrous oxide may be available in a single-tank mixture known as Entonox.

PATIENT PREPARATION

1. Assess and document vital signs.
2. Initiate pulse oximetry monitoring (see Procedure 23).
3. Instruct the patient to do the following:
   a. Form a tight seal with the mask or mouthpiece and take slow, deep breaths. A sucking sound will be heard when the demand valve is tripped—this is expected.
   b. Exhale into the mask or mouthpiece so that the exhaled gas is removed by the scavenger.
   c. Avoid unnecessary conversation to limit exhalation of nitrous oxide into the room.
   d. Discontinue use if nausea, light-headedness, or other side effects occur.

PROCEDURAL STEPS

1. Turn on the nitrous oxide and oxygen tanks by opening the cylinder valves with a wrench. Check that the mixture pressure is within the safe level per manufacturer's specifications (30-35 psi for Nitronox by Matrx Medical, Inc. [1996]). Do not use the unit if the mixture pressure is not within the safe level.

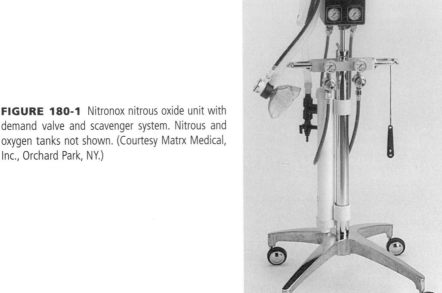

FIGURE 180-1 Nitronox nitrous oxide unit with demand valve and scavenger system. Nitrous and oxygen tanks not shown. (Courtesy Matrx Medical, Inc., Orchard Park, NY.)

Check the pressure of each cylinder, and replace any cylinder with a pressure less than 300 psi (see Procedure 28).

2. Connect the scavenger to the wall suction and turn the suction on. Turn the ball valve lever on the scavenger tube to the on position. Adjust the suction to 30-60 L/min.

3. Attach mask or mouthpiece to the demand valve.

4. Allow the patient to inhale the gas for 3 or 4 minutes before beginning any procedures. Some patients may require up to 6 minutes for adequate induction.

5. Monitor pulse oximetry continuously, and document it frequently (i.e., every 5 minutes) throughout the procedure.

6. As the patient becomes relaxed, he or she will be unable to create an adequate amount of negative pressure to trip the demand valve. This prevents excessive sedation.

7. When the patient drops the mask or mouthpiece, position or hold it so that the exhaled gas can be taken up by the scavenger.

8. Allow the patient to resume gas inhalation when he or she is able to hold the mask or mouthpiece.

9. Nitrous oxide administration is usually limited to a maximum of 30 minutes.

10. Assess and document vital signs and pulse oximetry.
11. When the procedure is completed, turn off the suction and nitrous and oxygen tanks. Clear the lines by blowing forcefully through the small holes on the back of the demand valve until all pressure gauges read zero. If the oxygen line bleeds before the nitrous line, you will not be able to remove the nitrous. Open and close the oxygen line and try again.
12. Monitor pulse oximetry and heart rate for 5-15 minutes after procedure.

NOTE: Some sources recommend that the patient receives upplemental oxygen for a period of time after receiving nitrous oxide to counteract the effects of diffusion hypoxia caused by the diffusion of nitrous oxide from the arterial blood into the alveoli, which dilutes alveolar oxygen levels. Research has demonstrated that diffusion hypoxia does not occur in healthy subjects after self-administration of nitrous oxide analgesia (Holcomb et al., 1976; Nieto & Rosen, 1980; Stewart et al., 1986).

AGE-SPECIFIC CONSIDERATIONS
Nitrous oxide can be used by children and elderly patients as long as they can cooperate and self-administer the nitrous oxide as described previously. The mask should never be held on the patient's face.

COMPLICATIONS
1. Side effects are unusual but may require termination of nitrous oxide administration. Side effects may include vomiting, shortness of breath, excitement, drowsiness, confusion, and light-headedness.
2. Propping or holding the mask against the patient's face may result in excessive sedation. The patient must hold the mask to prevent overdosage.
3. Aspiration may occur if the patient vomits with the mask in place.
4. The Nitronox unit has a mixer pressure whistle alarm that sounds if there is a disruption in gas pressures resulting in a low oxygen concentration. Discontinue use immediately and notify the manufacturer (Matrx, 1996).

PATIENT TEACHING
1. Report immediately any uncomfortable sensations during nitrous oxide use.
2. Keep conversation to a minimum, and exhale into the mask or mouthpiece.

REFERENCES
Holcomb, C., Erdmann, W., & Corssen, G. (1976). The significance of diffusion hypoxemia. *Southern Medical Journal, 69,* 1282-1284.
Matrx Medical, Inc. (1996). *Instructions Nitronox hospital model.* Orchard Park, NY: Author.
Nieto, J., & Rosen, P. (1980). Nitrous oxide at higher elevations. *Annals of Emergency Medicine, 9,* 610-612.
Stewart, R.D., Gorayeb, M.J., & Pelton, G.H. (1986). Arterial blood gases before, during, and after nitrous oxide administration. *Annals of Emergency Medicine, 1,* 1177-1180.

Sedation

Jean A. Proehl, RN, MN, CEN, CCRN
and Daun A. Smith, RN, MS, CEN

Sedation is also known as conscious sedation. The current term for conscious sedation is moderate sedation.

INDICATION

To allay patient fear, anxiety, and pain and to improve the patient's ability to cooperate during painful therapeutic, diagnostic, or surgical procedures. Moderate sedation is a minimally depressed level of consciousness wherein a patient retains the ability to maintain a patent airway and respond appropriately to verbal and tactile stimulation (American Society of Anesthesiologists [ASA], 2002; Association of Operating Room Nurses [AORN], 2002).

NOTE: The Joint Commission on Accreditation of Healthcare Organizations standards specifically address sedation practices; consult the current standards and your institutional policy for up-to-date requirements and recommendations.

ABSOLUTE CONTRAINDICATIONS

1. Hemodynamic or respiratory instability that requires immediate intervention
2. Refusal of a competent patient
3. Allergy to drug class

POTENTIAL CONTRAINDICATIONS AND CAUTIONS

If any of the following conditions are present, use of sedation must be approached with caution—consult with the physician about the risks and plan for sedation before medication administration. An anesthesia consultation may be indicated.

1. Intoxicated with central nervous system depressants
2. Neurologically impaired
3. Concurrent shock or myocardial infarction
4. Adrenal insufficiency or long-term steroid use (premedicate with intravenous steroid)
5. Moderate-to-severe liver or renal insufficiency
6. Pregnancy
7. Monoamine oxidase inhibitor use within the previous 2 weeks
8. Any condition that could make intubation difficult (e.g., facial or neck trauma, large tongue, short neck, congenital malformation of upper airway structures)
9. ASA Patient Physical Status Classification greater than class 2.

EQUIPMENT

Oral and nasopharyngeal airways (appropriate size for patient)
Suction equipment

Supplemental oxygen source, oxygen cannula, and mask (appropriate size for patient)

Bag-valve-mask (appropriate size for patient)

Cardiac monitor (if indicated by patient's condition)

Blood pressure monitoring equipment

Pulse oximeter

Crash cart with defibrillator

Reversal agent(s) for medications to be administered (naloxone, nalmefene, and/or flumazenil)

PATIENT PREPARATION

1. *Explain the procedure to the patient and obtain informed consent as required by institutional policy.
2. Establish intravenous access (see Procedure 63). Intravenous access must be continuously maintained to provide a method of administering sedatives and initiating corrective action for adverse effects. For oral administration of medications, you must have the ability to obtain intravenous access immediately (ASA, 2002).

PROCEDURAL STEPS

1. *Before the administration of sedatives, complete a preanesthesia assessment, with documentation, to include at least the following (ASA, 2002):
   a. Past and present medical history
   b. Drug allergies or sensitivities
   c. Current medications, tobacco, ethanol, or illicit drug use
   d. Last oral intake (liquid and solid)
   e. Previous anesthesia or sedation experience
   f. Patient physical status classification (Box 181-1)
   g. Results of relevant diagnostic studies
   h. Plan (choice) of anesthesia
2. Assess baseline physiologic status of patient including, but not limited to, the following:
   a. Blood pressure
   b. Heart rate
   c. Respiratory rate and status
   d. Level of consciousness
   e. Pulse oximetry
   f. Cardiac rhythm (optional)
   g. Skin color and temperature
   h. Ability to communicate
3. Have the following available in the procedure area before the administration of any medications: an emergency cart with defibrillator, suction, airway management devices, and reversal agents for the medications being administered.
4. Have supplemental oxygen and suction immediately available.
5. Establish provisions for backup personnel who are experts in airway management and cardiopulmonary resuscitation in the event that complications arise.

---

*Indicates portions of the procedure usually performed by a physician or an advanced practice nurse.

BOX 181-1

AMERICAN SOCIETY OF ANESTHESIOLOGY (ASA) PHYSICAL
STATUS CLASSIFICATION

1. Normal healthy patient
2. Patient with mild systemic disease
3. Patient with severe systemic disease
4. Patient with severe systemic disease that is a constant threat to life
5. Moribund patient who has little chance of survival but is submitted to surgery as a last resort
   (resuscitative effort)
6. (Emergency operation) Any patient in whom any emergency operation is required

---

From American Society of Anesthesiology (1963). A new classification of physical status. *Anesthesiology, 24,* 111.

6. Maintain a sedation checklist to complete all requirements and record frequently monitored physiologic parameters. Documentation should include the following (AORN, 2002):
   a. Dosage, route, time, and effects of medications
   b. Type and amount of fluids administered
   c. Any interventions and the patient's response
   d. Any untoward reaction and interventions
7. Monitor the patient carefully from the administration of the medications until recovery. The nurse monitoring the patient should have no other responsibilities during or after the procedure that will interfere the nurse's ability to adequately monitor the patient (ASA, 2002; AORN, 2002; Emergency Nurses Association, 2000).
8. During the procedure, document the following physiologic parameters at regular intervals (usually every 5-15 minutes, consult your institutional policy) (ASA, 2002):
   a. Respiratory rate
   b. Oxygen saturation
   c. Heart rate
   d. Blood pressure (unless it will interfere with sedation such as in a pediatric patient)
   e. Level of consciousness
   f. Cardiac rhythm (optional)
9. After the procedure, document the patient's level of consciousness, vital signs, and pulse oximetry every 15 minutes until he or she has recovered. Recovery is indicated by stable vital signs and oxygen saturation and alert and oriented state (or return to baseline mental status). Before discharge, the patient should be able to sit and ambulate (age appropriate) and tolerate oral fluids (ASA, 2002).

SAMPLE QUALIFICATIONS FOR ADMINISTERING AND MONITORING SEDATION

The nurse monitoring the patient must be competent in the use of resuscitation and monitoring equipment and should be able to interpret the data obtained (Emergency Nurses Association, 2000; AORN, 2002). This includes the ability to identify, rescue, and support a patient who slips into deep sedation and who may not be able to maintain a patent airway and adequate ventilation without assistance. Education in and demonstration of these competencies may be accomplished via the following:

1. Advanced Cardiac Life Support (ACLS)
2. Basic Life Support (BLS)
3. Training in the recognition of the cardiovascular and respiratory side effects of sedatives as well as the variability of patient response
4. Training in airway management
5. Emergency Nursing Pediatric Course (ENPC) or Pediatric Advanced Life Support (PALS) for sedation of children
6. Knowledge of the pharmacology of the medications administered

AGE-SPECIFIC CONSIDERATIONS

1. Consider dosage reduction in the elderly and chronically ill.
2. When selecting the medications for a pediatric patient, consider the nature of the procedure (painful or nonpainful), the desired onset and duration of action, and the route of administration. In children, *moderate sedation* may not be adequate, and *deep sedation* may be the goal. Careful monitoring is indicated.

COMPLICATIONS

1. Respiratory depression or apnea
2. Increase in untoward side effects with the dose and the number of different agents used
3. Paradoxical excitement occasionally caused by some drugs instead of the desired effect
4. Side effects as related to specific drug administered
5. Airway obstruction
6. Cardiopulmonary impairment

PATIENT TEACHING

1. Stay with a responsible adult for 12 hours after the procedure.
2. Do not drive an automobile or operate dangerous machinery for at least 6-12 hours. Children should not climb stairs unassisted, ride bikes, or play on playground equipment.
3. Return to the emergency department or call an ambulance for difficulty in breathing, pale or gray skin, or difficulty arousing.
4. Call the physician if vomiting is persistent and fluids do not stay down.

REFERENCES

American Society of Anesthesiology. (1963). A new classification of physical status. *Anesthesiology, 24,* 111.
American Society of Anesthesiologists (ASA). (2002). Practice guidelines for sedation and analgesia by non-anesthesiologists. *Anesthesiology, 96,* 1004-1017.
Association of Operating Room Nurses (AORN). (2002). Recommended practices for managing the patient receiving moderate sedation. *AORN Journal, 75,* 642-652.
Emergency Nurses Association (ENA). (2000). *Conscious sedation (position statement).* Des Plaines, IL: Author. Retrieved from www.ena.org, June 8, 2003; last updated December, 2000.

Streptokinase Administration

Teresa L. Will, RN, MSN, CEN

Streptokinase is also known as SK, STK, Streptase, or Kabikinase.

INDICATIONS
To lyse thromboses in the presence of:
1. Acute myocardial infarction (AMI) diagnosed by the following:
   a. Typical ischemic chest pain lasting for at least 30 minutes and less than 12 hours' duration, which is unresponsive to sublingual nitroglycerin
   b. ST-segment elevation of more than 1 mm in two of the three inferior leads (II, III, aVF), two of the six precordial leads (V1 through V6); or lateral leads I and aVL
   c. New-onset bundle-branch block
2. Pulmonary embolism diagnosed by angiography or lung scan, involving obstruction of blood flow to a lobe or multiple segments, with or without unstable hemodynamics
3. Deep vein thrombosis
4. Arterial thrombosis or embolism
5. Occlusion of arteriovenous cannulae

ABSOLUTE CONTRAINDICATIONS
1. Active internal bleeding
2. Recent (within 2 months) cerebrovascular accident or intracranial or intraspinal surgery
3. Intracranial neoplasm
4. Severe uncontrolled hypertension
5. History of allergic reactions to streptokinase (Astra USA, 1994)

CAUTIONS
Caution in the use of streptokinase is indicated in the presence of events or conditions that either in isolation or combination may increase the potential risk of streptokinase therapy and include the following:
1. Previous treatment with streptokinase or exposure to streptococcus infection in the past 6 months (this could result in the formation of antibodies and create resistance to the drug)
2. Recent (within 10 days) major surgery, obstetrical delivery, or organ biopsy
3. Recent (within 10 days) gastrointestinal bleeding
4. Recent (within 10 days) trauma, including cardiopulmonary resuscitation
5. Recent (within 10 days) puncture of subclavian or internal jugular vessel
6. Hypertension: systolic blood pressure greater than 180 mm Hg or diastolic blood pressure greater than 110 mm Hg

7. High likelihood of left-sided heart thrombus (e.g., mitral stenosis with atrial fibrillation)
8. Subacute bacterial endocarditis
9. Hemostatic defects, including those secondary to severe hepatic or renal disease
10. Pregnancy
11. Age greater than 75 years
12. Cerebrovascular disease
13. Diabetic hemorrhagic retinopathy
14. Septic thrombophlebitis or occluded arteriovenous cannula at a seriously infected site
15. Current treatment with oral anticoagulants
16. Any other condition in which bleeding constitutes a significant hazard or would be particularly difficult to manage because of its location.

EQUIPMENT

Streptokinase vial (1,500,000 international units)
Normal saline (NS) or dextrose 5% in water (D_5W) solution for reconstitution, 5 ml NS or D_5W solution for further dilution, 40-90 ml
Syringes: two 5 ml and one 50 ml
18-G needles
Catheter plug (also known as click lock, PRN adapter, heparin or saline lock, buffalo cap)
Volumetric intravenous (IV) infusion pump and tubing

PATIENT PREPARATION

1. Perform a thorough assessment, including:
   a. 12-lead electrocardiogram (see Procedure 59).
   b. Complete history and physical examination, including time of onset of chest pain.
   c. Review of selection criteria for streptokinase therapy.
2. Establish continuous cardiac monitoring (see Procedure 58).
3. Establish IV access with a minimum of two to three sites using 18- to 20-G catheters. The use of a double-lumen peripheral IV catheter may reduce the number of punctures (see Procedure 63).
4. Provide routine AMI care as prescribed, which may include but is not limited to the following:
   a. Oxygen therapy
   b. Aspirin
   c. IV nitroglycerin
   d. IV narcotic analgesia
   e. IV beta-blocker therapy
5. Administer pretreatment corticosteroids or diphenhydramine as prescribed.
6. Obtain laboratory studies, including the following:
   a. Cardiac markers (myoglobin, troponin, creatine kinase-MB)
   b. Chemistry profile
   c. Electrolyte profile
   d. Prothrombin time (PT), partial thromboplastin time (PTT)
   e. Complete blood count with platelets

PROCEDURAL STEPS

1. Mix streptokinase for administration. In some institutions, the pharmacy prepares the streptokinase solution.
   a. Add 5 ml of NS or D_5W solution for injection slowly to the streptokinase vial, directing the fluid stream against the side of the vial rather than into the powder. Roll and tilt the vial gently to mix the contents. To prevent further foaming, do not shake the vial.
   b. Withdraw the reconstituted solution from the vial slowly, and dilute carefully to a total volume as listed in Table 182-1.
2. When diluting the 1,500,000 International Units infusion bottle (50 ml), as in the AMI dose, follow the same procedure as in step 1a, but after the initial reconstitution, the drug can be further diluted in the same vial with an additional 40 ml of NS or D_5W.
3. Assemble IV tubing. An in-line IV filter size of 0.8 micron or larger may be used.
4. Because streptokinase contains no preservatives, it must be reconstituted just before use. It may be stored up to 8 hours at 2°-8° C (36°-46° F) if necessary.
5. Because of the limited availability of compatibility information, no other medications should be added to the container of streptokinase.
6. Administer the loading dose and initiate the maintenance dose as outlined in Table 182-1. Note that there is no loading dose for use with AMI.
7. Anticoagulation with heparin sodium may or may not be required after streptokinase administration (Astra USA, 1994). If heparin sodium is used intravenously, a bolus dose is not administered, and the continuous heparin infusion is begun only after the PTT falls to two times the normal control value. This can take several hours to occur after the conclusion of the streptokinase infusion. Therefore the PTT should be monitored every 2 hours to

TABLE 182-1
RECOMMENDED DOSAGES OF INTRAVENOUS STREPTOKINASE

Indication	Vial Size	Total Solution Volume (ml)	Infusion Rate
Acute myocardial infarction	1,500,000 Intenational Units	45	Infuse 45 ml within 60 min
Pulmonary embolism Deep vein thrombosis Embolism	1,500,000 Intenational Units	90	Loading dose 250,000 Intenational Units/hr Infuse 30 ml/hr for 30 min Maintenance infusion 100,000 Intenational Units/hr Infuse 6 ml/hr
	1,500,000 Intenational Units	45 (use when a more concentrated solution is desired)	Loading dose 250,000 Intenational Units Infuse 15 ml/hr for 30 min Maintenance infusion 100,000 Intenational Units/hr Infuse 3 ml/hr

Data from Astra USA (1994). *Streptase (streptokinase) prescribing information.* Westborough, MA: Author.

determine when it falls in that range. Subcutaneous heparin may be administered in lieu of IV heparin (GUSTO, 1993).

PATIENT MANAGEMENT

1. Monitor cardiac rhythm and neurologic status continuously.
2. Monitor for signs of allergic response, which can vary from a low-grade fever to an anaphylactic reaction. For a mild-to-moderate reaction, the physician may prescribe a corticosteroid and an antihistamine, but the streptokinase infusion may be continued. For a severe allergic reaction, the streptokinase infusion should be stopped and anaphylaxis treatment initiated.
3. Assess and document the vital signs every 5-10 minutes during streptokinase infusion. Be alert for a precipitous drop in blood pressure. Decrease the rate of streptokinase infusion if hypotension occurs. Hypotension may require volume replacement, pressor therapy, or both.
4. Monitor and document clinical signs of reperfusion, which include cardiac dysrhythmias, resolution of chest pain, and normalization of the ST segments. The dysrhythmias seen are the same as those seen in many patients having an MI and may include ventricular tachycardia, ventricular fibrillation, sinus bradycardia, accelerated idioventricular rhythm, and heart block. Any dysrhythmias that occur are treated according to advanced cardiac life support guidelines.
5. Assess for signs of bleeding complications and coronary artery reocclusion (e.g., recurrence of chest pain or ST-segment elevation) every 15 minutes during the infusion and every 2 hours thereafter until 2 hours after the heparin is discontinued.
6. Document the time the chest pain resolves and the time the streptokinase infusion ends.
7. Monitor the PTT every 2 hours. When the PTT falls to less than two times the normal control, a continuous heparin infusion may be initiated.
8. Institute thrombolytic bleeding precautions, which include the following:
    a. Avoid the use of automatic blood pressure cuffs if possible. If automatic blood pressure cuffs are used, monitor them carefully to ensure that they are not repeatedly inflating to high pressures, which may cause underlying bruising and bleeding into the extremity.
    b. Avoid unnecessary arterial and venous punctures. All puncture sites should be compressed manually for a minimum of 10 minutes for venous punctures and 20 minutes for arterial punctures. Apply pressure dressings after discontinuation of lines and after vessel puncture.
    c. Use a heparin or saline lock for blood draws, and consolidate blood draws when possible.
    d. Monitor all puncture sites and the gingivae for bleeding.
    e. Use a draw sheet to move and position the patient to avoid contusions. Instruct the patient to request assistance when changing positions.
    f. Observe for frank blood, and test urine, stools, and emesis for occult blood.
    g. Avoid intramuscular injections.
    h. Monitor hemoglobin and hematocrit for evidence of acute blood loss.

COMPLICATIONS

1. Bleeding should be expected to occur after streptokinase therapy. The goal is to avoid significant bleeding through careful screening and observation of

precautions pertaining to thrombolytic therapy bleeding. Careful monitoring and prompt treatment are critical in minimizing the effects of bleeding if it does occur. Types of bleeding seen with streptokinase therapy include the following:
  a. Intracranial
  b. Gastrointestinal
  c. Genitourinary
  d. Epistaxis
  e. Retroperitoneal
  f. Venous and arterial puncture sites
  g. Femoral artery catheter
  h. Gingival
  i. Ecchymosis
Intracranial bleeding is the most serious form of bleeding that can occur after thrombolytic therapy. Although intracranial bleeding is rare (<1%), it is so potentially devastating that care must be taken to exclude patients at risk for intracranial hemorrhage and to recognize and treat changes in neurologic status without delay.
  2. Allergic reaction
  3. Fever

PATIENT TEACHING
  1. Request assistance when moving.
  2. Report any bleeding, although some minor bleeding and bruising are normal.
  3. Report any changes in chest pain or other symptoms immediately.

REFERENCES
Astra USA. (1994). *Streptase (streptokinase) prescribing information.* Westborough, MA: Author.
GUSTO. (1993). An international randomized trial comparing four thrombolytic strategies for acute myocardial infarction. *New England Journal of Medicine, 329,* 673-682.

PROCEDURE 183

TNK-tPA Administration for Acute Myocardial Infarction

Ruth Altherr Rench, MS, RN
and Teresa L. Will, RN, MSN, CEN

TNK-tPA is also known as tissue plasminogen activator, TNK, tenecteplase, or TNKase.

INDICATION
To lyse thromboses in the presence of acute myocardial infarction diagnosed by:
1. Typical ischemic chest pain lasting for at least 30 minutes and less than 12 hours' duration, which is unresponsive to sublingual nitroglycerin.
2. ST-segment elevation of more than 1 mm in one of the following locations: two of the three inferior leads (II, III, aVF), two of the six precordial leads (V1 through V6), or lateral leads I and aVL.
3. New-onset bundle-branch block.

CONTRAINDICATIONS
1. Active internal bleeding
2. Any history of cerebrovascular accident
3. Recent (within 2 months) intracranial or intraspinal surgery or trauma
4. Intracranial neoplasm, arteriovenous malformation, or aneurysm
5. Known bleeding disorder
6. Severe uncontrolled hypertension

CAUTIONS
Cautions or relative contraindications to the use of TNK-tPA are those events or conditions that either in isolation or combination may increase the potential risk of TNK-tPA therapy and include the following:
1. Recent major surgery
2. Cerebrovascular disease
3. Recent gastrointestinal or genitourinary bleeding
4. Recent trauma
5. Recent puncture of subclavian, internal jugular, or other noncompressible vessel
6. Uncontrolled hypertension: systolic blood pressure greater than or equal to 180 mm Hg or diastolic blood pressure greater than or equal to 110 mm Hg
7. High likelihood of left-sided heart thrombus (e.g., mitral stenosis with atrial fibrillation)
8. Acute pericarditis
9. Subacute bacterial endocarditis
10. Hemostatic disorders, including those secondary to severe hepatic and renal disease
11. Pregnancy
12. Diabetic hemorrhagic retinopathy or other hemorrhagic ophthalmic conditions
13. Septic thrombophlebitis or occluded arteriovenous cannula at seriously infected site
14. Age greater than 75 years
15. Current treatment with oral anticoagulants (e.g., warfarin sodium)
16. Any condition in which bleeding constitutes a significant hazard or would be particularly difficult to manage because of its location

EQUIPMENT
50-mg TNK-tPA kit (contains one 50-mg vial of TNK-tPA powder, one 10-ml vial of sterile water, and one 10-ml syringe with TwinPak dual-cannula device)

10-ml syringe for flush
10 ml of normal saline
Intravenous (IV) starting equipment
IV catheter plug (also known as PRN adapter, heparin or saline lock, buffalo
    cap)

PATIENT PREPARATION

1. Perform a thorough assessment, including:
   a. 12-lead electrocardiogram (see Procedure 59)
   b. Complete history and physical examination, including time of onset of
      chest pain
   c. Review of selection criteria for TNK-tPA therapy
2. Establish continuous cardiac monitoring (see Procedure 58).
3. Establish IV access with a minimum of one to two sites using 18- to 20-G
   catheters. The use of a double-lumen peripheral IV catheter may reduce the
   number of punctures (see Procedure 63).
4. Provide routine acute myocardial infarction care as prescribed, which may
   include but is not limited to the following:
   a. Oxygen therapy
   b. Aspirin
   c. Intravenous nitroglycerin
   d. Intravenous narcotic analgesia
   e. Intravenous beta-blocker therapy
5. Obtain laboratory studies, including:
   a. Cardiac markers (myoglobin, troponin, creatine kinase-MB)
   b. Chemistry profile
   c. Electrolyte profile
   d. Prothrombin time, partial thromboplastin time
   e. Complete blood count with platelets

TNK-tPA RECONSTITUTION

1. Reconstitute TNK-tPA using a 50-mg vial.
   a. Remove the shield assembly from the supplied 10 ml syringe with
      TwinPak dual-cannula device and aseptically withdraw 10 ml of sterile
      water for injection, from the supplied diluent vial using the red hub can-
      nula syringe filling device. Do not use bacteriostatic water. NOTE: Do not
      discard the shield assembly.
   b. Inject the entire contents of the syringe (10 ml) into the TNKase vial,
      directing the diluent stream into the powder. Slight foaming upon recon-
      stitution is not unusual; any large bubbles will dissipate if the product is
      allowed to stand undisturbed for several minutes.
   c. Gently swirl until contents are completely dissolved. DO NOT SHAKE.
      The reconstituted preparation results in a colorless to pale yellow trans-
      parent solution that contains TNK-tPA at 5 mg/ml.
2. Once reconstituted, the TNK-tPA solution (5 mg/ml) may be used for direct
   administration. Determine the appropriate dose of TNK-tPA using Table 183-
   1 and withdraw this volume (in milliliters) from the reconstituted vial with
   the syringe. Any unused solution should be discarded.

TABLE 183-1
TNKase DOSING INFORMATION

Patient Weight (kg)	TNKase (mg)	Volume TNKase To Be Administered (ml)
<60	30 mg	6
≥60 <70	35 mg	7
≥70 <80	40 mg	8
≥80 <90	45 mg	9
≥90	50 mg	10

Modified from Genentech (2000). TNKase (tenecteplase, recombinant) prescribing information. San Francisco: Author.

3. Once the appropriate dose of TNK-tPA is drawn into the syringe, stand the shield vertically on a flat surface (with green side down) and passively recap the red hub cannula. Remove the entire shield assembly, including the red hub cannula, by twisting counterclockwise. NOTE: The shield assembly also contains the clear-ended blunt plastic cannula; retain for split-septum IV access.
4. Once reconstituted, TNK-tPA solution may be stored for 8 hours at 2°-30° C (36°-86° F). After 8 hours, any unused portion should be discarded.
5. The reconstituted TNK-tPA is not light sensitive, and no special handling is required. Unreconstituted TNK-tPA may be sensitive to light and therefore should be stored in its carton until use.
6. TNK-tPA is not compatible with other medications; use a separate IV line for TNK-tPA administration.

ADMINISTRATION OF TNK-tPA FOR ACUTE MYOCARDIAL INFARCTION
Procedural Steps
1. Visually inspect the product for particulate matter and discoloration before administration. TNK-tPA may be administered as reconstituted at 5 mg/ml.
2. Precipitation may occur when TNK-tPA is administered in an IV line containing dextrose. Dextrose-containing lines should be flushed with a saline-containing solution before and after single-bolus administration of TNK-tPA.
3. Reconstituted TNK-tPA should be administered as a single IV bolus over 5 seconds. Flush IV line with normal saline to ensure complete dose delivery.
4. Although the supplied syringe is compatible with a conventional needle, the supplied syringe is designed to be used with needleless IV systems. See Table 183-2 for information applicable to the IV system in use.
5. Dispose of the syringe, cannula, and shield per established procedures.

Patient Management for Acute Myocardial Infarction
1. Continuously monitor the cardiac rhythm and neurologic status.
2. Assess and document vital signs and status for clinical signs of reperfusion, bleeding complications (e.g., neurologic checks), and signs of coronary artery reocclusion (e.g., recurrence of chest pain or ST-segment elevation) every 15 minutes during TNK-tPA infusion and every 2 hours thereafter until 2 hours after heparin is discontinued. Clinical signs of reperfusion may include cardiac dysrhythmias, resolution of chest pain, and resolution of ST-segment elevation. These signs may indicate that TNK-tPA has been successful; however,

TABLE 183-2

IV SYSTEM COMPATIBILITY

System In Use	Instructions
Split septum IV system	1. Remove the green cap. 2. Attach the clear-ended blunt plastic cannula to the syringe. 3. Remove the shield and use the blunt plastic cannula to access the split-septum injection port. 4. Because the blunt plastic cannula has two side ports, air or fluid expelled through the cannula exits in two sideways directions; direct away from face or mucous membranes.
Luer-Lok system	Connect the syringe directly to the IV port.
Conventional needle	Attach a large-bore needle, e.g., 18 G (not supplied in TNKase kit), to the syringe's universal Luer-Lok.

Modified from Genentech (2000). TNKase (tenecteplase, recombinant) prescribing information. San Francisco: Author.
IV, Intravenous.

absence of these signs does not indicate that TNK-tPA has failed. The dysrhythmias seen are the same as those seen in many myocardial infarction patients and may include accelerated idioventricular rhythm, sinus bradycardia, ventricular tachycardia, ventricular fibrillation, and heart block. Any dysrhythmias that occur are treated according to advanced cardiac life support guidelines.

3. Document the time the chest pain resolves.
4. Maintain heparin infusion and monitor the partial thromboplastin time to maintain it at 1.5 to 2 times the control. Heparin may be continued for 24-72 hours until time of cardiac catheterization or other diagnostic tests.
5. Institute thrombolytic bleeding precautions as described subsequently.

THROMBOLYTIC BLEEDING PRECAUTIONS

1. Avoid the use of automatic blood pressure cuffs if possible. If automatic blood pressure cuffs are used, monitor them carefully to ensure that they are not repeatedly inflating to high pressures, which may cause underlying bruising and bleeding into the extremity.
2. Avoid unnecessary arterial and venous punctures. Puncture sites should be compressed manually for a minimum of 10 minutes for venous punctures and 20 minutes for arterial punctures. Apply pressure dressings after discontinuation of lines and vessel punctures.
3. Use a saline or heparin lock for blood draws, and consolidate blood draws.
4. Monitor all puncture sites and the gingivae for evidence of bleeding.
5. To avoid contusions, use a draw sheet to move and position the patient. Instruct the patient to request assistance in changing positions.
6. Observe for frank blood, and test urine, stools, and emesis for occult blood.
7. Avoid intramuscular injections.
8. Monitor hemoglobin and hematocrit for evidence of acute blood loss.
9. Suggest the use of antecubital or femoral sites for placement of central lines if needed.

COMPLICATIONS

The only adverse reactions attributable to TNK-tPA therapy are due to bleeding that occurs after TNK-tPA therapy. Bleeding should be expected to occur during and after TNK-tPA infusion. The goal is to prevent serious bleeding through careful screening and by observation of thrombolytic bleeding precautions. Thorough assessment and prompt treatment are also critical to minimize the effects of bleeding when it does occur. Most bleeding can be divided into two categories: surface bleeding and internal bleeding. Examples of the types of bleeding seen with TNK-tPA include the following:

1. Intracranial
2. Gastrointestinal
3. Genitourinary
4. Epistaxis
5. Retroperitoneal
6. Venous arterial puncture
7. Femoral artery catheter sites
8. Gingival
9. Ecchymosis

Intracranial bleeding is the most serious form of bleeding that can occur after thrombolytic therapy. Although intracranial bleeding is rare (<1%) (Genentech, 2000), it is so potentially devastating that care must be taken to exclude patients at risk for intracranial hemorrhage and to recognize and treat changes in neurologic status without delay.

PATIENT TEACHING

1. Ask for assistance before moving.
2. Report any bleeding.
3. Report any change in symptoms immediately.

REFERENCE

Genentech. (2000). TNKase (tenecteplase, recombinant) prescribing information. San Francisco: Author.

tPA Administration for Acute Myocardial Infarction or Pulmonary Embolus

Ruth Altherr Rench, MS, RN
and Teresa L. Will, RN, MSN, CEN

tPA is also known as tissue plasminogen activator, TPA, r-tPA, alteplase, or Activase.

INDICATIONS

To lyse thromboses in the presence of:
1. Acute myocardial infarction diagnosed by
   a. Typical ischemic chest pain lasting for at least 30 minutes and less than 12 hours' duration, which is unresponsive to sublingual nitroglycerin.
   b. ST-segment elevation of more than 1 mm in one of the following locations: two of the three inferior leads (II, III, aVF), two of the six precordial leads (V1 through V6), or lateral leads I and aVL.
   c. New-onset bundle-branch block.
2. Acute massive pulmonary embolus in which there is either obstruction of blood flow to a lobe or multiple lung segments or when accompanied by unstable hemodynamics. The diagnosis should be confirmed by objective means, such as pulmonary angiography, or noninvasive procedures, such as lung scanning.

CONTRAINDICATIONS

1. Active internal bleeding
2. Any history of cerebrovascular accident
3. Recent (within 2 months) intracranial or intraspinal surgery or trauma
4. Intracranial neoplasm, arteriovenous malformation, or aneurysm
5. Known bleeding disorder
6. Severe uncontrolled hypertension

CAUTIONS

Cautions or relative contraindications to the use of tPA are those events or conditions that either in isolation or combination may increase the potential risk of tPA therapy and include the following:
1. Recent major surgery
2. Cerebrovascular disease
3. Recent gastrointestinal or genitourinary bleeding
4. Recent trauma

5. Recent puncture of subclavian, internal jugular, or other noncompressible vessel
6. Uncontrolled hypertension: systolic blood pressure greater than or equal to 180 mm Hg or diastolic blood pressure greater than or equal to 110 mm Hg
7. High likelihood of left-sided heart thrombus (e.g., mitral stenosis with atrial fibrillation)
8. Acute pericarditis
9. Subacute bacterial endocarditis
10. Hemostatic disorders, including those secondary to severe hepatic and renal disease
11. Pregnancy
12. Diabetic hemorrhagic retinopathy or other hemorrhagic ophthalmic conditions
13. Septic thrombophlebitis or occluded arteriovenous cannula at seriously infected site
14. Age greater than 75 years
15. Current treatment with oral anticoagulants (e.g., warfarin sodium)
16. Any condition in which bleeding constitutes a significant hazard or would be particularly difficult to manage because of its location

EQUIPMENT

100-mg tPA kit (contains one 100-mg vial of tPA powder, one 100-ml vial of sterile water, and one double-sided transfer device)
Two 20-ml syringes
25 ml of normal saline (NS) or dextrose 5% in water (D_5W)
Intravenous (IV) starting equipment
IV catheter plug (also known as PRN adapter, heparin or saline lock, buffalo cap)
Volumetric IV pump and tubing (vented tubing preferred)

PATIENT PREPARATION

1. Perform a thorough assessment, including
   a. 12-lead electrocardiogram (see Procedure 59)
   b. Complete history and physical examination, including time of onset of chest pain
   c. Review of selection criteria for tPA therapy
2. Establish continuous cardiac monitoring (see Procedure 58).
3. Establish IV access with a minimum of two to three sites using 18- to 20-G catheters. The use of a double-lumen peripheral IV catheter may reduce the number of punctures (see Procedure 63).
4. Provide routine acute myocardial infarction care as prescribed, which may include but is not limited to the following:
   a. Oxygen therapy
   b. Aspirin
   c. Intravenous nitroglycerin
   d. Intravenous narcotic analgesia
   e. Intravenous beta-blocker therapy
5. Obtain laboratory studies, including
   a. Cardiac markers (myoglobin, troponin, creatine kinase-MB)
   b. Chemistry profile
   c. Electrolyte profile

    d. Prothrombin time (PT), partial thromboplastin time (PTT)
    e. Complete blood count with platelets

tPA RECONSTITUTION

NOTE: tPA is available in 50-mg and 100-mg vials. This procedure describes use of the 100-mg vial. The reconstitution is different for the 50-mg vial. Refer to the package insert for information.

1. Reconstitute tPA using a 100-mg vial.
    a. Insert one end of the transfer device into the vial containing the diluent. Hold the tPA vial upside-down, and insert the other end of the transfer device into the center of the stopper. Invert the vials.
    b. After transferring the sterile water, gently swirl or invert the vial to mix the contents. Do not shake. If foaming occurs, allow the vial to stand for 2-5 minutes for the foam to dissipate.
2. Assemble IV tubing without the use of an in-line filter. An in-line filter is not used because it can trap the tPA molecule and prevent it from reaching the patient. Vented pump tubing must be used to administer the solution directly from the 100-mg vial.
3. Once reconstituted, the tPA solution (1 mg/ml) may be used for direct administration. Although it may be further diluted with either NS or D_5W, most institutions prefer 1:1 dilution for ease of calculation and to limit fluids.
4. Hang the vial for direct infusion, or transfer the contents of the vial to an IV bag, bottle, or volume control chamber.
5. Set up infusion pump with the IV tubing and prime the tubing with the tPA solution, being careful not to discard any of the solution.
6. Once reconstituted, tPA solution may be stored for 8 hours at 2°-30° C (36°-86° F). After 8 hours, any unused portion should be discarded.
7. The reconstituted tPA is not light sensitive, and no special handling is required. Unreconstituted tPA may be sensitive to light and therefore should be stored in its carton until use.
8. tPA is not compatible with other medications; use a separate IV line for tPA administration.

ACCELERATED INFUSION (90 MINUTES) FOR ACUTE MYOCARDIAL INFARCTION
Procedural Steps

1. Bolus dose:
    a. Withdraw 15 mg from the tPA bag or vial, and administer over 1-2 minutes, *or*
    b. Administer the 15-mg bolus by setting the infusion pump at 450 ml/hr to deliver 15 ml over 2 minutes. NOTE: Careful attention to pump programming is warranted if this option is chosen.
2. After the bolus has infused, set the infusion pump at 100 ml/hr to deliver 50 mg over the first 30 minutes (see Step 6 for patients weighing <67 kg).
3. At the end of 30 minutes, decrease the IV rate to 35 ml/hr and continue until the infusion is complete. Remember to decrease the rate at the end of the first 30 minutes.
4. When the pump alarm sounds indicating the vial is empty, hang 25 ml of NS, or D_5W solution, and continue to infuse at the same rate until the pump alarm

sounds that the infusion is complete. This step ensures that the complete dose has been administered. After the full dose has been infused, convert the tPA line to a heparin or saline lock to use for blood draws.

5. The tPA dosing described here is based on the United States Food and Drug Administration–recommended dose of 100 mg, which is given over a 90-minute period (Table 184-1).

NOTE: A 3-hour infusion dose of tPA is also considered acceptable and is described more fully in the tPA prescribing information.

6. If a patient weighs 67 kg or less, administer a dose to the patient based on a milligram per kilogram schedule. The total dose approved by the United States Food and Drug Administration is 1.25 mg/kg, and the total tPA dose should never exceed 100 mg. Table 184-2 lists specific doses and infusion rates.

7. It is generally accepted that a loading dose of heparin should be administered and a continuous infusion started before the end of the tPA administration period. The PTT is then maintained at 1.5 times the control to prevent reocclusion.

Patient Management for Acute Myocardial Infarction

1. Continuously monitor the cardiac rhythm and neurologic status.

2. Assess and document vital signs and status for clinical signs of reperfusion, bleeding complications (e.g., neurologic checks), and signs of coronary artery reocclusion (e.g., recurrence of chest pain or ST-segment elevation) every 15 minutes during tPA infusion and every 2 hours thereafter until 2 hours after heparin administration is discontinued. Clinical signs of reperfusion may include cardiac dysrhythmias, resolution of chest pain, and resolution of ST-segment elevation. These signs may indicate that tPA has been successful; however, absence of these signs does not indicate that tPA has failed. The dysrhythmias seen are the same as those seen in many myocardial infarction patients and may include accelerated idioventricular rhythm, sinus bradycardia, ventricular tachycardia, ventricular fibrillation, and heart block. Any dysrhythmias that occur are treated according to advanced cardiac life support guidelines.

3. Document the time the chest pain resolves.

4. Be sure to turn down the tPA infusion and document the time at exactly 30 minutes into the infusion or 60 minutes into the infusion, depending on whether the accelerated 90-minute infusion or the 3-hour infusion is used.

5. Monitor the tPA infusion closely to ensure that it is infusing at the correct rate.

TABLE 184-1
ACCELERATED 90-MINUTE tPA INFUSION, tPA CONCENTRATION 1 mg/ml

	Dose (mg)	Pump Rate (ml/hr)
Bolus (over 2 min)	15	450
First 30 min	50	100
Next 60 min	35	35
Total dose	100	

From Genentech (1996). *Activase (alteplase, recombinant) prescribing information.* San Francisco: Author

TABLE 184-2

WEIGHT-BASED tPA DOSAGE CALCULATION CHART,
tPA CONCENTRATION 1 mg/ml

Weight (lb)	Weight (kg)	15-mg Bolus (ml)	30-Minute Infusion Rate (ml/hr) 0.75 mg/kg	60-Minute Infusion Rate (ml/hr) 0.5 mg/kg	Total Dose (mg)
90	41	15	62	20.5	66.5
92.5	42	15	63	21	67.5
94.5	43	15	64	21.5	68.5
97	44	15	66	22	70
99	45	15	68	22.5	71.5
101	46	15	69	23	72.5
103.5	47	15	70	23.5	73.5
105.5	48	15	72	24	75
108	49	15	74	24.5	76.5
110	50	15	75	25	77.5
112	51	15	76	25.5	78.5
114.5	52	15	78	26	80
116.5	53	15	80	26.5	81.5
119	54	15	81	27	82.5
121	55	15	82	27.5	83.5
123	56	15	84	28	85
125.5	57	15	86	28.5	86.5
127.5	58	15	87	29	87.5
130	59	15	88	29.5	88.5
132	60	15	90	30	90
134	61	15	92	30.5	91.5
136.5	62	15	93	31	92.5
138.5	63	15	94	31.5	93.5
141	64	15	96	32	95
143	65	15	98	32.5	96.5
145	66	15	99	33	97.5
147.5	67	15	100	33.5	98.5
>147.5	>67	15	100	35	100

Data from Genentech (1996). *Activase (alteplase, recombinant) prescribing information.* San Francisco: Author.

6. Maintain heparin infusion and monitor the PTT to maintain it at 1.5 to 2 times the control. Heparin may be continued for 24-72 hours until time of cardiac catheterization or other diagnostic tests.
7. Institute thrombolytic bleeding precautions as described subsequently.

DOSING AND ADMINISTRATION FOR PULMONARY EMBOLUS
Procedural Steps

1. The recommended dose of tPA for pulmonary embolus is 100 mg over 2 hours. Administer via volumetric pump at 50 ml/hr.

2. Heparin therapy should be instituted near the end or immediately after the tPA infusion when the PTT returns to twice normal or less.

Patient Management for Pulmonary Embolus

1. Monitor the cardiac rhythm and pulmonary and neurologic status continuously.
2. Assess and document vital signs, pulmonary status, and neurologic status, and check for evidence of bleeding every 15 minutes during tPA infusion and every 2 hours thereafter until the patient is stable.
3. Monitor the tPA infusion closely to ensure that it is infusing at the correct rate.
4. Institute heparin therapy when PTT returns to twice normal or less.
5. Repeat baseline laboratory and diagnostic tests to assess results of treatment.
6. Institute thrombolytic bleeding precautions as described subsequently.

THROMBOLYTIC BLEEDING PRECAUTIONS

1. Avoid the use of automatic blood pressure cuffs if possible. If automatic blood pressure cuffs are used, monitor them carefully to ensure that they are not repeatedly inflating to high pressures, which may cause underlying bruising and bleeding into the extremity.
2. Avoid unnecessary arterial and venous punctures. Puncture sites should be compressed manually for a minimum of 10 minutes for venous punctures and 20 minutes for arterial punctures. Apply pressure dressings after discontinuation of lines and vessel punctures.
3. Use a saline or heparin lock for blood draws, and consolidate blood draws.
4. Monitor all puncture sites and the gingivae for evidence of bleeding.
5. To avoid contusions, use a draw sheet to move and position the patient. Instruct the patient to request assistance in changing positions.
6. Observe for frank blood, and test urine, stools, and emesis for occult blood.
7. Avoid intramuscular injections.
8. Monitor hemoglobin and hematocrit for evidence of acute blood loss.
9. Suggest the use of antecubital or femoral sites for placement of central lines if needed.

COMPLICATIONS

The only adverse reactions attributable to tPA therapy are due to bleeding that occurs after tPA therapy. Bleeding should be expected to occur during and after tPA infusion. The goal is to prevent serious bleeding through careful screening and by observation of thrombolytic bleeding precautions. Thorough assessment and prompt treatment are also critical to minimize the effects of bleeding when it does occur. Most bleeding can be divided into two categories: surface bleeding and internal bleeding. Examples of the types of bleeding occurring with tPA include the following:

1. Intracranial
2. Gastrointestinal
3. Genitourinary
4. Epistaxis
5. Retroperitoneal
6. Venous arterial puncture
7. Femoral artery catheter sites

8. Gingival

9. Ecchymosis

Intracranial bleeding is the most serious form of bleeding that can occur after thrombolytic therapy. Although intracranial bleeding is rare (<1%) (Genentech, 1996), it is so potentially devastating that care must be taken to exclude patients at risk for intracranial hemorrhage and to recognize and treat changes in neurologic status without delay.

PATIENT TEACHING

1. Ask for assistance before moving.

2. Report any bleeding.

3. Report any change in symptoms immediately.

REFERENCE

Genentech (1996). *Activase (alteplase, recombinant) prescribing information.* San Francisco: Author.

---

tPA Administration for Acute Ischemic Stroke

Ruth Altherr Rench, MS, RN
and Teresa L. Will, RN, MSN, CEN

tPA is also known as tissue plasminogen activator, TPA, r-tPA, alteplase, or Activase. Acute ischemic stroke is one type of cerebrovascular accident.

INDICATIONS

tPA is indicated for the management of acute ischemic stroke in adults for improving neurologic recovery and reducing the incidence of disability when the following situations exist:

1. Identification of a focal neurologic deficit indicating a probability of acute ischemic stroke

2. Treatment can be initiated within 3 hours after stroke symptom onset

3. Exclusion of intracranial hemorrhage by a cranial computed tomography (CT) scan or other diagnostic imaging method sensitive for the presence of hemorrhage

CONTRAINDICATIONS

1. Evidence of intracranial hemorrhage on pretreatment evaluation
2. Suspicion of subarachnoid hemorrhage
3. Recent intracranial surgery, serious head trauma, or recent previous stroke
4. History of intracranial hemorrhage
5. Uncontrolled hypertension at time of treatment (e.g., >185 mm Hg systolic blood pressure or >110 mm Hg diastolic blood pressure)
6. Seizure at the onset of stroke
7. Active internal bleeding
8. Intracranial neoplasm, arteriovenous malformation, or aneurysm
9. Known bleeding diathesis including but not limited to the following:
   a. Current use of oral anticoagulants (e.g., warfarin sodium) with prothrombin time greater than 15 seconds
   b. Administration of heparin within 48 hours preceding the onset of stroke with an elevated activated partial thromboplastin time at presentation
   c. Platelet count less than 100,000/mm^3
10. Symptom onset greater than 3 hours before administration of medication. If the patient awoke from sleep with symptoms, the time he/she went to sleep is regarded as the time of symptom onset.

CAUTIONS

The following are cautions for using tPA to treat acute ischemic stroke. In these situations, the risk of treatment with tPA may be increased and should be weighed against the anticipated benefits.

1. Patients with severe neurologic deficit at presentation who have an increased risk of intracranial hemorrhage
2. Patients with major early infarct signs on a cranial CT scan
3. Events or conditions that either in isolation or in combination may increase the potential risk of tPA therapy include:
   a. Recent major surgery
   b. Cerebrovascular disease
   c. Recent gastrointestinal or genitourinary bleeding
   d. Recent trauma
   e. Recent puncture of subclavian, internal jugular, or other noncompressible vessel
   f. Hypertension: systolic blood pressure greater than or equal to 180 mm Hg or diastolic blood pressure greater than or equal to 110 mm Hg
   g. High likelihood of left-sided heart thrombus (e.g., mitral stenosis with atrial fibrillation)
   h. Acute pericarditis
   i. Subacute bacterial endocarditis
   j. Hemostatic disorders, including those secondary to severe hepatic and renal disease
   k. Pregnancy
   l. Diabetic hemorrhagic retinopathy or other hemorrhagic ophthalmic conditions
   m. Septic thrombophlebitis or occluded arteriovenous cannula at seriously infected site
   n. Age greater than 75 years

o. Current treatment with oral anticoagulants (e.g., warfarin sodium)

p. Any condition in which bleeding constitutes a significant hazard or would be particularly difficult to manage because of its location

EQUIPMENT

One 100-mg tPA kit (contains one 100-mg vial of tPA powder, one 100-ml vial of sterile water, and one double-sided transfer device)

Two 20- to 30-ml syringes

25 ml normal saline or dextrose 5% water solution

Intravenous (IV) catheter plug (also known as PRN adapter, heparin lock or saline lock, buffalo cap)

Volumetric intravenous pump and tubing

20-ml syringe with needle for discard solution

PATIENT PREPARATION

1. Provide critical care measures as prescribed, which may include but are not limited to:
   a. Oxygen therapy (see Procedure 27)
   b. 12-Lead electrocardiogram (see Procedure 59)
   c. Continuous cardiac monitoring (see Procedure 58)
   d. Establishment of IV access with a minimum of two to three sites using 18- to 20-G catheters (see Procedure 63)
   e. Complete history and physical examination, including time of stroke symptom onset
   f. Review of selection criteria for tPA therapy
2. *Do not administer heparin or aspirin for the first 24 hours after tPA treatment for acute ischemic stroke.*
3. Obtain laboratory studies, including the following:
   a. Chemistry profile
   b. Electrolyte profile
   c. Prothrombin time, partial thromboplastin time
   d. Complete blood count with platelets
4. Monitor blood pressure every 15 minutes.
5. Administer medications as ordered to maintain systolic blood pressure at 185 mm Hg or less and diastolic blood pressure at 115 mm Hg or less.

PROCEDURAL STEPS

NOTE: tPA is available in 50- and 100-mg vials. This procedure describes use of the 100-mg vial. The reconstitution is different for the 50-mg vial. Refer to the package insert for information.

1. Reconstitute tPA using a 100-mg vial:
   a. Insert one end of transfer device into the vial containing diluent. Hold the tPA vial upside-down, and insert the other end of the transfer device into the center of the stopper. Invert the vials.
   b. After transferring the sterile water, gently swirl or invert the vial to mix the contents. Do not shake. If foaming occurs, allow the vial to stand for 2-5 minutes for the foam to dissipate.
2. Assemble IV tubing without the use of an in-line filter. An in-line filter is not used because it can trap the tPA molecule and prevent it from reaching the

patient. Vented pump tubing must be used to administer the solution directly from the 100-mg vial.
3. Once reconstituted, the tPA solution (1 mg/ml) may be used for direct administration. Although it may be further diluted with either normal saline or dextrose 5% water solution, most institutions prefer 1:1 dilution for ease of calculation and to limit fluids.
4. Withdraw any tPA to be discarded and the bolus dose (Table 185-1).
5. Hang the vial for direct infusion or transfer the contents of the vial to an IV bag, bottle, or volume control chamber.
6. Set up infusion pump with the IV tubing, and prime the tubing with the tPA solution, being careful not to discard any of the solution.

TABLE 185-1
WEIGHT-BASED tPA DOSAGE CALCULATION CHART FOR ACUTE ISCHEMIC STROKE, tPA CONCENTRATION 1 mg/ml

Weight (lb)	Weight (kg)	Bolus Over 1 min (ml)	1-Hour Infusion Rate (ml/hr)	Total Dose (mg) 0.9 mg/kg
90	41	3.7	33.2	36.9
95	43	3.8	34.9	38.7
99	45	4.1	36.4	40.5
106	48	4.3	38.9	43.2
110	50	4.5	40.5	45
114	52	4.7	42.1	46.8
121	55	5	44.5	49.5
125	57	5.1	46.2	51.3
130	59	5.3	47.8	53.1
134	61	5.5	49.4	54.9
141	64	5.8	51.8	57.6
145	66	5.9	53.5	59.4
150	68	6.1	55.1	61.2
154	70	6.3	56.7	63
161	73	6.6	59.1	65.7
165	75	6.8	60.7	67.5
172	78	7	63.2	70.2
176	80	7.2	64.8	72
183	83	7.5	67.2	74.7
187	85	7.7	68.8	76.5
194	88	7.9	71.3	79.2
198	90	8.1	72.9	81
202	92	8.3	74.5	82.8
207	94	8.5	76.1	84.6
211	96	8.6	77.8	86.4
216	98	8.8	79.4	88.2
≥220	≥100	9	81	90

tPA, Tissue plasminogen activator.

7. Once reconstituted, tPA solution may be stored for 8 hours at 2°-30° C (36°-86° F). After 8 hours, any unused portion should be discarded.

8. The reconstituted tPA is not light sensitive, and no special handling is required. Unreconstituted tPA may be sensitive to light and therefore should be stored in its carton until use.

9. tPA is not compatible with other medications; use a separate IV line for tPA administration.

10. tPA dosing for acute ischemic stroke is always based on patient weight (see Table 185-1). The United States Food and Drug Administration–recommended total dose is 0.9 mg/kg. Never exceed 90 mg for the total dose of tPA for acute ischemic stroke (Genentech, 1996).
    a. Administer 10% of the total dose as an IV bolus over 1 minute.
    b. Administer the remainder of the dose as a continuous infusion over 1 hour.

PATIENT MANAGEMENT

1. Continuously monitor the patient's condition, cardiac rhythm, and neurologic status. Assess and document vital signs, neurologic status, and bleeding every 15 minutes for the first 2 hours after starting the tPA infusion, then every 30 minutes for 6 hours, then every hour for 16 hours.

2. Monitor the tPA infusion closely to ensure that it is infusing at the correct rate.

3. Do not give heparin, aspirin, or warfarin sodium for 24 hours after the tPA infusion. If heparin or any other anticoagulant is indicated after 24 hours, it is recommended that a CT scan be performed to rule out intracranial hemorrhage first.

4. Administer medications as ordered to maintain blood pressure at less than 185/110 mm Hg.

5. Institute thrombolytic bleeding precautions, which include the following:
    a. Avoid the use of automatic blood pressure cuffs if possible. If automatic blood pressure cuffs are used, monitor them carefully to ensure that they are not repeatedly inflating to high pressures, which may cause underlying bruising and bleeding into the extremity.
    b. Avoid unnecessary arterial and venous punctures. All puncture sites should be compressed manually for a minimum of 10 minutes for venous punctures and 20 minutes for arterial punctures. Apply pressure dressings after discontinuation of lines and vessel punctures.
    c. Use a saline or heparin lock for blood draws, and consolidate blood draws.
    d. Monitor all puncture sites and the gingivae for evidence of bleeding.
    e. To avoid contusions, use a draw sheet to move and position the patient. Instruct the patient to request assistance in changing positions.
    f. Observe for frank blood, and test urine, stools, and emesis for occult blood.
    g. Avoid intramuscular injections.
    h. Monitor hemoglobin and hematocrit for evidence of acute blood loss.
    i. Suggest the use of antecubital or femoral sites for placement of central lines if needed.

6. Observe for signs of intracranial hemorrhage, such as any acute neurologic deterioration, new headache, acute hypertension, or nausea and vomiting. If intracranial hemorrhage is suspected, discontinue the tPA infusion and obtain an emergency CT scan.

COMPLICATIONS

The only adverse reactions attributable to tPA therapy are due to bleeding that occurs after tPA therapy. Cholesterol embolization has been reported but is a rare complication. Bleeding should be expected to occur during and after tPA infusion. The goal is to prevent serious bleeding through careful screening and by observation of thrombolytic bleeding precautions. Thorough assessment and prompt treatment are also critical to minimize the effects of bleeding when it does occur. Most bleeding can be divided into two categories: surface bleeding and internal bleeding. Examples of the types of bleeding occurring with tPA include the following:

1. Intracranial
2. Gastrointestinal
3. Genitourinary
4. Epistaxis
5. Retroperitoneal
6. Venous or arterial puncture
7. Femoral artery catheter sites
8. Gingival
9. Ecchymosis

Intracranial bleeding is the most serious form of bleeding that can occur after thrombolytic therapy. It is so potentially devastating that care must be taken to exclude patients at risk for intracranial hemorrhage and to recognize and treat changes in neurologic status without delay.

PATIENT TEACHING

1. Ask for assistance before moving.
2. Report any bleeding.
3. Report any changes in symptoms immediately.

REFERENCE

Genentech (1996). Activase, alteplase, recombinant prescribing information. San Francisco: Author.

Reteplase Administration for Acute Myocardial Infarction

Teresa L. Will, RN, MSN, CEN

Reteplase recombinant is also known as Retavase, recombinant plasminogen activator, RPA, and rPA.

INDICATIONS
To lyse thromboses in the presence of acute myocardial infarction diagnosed by
1. Typical ischemic chest pain lasting for at least 30 minutes and less than 12 hours' duration, which is unresponsive to sublingual nitroglycerin
2. ST-segment elevation of more than 1 mm in one of the following locations: two of three inferior leads (II, III, aVF), two of six precordial leads (V1 through V6), or lateral leads I and aVL
3. New-onset bundle-branch block

CONTRAINDICATIONS
1. Active internal bleeding
2. Any history of cerebrovascular accident
3. Recent (within 2 months) intracranial or intraspinal surgery or trauma
4. Intracranial neoplasm, arteriovenous malformation, or aneurysm
5. Known bleeding disorder
6. Severe uncontrolled hypertension

CAUTIONS
Cautions or relative contraindications to the use of reteplase are those events or conditions that either in isolation or combination may increase the potential risk of reteplase therapy, including the following:
1. Recent major surgery
2. Cerebrovascular disease
3. Recent gastrointestinal or genitourinary bleeding
4. Recent trauma
5. Recent puncture of subclavian, internal jugular, or other noncompressible vessel
6. Hypertension: systolic blood pressure greater than or equal to 180 mm Hg or diastolic blood pressure greater than or equal to 110 mm Hg
7. High likelihood of left-sided heart thrombus (e.g., mitral stenosis with atrial fibrillation)
8. Acute pericarditis
9. Subacute bacterial endocarditis
10. Hemostatic disorders, including those secondary to severe hepatic and renal disease

11. Pregnancy
12. Diabetic hemorrhagic retinopathy or other hemorrhagic ophthalmic conditions
13. Septic thrombophlebitis or occluded arteriovenous cannula at seriously infected site
14. Age greater than 75 years
15. Current treatment with oral anticoagulants (e.g., warfarin sodium)
16. Any condition in which bleeding constitutes a significant hazard or would be particularly difficult to manage because of its location

EQUIPMENT

Reteplase administration kit (contains two vials of reteplase 10.8 units each and two vials of sterile water for injection, two dispensing pins, two 10-ml syringes, and two 20-G needles)
Intravenous (IV) starting equipment
IV catheter plug (also known as PRN adapter, heparin or saline lock, buffalo cap)

PATIENT PREPARATION

1. Perform a thorough assessment including:
   a. 12-lead electrocardiogram (see Procedure 59)
   b. Complete history and physical examination, including time of onset of chest pain
   c. Review of selection criteria for thrombolytic therapy
2. Establish continuous cardiac monitoring (see Procedure 58).
3. Establish IV access with a minimum of two to three sites, using 18- to 20-G catheters. The use of a double-lumen peripheral IV catheter may reduce the number of punctures (see Procedure 63).
4. Provide routine acute myocardial infarction care as prescribed, which may include but is not limited to the following:
   a. Oxygen therapy
   b. Aspirin (administered concomitantly in >99% of patients studied [Boehringer Mannheim, 1996])
   c. IV nitroglycerin
   d. IV narcotic analgesia
   e. IV beta-blocker therapy
   f. Heparin therapy (administered concomitantly in >99% of patients studied [Boehringer Mannheim, 1996])
5. Obtain laboratory studies, including
   a. Cardiac markers (myoglobin, troponin, creatine kinase-MB)
   b. Chemistry profile
   c. Electrolyte profile
   d. Prothrombin time, partial thromboplastin time
   e. Complete blood count with platelets

PROCEDURAL STEPS

1. Reconstitute a 10 unit/10 ml dose of reteplase (Boehringer Mannheim, 1996):
   a. Use the 10-ml syringe with attached needle to withdraw 10 ml of sterile water for injection.

   b. Remove the needle from the syringe, and discard the needle. Remove the protective cap from the Luer-Lok port of the dispensing pin, and connect the syringe to the dispensing pin.

   c. Insert the spike of the dispensing pin into the vial of reteplase. Transfer the 10 ml of sterile water for injection through the dispensing pin into the vial of reteplase.

   d. With the dispensing pin and syringe still attached to the vial, swirl the vial gently to dissolve the reteplase. Do not shake.

   e. Withdraw 10 ml of reconstituted reteplase back into the syringe. A small amount of solution (0.7 ml) remains in the vial because of overfill.

   f. Detach the syringe from the dispensing pin, and attach the sterile 20-G needle provided.

2. Administer the 10-ml bolus of reteplase over 2 minutes. No other medications should be infusing through the IV line or the line must be flushed before reteplase administration. Flush the line again after reteplase administration.

3. The second bolus of 10 units of reteplase must be administered 30 minutes after the first bolus. Repeat steps 1 and 2 for the second bolus.

4. Heparin and aspirin should be administered concomitantly.

PATIENT MANAGEMENT FOR ACUTE MYOCARDIAL INFARCTION

1. Continuously monitor the cardiac rhythm and neurologic status.

2. Assess and document vital signs and status for clinical signs of reperfusion, bleeding complications (e.g., neurologic checks), and signs of coronary artery reocclusion (e.g., recurrence of chest pain or ST-segment elevation) every 15 minutes for the first 2 hours after administration of the first reteplase bolus, then every 2 hours thereafter until 2 hours after heparin is discontinued. Clinical signs of reperfusion include cardiac dysrhythmias, resolution of chest pain, and resolution of ST-segment elevation. These signs may indicate the thrombolytic has been successful; however, absence of these signs does not indicate the thrombolytic has failed. The dysrhythmias seen are the same as those seen in many myocardial infarction patients and may include accelerated ventricular rhythm, sinus bradycardia, ventricular tachycardia, ventricular fibrillation, and heart block. Any dysrhythmias that occur are treated according to advanced cardiac life support guidelines.

3. Document the time the chest pain resolves.

4. Do not forget to give the second bolus of reteplase at precisely 30 minutes after the first dose. Remember to flush the line completely before and after the reteplase administration so that reteplase does not mix with other medications. Heparin and reteplase are incompatible when they are combined in solution.

5. Maintain heparin infusion and monitor partial thromboplastin time levels closely. The patient may be on heparin for 24-72 hours until time of cardiac catheterization or other diagnostic tests.

6. Institute thrombolytic bleeding precautions, including the following:

   a. Avoid the use of automatic blood pressure cuffs if possible. If automatic blood pressure cuffs are used, monitor them carefully to ensure that they are not repeatedly inflating to high pressures, which may cause underlying bruising and bleeding into the extremity.

   b. Avoid unnecessary arterial and venous punctures. Puncture sites should be compressed manually for a minimum of 10 minutes for venous punc-

tures and 20 minutes for arterial punctures. Apply pressure dressings after discontinuation of lines and vessel punctures.
   c. Use a saline or heparin lock for blood draws, and consolidate blood draws.
   d. Monitor all puncture sites and the gingivae for evidence of bleeding.
   e. To avoid contusions, use a draw sheet to move and position the patient. Instruct the patient to request assistance in changing positions.
   f. Observe for frank blood, and test urine, stools, and emesis for occult blood.
   g. Avoid intramuscular injections.
   h. Monitor hemoglobin and hematocrit for evidence of acute blood loss.
   i. Suggest the use of antecubital or femoral sites for placement of central lines if needed.

COMPLICATIONS

1. The major adverse reactions attributable to reteplase therapy are due to bleeding that occurs after therapy. Bleeding should be expected to occur during and after reteplase infusion. The goal is to prevent serious bleeding through careful screening and by observation of thrombolytic bleeding precautions. Thorough assessment and prompt treatment are also critical to minimize the effects of bleeding when it does occur. Most bleeding can be divided into two categories: surface bleeding and internal bleeding. Examples of the types of bleeding occurring with reteplase include the following:
   a. Intracranial
   b. Gastrointestinal
   c. Genitourinary
   d. Epistaxis
   e. Retroperitoneal
   f. Venous or arterial punctures
   g. Femoral artery catheter sites
   h. Gingival
   i. Ecchymosis
   Intracranial bleeding is the most serious form of bleeding that can occur after thrombolytic therapy. Although intracranial bleeding is rare (<1%), it is so potentially devastating that care must be taken to exclude patients at risk for intracranial hemorrhage and to recognize and treat changes in neurologic status without delay (Boehringer Mannheim, 1996). The effective half-life of reteplase is 13-16 minutes. In the event of serious bleeding, the second reteplase bolus should not be given, and heparin should be stopped immediately (Boehringer Mannheim, 1996). Heparin effects can be reversed by protamine.
2. Allergic reaction (Boehringer Mannheim, 1996)
3. Nausea, vomiting (Boehringer Mannheim, 1996)
4. Fever, hypotension (Boehringer Mannheim, 1996)

PATIENT TEACHING

1. Ask for assistance before moving.
2. Report any bleeding.
3. Report any change in symptoms immediately.

REFERENCE

Boehringer Mannheim. (1996). Retavase (reteplase recombinant) prescribing information. Gaithersburg, MD: Author.

PROCEDURE 187

High-Dose Steroids for Spinal Cord Injury

Daun A. Smith, RN, MS, CEN

INDICATION

High-dose steroids are indicated for symptomatic (motor and sensory) spinal cord–injured patients. Although the mechanism of action is yet unknown, high-dose steroid therapy (methylprednisolone sodium succinate), initiated within 8 hours of a spinal cord injury, has been shown to improve the neurologic outcome (motor function and response to pinprick and light touch) (Bracken et al., 1990). Another study (Bracken, et al., 1997) showed that if treatment was begun 3-8 hours after injury, treatment with methylprednisolone for 48 hours was likely to show improvement.

CONTRAINDICATIONS AND CAUTIONS

1. Methylprednisolone therapy must be initiated within 8 hours of injury to have any positive neurologic effects in spinal cord–injured patients (Bracken et al., 1990).
2. Although methylprednisolone has been shown to be compatible with many medications, compatibility should be checked before infusing methylprednisolone with any medication.
3. Methylprednisolone is available in two forms: methylprednisolone sodium succinate and methylprednisolone acetate. Only methylprednisolone sodium succinate may be given intravenously.

EQUIPMENT

Methylprednisolone sodium succinate, 4 g
Normal saline solution (for intravenous [IV] use), 250 ml
IV infusion pump and tubing

PATIENT PREPARATION

1. Initiate and maintain spinal immobilization (see Procedure 115).
2. Initiate IV access (see Procedure 63).
3. Assess baseline neurologic status, including motor and sensory levels.

PROCEDURAL STEPS
Preparation of the Infusion

1. Withdraw enough fluid from the bag of normal saline to account for the volume of medication to be added and the manufacturer's overfill of the IV fluid bag (contact manufacturer for specific information).
2. Mix and add 4 g of methylprednisolone sodium succinate to the prepared 250-ml IV bag (this provides a concentration of 16 mg/ml).

Loading Dose

1. A loading dose of 30 mg/kg is given over 15 minutes.
2. Prime the tubing with the prepared mixture before starting the infusion.
3. Infuse the loading dose at the appropriate rate for the patient's weight (Table 187-1). Rate is in ml/hr, but infuse for 15 minutes only.
4. After the loading dose has infused, turn off the methylprednisolone for 45 minutes, and run IV fluid at a keep-open rate.

TABLE 187-1
DOSING OF METHYLPREDNISOLONE*

Patient Weight (kg)	Loading Dose (30 mg/kg)	Rate of Loading Dose in ml/hr for 15 min only	Maintenance Dose per Hour (5.4 mg/kg/hr)	Maintenance Dose (Rate in ml/hr for 23 Hours)
30	900 mg/56 ml	225	162	10
35	1050 mg/66 ml	262	189	12
40	1200 mg/75 ml	300	216	14
45	1350 mg/84 ml	338	243	15
50	1500 mg/94 ml	375	270	17
55	1650 mg/103 ml	412	297	19
60	1800 mg/113 ml	450	324	20
65	1950 mg/122 ml	488	351	22
70	2100 mg/131 ml	525	378	24
75	2250 mg/141 ml	562	405	25
80	2400 mg/150 ml	600	432	27
85	2550 mg/159 ml	638	459	29
90	2700 mg/169 ml	675	486	30
95	2850 mg/178 ml	712	513	32
100	3000 mg/188 ml	750	540	34

*Table reflects preparation of methylprednisolone as a 16-mg/ml solution. Loading dose rate is in ml/hr; total loading dose is run in over 15 minutes. Then the infusion is stopped for 45 minutes before the maintenance infusion is initiated.

Maintenance Dose

1. Over the next 23 hours, infuse the above-prepared solution at a rate to provide a dose of 5.4 mg/kg per hour (see Table 187-1).
2. If treatment is initiated 3-8 hours after injury, continue the infusion for 27 hours at the 5.4 mg/kg per hour rate (see Table 187-1).

AGE-SPECIFIC CONSIDERATIONS

1. Studies have not yet addressed either the pediatric or the geriatric populations.
2. If it is necessary to restrict IV fluids, mix the solution in a more concentrated form and recalculate infusion rates based on the new concentration.

COMPLICATIONS

1. Impaired wound healing
2. Gastrointestinal bleeding
3. Infection

PATIENT TEACHING

1. Report any signs of infection.
2. Report any signs of gastrointestinal bleeding.
3. Results of the steroid infusion are not dramatic; however, even small gains in neurologic status can make a large difference in postinjury function.

REFERENCES

Bracken, M.B., Shepard, M.J., Collins, W.F., et al. (1990). A randomized controlled trial of methylprednisolone or naloxone in the treatment of acute spinal cord injury. *New England Journal of Medicine, 322,* 1405-1411.

Bracken, M.B., Shephard, M.J., Holford, T.R., et al (1997). Administration of methylprednisolone for 24 or 48 hours or tirilazad mesylate for 48 hours in the treatment of acute spinal cord injury. *Journal of the American Medical Association, 277*(20), 1597-1604.

Miscellaneous Procedures

Drug and Alcohol Specimen Collection

Reneé Semonin Holleran, RN, PhD, CEN, CCRN, CFRN, SANE

INDICATIONS

1. To identify whether the patient is intoxicated by a drug or alcohol
2. To obtain evidence in a criminal case
3. To obtain laboratory data for a differential diagnosis for an altered mental status or specific signs and symptoms, such as (Ohio Chapter of the International Association of Forensic Nurses, 2002):
   a. Slurred speech
   b. Dizziness
   c. Confusion
   d. Blurred vision
   e. Anxiety
   f. Euphoria
   g. Hallucinations
   h. Amnesia/memory impairment
   i. Lack of muscle coordination
   j. Hyperthermia

CONTRAINDICATIONS AND CAUTIONS

1. Life-threatening conditions should be managed before evidence collection.
2. Blood or body fluid specimen collection for evidence in an alleged crime generally requires patient consent or a court order. Each emergency department should have protocols that govern the collection of blood and/or urine for alcohol and drug screening. Some states have laws or regulations that stipulate that specimens can be obtained without the patient's consent in specified circumstances, such as a motor-vehicle crash resulting in serious injury or death.
3. Collection of blood/urine for alcohol or drug screening for an alleged crime without patient permission may be considered assault and battery (Nettina, 2001).
4. If the patient is exhibiting altered mental status, always rule out organic causes for the patient's behavior, signs, and symptoms. Hypoglycemia, shock, traumatic brain injury, or drug interactions are only a few of the disease processes that can cause signs and symptoms similar to those of drug and alcohol intoxication.

EQUIPMENT

Most states have a specific kit that is used for the collection of blood/urine for legal purposes. These kits may be stored in the emergency department or brought by the law enforcement agency requesting the test.

The following lists an example of the contents of an alcohol/drug determination kit:

One 10-ml blood tube containing sodium fluoride and potassium oxalate
Two 7-ml blood tubes containing EDTA
Two 40-ml plastic screw-cap containers
One direction sheet
Two police evidence seals for resealing kit box after collection of evidence
One biohazard bag for transportation of specimens

PATIENT PREPARATION

1. If not covered by state law/regulation or court order, obtain patient consent according to institutional policy.
2. Ensure that the law-enforcement agency requesting the test has explained the procedure and the patient's rights before the blood or urine is collected.
3. The law enforcement officer should witness the collection of the specimens whenever possible.

PROCEDURAL STEPS

1. For blood specimens:
   a. Clean the skin with a nonalcohol disinfectant.
   b. Draw blood as per Procedure 61.
   c. Label the evidence with the patient's name, area of collection, date, time, and the person collecting the evidence. In some cases, the label must be placed across the stopper of the blood tube.
2. For urine specimens:
   a. Have the patient place the specimen in a urine cup. For legal specimens, the patient is usually monitored during urination or placed in an area where no water or other fluid is available with which the specimen can be diluted.
   b. The more urine, the better, but at least 30 ml is required. Some drug screens require at least 100 ml of urine.
   c. For some legal samples, the temperature of the urine must be taken and documented as soon as the specimen is received. In this case, the patient's temperature should also be taken and documented.
3. Follow and document chain of custody procedures carefully.
4. Blood and urine may require refrigeration if they are not immediately transported by law enforcement or taken to the laboratory.
5. If the specimen must be sent to a laboratory, the laboratory should provide directions for packaging, chain-of-custody maintenance, temperature control, and shipment.
6. Provide the toxicologist with information concerning the suspected drugs, the time the drugs were ingested, how were they ingested, and if the patient has been given any medications in the emergency department.

AGE-SPECIFIC CONSIDERATION

Minors require parental/legal guardian permission for specimen collection unless institutional or state laws or regulations stipulate otherwise.

COMPLICATIONS

1. If only legal specimens are requested and no medical screening examination is performed, the patient may not be appropriately evaluated and could suffer serious injury or even death.
2. If the specimens are not appropriately collected and handled, they may be considered contaminated and ruled inadmissible.
3. If the chain of custody is not preserved and documented, the evidence may be ruled inadmissible.

PATIENT TEACHING

1. Provide the patient with information related to the law enforcement agency that requested the specimens for follow-up regarding legal procedures.
2. Instruct the patient/family when to return to the emergency department or call 911 for problems related to alcohol or drug intoxication.
3. Refer the patient/family to the appropriate agency for substance abuse counseling as indicated.

REFERENCES

Nettina, S. (2001). *The Lippincott manual of nursing practice*, 7th ed. Philadelphia: Lippincott.
Ohio Chapter of the International Association of Forensic Nurses. (2002). *The Ohio adolescent and adult sexual assault nurse examiner training manual.* Columbus: Author.

PROCEDURE 189

Preservation of Evidence

Reneé Semonin Holleran, RN, PhD, CEN, CCRN, CFRN

Evidence is something legally submitted to a court of law as a means of determining the truth related to an alleged crime (Doyle, 2001). The sources of evidence are the victim, the suspect, and the scene of the crime (Burgess, 2000). Every emergency department should have a protocol for evidence collection and preservation. The most common types of evidence collected include clothing; bullets; hairs; fibers; blood stains; fragments of materials such as paint, glass, and wood; dirt; or plants.

INDICATIONS

1. To properly preserve evidence that has been collected from the victim of an alleged crime or a suspected perpetrator. Evidence should be collected for (Lynch, 1995):

    a. A medicolegal case or when there is a treatment situation with legal implications
    b. Suspicious deaths
    c. Crime-related injuries: child maltreatment, sexual assault
    d. Motor vehicle crashes

2. To properly store evidence so that it may not be altered.
3. See specific procedures on collection of evidence for drug and alcohol testing (Procedure 188), sexual assaults (Procedure 190), and bite marks (Procedure 191).

CONTRAINDICATIONS AND CAUTIONS

1. Interventions may destroy evidence. Emergency care providers should recognize and preserve evidence whenever possible. For example, placing paper bags over the hands of gunshot victim can help preserve trace evidence of gunpowder and identify whether it is a self-inflicted wound (Figure 189-1). Also, try not to cut through bullet or knife holes in clothing.
2. Some evidence may be misinterpreted. The role of the emergency care provider is one of observation, collection, labeling, storing, and maintaining chain of custody, not interpretation (Lynch, 1995). For example, do not describe bullet wounds as per your interpretation of "entrance" and "exit." Instead, limit your documentation to objective information, such as wound location, size, and appearance.
3. In order to ensure good evidence collection, emergency care providers should possess accurate knowledge about what may or may not be evidence. Emergency departments should have protocols that indicate when evidence should be collected.
4. If photographic evidence is being collected, photographs should be taken before any treatment whenever possible.
5. All evidence must be properly collected, identified, and stored. The chain of custody must be maintained or the evidence may not be admissible in a court of law.
6. Do not handle bullets with forceps, because scratches on the bullet may interfere with ballistics analysis.

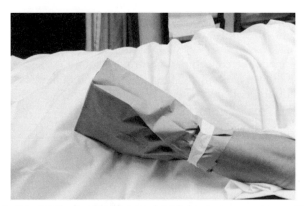

FIGURE 189-1 Covering the hands with paper bags helps preserve any trace evidence of gunpowder for wounds that may be self-inflicted. (Courtesy R.A. De Jarnette.)

EQUIPMENT

Sterile gloves

Evidence collection kit (There are kits available for specific crimes, such as sexual assault or driving under the influence of alcohol. See Procedures 188 and 190 for specific information.)

Suitable containers and sample contents if an evidence collection kit is not available (Containers need to be puncture resistant or tamper evident and prevent exposure to blood and body fluids.)

Glass or plastic vials—foreign objects, like bullets or rocks, sharp objects

Paper bags—clothing

Cardboard boxes—larger items, like boots or heavy coats

Envelopes—fingernail cuttings or scrapings, hair combings or pluckings

Evidence tape (provides tamper-evident seal)

Camera and film (instant camera with close-up capability or high-resolution digital camera)

Metric ruler (rigid)

Labels

Locked box or area where evidence can be stored until law enforcement assumes custody

PATIENT PREPARATION

1. Obtain consent for evidence collected based on institutional policy.
2. Obtain and document history related to the incident or alleged crime.

PROCEDURAL STEPS

1. Identify the indication for evidence collection and consult with law enforcement if you have any questions about what to collect. DNA profiling can be performed on saliva, bone, soft tissue, hair with roots, nasal secretions, blood or blood stains, semen or semen stains, vaginal secretions, skin and sweat, vomit, feces, and properly stored urine.
2. Obtain the appropriate evidence collection kit (e.g., sexual assault kit) (see Procedure 190).
3. Obtain patient consent for evidence collection according to institutional policy. Note that in some cases, such as homicide or suicide, no consent is required for evidence collection. Refer to your state laws and regulations.
4. Check the patient's clothing for the following and collect clothing as appropriate. If in doubt, collect the item.
   a. Blood
   b. Semen
   c. Gunshot residue
   d. Hair
   e. Dirt
   f. Debris
5. Change gloves frequently to prevent cross contamination (Ohio Chapter of the International Association of Forensic Nurses, 2002).
6. Do not perform wound care until injuries have been photographed.

7. Place all collected evidence in appropriate, separate containers. Each article of clothing should be placed in an individual bag or envelope.
8. Wet evidence should always be dried before packaging. Evidence should always be placed in a paper bag. If you need to submit blood-soaked clothing, place the paper bags in open plastic bags to prevent exposure to blood and fluids. Notify the receiving law enforcement officer that it should be removed from the plastic and allowed to dry in a secure evidence room as soon as possible.
9. Label all evidence with:
   a. Patient's name
   b. Source of collection
   c. Date
   d. Time
   e. Person collecting the evidence
10. Evidence should be sealed with evidence tape. Never lick envelopes or use staples. Licking envelopes may contaminate the evidence with your saliva and DNA.
11. A professional forensic photographer is preferred for evidentiary photography. However, photographs taken by emergency nurses are often helpful.
    a. Take a wide-angle picture of the victim to establish identity.
    b. Clearly label each picture with the date, time, patient's name, photographer's name, and location on victim's body (for close-ups).
    c. Include a rigid measuring device when taking close-up pictures of wounds or other small areas. If such a device is not available, a coin can be included in the photograph to provide a frame of reference for size.
    d. Film, negatives, photographs, or computer discs must be safely stored in a secure area until retrieved by law enforcement.
12. Document the evidence collection procedure. A checklist may useful to ensure that all of the steps have been correctly followed (Johnson, 2003). Document any interventions that may have interfered with evidence collection, for example, cutting off clothing.
13. Place evidence in a locked, secured area. Maintain chain of custody and only release the evidence to the appropriate law enforcement agency.
14. Notify the appropriate law enforcement agency per institutional protocols.
15. Complete the chart and ensure that all pertinent documentation is completed, including a list of what was given to the law enforcement agency, the name of the receiving officer, and the date and time that the evidence was released.

AGE-SPECIFIC CONSIDERATION

For every infant death, all clothing, including soiled diapers, should be saved for the medical examiner.

COMPLICATIONS

1. Essential medical interventions may interfere with evidence collection and preservation.
2. The chain of custody may be violated, interfering with the admissibility of the evidence.
3. Evidence stored in an inappropriate container may be altered or ruled inadmissible.

PATIENT TEACHING

1. Provide the patient/family with the appropriate legal agency to follow-up with regarding legal procedures.
2. Provide information about care specific to the injuries that the patient sustained.

REFERENCES

Burgess, A. (2000). *Violence through a forensic lens.* King of Prussia, PA: Nursing Spectrum.
Doyle, J.S. (2001). Evidence collection handbook from the Kentucky State Police. *www.firearmsID.com.* Web site accessed July 7, 2003. Last updated June 29, 2003.
Johnson, M. (2003). Child sexual abuse (pp. 585-592). In Thomas, D., Bernardo, L., & Herman, B. (Eds). *Core curriculum for pediatric emergency nursing.* Boston: Jones & Bartlett Publishers.
Lynch, V. (1995). Clinical forensic nursing. *Critical Care Nursing Clinics of North America 7,* 489-507.
Ohio Chapter of the International Association of Forensic Nurses. (2002). *The Ohio adolescent and adult sexual assault nurse examiner training manual.* Columbus, Ohio: Author.

PROCEDURE 190

Sexual Assault Examination

Reneé Semonin Holleran, RN, PhD, CEN, CCRN, CFRN, SANE and Linda A. Hutson, RN, SANE

INDICATIONS

1. To provide the physical and psychosocial assessment and management for the survivor of sexual assault (Emergency Nurses Association [ENA], 2001).
2. To provide nonjudgmental documentation of the history of the crime.
3. To collect, preserve, and document forensic evidence.
4. To prevent some of the physical and psychological health risks that may be associated with the sexual assault.
5. To prepare documentation so that expert testimony can be given in a court of law (Hutson, 2002).

CONTRAINIDCATIONS AND CAUTIONS

1. Consult state laws and regulations. In some states, sexual assault is a felony and must be reported to law enforcement authorities even if the victim

decides she/he is not interested in talking to the police. Also, some states have procedures that allow evidence to be collected and held anonymously by the state crime laboratory for a period of time while the victim decides whether or not to report the assault.

2. Improper interventions may destroy or alter potential evidence. If sexual assault is suspected, every effort should be made to collect according to local law enforcement requirements.

3. Improper or incomplete evidence collection, preservation, and documentation may result in evidence that is inadmissible in a court of law. Survivors of sexual assault are best served by a sexual assault nurse examiner (SANE) (ENA, 2001; Ledray, Faugno, & Speck, 1997). SANEs are specially trained in evidence collection and management as well as in documentation and testimony related to sexual assault.

4. Survivors of sexual assault should be triaged as emergent and taken to a private area for assessment as soon as they present to the emergency department.

5. Emergency care providers should receive additional training approved by the International Association of Forensic Nurses (IAFN) before performing pediatric sexual assault examinations (IAFN, 2002; ENA, 2001).

6. Research has demonstrated that the standardized collection of evidence contributes to easier identification of the perpetrator, improved testimony in court, and eventual conviction. Each state has its own legal definitions of sexual assault, and evidence should be collected according to state protocol. State protocols should comply with IAFN guidelines.

7. See Procedure 188 and your local laboratory/crime lab procedures if testing for "date rape" or other drugs is indicated.

EQUIPMENT

Sexual assault kit. Where available, use the kit specific to your jurisdiction.
   The following contents are in the State of Ohio Rape Kit (Ohio Chapter of the International Association of Forensic Nurses, 2002).
   History and consent forms
   Swabs
   Glass slides and slide holders
   Fingernail scraper
   Paper sheet
   Paper bags for evidence storage
   Sterile saline or sterile water
   Comb
   Tweezers
   Scissors
   Filter paper
   Envelopes
   Labels
   Evidence tape
   Blood tubes
   Urine tubes
Speculum
Wood's lamp (black light)

Camera
Colposcope
Toiletries
Change of clothing

PROCEDURAL STEPS

1. Perform a primary and secondary assessment to identify any life-threatening injuries that must be managed before evidence collection can begin. In critical situations, the forensic evidence may need to be collected in the operating room or critical care unit. A protocol should be developed and approved jointly by the medical and SANE staff for the management of these patients.
2. The sexual assault examination should be carried out in a private area. Many emergency departments have specific rooms used only for sexual assault patients (Figure 190-1). A patient advocate should be called to talk to the survivor. Some patients may request that a family member or friend accompany them during the examination. The patient's request should be honored to encourage their attempts to regain control.
3. Explain the procedures to the patient and have the victim sign the consent forms for evidence collection and photographs. Also have the victim sign consent for release of evidence to law enforcement.
4. Document the history of the assault using a standard form (Figure 190-2). If the patient has showered or changed clothing since the assault, document this and collect evidence regardless. It is suggested that the history be taken with law enforcement present if they have not already interviewed the patient to decrease the need to repeat the history of the assault multiple times. Take pictures of obvious injury at this time. Also take an orientation picture of the victim at this time. Label all pictures per protocol.
5. Unfold the paper sheet on the floor and have the patient remove all clothing. Be sure to give the patient a gown for cover and have her/him sit on the stretcher. At this time, observe the victim for signs of injury, such as bruising, bleeding, swelling, redness, or bite marks. Collect all pertinent clothing worn

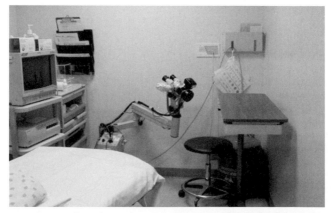

FIGURE 190-1 Sexual assault examination room. (Courtesy R.A. DeJarnette.)

SXASLT

THE UNIVERSITY HOSPITAL
CENTER FOR EMERGENCY CARE
EVIDENTIARY REPORT FOR REPORTED SEXUAL ASSAULT

Patient Name________________________________

Date___________ Sex _____ Age______

S. W.

Police __________________ Badge# ________ District/Agency _________

I voluntarily consent to this examination and the gathering of potential evidence including photographs of injured areas. In some cases, this may include the use of a magnifying camera called a colposcope to document internal vaginal injuries.

I authorize the hospital to release this record and all evidence collected to the police.

SIGNATURE ____

TUH-412, Rev. 9/99, Page 1 of 2

S A N E

Date of Exam:________________Time of Exam:_____________Hours Since Assault :___________LNMP: _____________

Bath/Shower: Yes____ No ____ Douche: Yes____ No ____ Urinated: Yes______ No _____ Defecated: Yes _____ No _____

Changed Clothes: Yes __ ____ No ______ Smoked/Ate: Yes ______ No ________ Mouthwash/Brushed Teeth: Yes _____ No _____

History as stated by patient: Patient's description of pertinent details of the assult: (oral, rectal vaginal, penetration: digital, penile, foreign objects), (oral contact), (ejaculation location, if known by the patient):

PHYSICAL EVIDENCE OF EXTRA-GENITAL TRAUMA: (Include all details of trauma—tears, lacerations, abrasions, ecchymosis, redness, bitemarks, presence of blood or other secretions.):

Photos Taken _______

Signature______________________________

Legend: T—tear, E—eechymosis, A—abrasion, R—redness, S—swelling

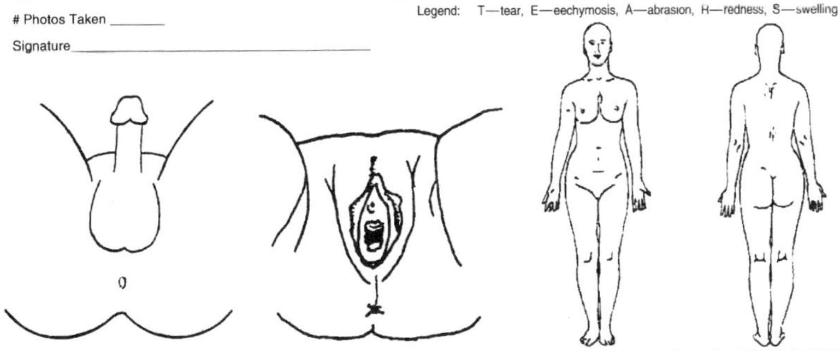

White - Medical Records, Yellow - Billing; Pink -SS; Goldenrod -Police

FIGURE 190-2 Sexual assault form. (Courtesy University Hospital, Center for Emergency Care, Cincinnati, OH.)

SXASLT

THE UNIVERSITY HOSPITAL
CENTER FOR EMERGENCY CARE
EVIDENTIARY REPORT FOR REPORTED SEXUAL ASSAULT

TUH-412, Rev. 9/99, Page 2 of 2

GENITAL EXAM: (Describe any trauma. Use common English terms): Trauma Visible: Yes ____ No ____

S

Labia Majora: _____

Labia Minora: _____

Posterior Fourchette: _____

Hymen: _____

Vagina _____

Cervix _____

A   Penis _____

Scrotum: _____

Rectal Exam: _____

c̄-with   s̄-without   NTN-no trauma noted   o-none   N/A-not applicable

EVIDENCE COLLECTION: (Collect and initial items below. Use stamped labels to seal envelopes. Use evidence tape to seal paper bags, blood and urine tubes. Collector dates and initials all labeled specimen envelopes; discard unused envelopes.)

N   Initial:

_____ **A. Clothing** Flouresce each item and place any stained clothing in a separate paper bag sealed with label and evidence tape.
_____   Articles submitted: _____
_____ **B. Saline swab of fluorescing body stains** (examine in dark room using Wood's lamp):
_____   Location _____
_____ **C. Tampons/Pads** (Dry and place in envelope - never in plastic)
E   _____ **D. Clipped Fingernails** (only if blood or tissue present or freshly broken)
_____ **E. Foreign Material** (e.g., burrs, grass, twigs)
_____ **F. Oral Swab** (roof of mouth and lower gum line) (four dry and smear)
_____ **G. Loose hair on body**
_____ **H. Bite Mark Swabs**
_____ **I. Combed Pubic Hair**
_____ **J. 10-15 pulled pubic hairs** from four different quadrants
_____ **K. 10-15 pulled head hairs** from various areas of head
_____ **L. Vaginal Swabs** (at least four dry)-smear
_____ **M. Rectal Swab** (four dry)-smear
_____ **N. Penile Swab** (four dry)
_____ **O. Other evidence:** _____
_____ **P. Photographs:** (Use ruler in photo to document size) # _____
_____ **Q. Colposcopy Exam**
_____ **R. #** _____ **Blood/Urine Tubes**

S
A   Examiner's Signature:_____ Initials: _____ Print Last Name: _____
N
E   Number of Evidence Parcels Secured: _____ Initials/Signature _____
/
S   Evidence Released By: _____ Date: _____ Time: _____
W
Evidence Released To: _____ Badge #: _____ Unit: _____

FIGURE 190-2 Cont'd Sexual assault form. (Courtesy University Hospital, Center for Emergency Care, Cincinnati, OH.)

during or immediately after the assault. Do not shake the clothing, and place each item in a separate paper bag. Seal with evidence tape.

6. Collect oral swabs regardless of the history given. Make a smear with a swab on a slide. Allow the swabs to air dry or place in a swab dryer. When the swab is dry, place it in an envelope and seal with evidence tape.

7. Collect hair standards. Allow the patient to pull 10-15 strands of hair from various spots on the head with gloved hands. Place the hairs in an envelope, seal with evidence tape, and label. (Protocols are different and may allow cutting or pulling hairs).

8. Scrape/swab under the patient's fingernails. If there are broken nails, cut a piece of the nail and place in the envelope, seal with evidence tape, and label.

9. Scan the patient's body with the Wood's lamp to identify any dried semen or saliva stains. Different fluids fluoresce under black light. Any areas that fluoresce should be swabbed. If the area is dry, use a moistened swab (water or saline) to sample. If the area if moist, use a dry swab. Dry the swabs and place them in an envelope, seal with evidence tape, and label. Swab injured areas only after a photograph has been taken.

10. Place the patient in the lithotomy position. Comb through the patient's pubic hair several times with an envelope or paper towel under the patient's buttocks. If there is an area of matted hair, cut the area out with scissors and place it in the envelope. Place comb in the envelope with the hair. Seal with evidence tape and label. If there is no pubic hair, document that on the envelope.

11. With a gloved hand, the patient should pull 10-15 stands of pubic hair. Place these in an envelope, seal with evidence tape, and label. Refer to your state protocol for the required amount.

12. *For female patients:* Inspect the genital area, photograph all injuries, and explain the speculum examination. Colposcopic photography may be performed at this time. Insert the speculum (plastic is recommended to provide better photography). Collect four swabs from the vaginal vault and cervix. Collect any foreign objects. If a tampon/pad is present, collect, dry, and seal in the kit. Make a slide from one of the swabs, dry, and seal in a labeled envelope. Allow the speculum to air dry and place in the evidence envelope.

13. *For male patients:* Inspect the genital area, and photograph all injuries using the colposcope. Moisten four swabs with saline or water. Swab the glans and shaft of the penis. Make a slide, dry, and place in the labeled evidence envelopes.

14. *Examine the anal area for injury and photograph all injuries. Collect four anal swabs regardless of the assault history. Make a smear with one of the swabs on a slide. Place this swab in a labeled evidence envelope.

15. Collect blood standard on filter paper provided in the kit. Wear gloves, label the filter paper, wipe patient's finger with alcohol, and place a drop of blood on each circle. Dry and place in the envelope. Alternatively, some jurisdictions require a tube of blood be drawn from the patient.

16. *Complete the assault history form (see Figure 190-2) documenting sites of injury and your findings during the examination. One set of photographs

---

*Indicates portions of the procedure usually performed by a physician or an advanced practice nurse if a SANE is not available.

should be given to law enforcement with the kit. One set of photographs should be kept with the medical record.

17. Administer sexually transmitted infection (STI) prophylaxis and pregnancy prophylaxis as prescribed and indicated. Explain to the patient about the need for follow-up with these treatments.

18. Make sure that all evidence is sealed correctly and that your documentation is completed according to protocol. The sealed completed kit and documentation should be immediately surrendered to a law enforcement to maintain chain of custody. If you are unable to give your kit to law enforcement immediately, a locked, secured cabinet should be available for storage until law enforcement retrieves the kit. It is critical to maintain your chain of custody with all evidence and documentation.

AGE-SPECIFIC CONSIDERATIONS

1. Pediatric sexual assault survivors should be evaluated only by those trained to care for pediatric patients (Johnson, 2003; ENA, 2001).

2. Postmenopausal women may incur vaginal tears and lacerations because of thinner skin due to hormonal changes.

COMPLICATIONS

1. The patient may decline specific parts of the sexual assault examination. Document "the patient declines" as indicated.

2. Improper collection or handling of the evidence or a break in the chain of custody could cause the evidence to be inadmissible in a court of law.

3. Patients may experience nausea and vomiting from the STI and/or pregnancy prophylaxis. Discuss this with the patient and offer suggestions for successful completion of the medication regimen. Written discharge instructions should be given to the victim so that the victim or a family member can review it at a later time. Because of the traumatic circumstances of the assault, victims may not comprehend the instructions at the time of discharge. Provide a phone number for any follow-up questions.

4. STI and pregnancy prophylaxis may not be effective. It is imperative that the patient be instructed about follow-up care.

5. Male survivors of sexual assault tend to suffer more physical injuries and should be carefully examined so a life-threatening injury is not missed (Burgess, 2000).

PATIENT TEACHING

1. The patient/family should receive clear instructions about the side effects of any medications given or prescribed. Antiemetics should be offered if pregnancy prophylaxis ("morning after" therapy) is prescribed.

2. The patient/family should be instructed about the importance of follow-up medical care. They should be given information about repeat STI testing and pregnancy testing because the specimens collected during this examination can diagnose preexisting conditions only, not infection or pregnancy that results from the assault.

3. The patient/family should be advised about local HIV and hepatitis testing and risks to the victim.

4. Provide information about sexual assault survivor advocacy groups and counseling opportunities.

REFERENCES

Burgess, A.W. (2000). *Violence through a forensic lens*. King of Prussia, PA: Nursing Spectrum.

Emergency Nurses Association (ENA). (2001). *Care of sexual assault victims* (position statement). Des Plaines, IL: Author.

Hutson, L. (2002). Development of sexual assault nurse examiner programs. *Nursing Clinics of North America, 37*, 79-88.

International Association of Forensic Nurses (IFAN). (2002). *Sexual assault nurse examiner standards of practice*. Pitman, NJ: Author.

Johnson, M. (2003). Child sexual abuse (pp. 585-592). In Thomas, D., Bernardo, L., & Herman, B. (Eds). *Core curriculum for pediatric emergency nursing*. Boston: Jones & Bartlett Publishers.

Ledray, L., Faugno, D., & Speck, P. (1997). Sexual assault: clinical issues. Efficacy of SANE evidence collection: a Minnesota study. *Journal of Emergency Nursing 23*, 182-186.

Ohio Chapter of the International Association of Forensic Nurses. (2002). *The Ohio adolescent and adult sexual assault nurse examiner training manual*. Columbus: Author.

PROCEDURE 191

Collection of Bite Mark Evidence*

Ruth L. Schaffler, PhD(c), CEN, ARNP

INDICATIONS

1. To obtain samples of saliva residue remaining on the patient's skin. It is nearly impossible to bite without leaving traces of saliva. More than 80% of the general population secrete substances in body fluids (e.g., saliva, perspiration, semen, and vaginal secretions) that identify their major blood type as well as other laboratory-detectable factors (e.g., DNA, gram-nega-

---

*Special thanks to Peter F. Hampl, DDS, Forensic Odontologist, of Tacoma, WA, for his assistance and contribution to the preparation of this material. His expertise is invaluable to the fields of medicine, nursing, law enforcement, and forensics.

tive and gram-positive bacteria, hepatitis B virus, and human immunodeficiency virus) (Barry, 1994; Hampl, 1997).
2. To obtain a sample of the patient's saliva as a control for comparison to skin samples.
3. To obtain blood samples from the patient as a comparison to samples obtained from the skin, if appropriate.
4. To obtain blood samples for baseline testing for blood-borne pathogens (e.g., human immunodeficiency virus).
5. To photograph wounds identified or suspected of being bite marks.
6. To collect, preserve, and surrender specimens according to local chain-of-custody protocols.
7. To document the original appearance of the patient, as well as all history, interventions, or pertinent observations. Identifiable patterns of injury should be documented with a diagram and photograph. If bite marks are incurred during the commission of a crime, law enforcement personnel and a forensic odontologist should be involved as soon as possible. For names and locations of forensic odontologists, contact the American Academy of Forensic Sciences, 410 North 21st, Suite 203, Colorado Springs, CO 80904-2798; phone (719) 636-1100; fax (719) 636-1993. The American Board of Forensic Odontologists, Inc. (ABFO) is located at the same address or can be contacted through their web site at http://www.abfo.org/bitemark.htm.

CONTRAINDICATIONS AND CAUTIONS
1. Saliva swabbings of the bite mark site should be obtained whenever possible. Interventions such as washing of the region destroy or alter potential evidence that could be sufficient to prove the identity of the attacker. Emergency personnel should be aware of forensic considerations to avoid loss of potentially valuable evidence, thus complicating criminal investigations.
2. Bite marks may be accompanied by contusions, abrasions, lacerations, ecchymosis, petechiae, avulsion, indentations, erythema, or punctures. Fingernail scratches may indicate a struggle with an assailant.
3. Bites can be located on any body part but are often found on the breasts, inner thighs, arms, buttocks, and genitalia (Bell, 2000). Because there is usually no eyewitness, a thorough inspection is necessary to look for bite marks (Nuckles et al., 1994). If one bite is present, others should be suspected as well. Look for representative patterns caused by the contact of teeth on the skin. Note the shape, color, and size of the wound(s).
4. Photograph the wound before treatment or sample collection is begun. It is important to determine whether the bite mark has been affected by cleaning, contamination, change in position, or lividity (Barry, 1994).
5. Improper collection, preservation, or labeling of specimens may result in the evidence being inadmissible in a court of law. Maintain chain-of-custody protocols for all evidence and photographic film.
6. Deceased persons should be refrigerated, but not embalmed, until evidence can be collected (Hampl, 1997).

EQUIPMENT
Sterile gloves
Distilled water or sterile water

Sterile cotton swabs for collecting samples and controls

One sterile no. 10 envelope or sterile test tube for each area swabbed (essential to avoid evidence contamination)

Lavender-topped blood collection tubes

1- × 1-inch gauze squares

Nonflexible metric ruler or scale; ABFO no. 2 scale is preferred (Lightning Powder Co., Eugene, OR)

Camera with black-and-white and color film, 35 mm or other nondistorting model for close-up views

PATIENT PREPARATION

1. Obtain and document a thorough history and description of the bite mark(s). Ask conscious patients if they were bitten or if they bit anyone. A suspect may have been bitten by the victim as well and may have identifiable bite marks that can be examined for evidence.
2. Document interventions that may interfere with evidence or produce other wounds, such as venipuncture or defibrillation.
3. Do not clean wounds until after photographs and samples are taken.
4. Obtain a written consent for photographs and evidence collection according to institutional policy.

PROCEDURAL STEPS
Photographing Bite Marks

Forensic photography is a specialty. The information supplied here is offered to assist with evidence collection when a specially trained photographer is not available. Law enforcement personnel should be involved with these cases as soon as possible, and they can determine the need for photography. Nurses who take evidentiary photographs may be required to testify in court and have their photography skills and training questioned by a defense attorney. Generally, it is preferable to have an experienced photographer or forensic dentist take the pictures (ABFO, 2002).

1. Place the area to be photographed on a firm flat surface.
2. Place the ABFO no. 2 scale as close to the bite mark as possible. The most critical photographs should be taken in such a way as to avoid distortion. A flexible ruler, such as a cloth tape measure, conforms to the body contours and distorts the dimensions of the bite in the photograph. Video or digital imaging can be used in addition to conventional photography (ABFO, 2002).
3. Off-angle lighting using a pointflash should be used whenever possible (Ramsland, 2000). A light source perpendicular to the bite site can be used in addition to off-angle lighting; however, care should be taken to prevent light reflection from obliterating bite mark details (ABFO, 2002).
4. Position the camera so that it is perpendicular to the bite mark. This is especially important if the bite is on a rounded surface, such as an extremity, a shoulder, or a breast (Figure 191-1).
5. Take photos with and without the scale from a close distance to show that there are no wound areas under the ruler.
6. Photograph wounds from several angles both before and after cleaning the area. Include close-up views from several angles as well as photos orienting

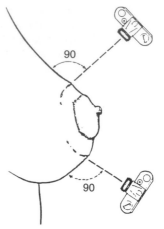

FIGURE 191-1 The camera is held perpendicular (at a 90-degree angle) to the bite mark when a forensic photograph is taken. (Courtesy P.F. Hampl, 1997.)

the relationship of the bite mark to the rest of the body. Change the lighting to show contours and shadows.

7. Take several pictures because this may be the only opportunity to photograph evidence (Hampl, 1997).

Collecting Swabs

1. To prepare the bite mark site for evidence collection, use a double-swab technique (Sweet et al., 1997). Wet a cotton swab with distilled or sterile water, shake off the excess, and moisten the tissues surrounding the bite using a circular motion from the periphery toward the center. Discard this swab.
2. Using a dry swab, rotate the tip over the moistened skin so that the sample from the bite area is equally distributed on the surface of the swab. Avoid contamination with blood.
3. Using the same two-swab technique, obtain a control sample by swabbing at least a 1- × 1-inch site that has not been bitten.
4. Air dry the swabs thoroughly.
5. Place each of the sample and control swabs in separate sterile no. 10 envelopes or sterile test tubes that are appropriately labeled with the name of the patient, site of the sample, date, time, and name of the collector (Hampl, 1997).
6. Collect a saliva sample by having the patient chew on a 1- × 1-inch square of gauze for 1 minute.
7. Air dry the gauze thoroughly and place it in a sterile envelope. CAUTION: Do not contaminate the gauze during the process of drying, which may take 1 full day. Seal the envelope with tape, do not lick the glue on the flap (Hampl, 1997).
8. Collect blood samples as needed (see Procedure 61). This may include fresh or dried blood on the skin as well as venipuncture.

COMPLICATIONS

1. A bite mark may not be recognized. The clarity and shape of a bite mark may change in a relatively short time in both living and dead victims (Rothwell, 1995).

2. Incisions, punctures, or other wounds made in close proximity to the bite mark during medical treatment may alter or destroy evidence.
3. Improper collection or preservation of evidence or a break in the chain of custody may result in the evidence's being declared inadmissible during legal proceedings.

PATIENT TEACHING

1. Follow up with law enforcement regarding legal proceedings and the possible need for additional photographs at a later date (e.g., after bruising is well developed).
2. Report any signs of infection (redness, swelling, pain or tenderness, draining pus) to your primary care provider.

REFERENCES

American Board of Forensic Odontologists (ABFO). (2002). Retrieved April 30, 2002, from http://www.abfo.org/bitemark.htm

Barry, L.A. (1994). Bite mark evidence collection in the United States. *Bulletin of the History of Dentistry, 42*, 21-27.

Bell, K. (2000). Identification and documentation of bite marks. *Journal of Emergency Nursing, 26*, 628-630.

Hampl, P.F. (1997). Personal communication, 1997, Tacoma, WA.

Nuckles, D.B., Herschaft, E.E., & Whatmough, L.N. (1994). Forensic odontology in solving crimes: dental techniques and bite mark evidence. *General Dentistry, 42*, 210-214.

Ramsland, K. (2000). Bite marks as evidence to convict: How it's done. Retrieved April 30, 2002 from http://crimelibrary.com/forensics/bitemarks/6.htm.

Rothwell, B.R. (1995). Bite marks in forensic dentistry: a review of legal, scientific issues. *Journal of the American Dental Association, 126*, 223-232.

Sweet, D., Lorente, M., Lorente, J.A., Valenzuela, A., Villanueva, E. (1997). An improved method to recover saliva from human skin: the double swab technique. *Journal of Forensic Science, 42*, 320-322.

PROCEDURE 192

Application of Restraints

Teresa L. Will, RN, MSN, CEN, and
Jean A. Proehl, RN, MN, CEN, CCRN

INDICATION

Restraint may be indicated because the patient is a danger to self or others or to protect the cognitively impaired patient from interfering with therapy that is medically necessary. The patient should be carefully assessed to determine whether other, less restrictive measures will control the behavior. Examples of less restrictive alternatives include:

Verbal intervention
Environmental modifications
Diversional activity
Family or patient sitter presence
Security presence
Show-of-force

CONTRAINDICATIONS AND CAUTIONS

1. Restraint use is addressed by both the Joint Commission on Accreditation of Healthcare Organizations (JCAHO, 2003) and the Centers for Medicare and Medicaid Services (CMS) (formerly the Health Care Financing Administration [HCFA], 2000). Refer to current standards and requirements from these bodies for specific requirements regarding the use of restraints.
2. The organizational culture must emphasize prevention and appropriate use of restraints and encourage less restrictive alternatives to restraints (JCAHO, 2003).
3. Review your institutional policy and procedure regarding restraint use, paying particular attention to:
   a. Required components of physician/nurse practitioner orders for restraints
   b. Indications for restraint application
   c. Identification of personnel who may place restraints. Staff must be trained, demonstrate competency, and have ongoing education about restraint use (JCAHO, 2003).
   d. Observation and assessment of patients in restraints and documentation of same
   e. Guidelines for removal of restraints or renewal of restraint orders
4. The competent patient's right to refuse treatment must be respected.
5. Restraints should never be used for convenience or because staffing is inadequate. An assessment process must be used to identify and prevent potential behavioral risk factors (JCAHO, 2003).
6. Restraints should not be used as fall prevention. Numerous devices are available to alert staff when patients are attempting to get out of bed. The use of restraints may actually increase the incidence of falls and patient injury.
7. The least restrictive restraint that affects a patient's ability to act in a manner harmful to self or others should be used after careful evaluation of the patient. The restrained patient should be frequently reassessed to determine whether restraints are still indicated.
8. Use only approved restraint devices. Gauze rolls, sheets, tape, and so on, are not intended to be used for restraint and have been associated with patient injury and death.
9. Avoid applying restraints to injured extremities whenever possible.
10. Beware of statements or actions that may escalate a violent patient. Paranoia and hostility are common reactions in a variety of medical conditions, when the patient is under the influence of drugs or alcohol, and when a patient is being treated against his or her will. Speak slowly and in a calm, low voice. Emphasize that violent behavior cannot be tolerated and that if the patient is

unable to control the behavior, the team will help him/her control the behavior to prevent injury to self or others.

11. Position yourself cautiously when dealing with a combative or violent patient.
    a. Stand to the side of the patient to protect your vulnerable zone. Never stand in front of the patient.
    b. Stand more than an arm's length from the patient to protect yourself from the patient who lunges or kicks.
    c. Never turn your back on the patient, and never precede the patient into a room.
    d. Always place yourself, not the patient, closest to the door to allow a means of escape. However, avoid standing where you "trap" the patient in the room.
    e. Stethoscopes worn around the neck, neck ties, jewelry, and scissors can all be used by the patient as weapons to hurt you. Be aware of what is on your body and in your pockets when caring for violent or potentially violent patients.

12. After restraints are discontinued, remove them from the room or lock them to the stretcher so that they cannot be used as weapons by the patient to harm himself or herself.

13. If the patient is in locked restraints, the patient should not be left unattended, and the key should be readily accessible to caregivers at the bedside, especially during emergencies, including fire alarms.

14. Patients in handcuffs per law enforcement should be attended and monitored by a law enforcement officer. In this circumstance, restraint orders and observation/reassessment as described below are not required. However, nursing assessment and documentation of the patient's behavior and clinical condition should still be performed as indicated by the patient's condition.

15. Leather cuffs cannot be adequately cleaned in the event of blood or body fluid contamination. They have largely been replaced by nylon with Velcro or hard plastic cuffs.

EQUIPMENT

Numerous devices are available; *always consult the manufacturer's instructions for application instructions*. Some devices commonly used in the emergency department include:

Vest Restraint (Figure 192-1)

Also known as Posey jacket or vest. For patients who require less restrictive restraint methods, a vest restraint may be adequate to remind the patient not to get out of the chair or bed. If used while the patient is in bed, all side rails should be up and any gap between split side rails covered as described below. A vest restraint is not appropriate for patients exhibiting violent, assaultive behavior.

Soft Limb Restraints, Locked or Unlocked (Figure 192-2, 192-3)

Used to prevent patients from pulling on IV lines, catheters, and so on. Stronger versions are used for patients who are combative and striking or kicking out at others.

Leather or Vinyl Limb Restraints (Figure 192-4)

Used for patients who are extremely combative or violent. These restraints are used for patients who are displaying aggressive assaultive behavior and present a danger

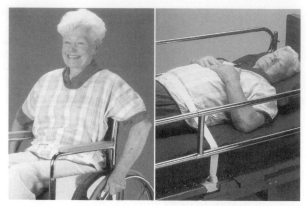

FIGURE 192-1 Vest restraint. (Posey jackets and vests, courtesy the Posey Company, Arcadia, CA.)

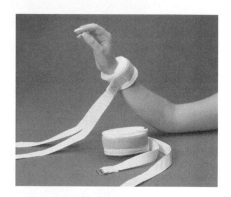

FIGURE 192-2 Soft limb restraint. (Limb holders, courtesy the Posey Company, Arcadia, CA.)

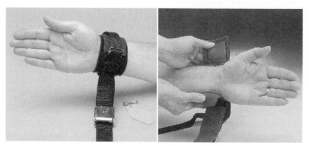

FIGURE 192-3 Nylon limb restraint with double hook and loop closure. (Twice-as-Tough Cuff-Keylock, courtesy the Posey Company, Arcadia, CA.)

to themselves or others. These restraints are used only as a last resort and for the minimal amount of time necessary for the patient to control his/her behavior.

Cloth Straps

Cloth straps secured with Velcro or other closures may be used across the patient's chest, hips, or knees if the patient continues to thrash and struggle when

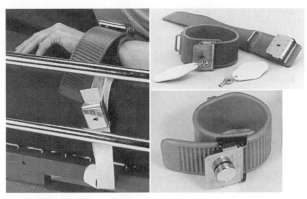

FIGURE 192-4 Locking vinyl limb restraint. (E.D. Security Cuffs, courtesy the Posey Company, Arcadia, CA.)

all extremities are restrained. Neither sheets nor tape should not be used because both are difficult to release quickly in an emergency.

Four Side Rails

The use of four side rails where the patient cannot lower the rails on his/her own is considered a restraint (HCFA, 2000). In some situations, full bed rails are considered a standard of care for the safety of all patients. Example: full bed rails may be considered a standard of care when a patient is transported from one unit of the hospital to another or for the patient who has received narcotics or sedatives. The gap or area between the bed rails is an area where patients have been known to entrap and injure themselves. The gap should be protected with a special gap protector, padded side rail, or pillow barrier to prevent the patient from slipping between the rails when all four rails are used.

PATIENT PREPARATION

1. If possible, undress the patient. At a minimum, attempt to remove the patient's belt and shoes to prevent their use as weapons.
2. Attempt voluntary restraint application, but do not bargain with the patient. Be prepared with adequate personnel to safely hold the patient down and apply restraints if necessary.
3. The patient should receive a thorough medical examination. Completion of the examination may need to be deferred until restraint application has been achieved if the patient is violent or combative. Consider the use of pharmacologic or chemical restraint if the patient continues to struggle and fight after physical restraints have been applied.
4. Consider obtaining alcohol and toxicology panels. Rule out organic and neurologic causes for the behavior, especially in the elderly.

PROCEDURAL STEPS

1. Ideally, four to five people should assist in the application of restraints to a violent, assaultive patient. One person should be assigned to the head and one

to each extremity. Holding the patient's head to the side with pressure on the forehead and mandible helps decrease the movement of the patient's body.

2. Apply all devices in accordance with manufacturer's directions.

3. Apply extremity cuffs snugly to prevent escape. To ensure that the cuff is not too tight, you should be able to insert one finger between the cuff and the patient's skin. Secure the restraints to the stretcher frame and never the side rails. Leave only enough slack to position the extremity safely.

   a. Full four-point arm and leg restraints should be used in patients who are a serious danger to self or others.

   b. Two-point restraints using an upper and lower extremity on opposite sides may be employed for less agitated patients or as an intermediate step when restraints are removed after the violent assaultive behavior has resolved. This prevents the patient from removing restraints, flipping off the stretcher, or tipping the stretcher over in an attempt to stand. For patients who are attempting to pull out tubes or lines, restraining both hands is appropriate.

   c. One-point restraint is not a safe option for patients with violent or assaultive behavior.

4. Consider a strap across the chest, hips, and knees in addition to four-point restraints to protect a patient from injury if the patient continues to thrash about. Be careful not to restrict chest excursion and impair ventilation with straps placed across the chest.

5. Position the restrained patient prone, on his or her side, or supine, with the head of the bed slightly elevated. Because restrained patients often are under the influence of drugs, alcohol, or both, suction and airway equipment should be readily available. Carefully monitor respiratory status in the prone patient because some patients, especially the obese, may not be able to breathe well when lying face down.

6. If necessary, apply restraint cuffs while the patient is on the floor. In this case, place the cuffs on the extremities while the patient is on the floor. Then, lift the patient to the stretcher in the prone position via a belt placed around the waist. This decreases the patient's ability to struggle while being transferred to the stretcher.

7. Search the patient thoroughly and remove all objects from pockets after applying restraints. Remove the patient's shoes and remove or loosen any constricting clothing.

8. Observe the patient as per institutional policy. Generally observations are documented every 15-30 minutes and indicate that the patient is in an appropriate position, the restraints are still appropriately placed, and the patient is in no obvious danger.

9. Obtain a written order for restraints if not previously obtained. Refer to your institution's policy regarding restraint orders. Components of the order include:

   a. Time limit for the use of restraints based on patient age

   b. Behavior leading to the use of restraints

   c. Alternative interventions attempted before restraint application

   d. Type of restraints used

10. Reassess the patient per institutional policy. Generally patients are reassessed every 15 minutes to 2 hours. Components of this reassessment include:

    a. Neurovascular assessment of restrained extremities
    b. Mental status and behavior
    c. Need for food, fluids, toileting
    d. Release for range of motion in restrained extremities
    e. Need for continued use of restraint

11. Restraint keys should be readily available to caregivers. A quick-release knot should be used for all restraints that are tied.

12. A debriefing with the patient and staff should occur after restraints are discontinued from the patient who was restrained because of violent or assaultive behavior. This debriefing should focus on the events that led to restraint and how future episodes of restraint could be avoided.

AGE-SPECIFIC CONSIDERATIONS

1. Therapeutic holding, comforting of children, and restraint associated with procedures (IV arm boards, and so on) are not considered restraint (JCAHO, 2003).

2. Requirements for time limits in the restraint of children are more restrictive. The order should not exceed two hours for children and adolescents aged 9-17 years. The order should not exceed 1 hour for children under age 9 (JCAHO, 2003).

3. Risks of restraint in the geriatric population include injury, death from strangulation, decline in functional status, altered skin integrity, sequelae of immobilization, and emotional desolation (Evans & Strumpf, 1989).

COMPLICATIONS

1. Circulatory compromise or altered skin integrity of restrained extremities

2. Respiratory compromise related to positioning or aspiration of vomitus

3. Vulnerability of the restrained patient to attack or abuse by other patients or family members. Close observation is warranted to ensure patient safety.

4. Compromised patient dignity, privacy, comfort, and rights

5. Injury to staff or patient during application of restraints

REFERENCES

Joint Commission on Accreditation of Health Care Organizations (JCAHO). (2003) *Comprehensive accreditation manual for hospitals.* Oakbrook Terrace, IL: Author.

Evans, L., & Strumpf, N. (1989). Tying down the elderly: a review of the literature of physical restraint. *Journal of the American Geriatrics Society, 37,* 65-74.

Health Care Financing Administration (HCFA). (2000). *Interpretive guidelines for hospital conditions of participation for patients rights.* Baltimore, MD: Author

Preparing and Restraining Children for Procedures

Daun A. Smith, RN, MS, CEN

INDICATIONS

1. All children need some form of preparation for a procedure to secure cooperation and in consideration of emotional well-being. This preparation should be performed in a manner appropriate to the child's developmental level.
2. Restraint may be indicated to facilitate examination or to perform interventions.
3. Positioning means to put the child in a position needed for a procedure; securing involves the use of physical, manual, or pharmacologic means to maintain the position (Bove, 1993).

CONTRAINDICATIONS AND CAUTIONS

1. Administration of sedatives and/or analgesics may be the most appropriate method of restraining a child for a procedure that is painful or takes more than just a few minutes (see Procedure 181).
2. Infants release tension by gross motor activity. Limiting this movement by restraints increases anxiety.
3. Preschoolers view restraints as a form of punishment.
4. Restraining a child for a procedure can cause feelings of powerlessness, anxiety, or anger.
5. Alternatives to physical restraints should be explored first (e.g., diversional activities) (Parnell, 2002).
6. Restraints should be kept to a minimum, both in the amount of restraint and in the length of time applied. The form of restraint chosen should be the least restrictive to accomplish the purpose (Parnell, 2002).
7. Whenever possible, the child should be restrained manually because this method provides human contact.
8. A child should never be restrained to accomplish a sexual assault examination. The child should be sedated or anesthetized if he or she is unable to cooperate with this examination.

PATIENT PREPARATION

All patient preparation for procedures should take place according to the child's developmental level and age-specific fears, concerns, and approaches.

Infants (birth-18 months)
Fears
1. Separation from parents
2. Stranger anxiety after 6 months

Approaches
1. Encourage parental presence.
2. Use touch, voice, and pacifiers to distract the infant.
3. Restrain the infant only as much and as long as is needed to accomplish the procedure. Infants cope with anxiety by movement; restraints increase anxiety. However, holding a young infant's flailing arms together and gently placing them on the child's chest may help the child calm down. Swaddling works in a similar fashion for neonates.
4. Return the infant to the parents immediately after the procedure for comforting and soothing.

Toddlers (18 months to 3 years)
Fears
1. Separation from parents
2. Strangers
3. Pain

Approaches
1. Toddlers learn through sensorimotor experiences. Let them handle equipment whenever possible.
2. Toddlers have limited coping abilities and need to be told that it is all right to cry. Allow them to keep a familiar object with them (e.g., blanket, stuffed animal).
3. Toddlers have limited language skills. Use simple, nonmedical language. Whenever possible, use their words for objects, body parts, and functions.
4. At this age, there is little conception of time. Toddlers need a brief explanation immediately before the procedure.
5. Some procedures (e.g., physical examination) can be accomplished with the child sitting on a parent's lap.

Preschool (3-5 years)
Fears
1. Body mutilation
2. The dark
3. Pain
4. The unknown
5. Loss of control

Approaches
1. Preschoolers learn through words, sight, motor, touch, and hearing. Let them play with equipment when possible. Focus your explanations on what they will hear, see, smell, and feel.
2. Preschoolers have a vivid imagination, which facilitates learning but also increases their fears. Clarify misconceptions and explain procedures in clear, simple language. Explain the procedure immediately before it occurs, so that the child does not have time to imagine the worst.
3. At this age, children want to please you. Praise all their efforts, whether successful or unsuccessful.
4. Preschoolers ask why continuously but are usually satisfied with clear, simple explanations.

5. Assure the child that this procedure is not a punishment for some imagined misbehavior.
6. Cover wounds, even injection sites, with a dressing or bandage.
7. Encourage parental presence.
8. Distract, encourage, and reward with colorful toys, crayons, or stickers.

School Age (6-11 years)
Fears
1. Loss of body parts
2. Disability
3. Loss of control

Approaches
1. The school-aged child wants to cooperate and to be seen as an adult. Praise all efforts to cooperate.
2. Abstract concepts are not understood. Encourage questions and clarify misconceptions.
3. Regression is not uncommon; be nonjudgmental.
4. The school-aged child understands rules and time limits. The child can bribe or bargain. Explain what needs to be done, and set time limits for cooperation (then allow a break if the procedure is not yet finished). Offer simple choices (e.g., which arm for the injection). Be careful not to offer a choice when there is no choice (e.g., "Can I give you this injection now?").
5. Peers are important. Allow for privacy so that a child does not have to be seen in a compromised situation (e.g., crying) in front of peers.

Adolescence (12-18 years)
Fears
1. Loss of control
2. Changes in body image

Approaches
1. Allow for privacy.
2. Encourage questions, clarify misconceptions, and explain carefully.
3. Be honest.
4. Accept any regression nonjudgmentally.
5. Peers are important to adolescents. Allow for privacy so that the child is not seen in a compromised situation (e.g., crying) in front of peers.

PROCEDURAL STEPS
Equipment
    Infant restraint board
    Sheet, blanket, pillowcase

Mummy Restraint (Parnell, 2002)
1. Fold down one corner of a sheet to form a triangle (Figure 193-1).
2. Place the infant or child on the sheet with his or her head on the middle of the folded edge.

Mummy restraint (body restraint)

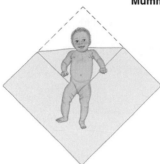

A restraint can be made from a sheet folded into a square of the appropriate size for the infant. Start by folding the top corner under the infant's shoulders and aligning the head with the folded edge.

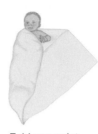

Fold one point of the sheet across the child and tuck it firmly behind his back.

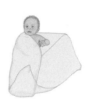

Fold the bottom corner of the sheet up to cover and restrain the infant's feet.

Fold the remaining corner over the child and tuck firmly behind his back.

FIGURE 193-1 Mummy restraint with a sheet. (From James, S.R., Ashwill, J.N., Droske, S.C. [Eds.] [2002]. *Nursing care of children: principles and practice,* 2nd ed. [p. 360]. Philadelphia: W.B. Saunders.)

3. Bring one side of the sheet firmly down across the child's shoulder and torso, and tuck securely under the opposite side of the body.
4. Fold the bottom corner of the sheet up. This secures the child's feet.
5. Bring the other side of the sheet down snugly across the remaining shoulder and across the torso, and tuck snugly under the infant.
6. The mummy restraint can be modified by tucking the sheet over each ipsilateral arm and under the child's body, leaving the chest exposed. Adhesive tape over the arms and chest makes this more secure.
7. Monitor respiratory status and distal neurovascular status during the procedure, to be certain that the restraint is not too tight.
8. Remove the child as soon as the procedure is completed.

Child Restraint Board (Olympic Medical, Seattle, WA)

A restraint board, also known as a papoose board, consists of a solid back, with nylon or cloth wrappings and Velcro fastenings. Three sizes are available: regular (2-6 years of age), large (6-12 years of age), and extra large (teenagers and adults).

1. Place the board on a solid surface (stretcher, bed) where the procedure is to be performed. Open the Velcro straps.
2. Place a sheet folded into a triangle over the board with the wide part of the triangle placed where the child's head will be.
3. Place the child in a supine position on the board with his or her arms at each side.
4. Wrap the child mummy-fashion with the sheet to facilitate secure restraint with the Velcro fasteners.
5. Place the wrappings snugly around the child, securing them with the Velcro fasteners (Figure 193-2).

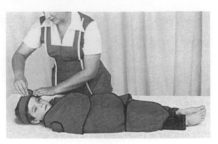

FIGURE 193-2 Child immobilized on a restraint board. (Courtesy Olympic Medical, Seattle, WA.)

6. Monitor respiratory status and distal neurovascular status during the procedure to be certain that the restraint is not too tight.
7. Remove the child as soon as the procedure is completed.

Pillowcase Restraint

This restraint can be used for a toddler, preschooler, or small, school-aged child (Emergency Nurses Association, 1999).
1. Slide a pillowcase up both arms behind the child to the axillae.
2. Have the child lie supine on the pillowcase. This restrains both arms with minimal restraint of the rest of the child's body.

COMPLICATIONS

1. Hypoventilation, vomiting, aspiration
2. Distal neurovascular compromise
3. Mistrust, fear
4. Soft tissue bruising

PATIENT TEACHING

1. Give age-appropriate explanations for the restraint and procedure.
2. Compliment the child on the positive aspects of his or her cooperation.
3. Reassure the child and the parents.

REFERENCES

Bove, M. (1993). Positioning and securing children for procedures (pp. 29-34). In Bernado, L.M., & Bove, M. (Eds.). *Emergency pediatric nursing procedures.* Boston: Jones & Bartlett Publishers.

Emergency Nurses Association (ENA). (1999). *Emergency nursing pediatric course: provider manual,* 2nd ed. Des Plaines, IL: Author.

Parnell, D.N. (2002). Application of nursing principles to pediatrics (pp. 430-485). In Ashwill, J.W., & Droske, S.C. (Eds.). *Nursing care of children: principles and practice,* 2nd ed. Philadelphia: W.B. Saunders.

Decontamination for Nuclear, Biologic, and Chemical Exposure

Alexis M. Newton, RN, MSN

Decontamination as defined by Hurst (1997) is the reduction or removal of chemical (or biologic) agents so that they are no longer hazards. Recent international situations have highlighted the need for hospitals to actively participate with their communities and medical agencies in the design and implementation of aggressive and comprehensive disaster planning. Because the emergency department (ED) is the gateway to the hospital, it is the most vulnerable area. ED staff must use sound judgment based on attainable information and react in a timely and efficient manner to protect themselves, their patients, and the hospital. This procedure is intended to provide general guidance only and should be used in conjunction with institutional and local protocols. Resources for current information are listed at the end of the procedure.

INDICATIONS
Nuclear, biologic, and chemical (NBC) decontamination is the first line of defense and treatment against the consequences of either the threat or the use of weapons of mass destruction. Patients *will* bypass emergency medical services as the result of panic. The ED will become the disaster scene, and this may overwhelm any ED, independent of size or location. Preparation of all ED nurses and support staff is vital. Whether a single or multiple patients are exposed, the following questions should be considered:
- What is the substance (if known)?
- What are the risks to yourself and others?
- When did contamination occur and is it a rapid-acting substance?
- Where outside of the hospital can you effectively decontaminate patients?
- How can this safely and efficiently occur during high-volume hours or during seasonal patient census fluctuations?

CONTRAINDICATIONS AND CAUTIONS
1. Do not become a victim by becoming contaminated yourself.
2. Look for signs of contamination among your peers.
3. Do not rush in to treat a contaminated patient without personal protection equipment (PPE).
4. Even with PPE, once you touch a patient, you are contaminated.
5. Establish an outer perimeter (Cold Zone). Do not let anyone who is not properly decontaminated enter the Cold Zone. Do not let anyone without PPE leave the Cold Zone to enter the Warm Zone (decontamination area).

6. Do not taste, smell, or touch anything.
7. Minimize the number of staff performing decontamination.
8. Do not transfer the patient to another facility if you can provide the necessary care. Transfer of patients can result in transfer of contamination (Treat et al., 2000.

EQUIPMENT
Staff Personal Protective Equipment
Full-face shield
Chemical-resistant suit with hood
Chemical-resistant rubber gloves
Waterproof chemical-resistant rubber boots
Air purifying respirator or self-contained breathing apparatus

Patient Identification and Belongings
Waterproof triage tags
Small and large plastic bags
Permanent marker/labels

Cleaning Supplies
Mild soap
Sponges
Long-handled brushes
Buckets

Water Source
Hoses with gentle flow, controlled nozzles
or
Shower with multiple heads
Drain
Plastic pallets for fall prevention

Patient Privacy
Gowns
Towels, blankets, or sheets
Portable modesty screens

Miscellaneous
Duct tape
Scissors
Traffic cones

PREPARATION (U.S. Department of Health and Human Services, 2000)
1. Establish a Hot Zone where contaminated patients are identified and undressed.
2. Establish a decontamination area (Warm Zone).
3. First aid and treatment takes place in a Cold Zone inside of the hospital.
4. Assign staff to each zone (with PPE in the Hot and Warm Zones).
5. Notify institutional administration, who should in turn notify the local public safety officials (health department, law enforcement, fire, and emergency

medical services), the Federal Bureau of Investigation, the Federal Emergency Management Administration, and the Centers for Disease Control (Richards et al., 1999).

6. Maintain a log of all patients decontaminated.

PROCEDURAL STEPS

1. With known biologic or radioactive agent, wet patient down from top to bottom using copious amounts of water before undressing. This prevents the agent from re-aerosolizing. With unknown or chemical agents, strip patients before wetting down because wetting clothing further contaminates skin. If mustard is the substance, blot (do not rub) first to remove liquid. Remember that pantyhose can maintain a large amount of contaminate close to skin and cover a large area. Attempts should be made to remove all clothing as soon as possible. Eighty percent of contamination should be removed with clothing.

2. Remove or cut clothing head to toe and front to back. Keep clothing away from face during removal to prevent inhalation and eye contamination. All clothing and valuables should be placed in a prelabeled plastic resealable bag. Label with the following information: name, date of birth, date, time, and type of contaminate, if known. Hospital security or police should handle this evidence if possible. Law enforcement agencies will determine whether or not clothing and valuables are needed as evidence. If this material is released to law enforcement agencies, they will be responsible for decontamination of bag contents. If not needed for evidence, valuables may be released to patient on discharge, according to hospital policy (after decontamination).

3. Wet patients from top to bottom. Have patient stand with arms and legs apart. Soap and water with a solution of dilute bleach of 5% is best, but do not wait. Using a large amount of water immediately is better than waiting for soap and water.

4. Maintain patient modesty at all times! Beware of the public and press who may be observing decontamination activities.

5. After thorough wet down, cover patient with gown, sheet, or blanket.

6. Assume that all patients in the Hot Zone are contaminated.

7. Leave contaminated equipment in Hot Zone until the situation is deemed over.

8. After all patients are decontaminated, contact hospital environmental services to begin clean-up.

9. After removing PPE, health-care providers should shower immediately with soap and water.

AGE-SPECIFIC CONSIDERATION

Pediatric and elderly patients are more prone to hypothermia, so pay close attention to preservation of body temperature.

COMPLICATIONS

1. Patients refusing to be decontaminated must remain isolated in the Hot Zone.

2. If exposed to contaminated patient before PPE, staff must perform a self-decontamination.

3. Limit the number of health-care providers on the decontamination team to prevent any further contamination.

4. Be watchful for contamination of yourself and your peers.

5. Ensure that nonconfined water run-off does not flow into clean areas.
6. If run-off flows into storm drainage, notify the proper authorities.
7. If run-off goes into sewer system, notify receiving waste water treatment facility.

PATIENT TEACHING
1. Continually explain the purpose and steps of decontamination.
2. Continually reinforce the rationale for PPE for health-care workers.
3. Reassure and calm patients.
4. Provide information regarding follow-up care if the patient is discharged.

Additional Resources Regarding NBC Agents
Centers for Disease Control and Prevention: www.cdc. gov. Federal Emergency Management Agency: www.fema.gov. Poison Control Center: 1-800-222-1222

REFERENCES
Hurst, C. (1997). Medical aspects of chemical and biological warfare (pp. 351-358). In Dsidell F.R., Takafuji, E.R., & Frans, D.R. (Eds.). *Textbook of military medicine*. Washington, DC: TMM Publications.
Richards, C., Burstein, J., Waeckerle, J .& Jutson, H. (1999). Emergency physicians and biological terrorism. *Annals of Emergency Medicine, 34*, 183-190.
Treat, K., Williams, J., Furbee, P., Manly, W., Russell, F., & Stamper, C. (2001). Hospital preparedness for weapons of mass destruction incidents: an initial assessment. *Annals of Emergency Medicine, 34*, 562-565.
US Department of Health and Human Services. *A planning guide for the management of contaminated patients, public health service, agency for toxic substances and disease registry*. www.greatlakesFPS.com/deconcnd.htm.

PROCEDURE 195

Preparation for Interfacility Ground or Air Transport

Reneé Semonin Holleran, RN, PhD, CEN, CCRN, CFRN, SANE

INDICATIONS
To prepare a patient for transport to another facility. Transfer may be necessary in the following situations:
1. When personnel and technology are not available at the referring facility to provide care to an ill or injured patient

2. Based on local or state protocols related to regional care of particular patient groups (e.g., trauma patients, neonatal patients, stroke patients, burn patients)
3. Per patient and/or family request

CONTRAINDICATIONS AND CAUTIONS

1. There is no contraindication for patient transfer; however, the referring facility must ensure that the patient is transported in a safe vehicle by skilled and competent transport care providers, or if they (the referring facility staff) are going to accompany the patient, they are educated about the type of transport vehicle being used and the care the patient requires during transport.
2. A combative, violent patient must be transported with caution and may require sedation, analgesia, and/or neuromuscular blockade before and during transport by air or ground to ensure patient and transport crew member safety.
3. Weather may prohibit safe transport by either air or ground.
4. A patient with an extreme fear of flying may require sedation for transport.
5. Patients with motion sickness may require antiemetics or sedatives for transport.

EQUIPMENT

Equipment needs are dictated by the patient's condition and current or potential interventions.

PROCEDURAL STEPS

1. Identify an indication for transport. Transport decisions should be based on local protocols and hospital or facility agreements and should be conducted in accordance with Consolidated Omnibus Reconciliation Act (COBRA) and Emergency Medical Treatment and Active Labor Act (EMTALA) requirements (Frew, 1995; Mitchiner & Yeh, 2002).
2. Decide which mode of transportation is appropriate for patient transport. Several factors influence this decision, including the following:
   a. Health care systems (e.g., trauma systems)
   b. Facility agreements
   c. The weather at the referring and receiving destinations
   d. The condition of the patient and the equipment required for care during transport
   e. The distance to the referring facility
   f. The location of the patient (e.g., rural, urban)
3. *Contact a physician at the receiving facility to accept the patient.
4. Contact the receiving facility and ensure that the referring facility has agreed to accept the patient.
5. *Obtain consent from the patient or family as required by institutional or local protocols.
6. Perform any critical interventions that the patient may require before transport (e.g., airway management, immobilization of the cervical spine, initiation of vasoactive drugs).

---

*Indicates portions of the procedure usually performed by a physician or an advanced practice nurse.

7. Prepare copies of all current medical records, radiology studies, and laboratory results for transfer with the patient.
8. Remove all valuables from the patient and give to family members when possible.
9. Allow the patient to see the family and significant others.
10. Check to see if a family member may accompany the patient and, if allowed, prepare the family for transport. If the family may not accompany the patient, provide written directions to the receiving facility.
11. Empty all containers before transport (e.g., urinary drainage bags, gastric contents, chest drainage units), and document output.
12. Provide sedation, analgesia, or antiemetics as indicated.
13. Contact the receiving nursing staff and provide pertinent patient information.

SAFETY
1. Beware of the potential safety hazards related to the transport vehicle (Semonin-Holleran, 2003).
2. Never approach a running vehicle (helicopter or ambulance) unless signaled by the transport team.
3. Always approach the transport vehicle from the front in view of the pilot or driver.
4. Protect hearing and vision by wearing earplugs and eye protection when approaching aircraft.
5. Learn to load and unload specific transport vehicles safely (Figure 195-1).
6. Always secure or remove loose objects (e.g., a stretcher mattress, oxygen tanks, gravel) around a helicopter landing area.

AGE-SPECIFIC CONSIDERATIONS
1. Ensure that the pediatric patient is placed in the appropriate safety device for transfer (e.g., pediatric board or age/weight appropriate safety seat).
2. When possible, allow a caregiver to accompany the child during transport.

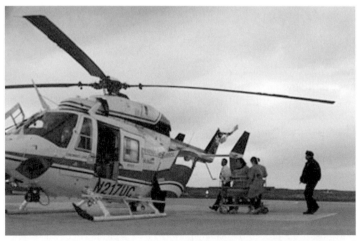

FIGURE 195-1 Example of a crew loading a helicopter after transport. (Courtesy R.A. DeJarnette.)

PATIENT TEACHING

1. Explain to the patient about the mode of transport he/she will be placed in for transfer (e.g., noise, where they will be placed, safety precautions).
2. When possible, introduce the patient to the entire transport team, including the pilot or driver.
3. Explain why family members may or may not accompany the patient during transport.

REFERENCES

Frew, S.A. (1995). *Patient transfers: how to comply with the law*, 2nd ed. Dallas: American College of Emergency Physicians.

Mitchiner, J. & Yeh, C. (2002). The Emergency Medical Treatment and Active Labor Act: what emergency nurses need to know. *Nursing Clinics of North America, 37*, 19-34.

Semonin-Holleran, R. (2003). *Air and surface patient transport: principles and practice*, 3rd ed. St. Louis: Mosby.

Index